D1823345

McGRAW-HILL SPECIALTY BOARD REVIEW

Internal Medicine/Pediatrics: Case-Based Review

Internal Medicine/Pediatrics: Case-Based Review

E. Allen Liles, Jr. MD
Program Director, Combined Internal Medicine and Pediatrics
    Residency Program
Associate Program Director, Internal Medicine Residency
    Program
Assistant Professor of Internal Medicine and Pediatrics
University of North Carolina School of Medicine
Chapel Hill, North Carolina

Richard M. Wardrop III, MD, PhD, FAAP
Director of Resident Research in Internal Medicine
Assistant Clinical Professor of Internal Medicine and Pediatrics
The Carilion Clinic and the Virginia Tech Carilion School
    of Medicine
Roanoke, Virginia

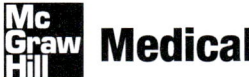

New York Chicago San Francisco Lisbon London Madrid Mexico City
Milan New Delhi San Juan Seoul Singapore Sydney Toronto

McGraw-Hill Specialty Board Review: Internal Medicine/Pediatrics: Case-Based Review

1 2 3 4 5 6 7 8 9 0   QPD/QPD   12 11 10 9 8

ISBN-13 978-0-07-148502-9
MHID-10 0-07-148502-3

The book was set in AGaramond by International Typesetting and Composition.
The editors were James Shanahan and Regina Y. Brown.
The production supervisor was Sherri Souffrance.
Project management was provided by International Typesetting and Composition.
The designer was Cathleen Elliott.
Quebecor Dubuque was printer and binder.

This book is printed on acid-free paper.

Catalog-in-Publication Data is on file for this title at the Library of Congress.

CASES

CONTRIBUTORS

Jennifer Andrews, MD
Clinical Fellow Pediatric Hematology-Onclogy
Emory University School of Medicine
Atlanta, GA

Alice Basinger, MD, PhD
Metabolism and Genetics
Cook children's Physician Network
Fort Worth, TX

Sonali Basu, MD
Clinical Fellow Pediatric Critical Care
Children's National Medical Center
Washington, DC

Andrew Bomback, MD, MPH
Clinical Fellow Adult, Nephrology
University of North Carolina Hospitals
Chapel Hill, North Carolina

Seuli Brill, MD
Resident Physician
University of North Carolina Hospitals
Chapel Hill, North Carolina

Tyler Buckner, MD
Resident Physician
University of North Carolina Hospitals
Chapel Hill, North Carolina

Harriett Burns, MD MPH
Chief Resident in Pediatrics
University of North Carolina Hospitals
Chapel Hill, North Carolina

Julie, Byerley, MD, MPH
Associate Professor of Pediatrics
North Carolina Children's Hospital
Chapel Hill, North Carolina

Alissa Clough, MD
Internal Medicine Hospitalist
Raleigh, North Carolina

Alissa Clough, MD
Internal Medicine Hospitalist
Raleigh, North Carolina

Don Coulter, MD
Clinical Fellow Pediatric Hematology-Oncology
North Carolina Children's Hospital
Chapel Hill, North Carolina

Carrie Cox, MD
Pediatric HIV Corps
Baylor Medical Center
Lilongwe, Malawi

Mary Elizabeth Cox, MD
Clinical Fellow Endocrinology
University of North Carolina Hospitals
Chapel Hill, North Carolina

Lisa DeCamp, MD
Robert Wood Johnson Clinical Scholar
University of Michigan
Ann Arbor, Michigan

Renee Dixon, MD
Private Practice
Cleveland, Ohio

Allison Dupont, MD
Clinical Fellow Adult Cardiology
University of North Carolina Hospitals
Chapel Hill, North Carolina

Lynne Fiscus, MD. MPH
Chief Resident in Internal Medicine
University of North Carolina Children's Hospital
Chapel Hill, North Carolina

Jamila Forte, MD
Pediatric Hospitalist
North Carolina Children's Hospital
Chapel Hill, North Carolina

Billy Hall, MD
Clinical Fellow Pulmonary and Critical Care
University of North Carolina Hospitals
Chapel Hill, North Carolina

Richard Hobbs, MD
Resident Physician
University of North Carolina Hospitals
Chapel Hill, North Carolina

Erin Hummert, MD
Pediatric HIV Corps
Baylor Medical Center
Mbabane, Swaziland

Holly Humprhey, MD
Resident Physician
University of North Carolina Hospitals
Chapel Hill, North Carolina

Jesse James, MD, MBA, MPH
Resident Physician
University of North Carolina Hospitals
Chapel Hill, North Carolina

Lynne Johnson, MD
Clinical Fellow Neonatology
North Carolina Children's Hospital
Chapel Hill, North Carolina

Michele Kautzman, MD, MPH
Assistant Professor of Internal Medicine and Pediatrics
Emory Medical Center
Atlanta, Georgia

Amber Khanna, MD
Clinical Fellow Adult Cardiology
Mayo Clinic
Rochester, Minnesota

Nathan Lambert, MD
Clinical Fellow Cardiology
Bowman-Grey Medical Center
Winston Salem, North Carolina

Kristi Lewis, MD
Clinical Fellow Pediatric Cardiology
Stanford Children's Hospital
Palo Alto, California

Morgan McDonald, MD
Assistant Professor of Internal Medicine and Pediatrics
Vanderbilt University
Nashville, Tennessee

David McSwain, MD, MPH
Clinical Fellow Pediatric Intensive Care
Duke University Medical Center
Durham, North Carolina

Renee Mapus, MD
Resident Physician
University of North Carolina Hospitals
Chapel Hill, North Carolina

Ansley Miller, MD
Pediatric Hospitalist
Mission Medical Center
Asheville, North Carolina

Lisa Parnell, MD
Pediatric Hospitalist
Moses Cone Health Care System
Greensboro, North Carolina

Grant Paulsen, MD
Resident Physician
University of North Carolina Hospitals
Chapel Hill, North Carolina

Eleanor Peterson, MD
Clinical Fellow Pediatric Critical Care
University of North Carolina Hospitals
Chapel Hill, North Carolina

Stacey Peterson-Carmichael, MD
Clinical Fellow Pediatric Critical Care and Pulmonology
North Carolina Children's Hospital
Chapel Hill, North Carolina

David Polisner, MD
Internal Medicine Hospitalist
University of North Carolina Hospitals
Chapel Hill, North Carolina

Sally Ravanos, MD
Resident Physician
University of North Carolina Hospitals
Chapel Hill, North Carolina

Kyle Rehder, MD
Clinical Fellow Pediatric Critical Care
Duke University Medical Center
Durham, North Carolina

Eric Riddle, MD
Internal Medicine Hospitalist
Lincoln, Nebraska

Kathryn Robinett, MD
Resident Physician
University of North Carolina Hospitals
Chapel Hill, North Carolina

Scott Sanhoff, MD, MPH
Clinical Fellow Adult Nephrology
University of North Carolina Hospitals
Chapel Hill, North Carolina

Leslie Scheuneman, MD
Clinical Fellow Geriatrics
University of North Carolina Hospitals
Chapel Hill, North Carolina

Sangeev Shah, MD
Clinical Fellow Adult Cardiology
University of North Carolina Hospitals
Chapel Hill, North Carolina

Sidharth Shah, MD
Cardiology Fellow
Wake Forest University
Winston-Salem, North Carolina

Adam Shapiro, MD
Clinical Fellow Pediatric Pulmonology
University of North Carolina Hospitals
Chapel Hill, North Carolina

Gretchen Shaughnessy, MD
Clinical Fellow Adult Infectious Diseases
University of North Carolina Hospitals
Chapel Hill, North Carolina

John Vavalle, MD
Clinical Fellow Adult Cardiology
Duke University Medical Center
Durham, North Carolina

Rebecca Vento, MD
Resident Physician
University of North Carolina Hospitals
Chapel Hill, North Carolina

Param Vidwan, MD
Resident Physician
University of North Carolina Hospitals
Chapel Hill, North Carolina

Jennifer Walsh, MD
Assistant Professor of Internal Medicine and Pediatrics
University of Texas – Southwestern
Dallas, Texas

To practice medicine is to continually learn. Every day on the wards and in the clinic is an opportunity to have our knowledge stretched and enhanced. Experience is the greatest teacher. Educators know this. Abraham Flexner knew this when he revamped medical education in the early twentieth century. William Osler knew this when he stated that *to know tuberculosis, is to know medicine*. The vast majority of our clinical learning as clinical medical students and house officers occurs in the care of patients and through thoughtful reflection and self-study afterward. There is something to learn from every patient.

With the cooperation of the departments of internal medicine and pediatrics, along with the combined internal medicine and pediatrics residency program, we have sought to compile our best learning cases. These case presentations are gathered from our experience at two community hospitals and one large tertiary care medical center. They represent a broad range of pathology among multiple disciplines and ages. The evidence-based review accompanying each case presentation contains high-yield information applicable to many specialties.

Through our presentation of interesting cases and informative discussions, we hope to create a valuable educational tool. We believe this tool will have broad appeal. Third-year medical students will find this helpful during several clerkships and as they prepare for their United States Medical Licensure Examination (USMLE). Residents will find the cases and discussions helpful to expand their knowledge base and as they prepare for the final USMLE test as well as certifying board examinations. Practitioners will find this review useful and thought-provoking even in the midst of a busy clinic. Attending physicians will find the cases useful for teaching exercises. Whatever stage you are in, we think you will enjoy working through these cases.

Richard M. Wardrop III, MD, PhD, FAAP
E. Allen Liles, Jr. MD

ACKNOWLEDGMENTS

Creating a book that crosses disciplines creates many unique challenges. There are many individuals whose effort and energy have made this process work, and at times even enjoyable.

We would like to thank our wives, Sarah Wardrop and Bonnie Liles, for their patience and encouragement. We would also like to thank our children, Mary Grace, Luke, Anna Claire, Anna, Clay, Beth, and Lida, for their constant inspiration, patience, and understanding.

The Chairs of the departments of Internal Medicine and Pediatrics at UNC, Drs. Marschall Runge and Alan Stiles have long been champions of graduate medical education.

Mrs. Denise Craig, the Program Coordinator for the Combined Internal Medicine and Pediatrics Residency Program, has provided tireless administrative support.

Finally, the contributing authors are an extremely talented group of individuals. Their intellect and energy has made this endeavor possible.

Evidence-Based Medicine

Difficult decisions are part of the practice of medicine. Combining your own experience and intuition with your patient's values is the beginning of resolving most clinical dilemmas. Using the best available evidence from the medical literature informs and enhances these decisions. Having a framework to approaching journal articles is essential. The two most important aspects are to understand the impact various study designs have on conclusions drawn from studies and to have a consistent method to reading individual articles. While many methods have been suggested and long lists of criteria proposed, we suggest a simple and effective method of asking "who, what, and what" of clinical trials.

Clinical Question	Hierarchy of study design
Causality	Clinical Trial, cohort, case control
Prognosis	Cohort
Diagnosis	Prevalence study
Risk	Cohort, case control
Treament	Clinical trial

Study Design

To use the medical literature to answer a clinical question, clinicians need to be familiar with various study designs. Each study design has inherent strengths. A hierarchy of study designs exists based on susceptibility to bias. Two broad categories are used to describe designs: descriptive

and analytic. Comparisons of groups of patients, therapeutic and diagnostic evaluations are more likely to be analytic designs, such as case control, cohort, clinical trials, or meta-analysis. Descriptive studies generate hypotheses. They are most often informational and describe associations at best. Descriptive studies include case reports/case series, ecological, or correlational or cross-sectional studies.

Before describing the individual types of study designs and their utility, it is important to understand the output to expect. In general, medical literature will provide measures of frequency and association. The primary measures of frequency are prevalence and incidence.

Prevalence is the proportion of cases (a particular disease, an exposure, or a risk factor) within a population at a given time. This is usually determined with a cross-sectional or ecological study. This can be thought of as a "census" or snapshot of a point in time. The early suggestion that stimulant treatment for attention-deficit hyperactivity disorder might impede linear growth arose from early cross-sectional studies showing a higher than expected prevalence of growth failure among children taking stimulant medications. Population studies have shown prevalence of coronary heart disease to be lower in groups who have a higher rate of red wine consumption. These two observations merely demonstrate the frequency of a finding at a point in time among a group at risk. They serve to generate hypotheses rather than answer a question.

Incidence measures cases developing over a period of time. Cohort, longitudinal, and follow-up studies generate incidence rates. A classic example is the Framingham cohort. The Framingham Heart Study was begun in 1948 to identify factors and characteristics that contribute to the development of cardiovascular disease over a long period of time. Our understanding of the classic risk factors (high blood pressure, diabetes, cigarette smoking, and high cholesterol) for coronary heart disease originated from observations of this cohort of individuals over time. Hearing loss as a sequela of meningitis was elucidated by follow-up studies of children who survived bacterial meningitis.

Incidence can be expressed as a cumulative incidence which represents new cases in a population over a period of time or incidence rate, new cases per person–time. Measures of association compare frequency measures. The *risk ratio,* or *relative risk,* is the ratio of incidence of a disease given a certain exposure or risk factor versus the lack of that exposure or risk factor. Cohort or clinical trials can provide this information. An odds ratio can be derived from a cohort or a case-control study. The ratio of odds of a disease given the presence or absence of an exposure will be shown with a cohort study. A case-control study will demonstrate the odds of an exposure given the presence or absence of a disease state.

Three types of study designs deserve special attention because of their high prevalence throughout the medical literature: cross-sectional, case-control, and cohort studies.

Cross Sectional

Cross-sectional studies measure exposure and outcomes at the same time. Groups or populations are chosen based on a certain exposure or commonality. To ascertain the differential diagnosis of a chronic cough in children, researchers could sample diagnoses of children attending a pediatric pulmonary clinic. To determine the prevalence of cancers in survivors of the Three Mile Island nuclear disaster, researchers could survey a sample of people living in that area. These studies are quick and easy to do, but significant bias is possible. Survey studies are limited by the difficulty of recall bias. In the hypothetical examples, referral and survivor bias would be present. The outcome of interest may change the exposure. It is difficult to generate conclusions about the relationship between outcomes and exposures.

Case Control

The selection of subjects in case-control studies is based on the presence or absence of a disease or an outcome. This concept is the key to understanding these studies.

Researchers start with the "answer" and seek to define an exposure or risk factor. These studies most frequently seek to answer questions of risk by defining associated exposures with a disease. Cases are selected based on presence of a disease state. Controls are selected to be representative of the population from which cases are derived. The similarity of the cases and controls is the key issue. Are they truly the same population? Would cases have been detected and included if they were part of the control population? Measures of frequency are not possible with case-control studies as proportions are determined by the investigator. The outcome measure is the ratio of exposure between the two groups. This is most often reported as an odds ratio (odds of exposure given the disease to odds of exposure without disease).

Case-control studies are excellent for investigation of rare diseases. They can be short and inexpensive to perform. With good sampling they may approximate a risk ratio. Several factors can bias these studies. Recall bias among subjects is difficult with this design. Factors unique to survivors of a disease will bias the results. Finally, it is difficult to determine the timing of exposure and outcome relationships.

Cohort

Subjects in a cohort study are selected based on an exposure status. An investigator will define and gather a group of subjects and longitudinally observe them. There is typically some sort of commonality among the population such as age, race, or geography. Measures of frequency and association are both possible with this design. A cohort study will provide the best estimate of risk and have the clearest estimate of temporal relationships between exposure and disease. This design also allows the simultaneous measurement of several outcomes and exposures. The Framingham study has provided a wealth of information regarding several risk factors for cardiovascular disease and prognosis. This design is very difficult to use with the study of a rare disease. The dropout of subjects during the follow-up period is also a problem. A clinical trial is essentially a special type of cohort study.

As an example, consider the influence television viewing exerts on early language development. In this example, preschool language development is the outcome of interest and the exposure to measure is quantity of television viewing. The easiest way to gather information regarding this question would be to conduct a cross-sectional survey within your clinical setting. A survey instrument could be developed to assess the quantity and type of television exposure of infants and toddlers. At the same time an assessment tool, parental report, or observation could be used to determine the level of language development. Outcome and exposure information are gathered simultaneously. This is an inexpensive and fast way to generate associations. However, the information is subject to recall bias of the reporter. Only one point in time is evaluated and temporal relationships are lost. Another approach is to collect cases of toddlers referred to speech pathologists for speech delay from your institution. The charts of these children can be reviewed for documentation of counseling regarding excessive television viewing and compared to toddlers in your practice without evidence of speech delay. This is a case-control method. Cases were defined and matched to controls. These cases and controls were then evaluated for an exposure. Finally, if time and organizational support are available, a cohort study can be conducted. Infants can be enrolled and followed for several years. Their exposure to television can be documented along the way, and at the conclusion of the study a language assessment instrument can be applied. This longitudinal study will provide the best information regarding the association of television exposure and early language development. The cohort design offers the least likelihood of bias in this example.

Does sickle cell trait lead to retarded growth and development? The impact of bias in study design can be seen when considering how this question was answered. In the early 1970s, several case series described children with sickle cell trait and delayed growth and development. Since there might be possible pathophysiologic explanations for this phenomenon, some felt this was a true cause and effect. Some felt that populations at risk for having sickle cell trait were more likely to have other risk factors for poor growth and development. These other risk factors such as socioeconomic factors may play a larger role in growth and development than sickle cell trait. Investigators decided to perform a careful cohort study. They identified newborns with sickle trait (AS). They then gathered a cohort of newborns without sickle trait (AA). AA infants were carefully matched to the AS infants for race, sex, birth date, birthweight, gestational age, 5-minute Apgar score, and socioeconomic status. Both groups of infants were followed and assessed for growth and development parameters for 3 to 5 years. At the end of this follow-up period, no differences were found in growth and development between AS and AA children.

The strength of studies can be understood when considering commonly asked questions. Questions of causality are best answered by clinical trials. Clinical trials offer the best demonstration of the temporal relationship, dose response, reversibility, and specificity. Cohort studies provide the best information to answer questions of risk and prognosis. Treatment decisions are best based upon clinical trial information.

The applicability of studies to answer clinical questions and inform patient decisions can be related to their susceptibility to bias. The ideal trial may not be available for every question. Informed use of the best available data is fundamental to the practice of evidence-based medicine. Working with patients and their families to understand the evidence and apply it to individual circumstances is a rewarding part of the practice of medicine.

Reading the Literature: The Who, What, and What of Studies

Armed with an understanding of common study designs and the impact of bias, you are ready to continue with a lifelong learning habit of consistent journal reading. However, even the most enthusiastic student will quickly be overwhelmed and intimidated by the volume of material available. A systematic approach to medical articles will help overcome these obstacles. It is often helpful to start with reading the methods section of an article. This will allow the reader to succinctly understand the purpose and framework of an article by answering two questions: Who did they study? What did they do to them? These two questions encompass most of the individual questions posed by the *Users' Guide to the Medical Literature* by Drs. Guyatt and Rennie. When a methods section is read with these two questions in mind, the applicability and design of the study are readily understood. The last step to understanding an article is to find from the results section, what did they find? Even the most complex article can be broken down into manageable parts by answering these questions.

Who did they study? This question is usually answered early in the methods section. This is a great opportunity to learn if your individual patient would be eligible for enrollment in a study. This is the critical question for applicability. Does your patient population look like the patient population in a particular study? Were the inclusion criteria likely to gather patients with any bias ? Are the diagnostic criteria consistent with your understanding of the disease process? It is also important to consider the exclusion criteria. Did the study miss a group you would consider important? Related to who did they study, surveying the table of demographics can illustrate factors thought to play a role in the entity being studied. This table is usually one of the first tables in the results section.

What did they do to them (the patients)? Critical appraisal of the study author's interventions or techniques reveals the design of the study and possible areas for bias. Within this question is the issue of reproducibility: Can you replicate the intervention in your practice? There is an expected difference between efficacy or the best possible situation seen in clinical trials and effectiveness seen in typical settings.

What did they find? To answer this question, the reader should pay close attention to the "primary outcome." The bias toward positive studies tends to produce journals full of possible interventions and associations. Statistical significance does not always translate into clinical significance. The magnitude of the findings should be easily discernable. Among the many questions to ask related to findings, the best initial question may be how clinically significant is any observed statistical significance. Understanding what leads to the observed findings will also help discern the appropriateness of any conclusions drawn from the results.

"You can't make silk out of a sow's ear." Most clinical questions are complex and not answered by the perfect long term randomized, controlled trial. Understanding the impact of study design and having a simple standard approach to medical literature will allow the integration of best available evidence with your expertise and a patient's desires into medical decision making.

Internal Medicine/Pediatrics: Case-Based Review

67-Year-Old Male with Anemia and Low Back Pain

C

1

CASE PRESENTATION

A 67-year-old male presented to the emergency department with a complaint of 1 month of worsening fatigue and lower back pain. The patient had coronary artery bypass (CAB) grafting 2 months prior to presentation. The surgery had been complicated by a sternal wound infection with methicillin-resistant *Staphylococcus aureus* (MRSA). The wound had been extensively debrided during his extensive hospitalization. He received 1 week of intravenous vancomycin and then transitioned to oral linezolid to complete a 6-week course. Since his surgery, he has developed worsening central low back pain which radiates to his right iliac crest. He had a history of mild chronic low back pain. A magnetic resonance image (MRI) 2 years earlier demonstrated mild canal stenosis at the level of L3-4 and L4-5. He has been treated conservatively with pain medication and stretching for his worsening pain. However, the pain had progressed to the point where the patient was unable to ambulate the day of presentation. The pain was present even while lying down, but worsened with any movement. There were no relieving factors. He denied any pain radiating to his legs. He had a history of benign prostatic hypertrophy requiring intermittent self-catheterization. He denied any new bowel or bladder dysfunction. He denied any lower extremity weakness or numbness. He had no recent fevers, chills, or night sweats. His weight was stable since the cardiac surgery. The rest of his medical history was significant for hypertension and hyperlipidemia.

Physical Examination

The patient was awake, alert, lying in bed, in no acute distress. Vital signs: temperature 36.2°C, pulse 70 beats/min, respiratory rate 20 breaths/min, blood pressure 168/94 mm Hg, oxygen saturation 99% on room air. Cardiac examination revealed regular rate and rhythm with a grade 2/6 systolic ejection murmur at the left upper sternal border. He had no jugular venous distention (JVD). His sternal wound was well healed without any erythema or tenderness. Lungs were clear to auscultation. Abdomen was soft, nontender, with normoactive bowel sounds. No rebound or guarding was present. Rectal examination demonstrated normal tone. On musculoskeletal examination, there was spinal tenderness over L3-4 and L4-5 area. Straight leg raise was performed with resultant back pain, but no radiation to legs. Neurologic examination revealed cranial nerves II through XII grossly intact. Strength is 5/5 in his bilateral upper extremities, 5/5 with plantar and dorsiflexion of this feet. Proximal strength examination is limited secondary to pain. Reflexes are symmetric. Sensation is intact. Babinski is going down bilaterally.

Laboratory Studies

White blood cells (WBC) 7.9, hematocrit (Hct) 21.9, platelets 213, Na 132, K 4.4, Cl 95, HCO_3 26, blood urea nitrogen (BUN) 23, creatinine (Cr) 1.3, glucose 99, erythrocyte sedimentation rate (ESR) 102, C-reactive protein (CRP) 26.4. Blood cultures were drawn. ECG and chest x-ray (CXR) were within normal limits. MRI of lumbar spine shown in Figs. 1-1a and 1-1b.

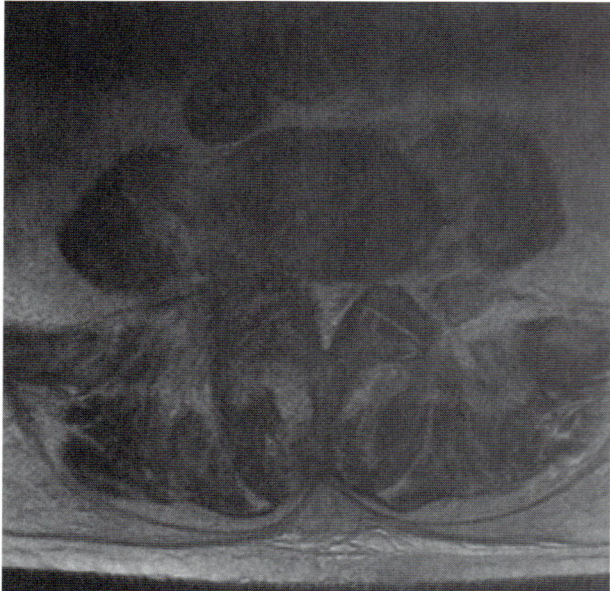 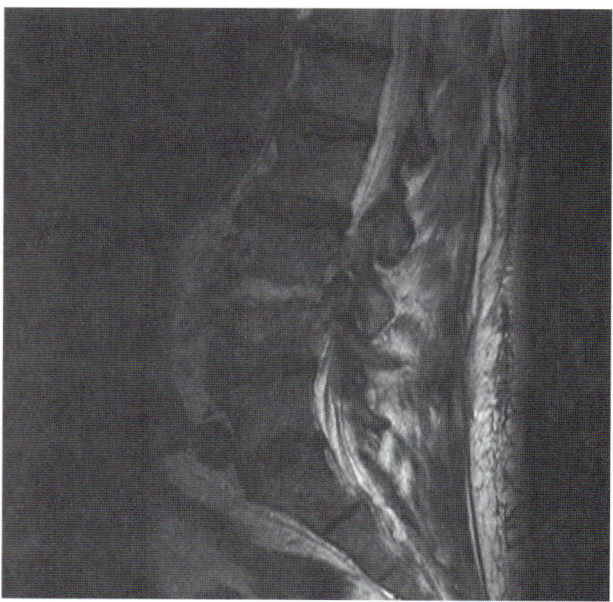

Figure 1-1 Axial and sagittal view of lumbar spinal MRI showing abnormal increased T2 signal centered at L3-4 disc space with extension into L3 and L4 vertebral bodies consistent with diskitis and osteomyelitis.

Case Resolution

The MRI of the lumbar spine showed changes consistent with diskitis and osteomyelitis of L3-4 and L4-5 with a small right psoas abscess. Blood cultures grew MRSA. It was felt that the patient had developed *S. aureus* bacteremia (SAB) secondary to this MRSA sternitis following his CABG. Complications of SAB are common with frequencies ranging from 11% to 53%. Common complications include endocarditis, infections of indwelling prosthesis, vertebral osteomyelitis, and septic arthritis. Transthoracic echocardiogram was negative for endocarditis. The patient had a peripherally inserted central venous catheter placed. He received a total of 4 months of intravenous vancomycin. His back pain improved and he did not suffer any neurologic sequelae.

Question

What were the red flags in the history and physical that made this patient's complaints of lower back pain more concerning for a serious underlying illness or infection?

Answer

In the history, the systemic complaints (fatigue) developing during the same time as the back pain is concerning for a

systemic illness as etiology of the back pain (Table 1-1). The degree of disability and the progression despite 6 weeks of conservative management is also concerning. On physical examination, there did not appear to be any neurologic deficits; however, complete strength examination was limited. The localized spinal tenderness is concerning for tumor or infection.

Discussion

Low back pain is consistently among the top 10 reasons for visits to primary care visits each year. Approximately

TABLE 1-1
"Red Flags" of Low Back Pain
Age > 50
History of cancer
Unexplained weight loss
Fever
No relief with mechanical unloading
Unresponsive to 6 weeks of conservative therapy
History of intravenous drug use
Abnormal neurologic examination

two-thirds of adults will be affected by low back pain at some time during their life. Typical age of onset is between 30 and 50 years. Men and women are affected equally. In the majority of cases, back pain is benign and self-limited. The challenge, however, is to recognize the 5% of cases that have associated neurologic deficits or represent systemic illnesses such as cancer or infection.

The differential for low back pain is broad. It can be divided into functional spinal etiologies, nonmechanical spinal etiologies, and visceral etiologies (Table 1-2). The most common causes are musculoligamentous injuries and degenerative processes. Close to 85% of patients with low back pain cannot be given a precise pathoanatomical diagnosis. The medical history and physical examination help physicians separate patients with systemic illness or neurologic compromise from isolated low back pain.

In the medical history, clues such as age of onset greater than 50, history of cancer, unexplained weight loss, symptoms lasting longer than 6 weeks, presence of nighttime pain or injection drug use should increase the suspicion for systemic illness. Often back pain caused by cancer or infection is not relieved by lying down. Involvement of hips and knees increases the likelihood of spondylitis. A history of sciatica or pseudoclaudication can suggest neurologic involvement. Sciatica is a pain that originates in the lower back or hip area and travels down the back of the leg. The pain can be described as shooting, numbing, or tingling. Sciatica produced by disc herniation often increases with coughing, sneezing, or lifting heavy objects. Pseudoclaudication is pain radiation down the legs with activity that is relieved with rest. This can mimic ischemic claudication. Classically, the pain of pseudoclaudication is relieved with sitting and exacerbated with standing. A history of bowel or bladder incontinence is concerning for cauda equina syndrome. Cauda equina syndrome is characterized by urinary retention with overflow incontinence, saddle paresthesias, bilateral sciatica, and leg weakness. This condition is usually caused by a tumor or massive midline disc herniation. Symptoms consistent with cauda equina syndrome are considered an emergency.

TABLE 1-2

Differential Diagnosis of Low Back Pain

Anatomic/functional low back pain (97%)	Nonmechanical spinal conditions (1%)	Visceral disease (2%)
Lumbar strain (70%)	Neoplasia (0.7%)	Nephrolithiasis
Degenerative disease (10%)	Multiple myeloma	Pyelonephritis
Herniated disk (4%)	Metastatic carcinoma	Perinephric abscess
Spinal stenosis (3%)	Lymphoma	Prostatitis
Osteoporotic compression fracture (4%)	Spinal cord	Aortic aneurysm
Spondylolisthesis (2%)	Tumors	Pancreatitis
Traumatic fracture (<1%)	Infection (0.01%)	Cholecystitis
Congenital disease (<1%)	Osteomyelitis	Penetrating peptic ulcer
	Septic diskitis	
	Paraspinous abscess	
	Epidural abscess	
	Shingles	
	Inflammatory arthritis (0.3%)	
	Ankylosing spondylitis	
	Psoriatic spondylitis	
	Reiters syndrome	
	Inflammatory bowel disease	
	Paget disease	

Table adapted from Jarvik JG, Deyo RA. Diagnostic evaluation of low back pain with emphasis on imaging. Ann Intern Med. 2002;137:586–597.

The physical examination including the vital signs is the next step in separating simple back pain from that with neurologic involvement because of a systemic etiology. Fever can suggest the presence of a spinal infection. Localized vertebral tenderness has sensitivity, but not specificity, for a spinal infection. Soft tissue tenderness, however, is poorly reproducible and varies with different examiners. Decreased spinal range of motion is not strongly associated with any specific diagnosis. A straight leg raising test should be performed on all patients with low back pain. The test is performed by the patient laying supine with the unaffected knee bent at 45°. The examiner cups the heel of the affected leg raising it straight up. A positive test is reproduction of pain that radiates below the knee. An elevation of less than 60° is abnormal, suggesting irritation or compression of the nerve roots. A positive ipsilateral straight leg raise test is sensitive, but not specific for disc herniation. A crossed straight leg raise test, in which symptoms are reproduced when the opposite leg is raised, is specific, but not sensitive, for a herniated disc. Further neurologic examination should focus on motor functions and dermatomal patterns of L4 through S1 nerve roots. Ninety-five percent of lumbar disk herniations involve L5 and S1 nerve roots. Ankle dorsiflexion and the patellar reflex reflect the function of L4. Ankle dorsiflexion and great toe extension are measures of L5. Plantar flexion and Achilles reflex represent S1 function.

The majority of patients presenting with low back pain do not require imaging. A suggested algorithm for diagnostic evaluation is presented in Fig. 1-2. Plain radiographs are indicated in patients older than 50, presence of systemic symptoms, history of cancer or IV drug use, or failure of conservative therapy for 6 weeks. ESR is also often obtained at this time as a marker for inflammation. Abnormal plain films, elevated ESR, neurologic symptoms, or persistence of pain despite conservative therapy are indications for an MRI.

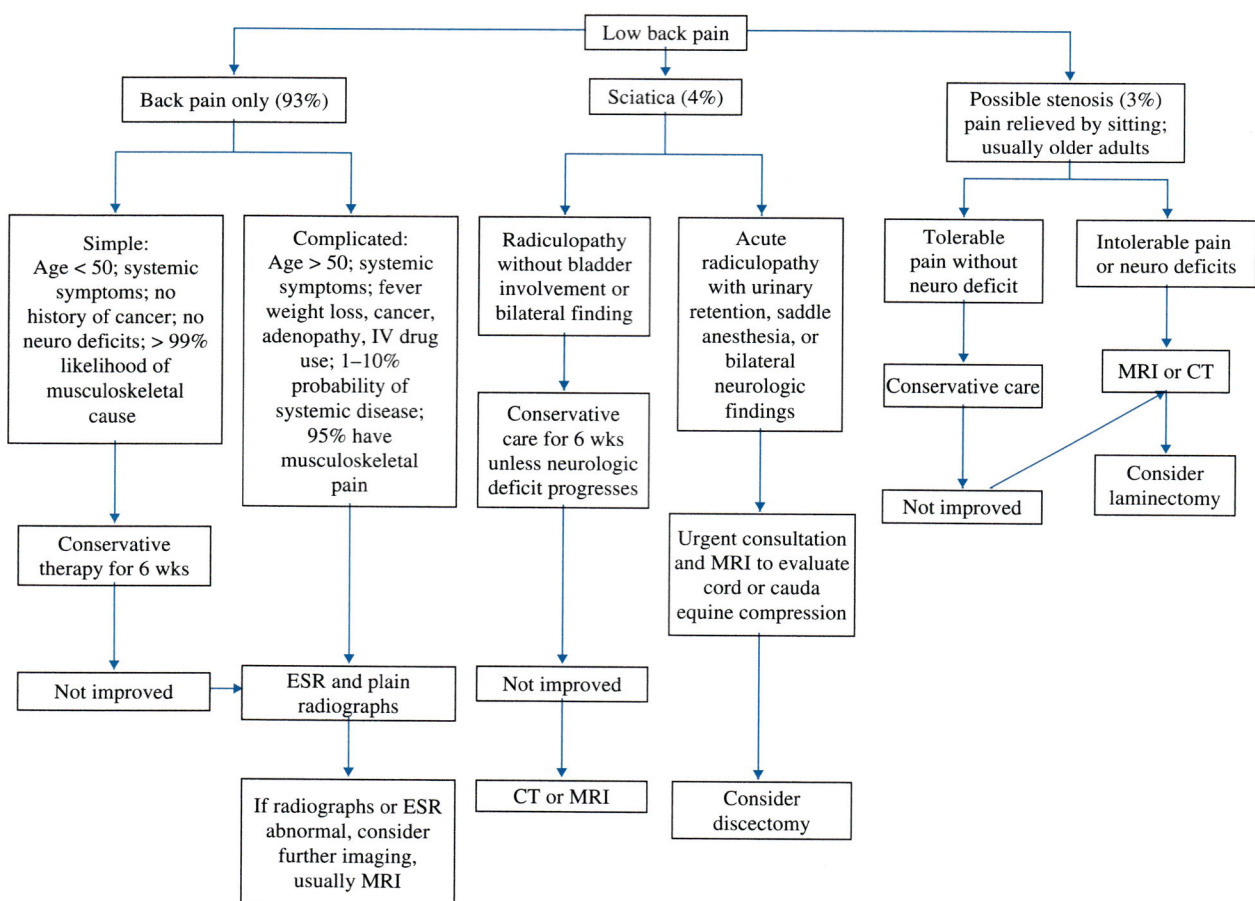

Figure 1-2 Diagnostic evaluation of low back pain. *Figure adapted from Deyo RA, Weinstein JN. Low back pain.* N Engl J Med. *2001;344:363–370.* CT, computed tomography; ESR, erythrocyte sedimentation rate; MRI, magnetic resonance imaging.

The mainstay therapies for nonspecific low back pain are nonsteroidal anti-inflammatory drugs and muscle relaxants for symptom relief. The majority of patients recover from nonspecific low back pain within 1 to 4 weeks. Physical therapy referrals can be of limited benefit for the patient whose pain has not improved after 3 to 4 weeks. Bed rest has not been shown to speed recovery. For most patients, the recommendation is made to return to normal activities as soon as tolerated.

Symptoms of cauda equina syndrome require urgent imaging and neurosurgical or orthopedic evaluation. Patients with suspected disc herniation without neurologic deficits should be treated nonsurgically for 4 to 6 weeks. Only 10% of patients continue to suffer from sufficient pain at 6 weeks to require surgical referrals. Patients with disc herniation may require narcotic medication or epidural corticosteroids for symptomatic relief during initial therapy; however, the time frame of narcotic use should be limited. A study of diskectomy showed improved pain relief at 4 years, but no difference at 10 years. Surgery is most appropriate for the small proportion of patients with intolerable sciatica or pseudoclaudication that persists after initial conservative therapy.

Selected References

1. Jarvik JG, Deyo RA. Diagnostic evaluation of low back pain with emphasis on imaging. *Ann Intern Med.* 2002;137:586–597.
2. Deyo RA, Weinstein JN. Low back pain. *N Engl J Med.* 2001;344:363–370.
3. Deyo RA, Rainvelle J, Kent DL. What can the history and physical examination tell us about low back pain? *JAMA.* 1992;268:760.
4. van Tulder MW, Koes BW, Bouter LM. Conservative treatment of acute and chronic nonspecific low back pain: a systematic review of randomized controlled trials of the most common interventions. *Spine.* 1997;22:2128–2156.
5. Weber H. Lumbar disc herniation: a controlled, prospective study with 10 years of observation. *Spine.* 1983;8:131–140.

33-Year-Old Male with Crushing Chest Pain

C
2

CASE PRESENTATION

A 33-year-old man called emergency medical services (EMS) to transport him to the hospital owing to a 2-day history of chest pain. He described the pain as a "crushing tightness" that radiated from his sternum across his shoulders bilaterally. The pain was rated 10 on a scale of 1 to 10. He had not noted any factors that alleviated or exacerbated the symptoms. He denied any nausea or vomiting, but did endorse dyspnea on exertion and subjective fevers and chills for the past week. He additionally noted that he had been sleeping on two pillows at night rather than his usual one pillow for the past week. He reported that he was diagnosed with a "heart condition" as a child and was formerly followed at a subspecialty hospital with annual echocardiograms. He did not remember when his last echocardiogram was performed or the name of his heart condition. He denied any past surgical procedures. He denied any alcohol or drug use, but did actively smoke cigarettes with an 18-pack/year smoking history. There was no family history of coronary artery disease. His father died from lung cancer. His mother was alive with hypertension and he had a healthy brother. He took no medications and reported no allergies.

Physical Examination

The patient was a diaphoretic, disheveled man in a moderate amount of distress. Vital signs: temperature 38.2°C, blood pressure of 94/58 mm Hg, pulse of 104 beats/min, respiratory rate 26 breaths/min. The oxygen saturation was 98% on 2 L of oxygen provided by EMS. Room air oxygen saturation was not recorded. The oropharyngeal examination revealed poor dentition. The cardiac examination revealed a harsh grade 4/6 late systolic crescendo/decrescendo murmur heard throughout the precordium, loudest at the right upper sternal border. The murmur radiated to his clavicles, the right side louder than the left. The point of maximal impulse on palpation was laterally displaced approximately 4 cm and a thrill was palpable over the sternum. Pulses were 2+ and symmetric at the posterior tibial artery bilaterally. The lungs were clear to auscultation; no rhonchi or wheezes were appreciated. The abdominal examination was unremarkable, without hepatomegaly. The skin revealed no rashes or lesions. He was anxious, but otherwise his neurological examination was unremarkable.

Laboratory Studies

Electrocardiogram revealed a rate of 84, normal sinus rhythm, with left ventricular hypertrophy. Portable chest radiograph revealed prominent heart shadow with pulmonary vascular congestion, no overt pulmonary edema, and no areas of consolidation or infiltrates. The peripheral blood white blood cell count was 16,000 with an absolute neutrophil count of 13.4, hemoglobin 12.8, hematocrit 36.1%, mean corpuscular volume (MCV) 88. Creatine kinase was 52 with MB of 2.5, troponin T was 0.212. Electrolytes were within normal limits including HCO_3 26, creatinine of 0.9, and normal liver function studies. Urine toxicology report was positive for cocaine. Urinalysis revealed elevated specific gravity of 1.100, but was otherwise unremarkable. Echocardiogram performed at the bedside revealed a severely calcified and stenotic bicuspid aortic valve with probable vegetation present, and a dilated aortic root. Further investigation with cardiac catheterization revealed no coronary artery disease, severe aortic stenosis with sinus of Valsalva aneurysm. Human immunodeficiency virus (HIV) antibody test was negative. Two out of two blood cultures drawn in the emergency department from different peripheral sites returned positive within 48 hours for *Streptococcus viridans*, sensitive to penicillin.

Case Resolution

The patient underwent cardiothoracic surgery with aortic root replacement, the Ross procedure (use of native pulmonary valves to replace damaged aortic valves with homograft valve placement at the pulmonary valves), repair of sinus of Valsalva fistula, and resection and replacement of ascending aorta. The patient recovered from the procedure well. He was discharged home 5 days following the procedure with a peripherally inserted central catheter to complete 4 weeks of ceftriaxone therapy. Three days following his discharge, his mother found the patient at his home, unresponsive. He was pronounced dead on the scene by EMS personnel. On autopsy, he was found to have a positive blood test for cocaine and to have ruptured the suture lines securing his new ascending aorta graft.

Question

What factors in this patient's history could cause him to be predisposed to the development of bacterial endocarditis?

Answer

Given that this patient had *S. viridans* (a bacteria common in the oropharynx) present in his bloodstream, pre-existing congenital heart disease (bicuspid aortic valve) in combination with poor dentition likely led to the development of endocarditis.

Discussion

An entity frequently listed on the differential diagnosis for prolonged, unexplained fever, infective endocarditis remains common with incidence estimates ranging from 1.7 to 7 cases per 100,000 persons/year. While this incidence rate has remained stable, the epidemiology of the patients affected and the pathogens have changed over the last several decades.

Important distinctions are made among patients with endocarditis between cases that rapidly progress from the time of the onset of symptoms to the development of complications ("acute") and those cases that are indolent and present with weeks to months of symptoms without much significant cardiac damage ("subacute–chronic"). A second important distinction is between native valve endocarditis and endocarditis that infects a prosthetic valve which have different presentations, causative organisms, and treatment strategies.

In order for a patient to develop bacterial endocarditis, bacteria must enter the blood stream, the body's immune system must fail to clear the organism, and the bacteria must be able to attach to the heart valve and begin to replicate. Risk factors for the development of endocarditis can be categorized to follow along this course. First, mechanisms that offer increased opportunities for bacteria to enter the blood stream will lead to a predisposition toward endocarditis. For example, poor dentition allows oropharyngeal flora to enter the blood stream and repeated venipunctures with hemodialysis or intravenous drug use also increased the likelihood that skin flora will enter the bloodstream. The second set of risk factors involves reduced ability of the body to clear bacteria once they enter the blood stream and include diabetes mellitus and HIV. The final category of risk factors includes conditions which make it easier for bacteria to attach to a structurally abnormal valve and develop into a collection of bacteria on the valve, called vegetation. These conditions include mitral valve prolapse in combination with mitral regurgitation or a thickened mitral leaflet, rheumatic heart disease, congenital heart disease (including bicuspid aortic valve), or presence of other intrinsic valvular disease.

The bacteriology of endocarditis has shifted in the last several decades. In the past, *S. viridans* was the most commonly isolated organism. Recent reviews, however, have found that *Staphylococcus aureus* is rivaling *S. viridans* as one of the most common causative organisms in infective endocarditis. This likely reflects an increasing portal of entry for bacteria through the skin (via intravenous drug use [IVDU], increasing population of individuals on hemodialysis, and increasing number of patients colonized with *S. aureus*) when compared to oral flora. Table 2-1 demonstrates the relative frequencies of different causative organisms for infective endocarditis.

The diagnosis of infective endocarditis can be a difficult one to make as many of the presenting symptoms are vague. To assist in the diagnosis, a group from Duke University in the early 1990s established criteria which have since been modified to aid in the diagnosis of infective endocarditis. Tables 2-2 and 2-3 illustrate the most recent

TABLE 2-1

Microbiologic Features of Native-Valve and Prosthetic-Valve Endocarditis

Pathogen	Native-valve endocarditis				Prosthetic-valve endocarditis		
	Neonates	2 mo–15 yr of age	16–60 yr or age	>60 yr of age	Early (<60 days after procedure)	Intermediate (60 days–12 mo after procedure)	Late (>12 mo after procedure)
	Approximate percentage of cases						
Streptococcus species	15–20	40–50	45–65	30–45	1	7–10	30–33
Staphylococcus aureus	40–50	22–27	30–40	25–30	20–24	10–15	15–20
Coagulase-negative staphylococci	8–12	4–7	4–8	3–5	30–35	30–35	10–12
Enterococcus species	<1	3–6	5–8	14–17	5–10	10–15	8–12
Gram-negative bacilli	8–12	4–6	4–10	5	10–15	2–4	4–7
Fungi	8–12	1–3	1–3	1–2	5–10	10–15	1
Culture-negative and HACEK organisms*	2–6	0–15	3–10	5	3–7	3–7	3–8
Diphtheroids	<1	<1	<1	<1	5–7	2–5	2–3
Polymicrobial	3–5	<1	1–2	1–3	2–4	4–7	3–7

*Patients whose blood cultures were rendered negative by prior antibiotic treatment are excluded. HACEK denotes haemophilus species (Haemophilus parainfluenzae, H. aphrophilus, and H. paraphrophilus), Actinobacillus actinomycetemcomitans, Cardiobacterium hominis, Eikenel-la corrodens, and Kingella kingae.

Mylonakis E, Calderwood SB. Infective endocarditis in adults. N Engl J Med. 2001;345(18):1318–1330.

TABLE 2-2

Modified Duke Criteria for the Diagnosis of Infective Endocarditis

Major criteria

Microbiologic	Blood culture positive for typical microorganisms consistent with IE from 2 separate blood cultures or persistently positive* blood cultures (*Viridans streptococci, Streptococcus bovis,* HACEK† group, *Staphylococcus aureus,* or community-acquired enterococcus, all in absence of a primary focus of infection) or single positive blood culture for *Coxiella burnetii* or IgG antibody titer to this organism of > 1:800
Endocardial involvement	New valvular regurgitation (increase or change in preexisting murmur not sufficient) or positive echocardiogram with vegetation

Minor criteria

Predisposing condition	Either cardiac condition or intravenous drug use
Fever	Temperature > 38°C
Vascular phenomena	Major arterial emboli, septic pulmonary infarct, intracranial hemorrhage, Janeway lesions, mycotic aneurysms, and conjunctival hemorrhages (petechiae and splinter hemorrhages are excluded)
Immunologic phenomena	Osler nodes, Roth spots, glomerulonephritis, rheumatoid factor
Microbiologic findings	Positive blood culture not meeting major criteria above or serological evidence of active infection with organisms noted in major criteria

Abbreviations: IE, infective endocarditis; IgG, immunoglobulin G.

*Persistently positive defined as at least 2 positive blood cultures drawn >12 hours apart or all of 3 or a majority of ≥ 4 drawn with at least 1 hour between first and last sample.

†HACEK − *Haemophilus* species, *Actinobacillus actinomycetemcomitans, Cardiobacterium hominis, Eikenella corrodens, Kingella kingae.*

Adapted from Li JS, Sexton DJ, Mick N, et al. Proposed modification to the Duke criteria for the diagnosis of infective endocarditis. Clin Infect Dis. *2000;30:633–638.*

TABLE 2-3

Classification of Clinical Cases Based on the Modified Duke Criteria

Definite case	(1) 2 major criteria
	(2) 1 major criterion and 3 minor criteria
	(3) 5 minor criteria
Probable case	(1) 1 major and 1 minor criteria
	(2) 3 minor criteria
Rejected case	(1) Firm alternate diagnosis explaining evidence of infective endocarditis
	(2) Resolution of infective endocarditis syndrome with ≤4 days of antimicrobial therapy
	(3) No pathological evidence of infective endocarditis at surgery or autopsy, with antimicrobial therapy for ≤4 days
	(4) Does not meet criteria for possible infective endocarditis as listed above

Adapted from Li JS, Sexton DJ, Mick N, et al. Proposed modification to the Duke criteria for the diagnosis of infective endocarditis. Clin Infect Dis. *2000;30:633–638.*

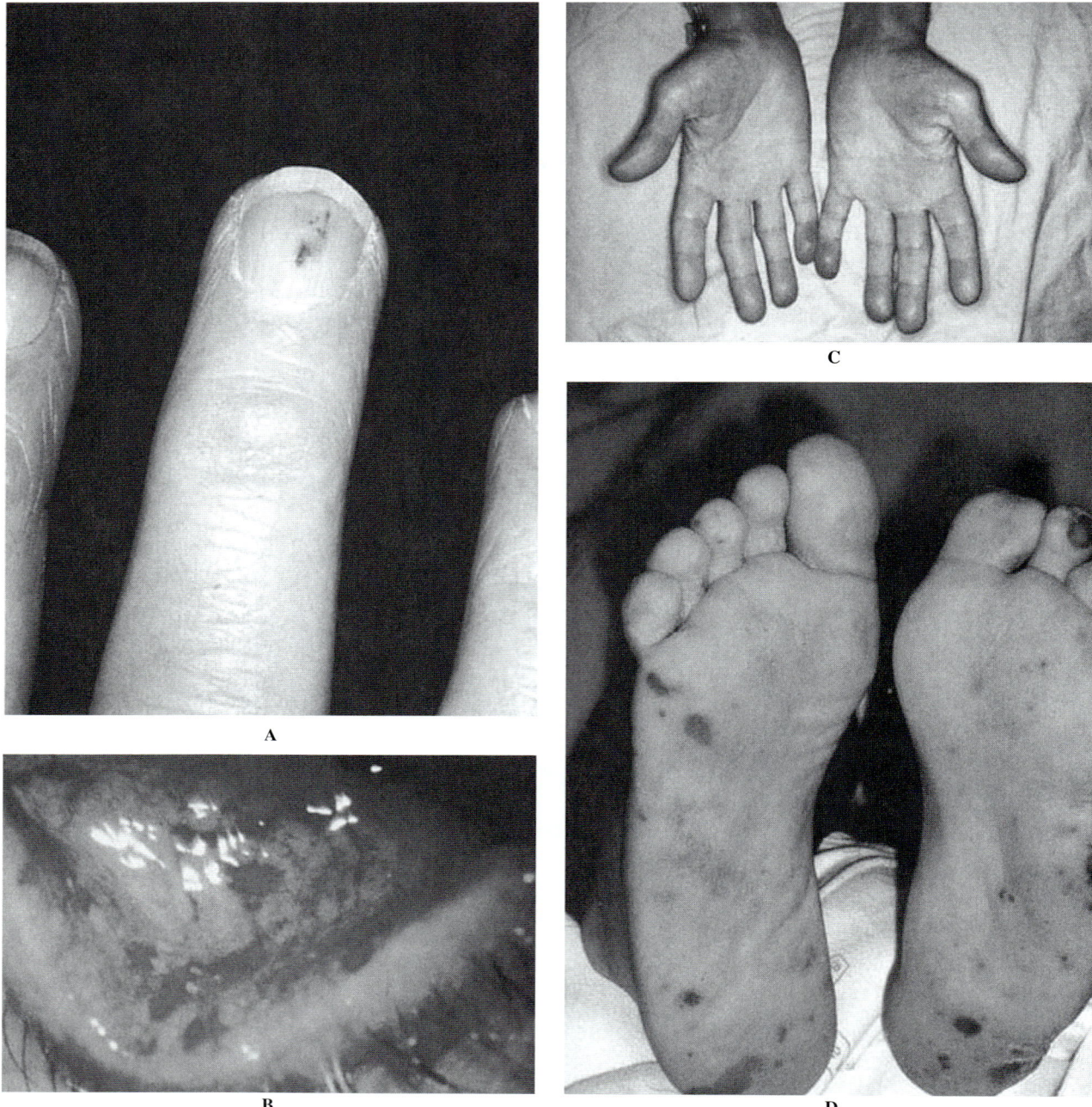

Figure 2-1 Common peripheral manifestations of infective endocarditis. Splinter hemorrhages (panel A) are normally seen under the fingernails or toenails. They are usually linear and red for the first 2–3 days and brownish thereafter. Panel B shows conjunctival petechiae. Osler nodes (panel C) are tender, subcutaneous nodules, often in the pulp of the digits or the thenar eminence. Janeway lesions (panel D) are nontender erythematous, hemorrhagic, or pustular lesions, often on the palms or soles. *Mylonakis E, SB Calderwood. Infective endocarditis in adults.* N Engl J Med. *2001;345(18):1318–1330.*

modifications to the Duke criteria. These criteria include microbiologic, radiographic, and clinical data. Figure 2-1 presents signs on physical examination that can point toward a diagnosis of infective endocarditis and fulfill minor

Duke criteria. Classically, Osler nodes, which are collections of immune complexes that are deposited in the skin and cause tender nodules, and Janeway lesions, nontender distal emboli, are seen in patients with endocarditis. As patients present earlier in the course with endocarditis, the less likely one is to discover these classic examination findings.

A common controversy regarding the diagnosis of infective endocarditis is under which circumstances a transesophageal echocardiogram should be performed in place of, or in addition to, a transthoracic echocardiogram. Guidelines for the use of echocardiography to aid in this diagnosis suggest a transthoracic echocardiogram should be initially performed for suspected cases, and if nondiagnostic, generally should be followed by a transesophageal echocardiogram. Transesophageal echocardiogram can be used as the initial test in patients with known prosthetic valves in whom infective endocarditis is suspected.

Initial antimicrobial therapy should be tailored to the organism identified and then narrowed as sensitivities return. Long-term antibiotic therapy is required, typically beginning in the hospital and then completed as an outpatient. Near the end of therapy, repeat blood cultures are required to document clearance of bacteremia prior to the discontinuation of therapy.

Antimicrobial prophylaxis prior to certain invasive procedures has recently been revised by the American Heart Asociation. In general, only those patients at highest risk of endocarditis and its complications who are undergoing invasive dental procedures should receive antibiotic prophylaxis. Patients at highest risk are those with previous bacterial endocarditis, prosthetic heart valves, or unrepaired cyanotic congenital heart disease. The dental procedures believed to justify prophylaxis are manipulation of the gingival tissue or periapical regions of teeth or perforation of the oral mucosa. This excludes routine anesthetic injections, dental radiographs, and orthodontic adjustments. A full listing of the procedures for which prophylactic antibiotics is recommended, the specific patients for whom prophylactic antibiotics are recommended, and the preferred antibiotic regimens can be found at the following Web site: http://www.americanheart.org.

Selected References

Bono RO, Carabello CA, Chatterjee K, et al. ACC/AHA 2006 guidelines for the management of patients with valvular heart disease: a report of the American College of Cardiology/American Heart Association task force on practice guidelines (Writing committee to revise the 1998 guidelines for the management of patients with valvular heart disease). *Circulation*. 2006;114(5):e84.

Dajani AS, Taubert KA, Wilson W. Prevention of bacterial endocarditis: recommendations of the American Heart Association. *Circulation*. 1997;96:358–366.

Hill EE, Herijgers P, Herregods MC, et al. Evolving trends in infective endocarditis. *Clin Microbiol Infect Dis*. 2006;12(1): 5–12.

Hoen B, Alla F, Selton-Suty C, et al. Changing profile of infective endocarditis: results of a 1-year survey in France. *N Engl J Med*. 2002;288(1):75–81.

Li JS, Sexton DJ, Mick N, et al. Proposed modification to the Duke criteria for the diagnosis of infective endocarditis. *Clin Infect Dis*. 2000;30:633–638.

Mylonakis E, Calderwood SB. Infective endocarditis in adults. *N Engl J Med*. 2001;345(18):1318–1330.

Tleyjeh IM, Steckelberg JM, Murad HS, et al. Temporal trends in infective endocarditis: a population-based cohort study in Olmsted County, Minnesota. *JAMA*. June 22/29, 2005;293: 3022–3028.

14-Year-Old Male with Fever, Abdominal Pain, and New Rash

CASE PRESENTATION

A 14-year-old male presented a 7-day history of a flu-like illness with fever, abdominal pain, progressive malaise, nonbloody diarrhea, increasing shortness of breath, orthopnea, and the appearance of two violaceous lesions on his forehead and arm. The patient had no past medical history per his parent's report but had suffered from a blistering sunburn the week before while swimming in a local pond. He had no history of tick bite or other known envenomations, no sick contacts, no recent travel, and no recent ingestion of undercooked meat. On the day of admission to our facility, the patient was seen first in his local emergency department (ED) and was found to be febrile with an exquisitely tender abdomen. His blood pressure remained low despite 60 mL/kg intravenous fluid resuscitation with normal saline. Because of his respiratory distress and ill appearance, he was transferred to our pediatric intensive care unit.

Physical Examination

The patient was a toxic-appearing male adolescent who had tachypnea, in moderate respiratory distress. Vital signs: temperature 38.4°C, pulse 120 beats/min, blood pressure (BP) 90/60 mm Hg, respiratory rate (RR) 40 breaths/min, with oxygen saturations of 95% on 100% oxygen. Lung fields had coarse rhonchi at both bases. The patient had mild distension of his abdomen with generalized tenderness to palpation and there was no guarding or rebound. He also had two purple-black lesions on his right arm and scalp, each measuring approximately 2.5 cm × 1 cm with a necrotic center. He had no petechiae. Cardiac examination revealed a hyperdynamic precordium with bounding pulses and a grade 3/6 murmur at the left upper sternal border (LUSB). Patient had flash capillary refill. The patient had no altered mental status and was alert and fully oriented. Remainder of the examination was unremarkable.

Laboratory Studies

Arterial blood gas (ABG) showed a pH of 7.40, P_{CO_2} of 30, PaO_2 of 58, and a calculated HCO_3 of 19.5, white blood cells (WBC) 11.0 with 23% bands, hematocrit (Hct) 32, platelets 145, aspartate aminotransferase (AST) 858, alanine aminotransferase (ALT) 310, Na^+ 130, K^+ 3.9, Cl^- 92, CO_2 19, blood urea nitrogen (BUN) 57, creatinine (Cr) 3.2, C-reactive protein (CRP) 28.2, prothrombin time (PT) 16.6, partial thromboplastin time (PTT) 36.7, international normalized ratio (INR) 1.4. Urinalysis (U/A) is anuric. Stool guaiac is positive. Chest radiograph shown with noncontrasted computed tomography (CT) scan of chest and abdomen (Fig. 3-1). Abdominal ultrasound (U/S) showed evidence for peritoneal and hepatic abscesses. Cultures of blood, stool, and skin were obtained.

Case Resolution

Bacterial cultures revealed infection with *Chromobacterium violaceum* as the cause of this patient's sepsis (Fig. 3-2). Human infection with *C. violaceum* is extremely rare; a handful of reports exist worldwide, although several exist from Maryland and South Carolina in children. Infection appears to be more common and more severe in those with certain kinds of immunodeficiency. After informing the patient's parents of the etiologic agent, new history

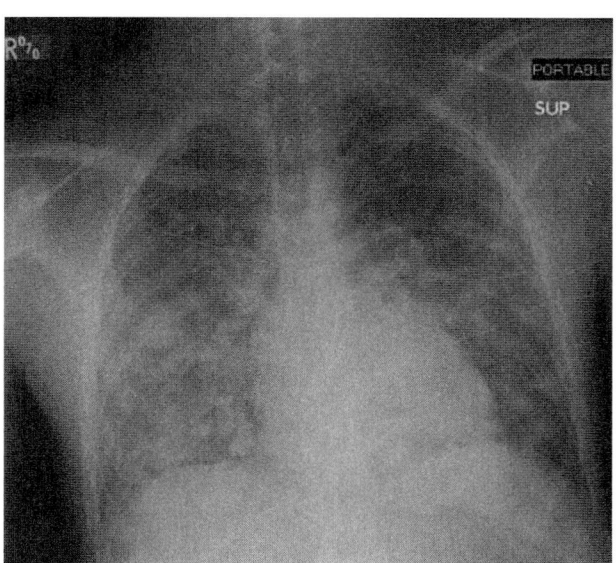
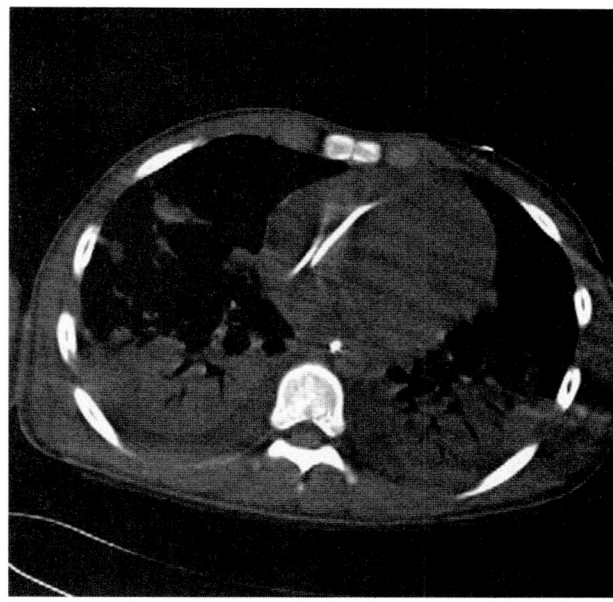

Figure 3-1 Portable chest radiograph shortly after admission notable for early ARDS and multiple opacities consistent with septic emboli of lung parenchyma. CT of chest and abdomen show bilateral infiltrates, effusions, ascites, and nodules of unknown etiology in the small bowel, consistent with disseminated septic emboli.
ARDS, acute respiratory distress syndrome; CT, computed tomography.

was obtained and it was learned that the patient had suffered from a case of suppurative lymphadenitis as a 4-year-old. Isolates of the infected lymph node 10 years prior grew *C. violaceum*. This fact was confirmed via the patient's primary care pediatrician, indicating that the ongoing infection was either a recurrence or a relapse. This led us to question the integrity of the patient's innate immune system. A screening immune workup was begun so that optimal therapy could be delivered should a lesion be identified in the patient's host defenses.

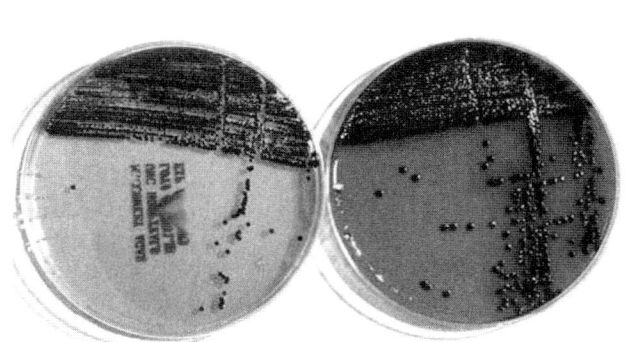
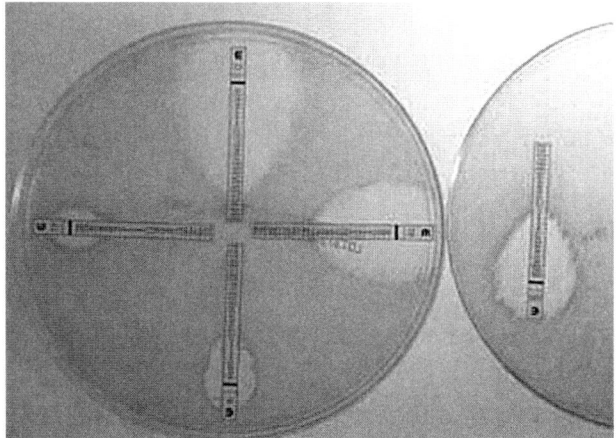

Figure 3-2 Culture of the catalase-positive facultative anaerobic soil and water bacterium *Chromobacterium violaceum* was obtained from cultures of skin and stool, but not blood, urine, or tracheal aspirate. Although nonsystemic disease occurs, infection with *C. violaceum* can be severe, leading to fulminate sepsis, multiorgan system failure, and death. Usually after a period of bacteremia, patients go on to develop deep tissue septic emboli. Sensitivities are not standardized for *C. violaceum* and specific antimicrobial therapy guidelines were acquired directly from the laboratory test as well as the literature.

Question

What kind of immunodeficiency could lead to this type of bacterial infection and sepsis?

Answer

A disorder of neutrophil function. Given the patient's age and history of past infections with catalase-positive organisms and history of suppurative lymphadenitis, a disorder such as chronic granulomatous disease (CGD) is certainly high in the differential diagnosis.

Discussion

A common problem encountered by practitioners is the patient, usually a child or adolescent with recurrent bacterial infections. Although often suspected, primary immunodeficiency is encountered much less often than expected. Oftentimes children and adolescents with recurrent infections do not have an underlying immune problem. There are more than 95 primary immunodeficiencies described, affecting persons of all ages. A description of all types is beyond the scope of this discussion, which is merely designed to direct the nonspecialist practitioner toward a rational approach to the evaluation of patients with suspected immunodeficiency.

Primary immunodeficiency refers to those disorders of the immune system of genetic origin in contrast to those that are acquired, such as HIV or the immunodeficiency of asplenia. As shown in Table 3-1, certain types of infections suggest defects in the immune system. In broad terms, the immune system can be broken down into four superficially distinct arms. Specifically, humoral immunity is mediated by B lymphocytes, cell-mediated immunity is mediated by T lymphocytes, the phagocytic cell system is mediated primarily by neutrophils and macrophages, and the complement system. It should be noted that, biologically speaking, all arms of the immune system are linked in vivo as B cells, T cells, macrophages, and neutrophils; all rely on the other cell types and proteins to most effectively mediate their effector functions in fighting disease. Nevertheless, most common immunodeficiency states can be classified into one of the four categories, and specific tests exist to evaluate both the presence and function of the component cells and proteins that make up each arm.

Certain clinical presentations behoove the practitioner to query the patient's immune function to ensure it is normal, because many immunodeficiency diseases are treatable, and treatment can prevent or make less likely life-threatening infections. As the above case demonstrates, certain infectious and clinical conditions warrant a high index of suspicion for underlying immune dysfunction. This point is even more relevant than in

TABLE 3-1

Classic Associations of Specific Recurrent Infectious Etiologies and Diseases of Immunity

Infectious agent	Suspect arm	History	Disease examples
Pneumocystis carinii, Cryptococcus neoformans, Herpesviruses (CMV, EBV, HSV, VZV, HHV 8)	T cells	Opportunistic infections, recurrent or persistent viral infections	Severe combined immunodeficiency of all types, AIDS
Hemophilus influenzae, Streptococcus pneumoniae, Giardia, Campylobacter jejuni, Enteroviruses	B cells	Respiratory infections from encapsulated organisms, chronic diarrhea, viral meningitis	X-linked agammaglobulinemia, common variable immune deficiency
Staphylococcus aureus, Burkholderia cepacia, Serratia, Aspergillus, Nocardia, Chromobacterium	Phagocytes	Delayed umbilical cord separation, gingivitis, aphthous ulcers, pyogenic infections	Chronic granulomatous disease, leukocyte adhesion deficiency, Chediak-Higashi syndrome
Neisseria species	Complement proteins	Recurrent bacteremia, recurrent meningitis	Late complement component deficiency

Adapted from Holland SM, Gallin JI. Evaluation of the patient with recurrent bacterial infections. Ann Rev Med. 1998;49:185–199.

CMV, cytomegalovirus; EBV, Epstein-Barr virus; HHV 8, human herpesvirus 8; HSV, herpes simplex virus; VZV, varicella-zoster virus.

the past as more and more children receive antibiotics for routine infections possibly masking underlying immune disorders. Moreover, screening for immunodeficiency states and syndromes is not routinely part of child care nor is it part of the state-sponsored screening in the United States or elsewhere. It is generally recommended that persons should undergo immune evaluation if they exhibit characteristics of known syndromes associated with immune dysfunction, have a family history of an immunodeficiency, demonstrate failure to thrive, or have recurrent infections that are unusual or chronic in combination with the preceding. The following may be used as a guide to help aid in judging what is unusual, chronic, or recurrent: (1) infections with unusual pathogens such as *Aspergillus, Nocardia, Serratia, or Burkholderia*; (2) infections occurring at unusual sites such as brain, liver, or other deep visceral sites; (3) severe infections with typical childhood pathogens; (4) two or more systemic or serious bacterial infections (such as meningitis, sepsis, or osteomyelitis); (5) three or more serious respiratory or soft tissue infections including recurrent sinopulmonary disease in 1 year; (6) patients with poor wound healing and periodontitis.

For those patients whose clinical course suggests immunodeficiency, a modest laboratory workup can exclude the majority of immune defects likely to be encountered in primary care settings. On top of a careful past medical, family, and developmental history, combined with careful physical examination, the laboratory studies suggested in Table 3-2 are widely available as screening tests for primary immune deficiency. Certainly referral to a specialist such as a hematologist or clinical immunologist is warranted if there is any question as to the interpretation of the results.

In the above case, this entire battery of testing was performed with the only detectable abnormality being a marked defect in the patient's neutrophil oxidative burst. As a result of the abnormal oxidative burst assay, the patient was given the presumptive diagnosis of CGD. This was not unexpected given the severity and recurrence of his infection with this rare organism. Moreover, despite the complex nature of his care in the intensive care unit, the nature of his immune dysfunction was of much more than just academic interest; it guided his therapy, rehabilitation, and follow-up care. Once the patient began to recover from

---

TABLE 3-2

Initial Screening Tests for Immune Function

Arm of immune system	Presence of arm	Function of arm
General screening for all arms	CBC with differential provides absolute lymphocyte count and absolute neutrophil count Erythrocyte sedimentation rate if normal reassures that chronic bacterial or fungal infection is unlikely	
Humoral (primarily B cells)	IgA measurement IgM and IgG if IgA is abnormal Measure isohemagglutinins If agammaglobulinemia is established, pursue flow cytometry for B cells' presence	Titers to diphtheria, tetanus, and *Haemophilus influenzae* and *Streptococcus pneumoniae*
Cell mediated (T cells)	Absolute lymphocyte count from CBC If lymphopenic, pursue flow cytometry to enumerate T-cell subsets	Candida skin testing T-cell proliferation assays
Phagocytic (neutrophils and macrophages)	Absolute neutrophil count from CBC	Oxidative burst assay via flow cytometry Neutrophil adhesion molecules via flow cytometry (CD11, CD18, and/or CD15)
Complement	Measure C3, C4	CH50

Adapted from Buckley, RH. Evaluation of suspected immunodeficiency. In: Behrman RE. Nelson Textbook of Pediatrics. *17th ed.* Philadelphia, PA: Saunders; 2004:112.

CBC, complete blood count; Ig, immunoglobulin.

his profound sepsis, this test was repeated and similar results were obtained. Interestingly the patient's mother was also tested, revealing that the patient's disease was not X-linked. The patient was started on IFN-gamma, which has been shown to be both effective and safe at preventing life-threatening infections and increasing survival in patients with CGD. Administering IFN-gamma in addition to antimicrobials in the acute phase of his illness likely improved his clearance of the infection and contributed to his survival and ultimate recovery. The patient now receives three weekly injections with IFN-gamma and prophylaxis with itraconazole and Keflex.

In this case, the diagnosis of CGD following the immune workup was of paramount importance to the care of this patient. Although this is a dramatic example given the profound septic shock of the patient, it brilliantly illustrates the importance of obtaining a complete infection history and combining that with a high index of suspicion for immunodeficiency diseases. Simple screening tests obtained while the patient was critically ill provided the insight to guide and optimize the therapy for the patient.

Selected References

1. Primary immunodeficiency diseases: report of an IUIS scientific committee. *Clin Exp Immunol.* 1999;118(suppl 1):1–28.

2. Macher AM, Casale TB, Fauci AS. Chronic granulomatous disease of childhood and *Chromobacterium violaceum* infections in the southeastern United States. *Ann Intern Med.* 1982;97(1):51–55.

3. Mouy R, Seger R, Bourquin JP, et al. Interferon gamma for chronic granulomatous disease. *N Engl J Med.* 1991;325:1516–1517.

4. Buckley, RH. Evaluation of suspected immunodeficiency. In: Behrman RE. *Nelson Textbook of Pediatrics.* 17th ed. Philadelphia, PA: Saunders; 2004:112.

5. Holland SM, Gallin JI. Evaluation of the patient with recurrent bacterial infections. *Ann Rev Med.* 1998;49:185–199.

6. Lekstrom-Himes JA, Gallin JI. Immunodeficiency diseases caused by defects in phagocytes. *N Engl J Med.* 2000;343: 1703–1714.

7. Buckley RH. Primary immunodeficiency diseases due to defects in lymphocytes. *N Engl J Med.* 2000;343:1313–1324.

36-Year-Old Female with Intermittent Crushing Chest Pain

C 4

CASE PRESENTATION

A 36-year-old Hispanic female presented to the emergency department with 4 days of intermittent crushing substernal chest pain. These episodes lasted 5 to 10 minutes and are reported as 10/10 pain. The pain was relieved with sublingual nitroglycerin in the emergency department. The pain has occurred at rest as well as during activity and eventually self-resolves. The pain radiates into the left jaw and down the left arm and is associated with nausea and diaphoresis. She occasionally reports light-headedness with the chest pain. She reports several years of this intermittent chest pain. She was told she had a myocardial infarction 5 years ago. Other past history is significant for anxiety and frequent headaches. These episodes of chest pain are worse and more frequent during episodes of migraine headaches. Her medicines include amlodipine, clonazepam, and venlafaxine. She does not smoke, drink, or use illicit drugs. She denies any history of hypertension, hyperlipidemia, or diabetes. She works at a day care and endorses frequent feelings of anxiety and stress. Her family history is negative for coronary artery disease (CAD).

Physical Examination

Vital signs: temperature 35.5°C, pulse 94 beats/min, respirations 20 breaths/min, blood pressure 119/74 mm Hg, weight 45 kg, and oxygen saturation 99% on room air. The patient is a very thin-appearing female in no distress. Head, eyes, ears, nose, and throat (medical) (HEENT): normocephalic and atraumatic. Pupils equal, round, reactive to light and accommodation (medical) (PERRLA), extraocular movement intact (EOMI). Mucous membranes are moist. Neck: supple. No lymphadenopathy, no jugular venous distention (JVD). Heart: regular rate and rhythm without murmur, rub, or gallop. Normal sounding S_1 and S_2, no S_3 or S_4 heard. Lungs: clear to auscultation. No crackles or wheezes. Skin: no rashes or lesions. Abdomen: soft, nontender, and nondistended. No hepatosplenomegaly. Extremities: no clubbing, cyanosis, or edema. Musculoskeletal: no joint deformities, effusions, or spinal tenderness. Neurologic: alert and oriented × 3. Cranial nerves: II to XII grossly intact. Muscle strength 5/5 throughout. Normal cerebellar function.

Laboratory Studies

White blood cells (WBC) 5.5, hemoglobin (Hgb) 15.4, platelets 261, cardiac enzymes: CK 71, CK-MB 1.1, troponin T <0.029. Thyroid-stimulating hormone (TSH) 1.04, international normalized ratio (INR) 1.1. Fasting lipid profile: total cholesterol 195, high-density lipoprotein (HDL) 69, low-density lipoprotein (LDL) 118. Urine toxicology: negative. Chest x-ray clear with no acute cardiac or pulmonary process. Electrocardiogram (ECG): rate of 82, rhythm sinus. Axis normal. Intervals are all within normal limits. No Q waves appreciated. No ischemic changes noted in ST segments. No signs of ventricular hypertrophy.

Case Resolution

Given the history of substernal chest symptoms that were relieved by nitroglycerin, but not consistently exacerbated by exertion, the patient was felt to have atypical angina symptoms. The absence of a gallop (S_3) provided physical examination evidence against an acute myocardial infarction. The normal serum biomarkers and ECG did not suggest an acute coronary syndrome. However given the history of a myocardial infarction, the patient was admitted to rule out myocardial infarction. Her cardiac enzymes were serially measured over the next 16 hours and were normal. Serial ECGs obtained 12 hours apart revealed no changes. She had no dysrhythmias on telemetry. She experienced no recurrence of her chest pain after the initial dose of sublingual nitroglycerin. Amlodipine, clonazepam, and venlafaxine were continued. Outside records were obtained to clarify the patient's reported history of myocardial infarction 5 years ago. Her admission ECG from that admission is given below (Fig. 4-1). Cardiac biomarkers during that hospitalization were strongly positive and a cardiac catheterization documented normal coronary arteries.

She was discharged home on continued amlodipine with the addition of nitroglycerin sublingual to be used as needed for chest pain and Ultram for severe headaches, which were thought to be migrainous in nature. The patient was advised to schedule an appointment with her mental health provider and follow up next week with her primary internist.

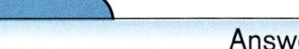

Question

What is the most likely cause of this patient's intermittent chest pain and prior myocardial infarction?

Answer

Given the patient's documented myocardial infarction by elevated biomarkers, normal coronary angiography, a history of recurrent chest pain, and migraine headaches, a presumptive diagnosis of variant angina was made.

Discussion

Variant angina (also called Prinzmetal angina) is characterized by spontaneous episodes of angina with ST elevation seen on ECG. It has typically been attributed to vasospasm in the coronary arteries. It occurs in both normal coronaries as well as those with atherosclerotic plaques. The disease has a higher prevalence in Japanese populations but has also shown predominance in younger

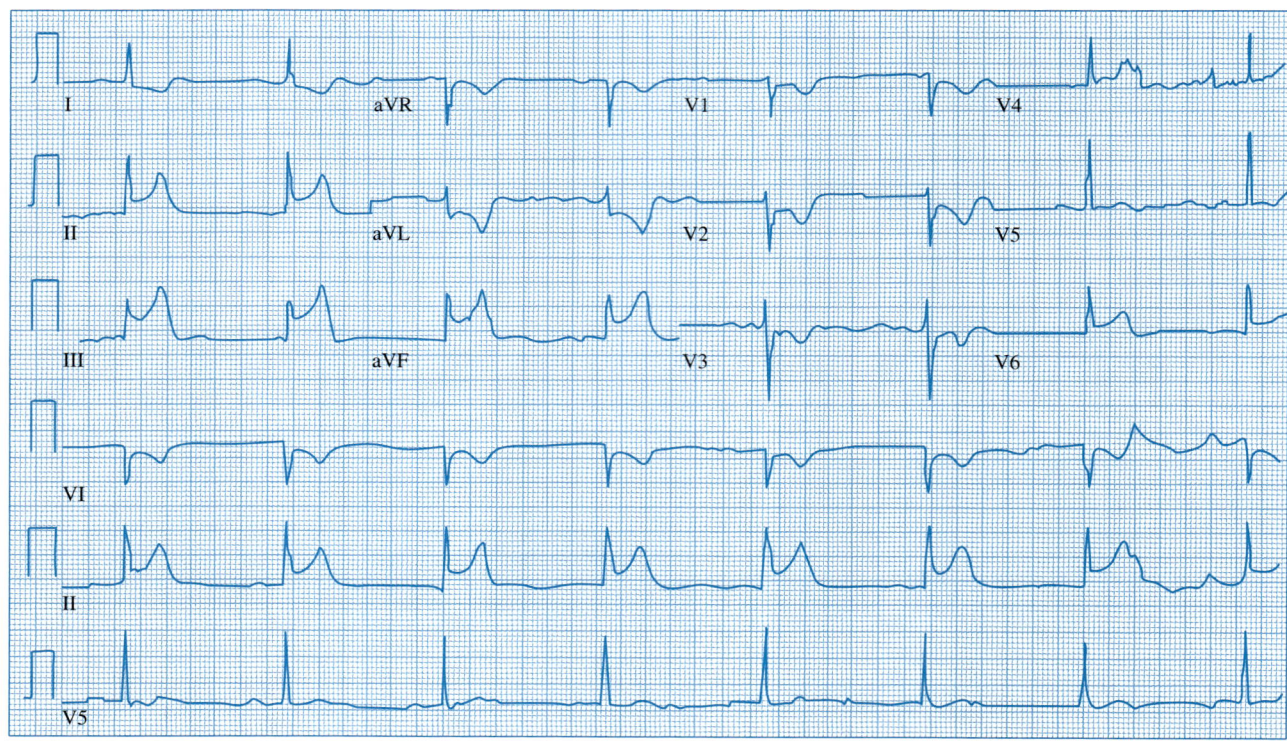

Figure 4-1 12-lead ECG obtained from prior admission with evidence of acute MI in inferior leads II, III, aVF. ST elevation in inferior leads, reciprocal ST depression in I, V1–V5.

women when compared with typical angina. There is frequently an association with other vasospastic conditions such as migraine headaches and Raynaud phenomenon.[1] Cigarette smoking is a major risk factor. In fact, smoking carries a higher association with variant angina than it does with atherosclerotic CAD.[2] Cocaine abusers are also at high risk for vasospasm. Symptoms may occur while at rest, with exercise, or during hyperventilation. Most episodes seem to occur in the morning hours.

The pathogenesis of variant angina is still under investigation but a higher prevalence among the Japanese suggests an important role of genetic factors.[3] Some proposed mechanisms include autonomic abnormalities such as increased sympathetic tone and inappropriate response to acetylcholine.[4] Endothelial dysfunction also plays a role likely because of a deficiency of nitric oxide synthesis/release in the coronary arteries.[2]

Variant angina should be suspected in patients with recurrent episodes of rest angina and no history of CAD. Acute ST elevation on ECG, which returns to baseline once the pain subsides, is the typical finding as compared to ST depression in flow-limiting CAD. Angiography frequently reveals normal coronaries although vasospasm within diseased vessels is also common. Provocative testing using ergonovine, acetylcholine, or hyperventilation can be performed during cardiac catheterization. Angiography shows induced spasm with resolution after intracoronary injection of nitroglycerin.[2] See Fig. 4-2. Myocardial infarction in patients with variant angina is well documented but is typically associated with concurrent atherosclerotic disease. Myocardial infarction most often occurs within the first 6 months to 1 year after diagnosis as the disease often has a "hot phase" initially with gradual improvement in symptoms over time.[1]

Calcium channel blockers and nitrates have been proven effective in preventing vasoconstriction in the coronary vasculature and are the mainstays of treatment.[4] Revascularization with angioplasty and stent placement can be beneficial in patients with plaques that serve as lead points for vasospasm. Coronary artery bypass grafting is unlikely to be beneficial unless there is severe underlying atherosclerotic disease.[1]

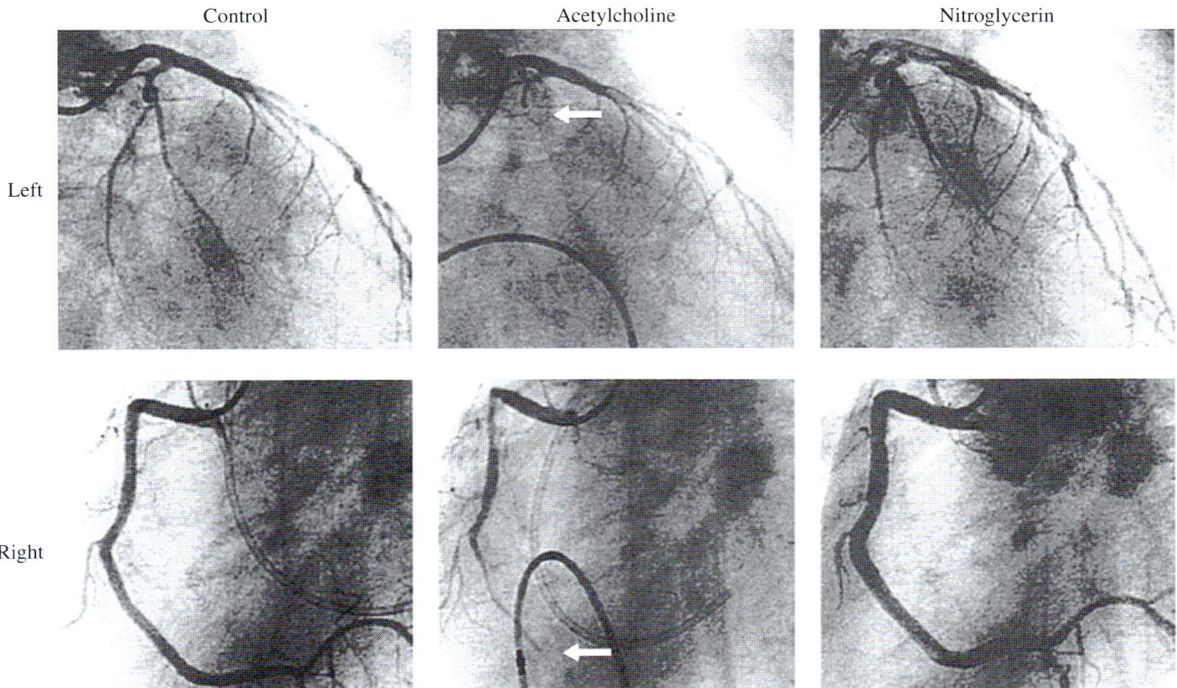

Figure 4-2 Representative case of coronary spasm. There is no coronary stenosis in the control angiography. After the intracoronary injection of acetylcholine, left circumflex artery and right coronary artery were occluded because of coronary spasm (white arrow). Coronary angiography did not show any stenosis after the intracoronary injection of nitroglycerin. Nitroglycerin relieved the coronary occlusion because of spasm. *Adapted from Kawano H, Ogawa H. Endothelial function and coronary spastic angina. Ann Intern Med. 2005;44:91–99.*

Selected References

1. Beltrame JF. Concise review: Prinzmetal's variant angina: current diagnostic and therapeutic strategies. In: Kasper DL, Fauci AS, Longo DL, Braunwald E, Hauser SL, Jameson JL, eds. *Harrison's Principles of Internal Medicine*. 16th ed. New York, NY: McGraw-Hill; 2005:226.

2. Kawano H, Ogawa H, et al. Endothelial function and coronary spastic angina. *Ann Intern Med*. 2005;44:91–99.

3. Mashiba J, Koike G, Kamiunten H, et al. Vasospastic angina and microvascular angina are differentially influenced by *PON1* A632G polymorphism in the Japanese. *Circ J*. 2005;69:1466–1471.

4. Yasue H, Kugiyama K, et al. Coronary spasm: clinical features and pathogenesis. *Ann Intern Med*. 1997;36:760–765.

3-Year-Old Female Child with Easy Bruising

CASE PRESENTATION

A 3-year-old female presented to the emergency room with increased bruising. Her mother noted that she had been having cold symptoms for about 1 week including cough and congestion. She was seen in the emergency room (ER) at that time and given an inhaler for presumed reactive airway disease. She seemed to have become weaker, progressively pale, and more lethargic over the 2 days prior to admission. On the day of presentation, her mother felt as though she was breathing faster and her lips were bluish in color. She stated that her daughter had had unusually easy bruising her entire life, which may have been worse over the past few weeks. Over the last week, she experienced fever to 100°C and intermittent chills. She has had no diarrhea. She had a dry cough with occasional post-tussive emesis which gets worse with agitation. She complained intermittently of chest pain and abdominal pain over the past week.

Past medical history was significant for thrombocytopenia at birth, which her mother was told was related to possible cytomegalovirus (CMV) infection. She had no history of asthma or significant illnesses. She was currently taking albuterol and prednisone. She had no known drug allergies. Family history was significant for lung and colon cancers in adult relatives, multiple kidney infections in the mother requiring numerous hospitalizations. There was no history of family members needing multiple blood transfusions, splenectomy, having had jaundice, or other problems. Her home situation was chaotic. There were other children and pets in the home but no known sick contacts.

C

5

Physical Examination

The patient was irritable and uncooperative, but in no distress when left alone. She was quite large, with a height of 106.8 cm and weight of 26.5 kg (both > 95th percentile). Vital signs: temperature 36.2°C, pulse 112 beats/min, respiratory rate 30 breaths/min, blood pressure 135/70 mm Hg. Head examinations revealed a mild soft tissue swelling on the left forehead where she had banged against a table last week. She had no palatal petechiae, and dry mucous membranes. Sclerae and conjunctivae were clear and without icterus. She did appear to have a left eye lid lag as well as some fleeting nystagmus of her left eye. Otherwise neurologic examination including speech and gait were normal. Lungs were clear to auscultation bilaterally. She had no retractions. Heart was regular without murmurs. Pulses were 1+ throughout and cap refill was less than 2 seconds. Abdomen was nontender and soft with normal abdominal bowel sounds. She had no masses or organomegaly. Genitalia were normal, and there was no lymphadenopathy. Skin examination showed multiple bruises, most of which appeared new. There were no petechiae or rashes.

Laboratory Studies

Complete blood count (CBC) showed hemoglobin 4.1, hematocrit 12.6, platelets 15, and white blood cell count of 39.9 (absolute neutrophil count [ANC] 26.3, acetyl-L-carnitine [ALC] 13.2, mean corpuscular volume [MCV] 96, mean corpuscular hemoglobin concentration [MCHC] 32).

Retic count was 22.3%. Blood smear showed 2+ schistocytes. Electrolytes included Na 141, K 4, Cl 106, HCO_3 23, blood urea nitrogen (BUN) 16, creatinine 0.6, glucose 108; Ca, Mg, and P were normal. Coagulation studies included prothrombin time (PT) 14.4, international normalized ratio (INR) 1.4, partial prothrombin time (PTT) 24.1, and D-dimer 2.4. Uric acid was elevated at 11.1. Total bilirubin was slightly elevated at 1.7 with 0.5 direct, aspartate aminotransferase (AST) 196, alanine aminotransferase (ALT) 29, gamma-glutamyltransferase (GGT) 47.

Chest x-ray showed a normal mediastinum with no infiltrates or masses. Head computed tomography (CT) showed no masses and no bleeding and was read as normal. Urinalysis showed a specific gravity 1.010, pH 6.5, 2+ protein, 4+ blood, 5 RBCs; no glucose, no ketones, no nitrites, no leukocyte esterase.

Case Resolution

This patient was found to have ADAMTS13 deficiency and no inhibitor activity. She was also found to have high levels of high-molecular-weight multimers of von Willebrand factor. She was treated with FFP (fresh frozen plasma) and improved. She had several relapses which usually seemed to be triggered by infection. These also responded to FFP. Relatives on her father's side were also found to have the enzyme deficiency.

Question

A prominent feature of this presentation is the presentation of fever and purpura. What are some of the causes of fever and purpura?

Answer

Three important causes of fever and purpura are Henoch-Schönlein purpura, rickettsial disease, and meningococcal infection. Henoch-Schönlein purpura is the most common form of vasculitis in children. It is usually self-limited. Its pathogenesis is immune-mediated vasculitis with deposition of immunoglobulin A. It is marked by the tetrad of palpable purpura without coagulopathy or thrombocytopenia, arthritis/arthralgia, abdominal pain, and renal disease. Rocky Mountain spotted fever is caused by a gram-negative bacterium *Rickettsia rickettsi,* which is tick-borne. This disease occurs primarily in the southeast and south central United States. The principal vector is the *Dermacentor* species of tick. More than 50% of patients with *Neisseria meningitidis* infection present with petechiae, which can coalesce into purpuric or ecchymotic lesions.

Discussion

The classic pentad of thrombotic thrombocytopenic purpura (TTP) consists of thrombocytopenia, hemolytic anemia (including schistocytes on peripheral blood smear), fever, acute renal failure, and neurologic abnormalities (confusion, altered sensorium, seizures). In children, it is not uncommon for the diagnosis to be made on less than the usual five criteria seen in adults. Most commonly, children present with thrombocytopenia, hemolytic anemia, schistocytes, and an elevated lactate dehydrogenase (LDH) (suggesting ischemic or necrotic tissue). The differential diagnosis for thrombocytopenia is presented in Table 5-1.

Schistocytes on blood smear can be associated with a multitude of disorders. Generally, schistocytes may be created by turbulent blood flow, intrinsic red blood cell abnormalities, and shearing by fibrin strands. Causes of turbulent blood flow may include congestive heart failure, valvular stenosis (or valve replacement), hemangiosarcoma, and malignant hypertension. Intrinsic abnormalities of red blood cells causing hemolysis include severe iron deficiency anemia, pyruvate kinase deficiency, and congenital and acquired dyserythropoiesis. Shearing by fibrin strands may be secondary to microangiopathic hemolytic anemia (as in TTP), disseminated intravascular coagulation (DIC), glomerulonephritis, hemolytic uremic syndrome (HUS), and hypersplenism.

The mechanism of TTP is presented in Fig. 5-1. The intravascular hemolysis seen in TTP in the peripheral blood smear in Fig. 5-2, in TTP is because of partial occlusion of the microcirculation by platelet aggregates. Ordinarily, ADAMTS13 (von Willebrand factor–cleaving metalloprotease) is responsible for the usual von Willebrand factor cleaving. In TTP, this cleaving does not happen, resulting in platelet thrombi which contain unusually large multimers of von Willebrand factor. These uncleaved multimers cling to endothelial cells and adhere to and activate platelets by the glycoprotein Ibα receptor pathway.

TTP may be either acquired or congenital/familial. Acquired TTP generally presents in older adolescents and

TABLE 5-1

Differential Diagnosis of Thrombocytopenia

Decreased production	Increased destruction
• Leukemia, lymphoma, histiocytosis	• ITP
• Storage disorders, myelofibrosis, granulomatous disorders	• Evans syndrome: hemolytic anemia, low plts because of autoantibodies
• Bone marrow aplasia: aplastic anemia, Fanconi anemia	• Kasabach-Merritt: giant hemangiomas
• Bernard-Soulier: large, dysfunctional platelets, mild thrombocytopenia	• Neonatal alloimmune thrombocytopenia
• Wiskott-Aldrich: thrombocytopenia, eczema, immunodeficiency	• Medications: heparin, Zantac, chemotherapy, penicillin, digoxin, antiepileptic drugs
• TAR: thrombocytopenia, absent radius	• TTP
• Marrow damage from radiation, medication, chemicals, or infection	• HUS
• Vitamin B_{12} or folate deficiency	• DIC and sepsis
	• Infections: CMV, RMSF, parvovirus, varicella, mononucleosis, sepsis

CMV, cytomegalovirus; DIC, disseminated intravascular coagulation; HUS, hemolytic uremic syndrome; ITP, idiopathic thrombocytopenic purpura; plts, platelets; RMSF, Rocky Mountain spotted fever.

adults. The recurrence rate is 11% to 36%, which is much lower than the rate of recurrence of congenital TTP. The mechanism of acquired TTP is felt to be dysfunctional or destroyed ADAMSTS13 or autoantibodies to ADAMSTS13.

It is associated with medications as well as diseases such as human immunodeficiency virus (HIV), lupus, and various neoplastic processes. It is felt that inflammatory conditions decrease ADAMSTS13 activity.

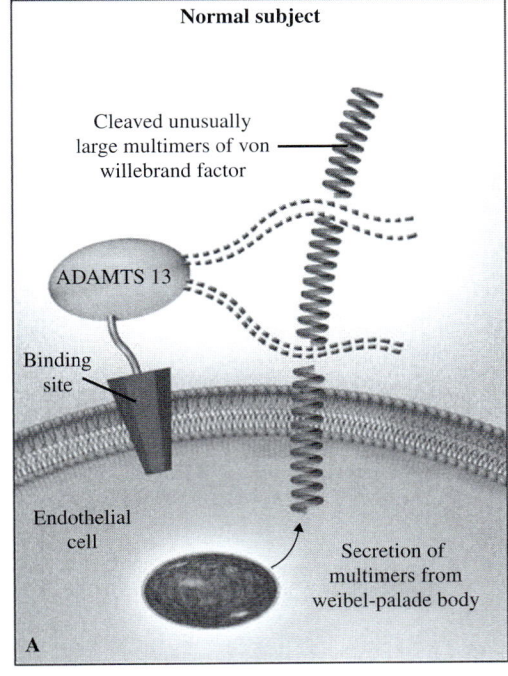
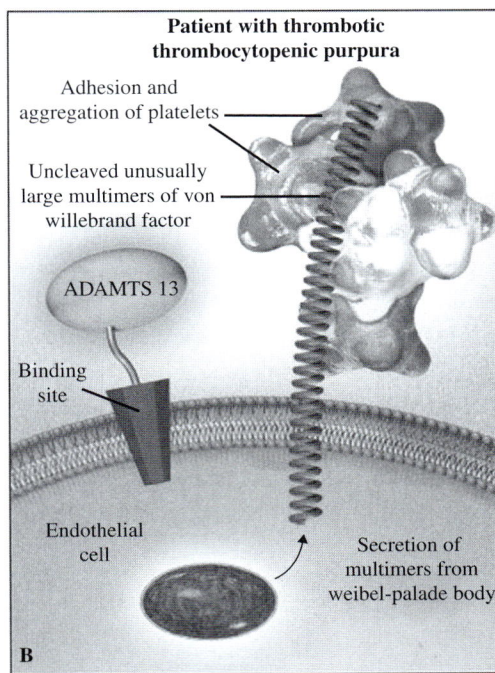

Figure 5-1 Mechanism of thrombotic thrombocytopenic purpura. (*Reproduced, with permission from George J Thrombotic Thrombocytopenic Purpura.* N Engl J Med *2006 May 4;354(18):1927–1935.*)

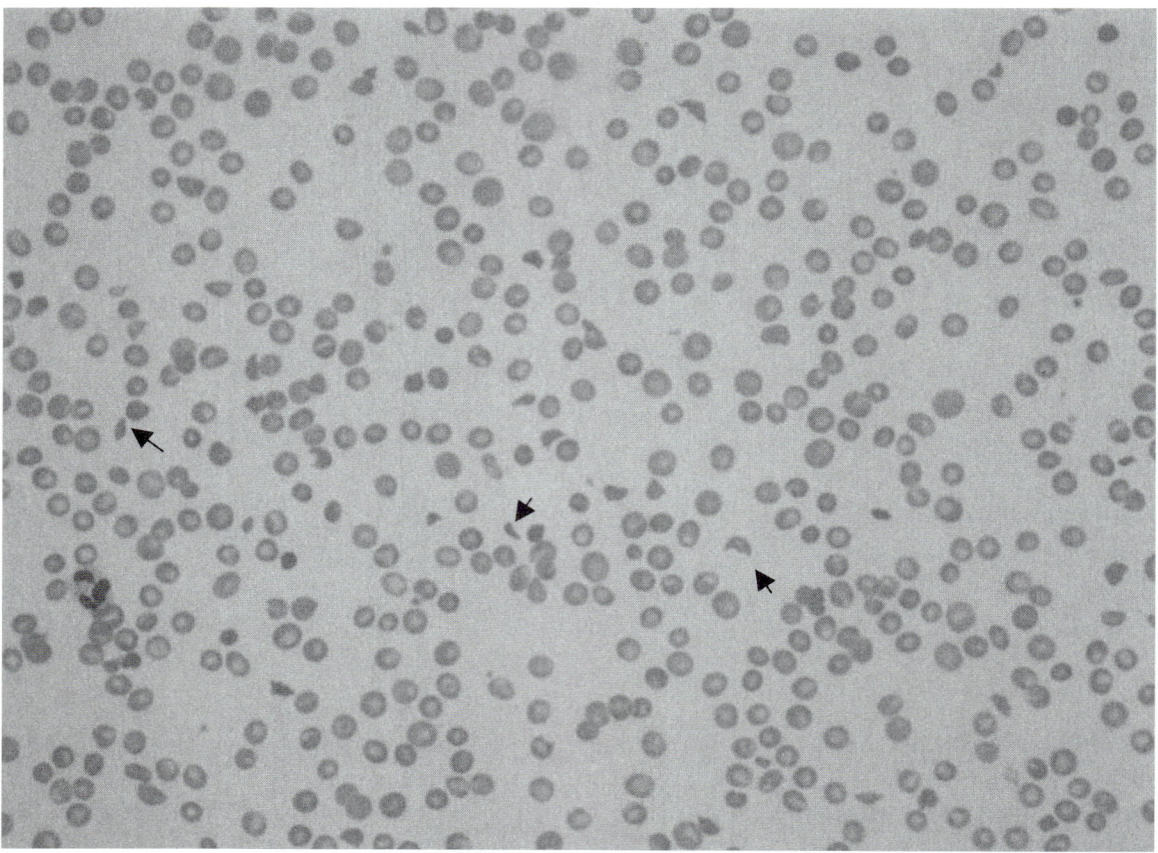

Figure 5-2 Multiple fragmented red blood cells (schistocytes).

Congenital TTP may present in infancy or childhood. After initial presentation, it often recurs at regular intervals (~3 weeks). It may be misdiagnosed as idiopathic thrombocytopenic purpura (ITP) or Evans syndrome. It is generally felt to be secondary to deficiency of ADAMSTS13 rather than an inhibition of enzyme activity as in acquired TTP. The familial form is generally autosomal recessive.

TTP is treated with emergent plasma exchange (PLEX). If the patient is not responsive or relapses, other treatments to interfere with autoantibody production may be utilized, including rituximab, splenectomy, and steroids. On the other hand, because of the difficulty of plasma exchange in younger patients and the theory that congenital TTP is often a result of ADAMSTS13 deficiency, these patients are often treated with fresh frozen plasma (FFP) infusion as needed, which may be as often as every 2 to 3 weeks.

Selected References

Miller D, Bachner R. *Blood Diseases of Infancy and Childhood.* 7th ed. Mosby Year Book. St. Louis, MO.1995.

George J. Thrombotic thrombocytopenic purpura. *N Engl J Med.* 2006 May 4;354(18):1927–1935.

Moake J. Thrombotic microangiopathies. *N Engl J Med.* 2002 Aug 22;647(8):589–600.

Schnepperhem R, Budde U, Oyen F, et al. von Willebrand factor cleaving protease and ADAMTS13 mutations in childhood TTP. *Blood.* 2003 Mar 1;101(5):1845–1850.

19-Year-Old Male with Malaise, Weight Loss, and Cough

CASE PRESENTATION

A 19-year-old African American male with no significant past medical history presented to urgent care with a 3-month history of generalized malaise, body aches, fevers, and increasing shortness of breath. He endorses a history of unintentional weight loss over that same period of time to a total of 40 lb. He also complained of a nonproductive cough. He denies hemoptysis. He also is complaining of a rash that is worse over his chest and back that has been present for 4 months. He was checked for human immunodeficiency virus (HIV) last month at an outside clinic but his results are unknown. He denies any sick contacts. He has never been in prison and has no known exposure to tuberculosis (TB).

The patient has no significant past medical history. He is currently taking Zyrtec and ibuprofen as needed. He is single with no children. He reports a history of six sexual partners over the last 5 years with condom use most of the time. He denies any illicit drug use but does smoke half a pack a day of cigarettes and drinks socially on weekends. Family history is negative for autoimmune diseases, cancer, or heart disease. Review of systems is positive for fevers, chills, and night sweats. He denies any easy bruising or bleeding gums. He denies headaches, chest pain, vomiting, or diarrhea. He does complain of some myalgias. All other systems reviewed are negative.

Physical Examination

Patient was alert and oriented, in no apparent distress. Vital signs: temperature 36.8°C, pulse 115 beats/min, respiratory rate 18 breaths/min, blood pressure 95/72 mm Hg, and oxygen saturations were 99% on room air while sitting and 89% with ambulation. Head, eyes, ears, nose, and throat (HEENT): normocephalic, atraumatic, pupils equal, round, reactive to light and accommodation (PERRLA), extraocular movement intact (EOMI), sclera nonicteric. His oropharynx was clear with no thrush. His neck was supple with a 1-cm anterior cervical lymph node on the left. No thyroid nodules or bruits. Lymphadenopathy: He had palpable nontender axilla and inguinal nodes bilaterally. Cardiovascular (CV): tachycardic with a grade 2/6 systolic ejection murmur heard best at the apex. Lungs: clear to auscultation bilaterally with a normal work of breathing. Abdomen (ABD): soft, nontender, normal bowel sounds, no hepatosplenomegaly. Extremities: no edema or cyanosis. Neurology: cranial nerves were intact. Strength equal and symmetric bilaterally. Skin: dry skin with patches of depigmentation and hyperpigmented plaques.

Initial Laboratory Studies

A complete blood count (CBC) revealed white blood cells (WBC) 4.6, hemoglobin 8.1, hematocrit 23.8, platelets 190. Absolute neutrophil count was 3.1 and absolute lymphocyte count was 1.2. Mean corpuscular volume (MCV) was 89. Reticulocyte count was 2.4%. Serum chemistries showed Na 136, K 4.0, Cl 109, HCO_3 25, blood urea nitrogen (BUN) 18, creatinine 1.9. Urinalysis showed a specific gravity of 1.015, 2+ protein, 4+ blood, and 266 red blood cells (RBCs). Microscopic urinalysis showed dysmorphic RBCs and red cell casts. Serum transaminases showed aspartate aminotransferase (AST) 84, alanine

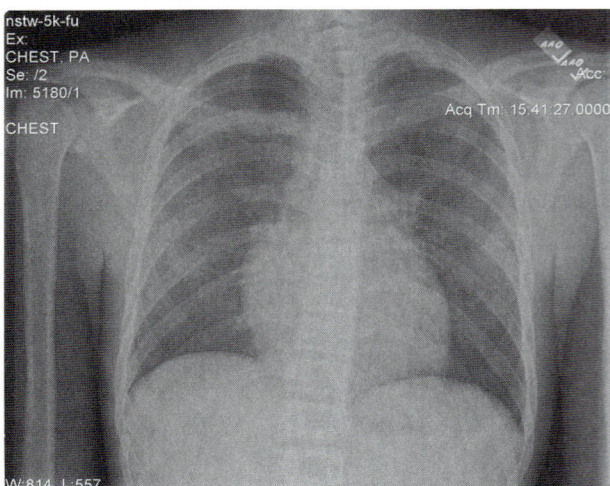

Figure 6-1 CXR of patient at admission showed multiple small rounded opacities which resulted from diffuse alveolar hemorrhage.
CXR, chest x-ray.

aminotransferase (ALT) 49, alkaline phosphatase 48, lactate dehydrogenase (LDH) 1074, albumin 2.3. Erythrocyte sedimentation rate (ESR) was 115. Monospot was negative. Chest x-ray (CXR) (Fig. 6-1) showed multiple small rounded opacities. Computed tomography (CT) of the chest with contrast showed marked bilateral axillary adenopathy, bilateral hilar adenopathy, and ground-glass airspace opacities.

Subsequent Laboratory Studies

HIV serology was negative. Hepatitis panel was negative. Urinary legionella negative. Bronchiolar lavage fluid was negative for *Pneumocystis carinii* pneumonia (PCP) and acid-fast bacillus (AFB). Lymph node biopsy showed a heterogeneous lymphoid population without evidence of granulomas or metastatic disease and no definitive evidence of a neoplastic population by flow cytometry. Anti–glomerular basement membrane (anti–GBM) was 66.3 EU/mL (normal 0–5).

Case Resolution

The patient underwent bronchoscopy on hospital day 3, which showed diffuse alveolar hemorrhage. This along with a positive anti–GBM antibody suggested Goodpasture

syndrome. Plasma exchange was initiated in addition to high-dose steroids and Cytoxan. Despite these aggressive measures, the patient developed overt pulmonary hemorrhage and respiratory failure with refractory hypoxia. He was subsequently intubated. Additionally, he received fresh frozen plasma, cryoprecipitate, and activated factor VIIa without improvement of his pulmonary hemorrhage. Despite aggressive fluid resuscitation, he went on to develop shock with metabolic acidosis and ultimately expired from multiorgan system dysfunction syndrome.

Question

What is the differential diagnosis of pulmonary renal syndrome?

Answer

Pulmonary renal syndrome refers to individuals with both diffuse alveolar hemorrhage and glomerulonephritis. The differential diagnosis includes Goodpasture syndrome, systemic lupus erythematosus (SLE), and antineutrophil cytoplasmic antibody (ANCA)–associated vasculitides comprising of Wegener granulomatosis (WG), microscopic polyangiitis, and Churg-Strauss syndrome (Table 6-1).

Discussion

Goodpasture syndrome, or anti–GBM disease, is a noninfectious small vessel vasculitis, and is characterized by glomerulonephritis, pulmonary hemorrhage, and the presence of anti–GBM antibodies which target an antigen in the GBM. It can be difficult to diagnose given its variable presentations and low prevalence in the general population.

The principal target for the anti–GBM antibody is the noncollagenous domain of the α_3 chain of type IV collagen. The α_3 chain is preferentially expressed in the glomerular and alveolar basement membranes. Although primarily idiopathic, it is believed that an environmental insult may stimulate production of antibodies and allow easier access of antibodies to the basement membrane. These insults include cigarette smoking, hydrocarbon

---

TABLE 6-1

Differential Diagnosis of Pulmonary Renal Syndromes

Disease	Clinical findings	Laboratory findings
Goodpasture syndrome	Characterized by pulmonary infiltrates, anemia, and rapidly progressing glomerulonephritis with or without hemoptysis. Constitutional symptoms are common	Anti−GBM+ p-ANCA (30%) (mostly anti−MPO+ but anti−PR3+ is described)
Wegener granulomatosis	Characterized by a triad of upper airway involvement, lower respiratory involvement, and glomerulonephritis. Chest radiographs often show infiltrates, nodular or cavitary disease	c-ANCA/anti−PR3+
Microscopic polyangiitis	RPGN is essentially universal although profound constitutional symptoms often precede the renal findings. Pulmonary complaints occur in a minority of patients	p-ANCA/anti−MPO+
Churg-Strauss syndrome	Characterized by asthma, hypereosinophilia, and necrotizing vasculitis. Cardiac and GI complications are common and often the cause of mortality	p-ANCA/anti−MPO+
Systemic lupus erythematosus	Fatigue, fever, and weight loss occur in nearly all patients. Pulmonary findings include pleural effusion, pneumonitis, and alveolar hemorrhage. Renal involvement is present in more than half of patients	ANA+, anti−dsDNA+

See references 1 to 7 at the end of the case.

ANA, antinuclear antibody; anti−dsDNA, anti−double-stranded DNA; anti−GBM, anti−glomerular basement membrane; anti−MPO, anti−myeloperoxidase; anti−PR3, anti−proteinase 3; p-ANCA, perinuclear neutrophil cytoplasmic antibody; RPGN, rapidly progressing glomerulonephritis.

---

exposure, and viral infections. As with many other autoimmune diseases, there is increasing evidence that different HLA types such as DRw15 and DR 4 may increase susceptibility and risk of anti–GBM disease while other alleles such as HLA DR1 may be associated with a lower risk.

The classic form of Goodpasture syndrome occurs primarily in young adult males. These individuals tend to present with both lung and kidney involvement. A more atypical form can occur in the elderly with women and men being affected equally. This group rarely suffers from pulmonary hemorrhage and manifests with a predominantly nephritic presentation.

The presentation of Goodpasture disease consists of renal, pulmonary, and systemic complaints. Individuals often present with other rapidly progressing glomerulonephritis with acute renal failure, non-nephrotic proteinuria, and nephritic sediment. Pulmonary manifestations

include hemoptysis, anemia secondary to prolonged pulmonary bleeding, abnormal chest x-ray, and an increased diffusing capacity. Systemic complaints are seen less than those with systemic vasculitis but include generalized malaise, fatigue, weight loss, and arthralgia. The differential diagnosis of hemoptysis is broad (Table 6-2), but in the setting of renal failure or nephritis should include other ANCA-positive vasculitides.

The clinical evaluation of a patient like that described above begins with a detailed history and physical examination. One must be aware of otherwise asymptomatic extrapulmonary disease. The initial laboratory evaluation should include a CBC, metabolic panel, and urinalysis with microscopic examination to identify hematologic and renal abnormalities. A careful examination looking for infections should also be carried out, especially before treatment with immunosuppressizve therapy is initiated.

TABLE 6-2

Common Causes of Hemoptysis

Airway disease

Acute or chronic bronchitis
Bronchogenic carcinoma or other tracheobronchial neoplasms
Bronchiectasis
Cystic fibrosis
Postbronchial biopsy
Airway trauma
Foreign body

Lung parenchymal disease

Pulmonary thromboembolism (infarction)
Infection
  Tuberculosis
  Aspergillus or other mycetoma
  Bacterial pneumonia
  Necrotizing pneumonia
  Lung abscess
Vasculitis
Goodpasture syndrome
Idiopathic pulmonary hemosiderosis

Vascular disorders

Pulmonary arteriovenous malformations
Hereditary telangiectasia

Cardiovascular

Left ventricular failure
Mitral stenosis

Miscellaneous

Coagulopathy
  Platelet dysfunction
  Thrombocytopenia
Cocaine use
Cryptogenic

Adapted from Sue D, Vintch JR. Pulmonary disease: life-threatening hemoptysis. In: Bongard F, ed. Current Critical Care: Diagnosis & Treatment. New York, NY: McGraw-Hill Companies Inc; 2003.

Hepatitis B and C and HIV should be ruled out. Initial rheumatologic serologies including antinuclear antibody (ANA) and rheumatoid factor (RF) should be obtained as well as ANCA including anti–PR3 and anti–myeloperoxidase (anti–MPO).

Goodpasture syndrome requires the demonstration of anti–GBM antibodies either in the serum or kidney. Several tests are available including tests by indirect immunofluorescence and direct enzyme-linked immunosorbent assay (ELISA). Serum tests are not perfect; therefore, a negative test does not exclude the diagnosis. For serum ELISA assays, the sensitivity ranges from about 65% to 100%. However, the use of native and recombinant human α_3 (IV) antigen substrates can reportedly provide a sensitivity of between 95% and 100% and specificity of between 90% and 100%.

Renal biopsy is generally indicated if the initial tests are negative and the diagnosis is still suspected. Light microscopy usually shows crescentic glomerulonephritis. The pathognomonic finding of linear deposition of immunoglobulin G (IgG) along the glomerular capillaries can be seen by immunofluorescence microscopy.

Imaging studies can also be important especially in identifying clinically occult pulmonary disease. Chest radiographs and CT scans of the chest can be helpful in identifying infiltrates, nodular or cavitary disease.

The treatment of choice in Goodpasture syndrome is plasmapheresis. This along with corticosteroids and/or cyclophosphamide removes circulating antibodies and minimizes new antibody formation. Plasmapheresis is usually performed daily or alternate days for a 2- or 3-week period. Therapy is often divided into two parts: an initial induction phase and a maintenance phase. Regardless of the phase, complications of immunosuppression therapy are common and can be severe. The degree of immunosuppression is tailored to the severity of disease as to limit side effects. Treatment recommendations often depend on the disease severity as some individuals with limited disease may respond to pulse corticosteroids alone. Immunosuppressive therapy is usually continued for 6 to 12 months. Additional therapies for patients with diffuse alveolar hemorrhage includes activated human factor VII, which has been used to induce hemostasis as well as extracorporeal membrane oxygenation (ECMO).

Prognosis often depends on the severity of renal impairment. Patients who survive the first year with minimal renal impairment tend to do well. Unlike our patient, individuals with pulmonary hemorrhage often respond well to plasmapheresis. It has also been shown that patients with anti–GBM disease who also have positive ANCA are more likely to have more treatable disease than those with anti–GBM antibodies alone; although relapses and recurrent disease can occur in any patient with a history of anti–GBM disease.

References

1. Frankel SK, Cosgrove GP, Fischer A, et al. Update in the diagnosis and management of pulmonary vasculitis. *Chest.* 2006;129:452–465.
2. Hudson BG, Tryggvason K, Sundaramoorthy M, et al. Alport's syndrome, Goodpasture's syndrome and type IV collagen. *N Engl J Med.* 2003;348:2543–2556.
3. Sinico RA, Radice A, Corace C, et al. Anti-glomerular basement membrane antibodies in the diagnosis of Goodpasture syndrome: a comparison of different assays. *Nephrol Dial Transplant.* 2006 Feb;21(2):397–401. Epub 2005 Oct 18.
4. Niles JL, Bottinger EP, Saurina GR. The syndrome of lung hemorrhage and nephritis is usually an ANCA-associated condition. *Arch Intern Med.* 1996 Feb 26;156(4):440–445.
5. Specks U. Diffuse alveolar hemorrhage syndromes. *Curr Opin Rheumatol.* 2001 Jan;13(1):12–17.
6. Jennette JC, Falk RJ. Small-vessel vasculitis. *N Engl J Med.* 1997 Nov 20;337(21):1512–1523.
7. Sue D, Vintch JR. Pulmonary disease: life-threatening hemoptysis. In: Bongard F, ed. *Current Critical Care: Diagnosis & Treatment.* New York, NY: McGraw-Hill Companies Inc; 2003.

2-Year-Old Female with Cyanosis and Lethargy

C
7

CASE PRESENTATION

A 2-year-old Caucasian female presented to the emergency room with the chief complaint of "turning blue" at home. This has never happened to her before. Per her parents' report, the patient also has a new intermittent cough and drooling that has become progressively worse throughout the day. She had been doing well until today, except for being fussy and gassy while teething with her 2-year molars. She has been previously healthy with normal development and no serious illnesses or hospitalizations. She has had no sick contacts and is not in day care, and has had no other prodromal symptoms. She is currently taking no medicines except Orajel and Hyland's teething tablets for her teething. The family denies any possible ingestion of household chemicals or any other medicines in the home except ibuprofen that had been dosed appropriately. At presentation in the emergency room, she is working harder to breathe and is sleepy.

Physical Examination

The patient is a lethargic-appearing but well-developed female toddler. She is markedly cyanotic with blue extremities and lips. Vital signs: temperature 36°C (orally), pulse 113 beats/min, respiratory rate 45 breaths/min, blood pressure 138/77 mm Hg, oxygen saturations 87% on room air. Other significant physical findings include excessive drooling with an otherwise normal oropharynx. Lungs are clear to auscultation despite tachypnea and mild retractions. Heart examination is normal except prolonged capillary refill (~5–6 seconds). Abdominal examination is benign.

Laboratory Studies

An arterial blood gas (ABG) was obtained and it is noted that the blood is rust colored rather than being bright red (Fig. 7-1). Bedside ABG analysis shows pH 7.2, P_{CO_2} 41.4, Pa_{O_2} 40.1. Complete blood count (CBC) shows a white blood cell (WBC) count of 12.9, hematocrit 35.4, and platelets 270. Electrolytes are essentially normal with Na^+ 139, K^+ 4.5, Cl^- 104, HCO_3^- 20, blood urea nitrogen (BUN) 20, creatinine (Cr) 0.3, and glucose 100. Urine toxin screen is negative. Chest radiograph shows

mild hyperinflation but is otherwise negative. Blood and urine cultures were obtained.

Case Resolution

An arterial blood sample sent to the laboratory showed 34% methemoglobinemia. The patient was admitted to the pediatric intensive care unit (ICU) because of her respiratory distress, and methylene blue 2 mg/kg was administered intravenously. The patient showed marked improvement overnight and was discharged home the next day.

Question

What in this patient's history puts her at risk for methemoglobinemia?

Answer

Orajel, a topical benzocaine solution, is one medicine on a long list of medications and toxins that can cause methemoglobinemia, along with a genetic disposition. Speaking

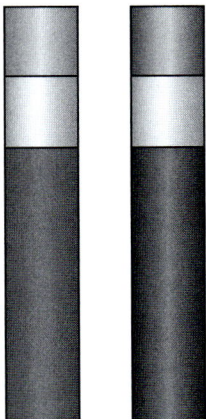

Figure 7-1 Approximate color of arterial blood in a patient with methemoglobinemia. Note the normal lighter arterial blood (left) contrasted with the darker color of the arterial blood in the patient with methemoglobinemia (right).

to the parents further, it was determined that the father had been liberally applying the benzocaine gel to all four posterior molars more frequently than recommended.

Discussion

Methemoglobinemia, or a state of increased ferric hemoglobin, can be a fatal complication of commonly used medicines (Table 7-1). To understand how systemic administration of methylene blue may help correct methemoglobinemia, it is important to review the pathogenesis of methemoglobinemia. Hemoglobin normally carries oxygen with its iron atom in its ferrous (or Fe^{+2}) state. Exposure to certain chemicals, such as benzocaine, can cause oxidation of the heme iron atom to its ferric (Fe^{+3}) state, or methemoglobin (Fig. 7-2). This is constantly happening in the human body, but at low-grade levels. Normally, at steady state, the body is able to maintain a low concentration of methemoglobin by reducing ferric heme back to ferrous heme via methemoglobin reductase, a naturally occurring enzyme in red blood cells. Under times of greater oxidative stress and increased production of methemoglobin, an alternative pathway may be utilized if an electron acceptor is available. Within red blood cells, there is usually not such an acceptor. However methylene blue will act as this electron acceptor, allowing the individual to reduce methemoglobin back to normal ferrous hemoglobin more rapidly. However, this is a nicotinamide adenosine dinucleotide phosphate (NADPH)–dependent reaction, and in individuals unable to make NADPH (specifically those

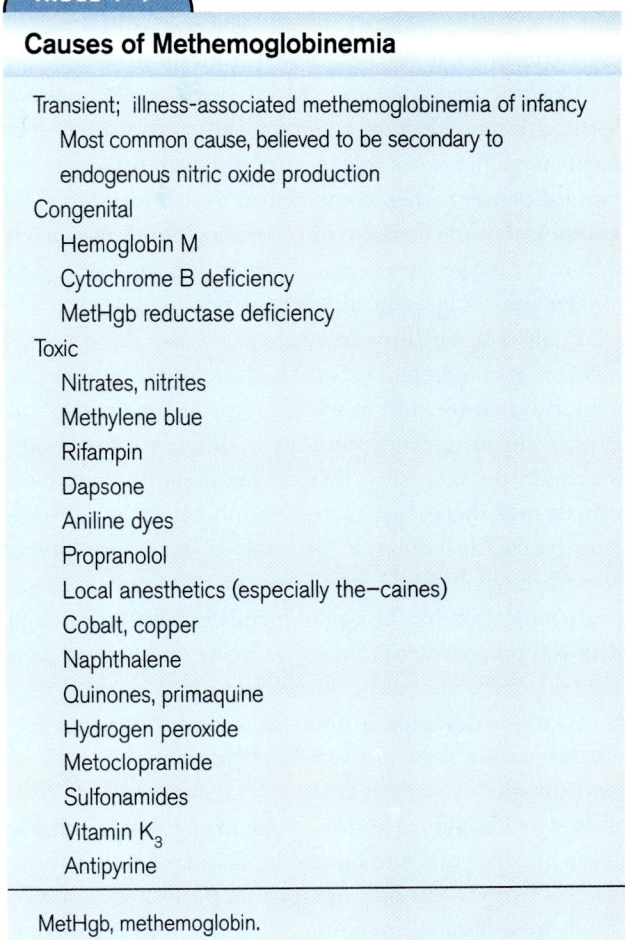

TABLE 7-1

Causes of Methemoglobinemia

Transient; illness-associated methemoglobinemia of infancy
    Most common cause, believed to be secondary to
    endogenous nitric oxide production
Congenital
    Hemoglobin M
    Cytochrome B deficiency
    MetHgb reductase deficiency
Toxic
    Nitrates, nitrites
    Methylene blue
    Rifampin
    Dapsone
    Aniline dyes
    Propranolol
    Local anesthetics (especially the–caines)
    Cobalt, copper
    Naphthalene
    Quinones, primaquine
    Hydrogen peroxide
    Metoclopramide
    Sulfonamides
    Vitamin K_3
    Antipyrine

MetHgb, methemoglobin.

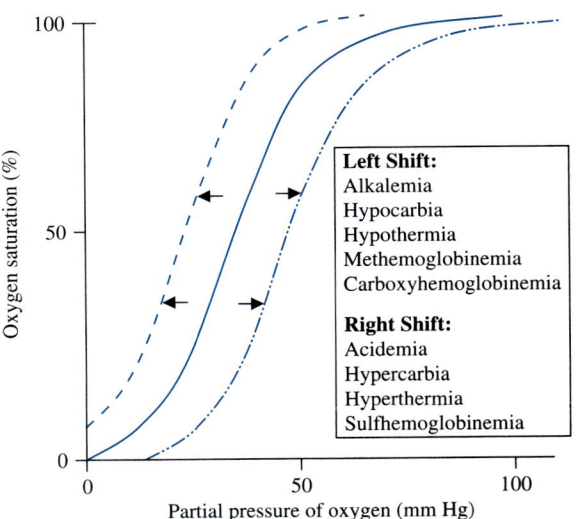

Left Shift:
Alkalemia
Hypocarbia
Hypothermia
Methemoglobinemia
Carboxyhemoglobinemia

Right Shift:
Acidemia
Hypercarbia
Hyperthermia
Sulfhemoglobinemia

Figure 7-2 Oxidation and reduction of hemoglobin and methemoglobin.

with glucose-6-phosphate dehydrogenase [G6PD] reductase deficiency), methylene blue is contraindicated.

During times of increased blood methemoglobin, tissue hypoxia is caused by two mechanisms. The first is that methemoglobin is less able to carry sufficient oxygen to tissues for delivery when compared to oxyhemoglobin. The second is that the presence of methemoglobin causes a left shift in the oxygen disassociation curve, leading to even less oxygen unloading in the microcirculation tissues (Fig. 7-3).

Predicting which patients are at risk for the development of methemoglobinemia is difficult. Complicating matters is that the shift to methemoglobinemia may occur at different drug concentrations in different individuals. Moreover, the same dose that has been safe in many individuals may then cause methemoglobinemia in a genetically susceptible individual. See Table 7-2 for the symptoms of methemoglobinemia at different concentrations of blood methemoglobin. Methemoglobinemia is common enough with topical anesthetics now that many endoscopy suites routinely carry methylene blue to be used as an antidote.

Cyanosis develops at lower concentrations in methemoglobinemia than in overt hypoxia, with 1.5 g/dL of methemoglobin causing cyanosis as compared to 5 g/dL of deoxyhemoglobin. Routine pulse oximetry is unreliable in the presence of methemoglobin. Standard pulse oximetry uses two wavelengths of lights, 660 nm and 904 nm, which are calibrated to monitor absorption by circulating

TABLE 7-2

Symptoms of Methemoglobinemia

Level of methemoglobin	Symptoms
<1.7%	Normal
10%–20%	Mild cyanosis (asymptomatic)
30%–40%	Headache, fatigue, tachycardia, weakness, dizziness, dyspnea, lethargy
50%–60%	Acidosis, arrhythmias, coma, convulsions, bradycardia, hypoxia, seizures
>70%	Death

oxygenated and deoxygenated hemoglobin. In the presence of a different hemoglobin configuration, such as methemoglobin or carboxyhemoglobin, any calculations done by the pulse oximeter will be incorrect. Methemoglobin skews the pulse oximeter toward 85% (while carboxyhemoglobin skews the pulse oximeter toward 90%). A cooximeter, however, may use more than 250 wavelengths of light, and can therefore accurately measure all the different hemoglobin configurations. A few bedside cooximeters are commercially available, but most laboratories capable of running ABG tests can also accurately measure methemoglobin and carboxyhemoglobin in the same sample, if asked to do so.

This case shows a rare, life-threatening complication of a relatively common over-the-counter medication. When faced with an unexplained case presentation, it is important to remember that any medicine is toxic at a high enough dose, and that individuals may react very differently to the same medicine.

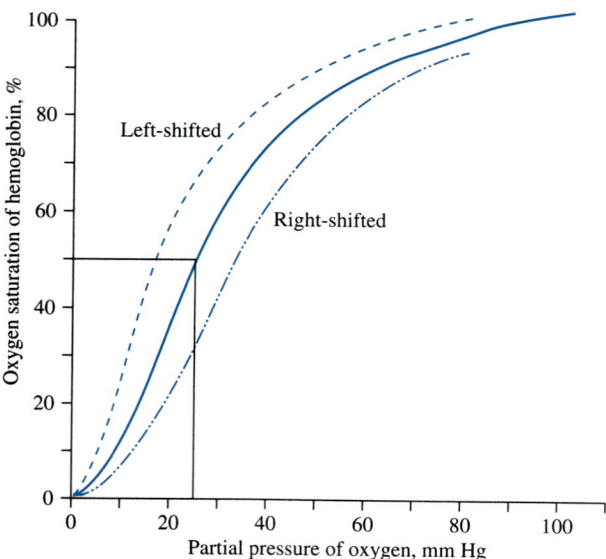

Figure 7-3 Presence of methemoglobin causes a left shift in the curve, such that the hemoglobin-carrying oxygen binds the oxygen more tightly. Because of this, at a given oxygen saturation, less oxygen is delivered to the tissues.

Selected References

1. Sigillito RJ. Evaluation and initial management of the patient in respiratory distress. *Emerg Med Clin North Am.* 2003;21(2):239–258.
2. Ford M, Dealney K, Ling L, et al. *Clinical Toxicology.* 1st ed. Philadelphia, PA: W.B. Churchill Livingstone. 2001.
3. Miller RD. *Miller's Anesthesia.* 6th ed. Philadelphia, PA: Churchill Livingstone. 2003.
4. Hoffman R, Benz E, Shattil S, et al. *Hematology: Basic Principles and Practice. 4th ed.* Philadelphia, PA: Churchill Livingstone. 2005.
5. Lukens JN. Methemoglobinemia and other disorders accompanied by cyanosis (Chapter 13). In: Lee GR, et al, eds. *Wintrobe's Clinical Hematology.* 10th ed. Philadelphia, PA: Lippincott, Williams and Wilkins; 1999:1046–1055.

8-Day-Old with Poor Feeding

CASE PRESENTATION

An 8-day-old infant was brought to the emergency department with a 10-hour history of poor feeding. His mother reported that he had been nursing vigorously with a good latch since discharge from the hospital until the day of presentation when he refused to feed. She reported five to six episodes of emesis during the day. The emesis was milk colored to light yellow. They were initially small volumes, but progressed to larger volumes.

Laboratory Studies

The infant was the product of a 38-week uncomplicated pregnancy born by spontaneous vaginal delivery to a 30-year-old gravida 7 para 6 (now 7) mother. Prenatal laboratories were unremarkable with the exception of unknown group B streptococcus (GBS) status. No antibiotics were given during delivery. The nursery course was unremarkable with the exception of moderate jaundice with a bilirubin of 12 on the third day of life. The bilirubin peaked at 14, declined to about 12, and had persisted at that level. He was gaining weight well and had no fever. Except for a mild rash on his scalp and legs, his mother reported no other symptoms or concerns. Family history was unremarkable, with no history of metabolic disorders, no consanguinity, and six healthy older siblings.

Physical Examination

The examination was remarkable for overlapping sutures with a soft, flat fontanelle; a grade 2/6 systolic murmur radiating throughout lung fields; erythema toxicum; and a very poor suck. The infant was active and alert. The abdomen was very soft, nondistended, and nontender to palpation. The liver edge was soft and palpable just below the right costal margin. He had scleral icterus and jaundice to the midabdomen. Electrolytes were within normal limits. The complete blood count (CBC) was appropriate for age (white blood cells [WBCs] 12 with atypical lymphocytes noted, hematocrit [Hct] 56, platelets 427).

Cerebrospinal fluid (CSF) was obtained with a WBC of 2 and red blood cells (RBCs) of 986 (traumatic tap documented), Gram stain was negative for organisms.

During the course of examination and the procurement of laboratory studies, the infant had a noticeable increase in the frequency of vomiting and a change in color from yellow tinged to bright yellow. An upper gastrointestinal (GI) study (Fig. 8-1) was obtained, confirming the diagnosis.

Question

Which diagnostic consideration warrants emergent surgical evaluation?

Answer and Case Resolution

The infant was taken to the operating room after an upper GI study confirmed the diagnosis of malrotation. Fortunately, he did not have midgut volvulus. Instead, the surgeon found complete obstruction of the third and fourth portion of the duodenum with collapsed jejunum. There was acute angulation of the jejunum because of an abnormal fibrous band replacing the ligament of Treitz. Bands were also seen between the duodenum and cecum. There was also narrowing of the base of the mesentery. The cecum was located in the left upper quadrant without fixation (Figs. 8-1 and 8-2). A Ladd procedure that includes ligation of Ladd bands (Fig 8-3), division of the mesentery

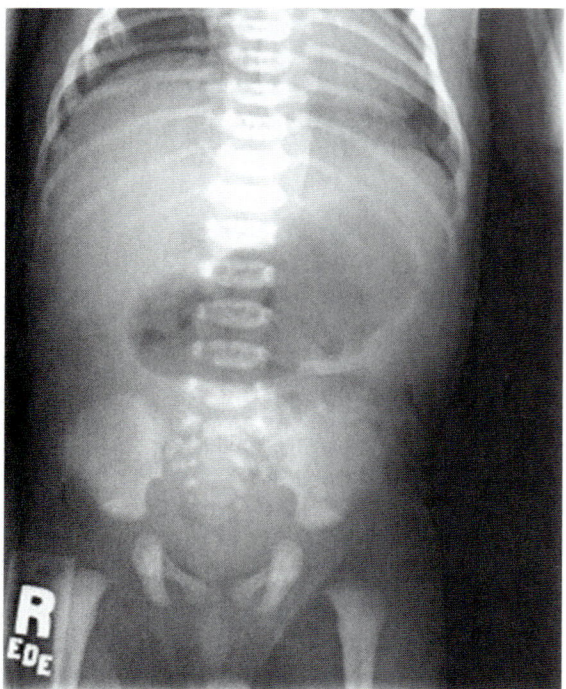

Figure 8-1 Scout film of upper GI series. The scout film demonstrates a small amount of gas in the small bowel, to the right of the midline. Minimal gas is seen in the transverse colon, which appears to be located in the midleft abdomen. GI, gastrointestinal.

to provide a more stable base, placement of cecum in right lower quadrant, and appendectomy was performed. He recovered uneventfully after the procedure.

Discussion

Malrotation results from a disruption of fetal development in the first trimester. Gut development begins as a straight tube from the stomach to the rectum. As the midbowel elongates, it protrudes into the umbilical cord, lying outside of the abdominal cavity. When the bowel returns to the abdominal cavity, it rotates around the superior mesenteric artery (SMA). The duodenum is positioned near the ligament of Treitz and the colon follows. The cecum rotates counterclockwise until it rests in the right lower quadrants. The duodenum becomes fixed to the posterior abdominal wall. Following rotation, the right and left colon and mesenteric root also become fixed to the posterior abdominal wall to provide support of the mesentery and prevent twisting of the mesenteric root that could compromise vascular supply.

Failure of proper rotation of the cecum is the most common type of malrotation. Instead of its usual position in the right lower quadrant, the cecum rests in the subhepatic area. This positioning disrupts the usual attachment of the bowel to the posterior abdominal wall, resulting in a narrow mesenteric stalk and ectopic fibrous tissue (Ladd bands). The narrow mesenteric stalk creates the potential for twisting of the bowel, disrupting the vascular supply and creating a midgut volvulus. Ladd bands may also compress the duodenum creating partial or complete obstruction.

Midgut volvulus is a life-threatening complication of malrotation and requires immediate clinical recognition and emergent surgical correction. Diagnosis can be made by

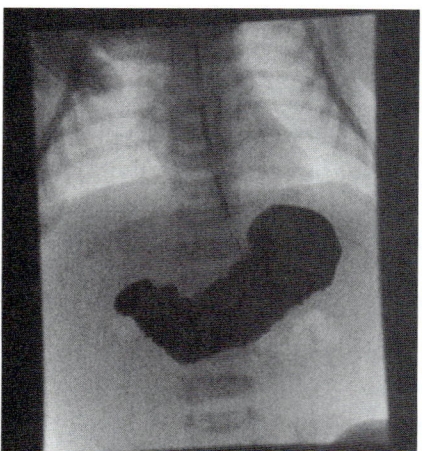
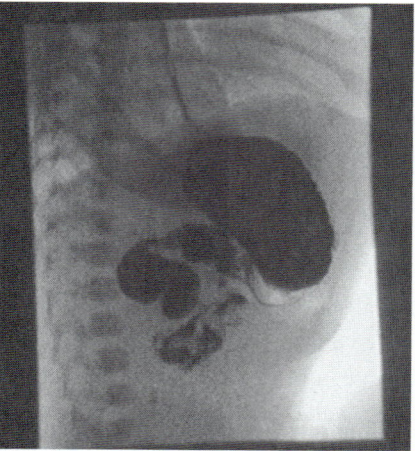
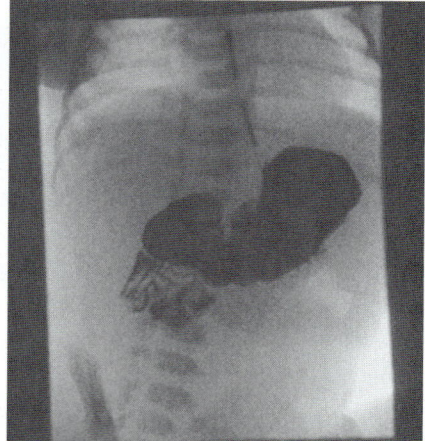

Figure 8-2 A. Serial films demonstrate mildly delayed gastric emptying. The proximal jejunum and small bowel are located to the right of midline, suggesting malrotation. Decompression of the more distal bowel beyond the third portion of the duodenum suggests partial obstruction at the third/fourth portions of the duodenum. Elapsed time is 17 minutes. Delayed study (1.5 hours) reveals some contrast within the proximal small bowel. No contrast is seen significantly past the midline. There is no contrast in the colon.

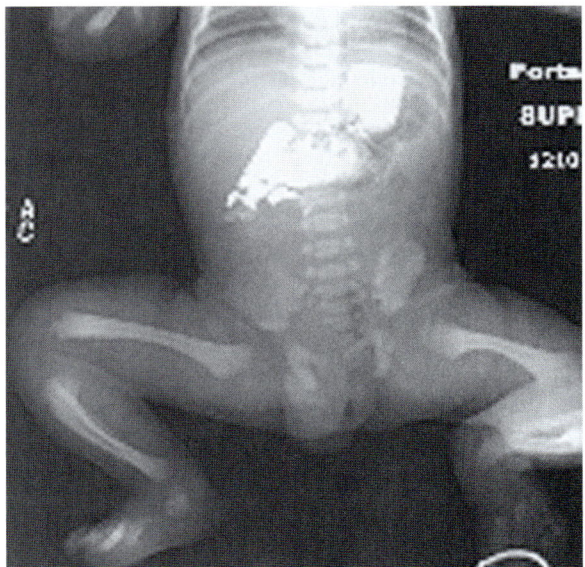

Figure 8-2 (*Cont.*) B. Overall impression: malrotation with obstructive Ladd bands.

abdominal ultrasound demonstrating an inversion of the relationship of the SMA and superior mesenteric vein (vein is usually located to the right) or by contrast study. Upper GI demonstrates malposition of the ligament of Treitz and

may reveal duodenal obstruction. Corroborative findings include obstruction, thickened bowel loops to the right of the spin, and free peritoneal fluid. Radiographic findings on abdominal x-ray may be misleading as there are several patterns of duodenal malrotation. Abdominal x-ray may show the "double bubble" of duodenal obstruction or cecum position in the right upper quadrant.

Clinical symptoms of malrotation are associated with volvulus (which may be intermittent), duodenal compression by Ladd bands, or compression of small and large bowel loops by ectopic adherent bands. The majority of patients present in the first year of life with symptoms of acute or chronic obstruction. Although most cases of symptomatic malrotation occur in infants, symptoms may occur at any age and patients may develop midgut volvulus without preceding symptoms. In a symptomatic patient, surgical intervention is required emergently. For asymptomatic patients with incidentally discovered malrotation, surgical correction is indicated owing to the risk of spontaneous midgut volvulus.

The true prevalence of malrotation is difficult to ascertain as a portion of patients with malrotation remain asymptomatic throughout life. Population-based studies have estimated the rate at 2.8 to 3.5/10,000 live births. In case series, 60% to 80% of identified patients with malrotation present with symptoms in the first year of life. In a population-based study of children greater than 1 year of age, the majority of patients presented in the second and third year of life, with an all-age estimation of 5.3 cases/1 million population. While the overall incidence is low, the substantial morbidity and mortality associated with delayed diagnosis requires that the practitioner strongly consider malrotation in any infant with bilious emesis.

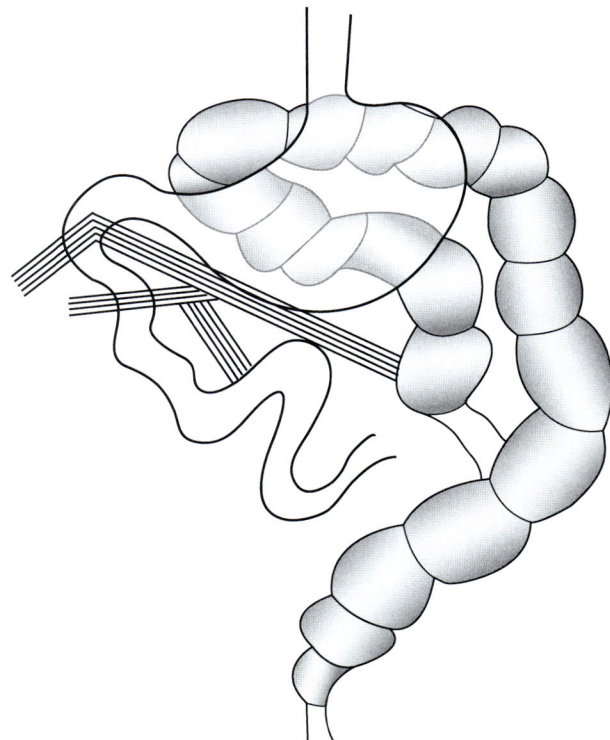

Figure 8-3 Operative findings of malrotation and duodenal compression by Ladd bands.

Selected References

1. Wyllie R. Intestinal Atreasia, Stenosis, and Malrotation. *Nelson Textbook of Pediatrics.* 17th ed. Elsevier Publishing; 2004: 1233–1236.
2. Forrester MB, Merz RD. Epidemiology of intestinal malrotation, Hawaii, 1986–1999. *Paediatr Perinat Epidemiol.* 2003;17: 195–200.
3. Kim WK, Kim H, Ahn DH, et al. Timetable for intestinal rotation in staged human embryos and fetuses. *Birth Defects Res A Clin Mol Teratol.* 2003 Nov;67(11):941–945.
4. Kluth D, Jaeschke-Melli S, Fiegel H. The embryology of gut rotation. *Semin Pediatr Surg.* 2003 Nov;12(4):275–279.
5. Malek MM, Burd RS. Surgical treatment of malrotation after infancy: a population-based study. *J Pediatr Surg.* 2005 Jan; 40(1):285–289.

6. Murphy FL, Sparnon AL. Long-term complications following intestinal malrotation and the Ladd's procedure: a 15-year review. *Pediatr Surg Int.* 2006 Apr;22(4):326–329.

7. Orzech N, Navarro OM, Langer JC. Is ultrasonography a good screening test for intestinal malrotation? *J Pediatr Surg.* 2006 May; 41(5):1005–1009.

8. Torres AM, Ziegler MM. Malrotation of the intestine. *World J Surg.* 1993 May;17(3):326–331.

9. Strouse PJ. Disorders of intestinal rotation and fixation ("malrotation"). *Pediatr Radiol.* 2004 Nov;34(11):837–851.

28-Year-Old Male with Fever after Return from Thailand

C 9

CASE PRESENTATION

A 28-year-old Caucasian male presents to urgent care 6 days after returning home from his honeymoon to Thailand. Four days prior to presentation, the patient developed fever 39°C, headache, chills, and sweats. The patient spent 3 weeks traveling throughout Thailand, where he predominantly visited the major cities along the coast staying in nice hotels. He also camped in remote areas. He enjoyed food from street vendors, drank tap water, swam in fresh water, and believes he may have swum downstream from people's refuse. He did not obtain any vaccinations prior to his trip and did not take any malaria prophylaxis. He denies any photophobia, neck pain, cough, shortness of breath, nausea, vomiting, diarrhea, bright red blood per rectum, dysuria, or myalgia. He and his wife have not noticed any changes in mentation or confusion. He denies any new sexual contacts or drug use. He does have some palpitations when he has fever. He has no past medical history. He is on no chronic medications, but has been taking acetaminophen for his fevers.

Physical Examination

Vital signs: temperature 38.6°C, pulse 111 beats/min, respiratory rate 16 breaths/min, blood pressure (BP) 153/80 mm Hg, with room air oxygen saturation of 100% on room air. Orthostatics: sitting BP 153/73 mm Hg and heart rate (HR) 96 beats/min, standing BP 131/75 mm Hg and HR 114 beats/min. Patient was flushed and ill appearing lying on the examination table. Head, eyes, ears, nose, and throat: normocephalic, atraumatic, pupils equal, round, reactive to light, extraocular movement intact, sclera anicteric, dry mucous membranes. Neck: supple, no lymphadenopathy. Cardiovascular: tachycardic; normal S_1, S_2; no murmur. Lungs: clear to auscultation bilaterally. Abdomen: soft, nontender, normal active bowel sounds. No hepatosplenomegaly. Skin: flushed with fine reticular pattern throughout his trunk and body, not on his palms or soles. Neurologic: cranial nerves II to XII grossly intact, strength 5/5 bilateral upper extremity and lower extremity; sensation intact to light touch throughout. Gait normal.

Laboratory Studies

White blood cells 5.3, hemoglobin 16.1, hematocrit 44, mean corpuscular volume 84, platelets (plts) 204 with giant platelets

Na 139, K 4.3, Cl 98, CO_2 29, blood urea nitrogen 10, creatinine 1.1, glucose 99, Ca 9, Mg 1.7, K 2.9

Aspartate aminotransferase 36, alanine aminotransferase 31

Malaria thick and thin smears: no parasites detected

Mononucleosis: negative.

Schistosoma immunoglobulin G antibody: negative

Blood culture × 2: no growth at 5 days. Urine culture: negative

Stool culture: *Salmonella* species

Chest x-ray: no cardiomegaly, infiltrate, or effusion

Case Resolution

The patient received an intravenous fluid bolus bolusin in the emergency room with resolution of his orthostasis. Therapy was initiated with ciprofloxacin, and the patient remained in the hospital overnight for observation. He defervesced and felt much better in the morning. He was discharged home and followed up in clinic 1 day after discharge at which time he continued to improve. The patient completed his course of ciprofloxacin and recovered completely. The stool culture sent to the state laboratory demonstrated *Salmonella virchow*.

Question

What is the most helpful aspect of the workup of fever in the international traveler?

Answer

A thorough history and physical examination with particular attention to destination and timing of travels and possible exposures allowing you to narrow the oftentimes broad differential.

Discussion

International travel is becoming exceedingly common, with many travelers now seeking even more remote and exotic destinations. According to the World Tourism Organization, international tourist arrivals reached an all time record of 763 million in 2004. More than 50 million people travel from industrialized to developing countries. The growth of ecotravel and visits to family and friend in areas off the typical tourist path increase the possibility of exposures. Although most reported illnesses are mild, 1% to 5% of travelers become ill enough to seek medical care either during or soon after their trip, 0.01% to 0.1% require medical evacuation, and 1 in 100,000 dies. While infectious pathogens cause significant morbidity, they account for only about 1% of deaths; cardiovascular events and accidents (automobile, aircraft, drowning, etc) actually cause most deaths.

A diagnostic framework based on geographical medicine may be helpful when evaluating the ill international

traveler. A careful history (See Table 9-1) with particular attention to the itinerary including specific dates of travel, destination (urban vs. remote), and style of travel (five-star hotels vs. camping); exposure history (foods, drinking water, freshwater contact, sexual history; drug use, medication or treatment received abroad; animal contact; and insect bites); immunization history and antimalarial chemoprophylaxis is the essential first step. This initial evaluation should focus on life-threatening, treatable, or contagious infections.

This detailed travel history will begin the process of identifying potential pathogens. Freedman et al (2006), with the GeoSentinel study group, recently published

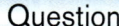

TABLE 9-1

Incubation Periods of Common Traveler-Related Illnesses

Short <7 days
- Arbovirus
- Enteric bacterial infections including paratyphoid
- Enteric viral infections
- Pneumonia
- Influenza
- Plague

Medium (11–21 days)
- Malaria
- Typhoid fever
- Rickettsial infections: spotted fever group, Q fever
- Enteric protozoal infections
- Enteric hepatitis
- Leptospirosis
- African trypsanomiasis
- Brucellosis
- Strongyloides

Long (>30 days)
- Malaria
- Viral hepatitis
- Enteric protozoal infections
- Enteric helminthic infections
- Tuberculosis
- Amebic liver abscess
- Filariasis

Adapted from Spira AM. Assessment of travelers who return home ill. Lancet. 2003 April 26;361:1459–1469.

the largest study to date detailing the regional differences in infectious etiologies among 17,353 ill travelers from 230 countries. Malaria was among the top three etiologies of undifferentiated fever in ill travelers from all regions. Moreover, it was the leading cause of undifferentiated fever in travelers from sub-Saharan Africa. Dengue fever was a common cause of fever and occurred more frequently than malaria, except as mentioned in sub-Saharan Africa and also in Central America. Travelers from south central Asia were often suffering from typhoid fever. These new data detailing regional differences in infectious etiologies in combination with travel resources from the Center for Disease Control (www.cdc.gov) will help quickly develop a broad differential.

Different exposures during travel may also significantly contribute to infection. Local food and water consumption may result in diarrheal illnesses, the most common illness associated with travel. Remote locales with associated insect bites and fresh water swimming make leptospirosis and schistosomiasis possible. New sexual contacts are common among travelers, especially among young, long-term travelers, for example, Peace Corps volunteers, who are often without reliable condom use. Any known sick contacts and consideration of any medical care or treatments obtained abroad may be revealing, as injections of medication are a common therapy.

Incubation periods of different infections may help to narrow the differential. As outlined in Table 9-2, fever less than 5 days after exposure would rule out malaria, as the incubation period is too short; however, fever 1 week to even up to 1 year after travel to a malarious region may certainly be a result of malaria infection.

Although the physical examination is often entirely benign even in those infected with *Plasmodium falciparum*, when present, certain physical findings may help make the diagnosis. Any signs of mental status changes, focal neurological

---

TABLE 9-2

Key Questions for History

1. Destinations and all places visited
2. Dates of travel and temporal relationship to symptoms
3. Exposure to insects and animals
4. Sexual activity
5. Medication and vaccination history
6. Quality and preparation of food and liquids consumed

---

signs, respiratory distress, hemorrhagic symptoms, or hemodynamic instability obviously require emergent treatment. In addition to consideration of rare causes of symptoms, always recall treatable infections that may exhibit the same findings. For example, while hemorrhage may result from viral hemorrhagic fevers, requiring supportive care and isolation, other diseases such as meningococcemia, leptospirosis, plague, rickettsial illness, or vibrio infection may produce similar findings and have available treatments.

Initial laboratory studies should include a complete blood count (CBC) and differential, blood cultures, blood smears for malaria, liver function tests, and chest radiograph with additional studies dictated by history.

For the 3% of travelers to developing countries who develop fever, this systematic approach will help identify the infections and treat them. Common infections with unusual presentations outside of the expected season, for example flu in the southern hemisphere in June must be considered. Malaria, dengue fever, mononucleosis (Epstein-Barr virus [EBV], cytomegalovirus [CMV]), rickettsial infection, and enteric fever were the most commonly identified infections in travelers with undifferentiated fever presenting to GeoSentinel study sites. Please see Table 9-3 for a summary of the frequency of fever and concomitant diagnoses in four series of returning travelers with fever.

Malaria

Early identification of travel to malarious destinations can be lifesaving. Malaria infection with *P. falciparum* can be quickly fatal and fever is an emergency in patients traveling in endemic regions. Even if afebrile at the time of presentation, a malaria smear should be performed on the same day. *Plasmodium falciparum* infections usually present within 1 month of returning from an endemic area while *Plasmodium malariae* and *Plasmodium ovale* infections may present up to 1 year after return. Chemoprophylaxis does not eliminate the possibility of infection, but may prolong the incubation time, and one negative malaria smear does not rule out the diagnosis. A longer length of stay in an endemic area increases the likelihood of infection.

Dengue

Dengue fever is the most common arboviral infection among travelers. It is common in tropical and subtropical regions. The urban, daytime-biting *Aedes* mosquito transmits the flavivirus. Children are reportedly most susceptible to infection and morbidity appears to worsen with repeated infection.

TABLE 9-3

Frequency of Fever and Diagnosis in Four Published Series of Returned Travelers

Diagnosis	Frequency of fever (%)			
	MacLean (n = 587)	Doherty (n = 195)	O'Brien (n = 587)	Hill (n = 822)
Malaria	32	42	27	2
Unknown	25	25	9	8
Hepatitis	6	3	3	2
Respiratory	11	2.5	24	24
Urinary tract	4	2.5	2	0
Dengue	2	6	8	1
Enteric fever	2	2	3	0
Diarrheal disease	4.5	6.5	14	31
Infectious mononucleosis	2	0.5	0.4	0
Pharyngitis	1	2	0	0
Rickettsia	1	0.5	2	1
Amoebic liver abscess	1	0	0	0
Tuberculosis	1	2	1	0
Meningitis	1	1	1	0
Acute HIV	0.3	1	0.4	0
Miscellaneous	6.3	5	5.2	33

Adapted from MacLean JD, Lalonde R, Ward B. Fever from the tropics. Travel Med Advisor. *1994;5:27.1–27.14. Doherty JF, Grant AD, Bryceson AD. Fever as the presenting complaint of travellers returning from the tropics.* QJM. *1995;88:277–281. O'Brien D, Tobin S, Brown G, et al. Fever in returned travelers: review of hospital admissions for a 3-year period.* Clin Infect Dis. *2001;33:603–609. Hill DR. Health problems in a large cohort of Americans traveling to developing countries.* J Trav Med. *2000;7:259–266.*
HIV, human immunodeficiency virus.

Diagnosis is most often clinical in patients presenting within 2 weeks of exposure with complaints of fever, chills, myalgias, and headache, often retro-orbital. Diagnosis may be confirmed with a fourfold increase in antibody titer between acute and convalescent titers drawn at least 4 weeks apart. Dengue does not respond to antivirals; however, supportive care can be lifesaving especially if patients develop hemorrhagic complications.

Rickettsial Illness

Rickettsial infections are probably underreported in patients and occur more frequently than we appreciate. The predominance of rickettsial infections in travelers is caused by tick-borne spotted fever. This tick typhus, also known as African tick typhus, Mediterranean spotted fever, or boutonneuse fever, caused by infection with *Rickettsia africae* and *Rickettsia conorii,* is the most common

rickettsial illness in travelers. Moreover, in the GeoSentinel sample, it was the only rickettsial infection seen, and only in travelers to sub-Saharan Africa. Q fever (*Coxiella burnetii*) represents a much less common rickettsial infection. Infection is spread through inhalation or consumption of unpasteurized dairy products and not by arthropod bites. While other rickettsial infections often present with persistent fever, headache, myalgia, arthralgia, and malaise with rash developing 5 to 6 days after fever, Q fever usually does not have any rash and may present with pneumonia symptoms or hepatitis. Diagnosis is oftentimes clinical and confirmed with serologic testing. Treatment is with doxycycline.

Enteric Fever

Infection with *Salmonella typhi* or *Salmonella paratyphi* from contaminated food and water causes enteric fever.

Patients often present with a 1- to 2-week history of progressively increasing fever, headache, abdominal pain, and constipation. Diarrhea may have occurred earlier in their course and is more common in children. Rose spots, blanching macular lesions on the trunk, may be present. Diagnosis is most commonly made by blood culture during the first week of illness, and then by either stool or bone marrow culture later in the course of the disease. However, culture yield may be affected by antibiotic treatment during travel. Recent vaccination does not exclude the possibility of infection as the oral vaccine is only 70% effective and does not cover *S. paratyphi* infection. Treatment is with ciprofloxacin; however, fluoroquinolone resistance is increasing.

While the list of possible etiologies of fever in the returned international traveler is daunting, a systemic approach with emphasis on a detailed, thorough history and physical examination will facilitate an efficient and potentially lifesaving diagnosis and subsequent treatment of patients.

References

Freedman DO, Weld LH, Kozarsky PE, et al. Spectrum of disease and relation to place of exposure among ill returned travelers. *N Engl J Med.* 2006 Jan 12;354(2):119–130.

Hill DR. Health problems in a large cohort of Americans traveling to developing countries. *J Travel Med.* 2000 Sept–Oct;7(5):259–266.

Ryan ET, Milson ME, Kain KC. Illness after international travel. *N Engl J Med.* 2002 Aug 15;347(7):505–516.

Re VL III, Gluckman SJ. Fever in the returned traveler. *Am Fam Physician.* 2003 Oct 1;68(7):1343–1350.

Spira AM. Assessment of travelers who return home ill. Lancet. 2003 April 26;361:1459–1469. *UNWTO Tourism Highlights* 2005 World Tourism Organization Publications, Madrid, Spain, 2005. Wilson M. Evaluation of fever in the returning traveler. Rose, BD, ed. *UpToDate.* Waltham, MA, 2007. Version 15.3. August 2007.

MacLean JD, Lalonde R, Ward B. Fever from the tropics. *Travel Med Advisor.* 1994;5:27.1–27.14.

Doherty JF, Grant AD, Bryceson AD. Fever as the presenting complaint of travellers returning from the tropics. *QJM.* 1995;88:277–281.

O'Brien D, Tobin S, Brown G, et al. Fever in returned travelers: review of hospital admissions for a 3-year period. *Clin Infect Dis.* 2001;33:603–609.

9-Year-Old African American Male with Juvenile Rheumatoid Arthritis and Progressive Dyspnea

CASE PRESENTATION

A 9-year-old African American male with a 4-year history of chronic right knee pain and persistent swelling presents with gradually worsening shortness of breath. The patient developed right knee pain and swelling at 5 years of age and was diagnosed with pauciarticular juvenile rheumatoid arthritis (JRA) (antinuclear antibody test [ANA] negative, rheumatoid factor negative). He has had no other affected joints or other symptoms until his current presentation. His treatment regimen includes daily prednisone and weekly methotrexate as well as several past steroid injections into the affected joint. Despite these therapies, his joint pain has been persistent. Ten days ago, the patient began to experience shortness of breath that has progressed over the past 24 hours to significant dyspnea while at rest. His mother reports that he has also had a mild dry cough and a 10-lb weight loss during this time period, but no fever, chills, night sweats, hemoptysis, or runny nose. His past medical history is significant only as noted above. He is doing well in the third grade. He has no significant travel history and no sick contacts. There is no family history of arthritis, lupus, or sarcoid.

Physical Examination

The patient is alert, anxious appearing, in moderate respiratory distress. Height and weight measurements are at the 25th percentile. Vital signs: temperature: 36.9°C, pulse 120 beats/min, blood pressure 94/71 mm Hg, respiratory rate 50 breaths/min, with room air oxygen saturation of 88%. Head, eyes, ears, nose, and throat: normocephalic, pupils equal, round, reactive to light, extraocular movement intact. Neck: supple with shotty bilateral cervical lymph nodes. Lungs: significant increased work of breathing with intercostal retractions, coarse bilateral breath sounds, scattered crackles, and decreased air movement at the bases bilaterally. Cardiovascular: regular rhythm and rate with a grade 1/6 systolic ejection murmur heard best at the left lower sternal border, 2+ pulses bilaterally. Abdomen: soft, nontender, nondistended, normal bowel sounds; no hepatosplenomegaly. Extremities: right knee is moderately swollen with slight warmth but no erythema, mild pain to palpation, and active/passive motion; no other joint abnormalities or gross bony abnormalities. Skin: no rashes. Neurologic: anxious appearing, cranial nerves (CN) II to XII intact, deep tendon reflexes brisk and symmetric, no focal neurologic deficits.

Laboratory Studies

White blood cells 7.7, hemoglobin 12.4, hematocrit 37. Mean corpuscular volume 77, platelets 273. Electrolytes, blood urea nitrogen, creatinine within normal limits. Aspartate aminotransferase 138, alanine aminotransferase 63, erythrocyte sedimentation rate 32. Prothrombin time/activated partial prothrombin time slightly elevated. Arterial blood gas on room air, pH 7.48, P_{CO_2} 35, P_{O_2} 55. Purified protein derivative (PPD) negative. Gastric aspirates × 3: negative acid-fast bacillus (AFB) smear. Posterior to anterior/lateral chest x-ray: diffuse nodular interstitial infiltrates, low lung volumes, normal mediastinal contour and heart size, no bony abnormalities (Fig. 10-1). Chest computed tomography (CT): diffuse bilateral interstitial airspace opacities, calcified

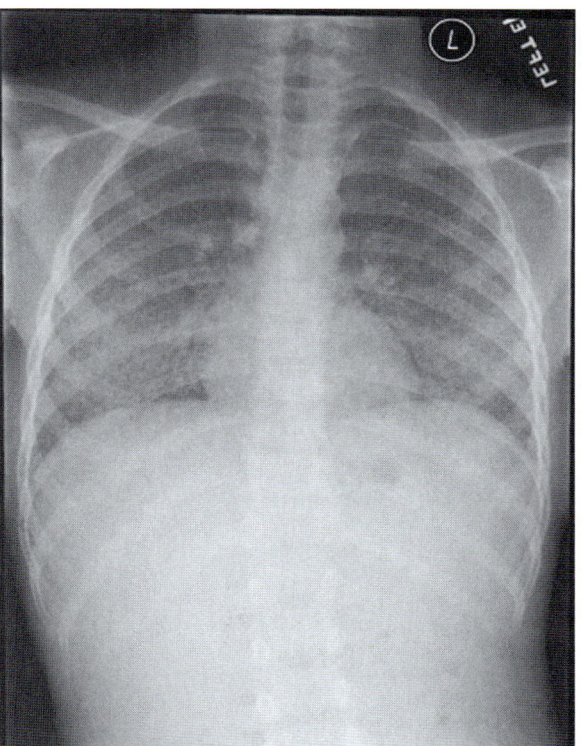 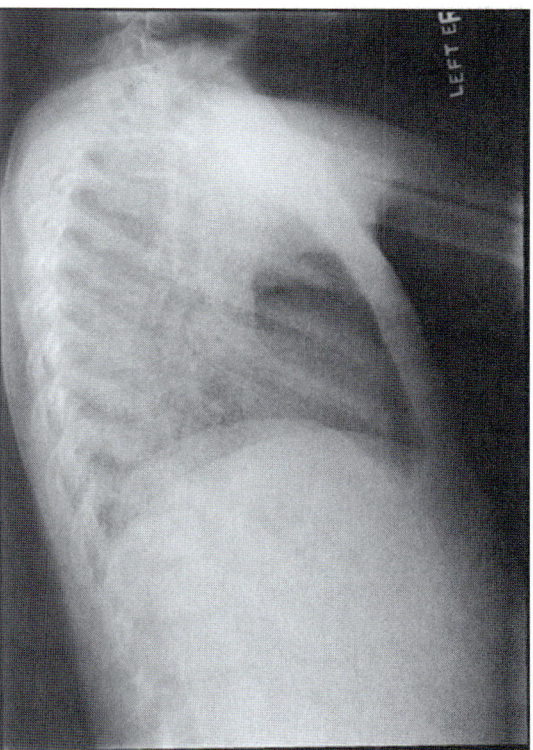

Figure 10-1 Chest x-ray showing diffuse nodular interstitial infiltrates without focal consolidation. The cardiac silhouette is within normal limits, and no bony abnormalities are seen.

right paratracheal and right hilar lymphadenopathy, calcified 2 mm right upper lobe nodule (Fig. 10-2).

Case Resolution

The patient was initially started on empiric antibacterial therapy with ceftriaxone, azithromycin, and trimethoprim/ sulfamethoxazole (TMP/SMX). His respiratory distress and pulmonary infiltrates worsened, requiring intubation and mechanical ventilation. Given the high index of suspicion for tuberculosis (TB), an open lung biopsy was performed, the pathology from which showed necrotizing granulomatous inflammation with histochemical stains positive for AFB. Cultures from the lung tissue were negative on AFB stain but eventually grew mycobacterium TB. The patient also underwent surgical exploration, debridement, and biopsy of his right knee after MRI was obtained (Fig. 10-3) and revealed extensive synovitis with severe erosion of cartilage and cyst formation in the medial femoral condyle. Histopathology from synovial and bony tissue revealed AFB (Fig. 10-4), and cultures from synovial tissue, bony tissue, and cyst fluid all grew mycobacterium TB. The patient was started

on a four-drug therapy for miliary tuberculosis (MTB) with isoniazid, rifampin, pyrazinamide, and ethambutol, once pathology results from the lung biopsy were available. His lung disease gradually improved on this regimen, and he was extubated after 2 weeks on mechanical ventilation. Attempts to feed the patient after extubation were complicated by complaints of abdominal pain and vomiting. Amylase and lipase at that time were moderately elevated and abdominal ultrasound was normal. Rifampin was held briefly without improvement in amylase/lipase, and the patient was given the presumptive diagnosis of pancreatic involvement with MTB. His symptoms and laboratory abnormalities slowly improved with TB therapy and tube feeding. Given the extensive destruction of the patient's right knee and young age for knee replacement, the patient was placed in a soft cast with plans for joint fusion once he fully recovered from his hospitalization.

Question

How do you diagnose extrapulmonary or disseminated mycobacterium TB?

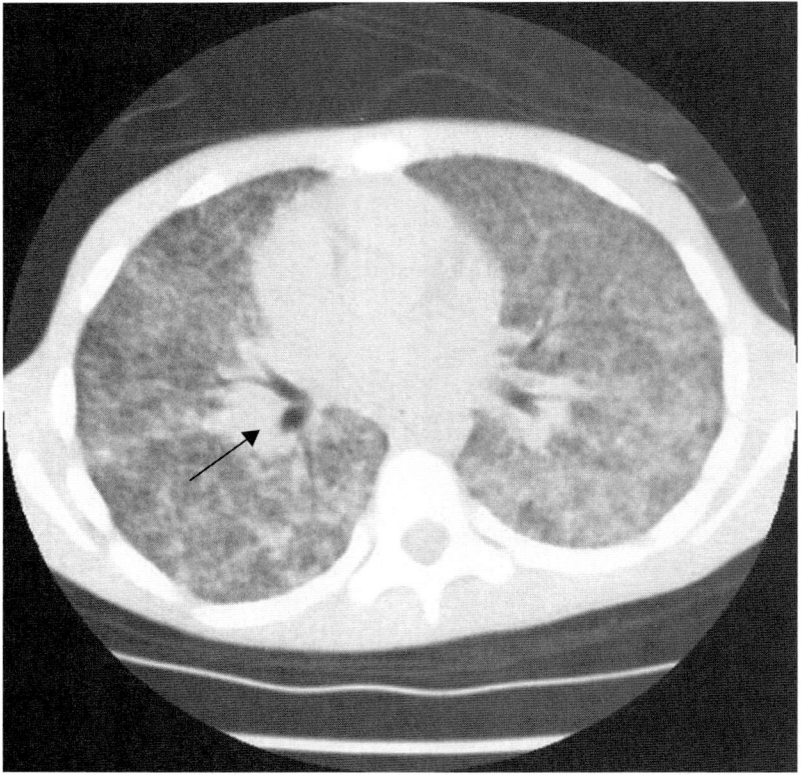

Figure 10-2 Chest CT showing miliary pattern with diffusely scattered 2- to 3-mm nodules and right hilar lymphadenopathy (black arrow). CT, computed tomography.

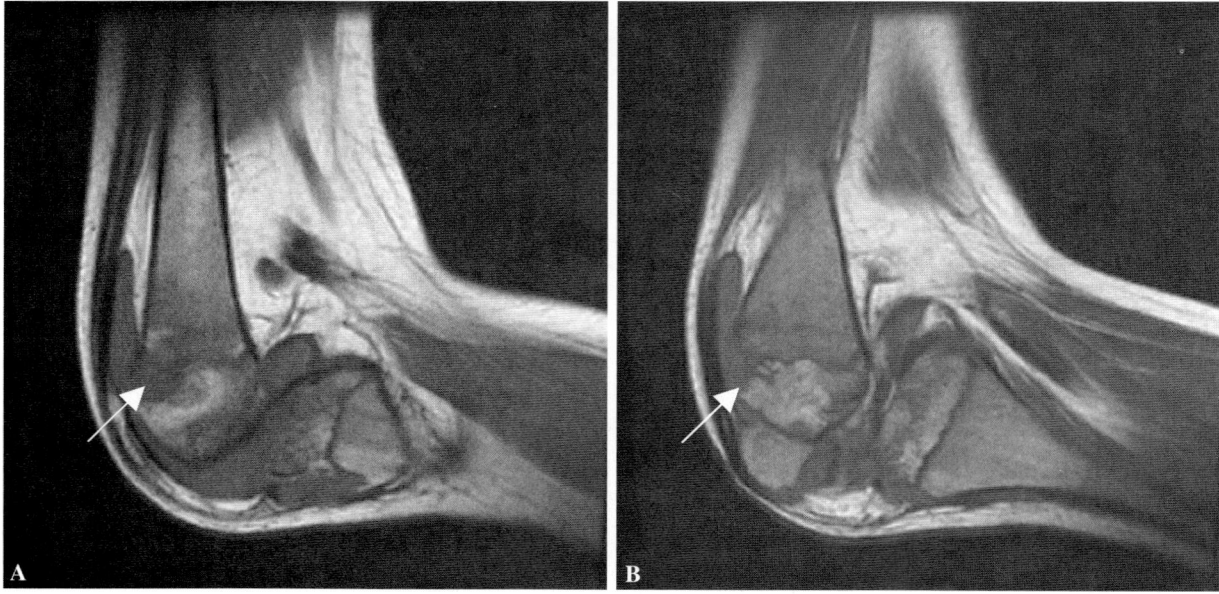

Figure 10-3 Sagittal T1-weighted images of the right knee following contrast administration demonstrate cartilage destruction and anterior subluxation of the femur upon the tibial plateau. A large bony erosion (white arrows) is seen anteriorly at the femoral growth plate, and joint effusions with mild synovial enhancement are seen both anteriorly and posteriorly.

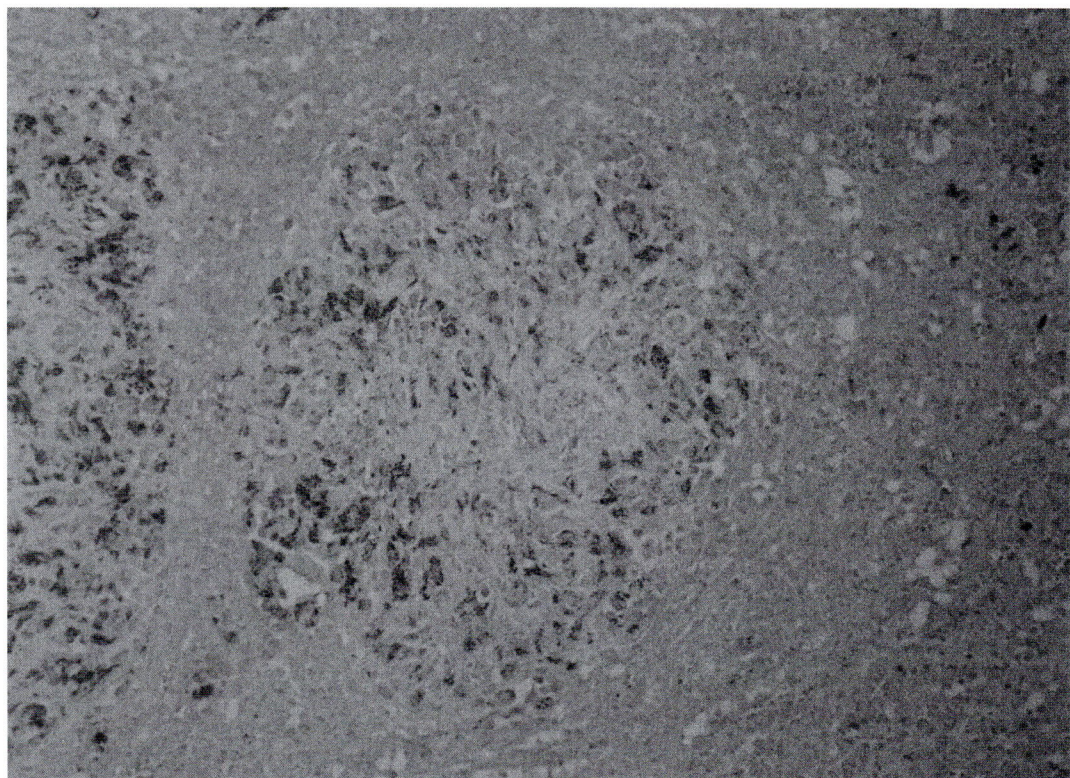

Figure 10-4 Acid-fast bacilli as seen in a lymph node biopsy from the index patient. Multiple red-stained bacilli are seen throughout.

Answer

The diagnosis of extrapulmonary or disseminated TB can be challenging, particularly in children who have a higher incidence of extrapulmonary TB (EPTB) and may be unable to produce induced sputum for culture. The most important aspect of diagnosing extrapulmonary TB is a high index of clinical suspicion (see Table 10-1). Obtaining tissue for histopathology and culture is the most effective method of diagnosing EPTB, but there are many other studies to consider.

Discussion

The incidence of TB in United States increased dramatically from 1985 to 1992 because of the HIV/AIDS epidemic. Since then, rates have declined each year, but the rate of decline is now slowing, due in part to the increasing proportion of the American population represented by foreign-born persons. The TB rate in foreign-born persons in 2005 was 8.7 times that of US-born persons. The TB rate in Hispanics, blacks, and Asians was 7.3, 8.3, and 19.6 times higher than that in whites, respectively.

TB in children represents 6% to 7% of all cases in United States from 1993 to 2005. Children are also at higher risk of developing active TB when initially infected, with 24% of children age 1 to 5 and 42% of children less than 1 year old developing active disease at the time of infection. Approximately 10% to 15% of children have a negative tuberculin skin test at the time of initial diagnosis. Smears for AFB are also less likely to be positive in children because they generally have paucibacillary disease. Finally, children are more likely than adults to present with extrapulmonary or atypical pulmonary disease.

EPTB and MTB are usually caused by hematogenous spread from the primary complex through the intrathoracic lymph node and thoracic duct. After infecting multiple sites, the infection is usually contained by cell-mediated immunity. It may then resurface later in life because of concurrent illness or immunosuppression. As expected, the risk of EPTB and MTB increases with increasing immunosuppression, and extrapulmonary disease can be seen in more than 50% of patients with AIDS and TB.

A high index of suspicion is necessary to diagnose EPTB, especially in the absence of obvious risk factors.

TABLE 10-1

Clinical Findings Suspicious for Extrapulmonary Tuberculosis

Fluid analyses showing evidence of inflammation with negative bacterial cultures
- Sterile pyuria
- Ascitic fluid with lymphocyte predominance
- Exudative pleural fluid with lymphocyte predominance and pleural thickening
- Monoarticular joint inflammation: Examination of synovial fluid is central to the management of monoarticular synovitis
- CSF with lymphocytic pleocytosis, elevated protein, and low glucose

Unexplained signs of chronic inflammation in other tissues
- Pericardial effusion, constrictive pericarditis, or pericardial calcification
- Vertebral osteomyelitis involving the thoracic spine
- Chronic lymphadenopathy (especially cervical)
- Differential diagnosis of Crohn disease and amebiasis
- HIV infection
- Tuberculosis: endemic country of origin

Adapted from Golden MP, Vikram HR. Extrapulmonary tuberculosis: an overview. Am Fam Physician. 2005;72(9):1761–1768.
CSF, cerebrospinal fluid; HIV, human immunodeficiency virus.

TABLE 10-2

Distribution of Anatomical Sites in Tuberculosis*

HIV-negative	
Pulmonary only	75%
Extrapulmonary only	20%
Both	5%
HIV-positive	
Pulmonary only	30%
Extrapulmonary only	20%
Both	50%
Extrapulmonary sites	
Lymph nodes	35%
Pleural effusion	20%
Bone and joint	10%
Genitourinary	9%
Miliary	8%
Meninges	5%
Abdominal	3%
Other	10%

Adapted from Sharma SK, Mohan A. Extrapulmonary tuberculosis. Indian J Med Res. 2004;120:316–353.
*These rates represent the general population and are not specific to adult or pediatric patients.

The most common sites of involvement in EPTB are listed in Table 10-2. This discussion will focus on the diagnosis of extrapulmonary and disseminated TB in the general population, with specific references to certain epidemiological differences in children.

Tuberculous lymphadenitis (scrofula) is most commonly found in cervical nodes, although any site can be involved. Previously thought to be a childhood illness, lymphadenitis actually peaks around age 20 to 40. While nontuberculous mycobacterial lymphadenitis is more common in children, tuberculous disease is the more common form in adults. The nodes are slow growing, firm and nontender, and may eventually become matted and discolored, with fluctuance and sinus tract formation. Most often, tuberculin skin testing is positive (74%–98%) and chest radiographs are usually negative. Diagnosis is by excisional biopsy with histology, AFB stain, and mycobacterial culture. Fine needle aspiration may be possible in HIV-positive patients because of the higher burden of organisms seen in these patients.

Pleural TB is considered a form of EPTB and can occur during any stage of infection, often presenting acutely with cough, dyspnea, fever, or pleuritic chest pain. About 20% of cases are associated with concurrent pulmonary lesions. CT of the chest may reveal other lesions not seen on CXR, and pleural thickening on CT of more than 1 cm is seen in most cases. PPD is positive in 73% to 93% of cases. Analysis of pleural fluid reveals a lymphocytic predominance later in the disease, although a neutrophil predominance can be seen in the first 2 weeks of illness. Fluid glucose and pH may be low or normal, and AFB smears of pleural fluid are rarely (<5%) positive in the absence of a tuberculous empyema. While pleural fluid cultures are positive in less than 40% of cases, pleural biopsy specimens for histology, smear, and culture have a combined sensitivity of more than 90%. Biochemical markers in the pleural fluid such as adenosine deaminase, interferon-gamma, and lysozyme are being studied, as is pleural fluid polymerase chain reaction (PCR).

Bone and joint EPTB is most often seen in the spine (Pott's disease), where it is usually thoracic. Other sites include large weight-bearing joints and extraspinal osteomyelitis, which can involve any bone. The classic palpable spinal prominence (gibbus) is formed by anterior wedging and angulation of the spine because of disc space obliteration and destruction of adjacent vertebrae. Presenting symptoms of spinal involvement include localized pain, constitutional symptoms, or paraplegia because of spinal cord compression (Pott's paraplegia, seen in 30% of patients). Involvement of the hip or knee joints presents without systemic symptoms as slowly progressive monoarthritis with pain, swelling, and decreased range of motion. Skin testing is usually positive in bone disease. Radiographic findings may include soft tissue swelling, joint space narrowing, subchondral erosions, and juxta-articular osteopenia. CXRs reveal pulmonary involvement in about 50% of patients with bone and joint disease. Synovial fluid culture is positive in about 80% of patients with arthritis, and synovial biopsy can also be diagnostic. Bone biopsy is necessary when tuberculous osteomyelitis is suspected.

Tuberculous meningitis is the most common form of central nervous system (CNS) disease and also represents the second most common form of extrapulmonary TB in children after lymphadenitis. It complicates 20% of cases of MTB in children and can be seen in 1% to 2% of all cases of untreated pediatric TB. Neurological involvement is five times more common in HIV-positive patients than in HIV-negative patients. It results from rupture of a subependymal tubercle into the subarachnoid space, causing intense inflammation of the arachnoid, which can in turn lead to CN palsies, focal neurologic deficits (from inflammation around penetrating vessels), and communicating hydrocephalus in addition to the classic features of meningitis. Progression of disease usually occurs over weeks, but the acuity can range from a rapidly progressive disease simulating acute bacterial meningitis to an indolent course presenting as cognitive decline. As opposed to adult cases, the majority of pediatric cases of TB meningitis occurs within 8 weeks of initial infection and may actually precede any CXR findings. CNS disease also includes intracranial tuberculomas, which can present as space-occupying lesions. Tuberculomas are usually infratentorial in patients less than 20 years old and supratentorial in older adults.

Cerebrospinal fluid (CSF) findings in CNS TB include a moderate lymphocytic pleocytosis, elevated protein, and low glucose. Sensitivity of the AFB smear ranges from 10% to 90%, and is improved with larger volumes of CSF, multiple taps, and centrifugation of samples. The use of adenosine deaminase concentrations in CSF is being studied. Head CT may reveal basilar arachnoiditis, tuberculomas, infarctions, or hydrocephalus. In children, as many as 50% of cases of tuberculous meningitis will have a negative PPD, because of the early development of the disease as noted above.

Tuberculous enteritis presents with nonspecific symptoms including fever, weight loss, abdominal pain, and diarrhea. Melena and rectal bleeding can also occur, and a palpable right lower quadrant mass is found in up to 50% of patients. Patients may develop fistulas, obstruction, perforation, anal fissures, or perirectal abscesses. Barium study and colonoscopy may show ulcerative or hypertrophic lesions, while abdominal CT may show extraluminal involvement such as lymphadenopathy. Biopsy by colonoscopy or laparotomy provides a definitive diagnosis. Since Crohn's disease presents in a similar fashion, it is essential to consider TB in the differential diagnosis of inflammatory bowel disease, because institution of immunosuppressive therapy can lead to dissemination of mycobacteria.

Tuberculous peritonitis presents with slowly developing abdominal pain, ascites, and fever. It is more common in patients with HIV or cirrhosis and in patients on peritoneal dialysis. The ascitic fluid is exudative and fluid findings mirror those seen in pleural and CNS disease, with a moderate lymphocytic pleocytosis. Centrifugation of more than 1 L of ascitic fluid enhances the yield of AFB smear and culture. Peritoneal biopsy has the highest diagnostic accuracy and should be performed if possible. Other forms of abdominal TB include hepatobiliary, pancreatic, and splenic disease, but these are rare in immunocompetent patients and usually associated with miliary disease.

Genitourinary tuberculosis (GUTB) includes renal TB and genital TB. GUTB most often develops 5 to 25 years after the primary infection because of rupture of previously formed tubercles into the urinary tract. Renal disease usually presents as sterile pyuria, but can also cause flank pain, hematuria, and dysuria. Mycobacterial culture of three morning urine specimens is 90% sensitive in diagnosing renal disease. Intravenous pyelography may show papillary necrosis. Male genital involvement usually presents as a scrotal mass in association with renal disease, and may involve the prostate, seminal vesicles, epididymis, or testes. Surgical biopsy may be required for diagnosis. Female genital disease originates in the endosalpinx and can spread from there to the ovaries, peritoneum, endometrium, cervix, or vagina. Patients present with pelvic pain, infertility, or vaginal bleeding. Abdominal CT can reveal a number of nonspecific findings in the genitourinary system in both renal and genital disease.

Tuberculous pericarditis can present acutely or insidiously, and may include inflammatory symptoms such as chest pain, fever, and pericardial friction rub or symptoms relating to a large pericardial effusion such as pulsus paradoxus, tachycardia, distended neck veins, cardiomegaly, and ankle edema. Pericardial biopsy has a higher yield than analysis of pericardial fluid.

MTB occurs when the organism disseminates through the bloodstream and is not controlled by the host immune system. It is more common in immunosuppressed patients, occurring in 10% of patients with AIDS and pulmonary disease and 38% of patients with AIDS and extrapulmonary disease. Clinical findings include nonspecific symptoms such as fever, chills, night sweats, weight loss, and anorexia as well as symptoms relating to any involved organ system. Fever may develop several weeks prior to radiographic changes. MTB gets its name from the typical CXR findings seen in the majority of cases, with 2- to 3-mm nodules seen diffusely throughout the lungs (millet seeds). Diagnosis depends on the involved systems, but may require analysis of sputum; gastric aspirates (particularly in children); bronchoalveolar lavage; CSF; blood culture; or biopsy of lymph nodes, liver, or bone marrow (see Table 10-3). The PPD is negative in more than 50% of patients with MTB.

In summary, extrapulmonary and disseminated tuberculosis can present in a number of different ways and mimic a number of other diseases. Therefore, it is important to have a high index of clinical suspicion and understand the limitations of various diagnostic modalities. In particular, TB cannot be ruled out on the basis of a negative skin test, especially in children and immunosuppressed patients. Analysis of pleural, ascitic, joint, pericardial, or CSF should be preformed on large volumes of centrifuged samples, and in most cases obtaining tissue for histopathology and culture is the most reliable means of diagnosis. The patient discussed above was treated for years for presumed JRA, and there is no history that his knee was ever aspirated for mycobacterial culture, despite his poor response

TABLE 10-3

Sensitivities of Diagnostic Methods in Diagnosing Miliary/Disseminated Tuberculosis

Method	Sensitivity
Sputum	41%
Bronchoscopy	36%
Gastric lavage	61%
CSF	21%
Urine	32%
Bone marrow	58%
Liver biopsy	89%
Lymph node biopsy	90%

Adapted from Sharma SK, Mohan A. Extrapulmonary tuberculosis. Indian J Med Res. 2004;120:316–353.
CSF, cerebrospinal fluid.

to aggressive therapy for rheumatologic disease. A more concerted attempt at diagnosing TB earlier in his course, despite his lack of risk factors and negative skin test, may have prevented a severe case of MTB and avoided a prolonged intensive care unit stay.

Selected References

1. CDC. *Reported Tuberculosis in the United States, 2005*. Atlanta, GA: U.S. Department of Health and Human Services, CDC; Sept 2005.
2. CDC. Trends in tuberculosis—United States, 2005. *MMWR.* 2006;55(11):305–308.
3. Golden MP, Vikram HR. Extrapulmonary tuberculosis: an overview. *Am Fam Physician.* 2005;72(9):1761–1768.
4. Loeffler AM. Pediatric tuberculosis. *Semin Respir Infect.* 2003;18(4):272–291.
5. Sharma SK, Mohan A. Extrapulmonary tuberculosis. *Indian J Med Res.* 2004;120:316–353.

1-Day-Old Female with Cyanosis

CASE PRESENTATION

The patient is a 1-day-old female, who is the product of a normal full-term pregnancy, born by spontaneous vaginal delivery. There are no complications with the delivery and the infant is sent to the normal newborn nursery. At 9 hours of age, on routine examination, the nurse notices the infant is dusky appearing and tachypneic. She immediately provides blow-by oxygen, and places the infant on pulse oximetry. The pulse oximeter is reading 82% despite continuation of the blow-by oxygen. The infant remains tachypneic, and her extremities begin to look gray and mottled. The neonatal intensive care unit (NICU) team is paged to evaluate the baby.

Physical Examination

Patient is a cyanotic-appearing term infant in mild respiratory distress. Vital signs: temperature 37.3°C, pulse 140 beats/min, blood pressure 58/34 mm Hg, respiration rate 54 breaths/min, and oxygen saturations of 78%. Cardiac examination reveals a harsh grade 3/6 systolic ejection murmur heard throughout the precordium. Regular rate and rhythm. Femoral pulses are present bilaterally. Respiratory examination reveals a tachypneic infant with mild subcostal retractions. Lungs are clear to auscultation bilaterally without crackles. Abdomen is soft and liver is non-palpable. Extremities are mildly mottled, with bluish nail beds. Capillary refill is about 3 seconds. Remainder of the examination is unremarkable.

Laboratory Studies

Arterial blood gas (ABG) on 100%, F_{IO_2}: 7.24/62/33/26.6/-0.2. Lactate is 1. Complete blood count is unremarkable. Chemistries are unremarkable. Blood cultures are drawn. A stat chest x-ray (CXR) is done and is shown below (Fig. 11-1). An echocardiogram was done and showed pulmonary atresia, ventricular septal defect (VSD), right ventricular hypertrophy (RVH), posterior descending artery (PDA), and an overriding aorta.

Case Resolution

Patient was started on a prostaglandin E1 drip until an echocardiogram was obtained to confirm the diagnosis of Tetralogy of Fallot (TOF). Because of the small size of the pulmonary arteries and the distance between the right ventricle and pulmonary trunk, the decision was made to perform a modified Blalock-Taussig shunt on day of life (DOL) 2 as a palliative procedure. Corrective surgery was done at 8 months of age.

Question

Will a hyperoxia test help in the diagnosis of this child's cyanosis?

Answer

Yes. A hyperoxia test is done by measuring the arterial oxygen tension in the right radial artery (preductal) while the patient breathes 100% oxygen concentration for 10 minutes. This test is used to help distinguish pulmonary from cardiac causes of cyanosis. The response of the arterial oxygen tension will be different, and minimal, in the presence of shunt physiology. If an intracardiac right-to-left shunt exists, the pulmonary veins are already fully saturated with

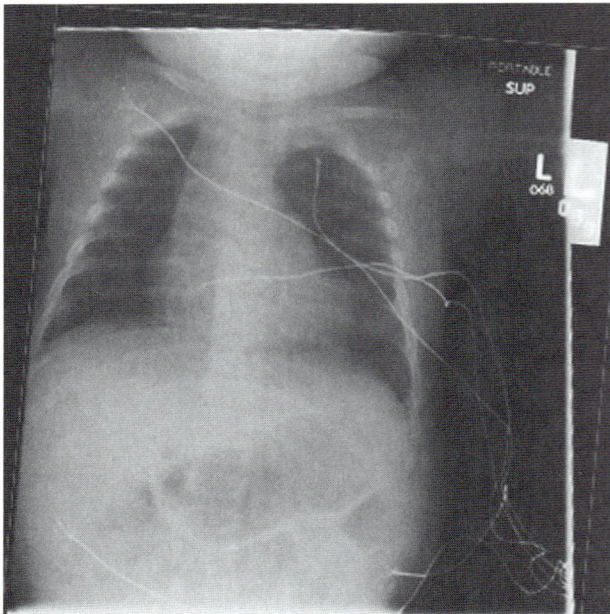

Figure 11-1 Chest roentgenogram in the cyanotic infant.

oxygen from breathing ambient air. The cyanosis in this situation arises from the mixing of deoxygenated blood with oxygenated blood within the heart. Increasing the amount of dissolved oxygen within the pulmonary veins will have little effect on arterial oxygen tension levels.

Discussion

The cyanotic infant in respiratory distress presents a diagnostic challenge to the general pediatrician. Speedy recognition of the cyanosis with a thorough physical examination is essential. The infant can then be stabilized, and further diagnostic studies can be performed. Ultimately, if a congenital cardiac anomaly is discovered, prompt referral to a tertiary care center for surgical intervention is indicated.

Cyanosis as a result of congenital heart disease may be caused by several different etiologies. Obstructions of the right ventricular outflow tract leading to intracardiac right-to-left shunting, or other anatomical anomalies causing a mixing of the pulmonary and systemic vascular return, is the most common cause of cyanosis in neonates (see Table 11-1). Cyanosis can also be seen with severe pulmonary edema from heart failure because of left-to-right shunting, or persistent fetal circulation pathways after birth. Delineation of the etiology of cyanosis in a neonate

should take place after initial stabilization. As seen in our patient, this evaluation includes an ABG on 100% oxygen, an electrocardiogram (ECG), a CXR, and an echocardiogram.

TOF is the most common form of cyanotic congenital heart disease. It involves a constellation of anatomic abnormalities that include a large ventricular septal defect, an overriding aorta over the defect, right ventricular outflow obstruction, and right ventricular hypertrophy. TOF was first correctly identified in the late nineteenth century by Etienne-Louis Arthur Fallot, and was initially termed *la maladie bleue*. Since that time, great advances have been made in the diagnosis and treatment of children with TOF. It is seen in 0.3 to 0.5/1000 live births, and accounts for about 10% of cases of congenital heart disease. Prevalence in males and females is about even. A large portion of children with TOF are found to be syndromic or have other chromosomal abnormalities (such as 22q11 deletion).

The lesions comprising TOF occur from abnormal development of the conotruncus in the fetal period. In order to develop a normal four-chamber heart, the pulmonary and aortic outflow tracts must orient and align over their prospective ventricles. In tetralogy, there is anterior and cephalad malalignment of the outlet septum relative to the muscular septum of the ventricles. There is also disproportionate division of the primitive truncus arteriosus into a small, atretic pulmonary component and a larger aortic component. This embryological defect results in the four morphological lesions that are characteristic of TOF: right ventricular outflow tract obstruction, ventricular septal defect, overriding aorta, and right ventricular hypertrophy (see Fig. 11-2). Other associated cardiac abnormalities that may be seen with TOF include a right-sided arch in 25% of the cases, and aortopulmonary collateral arteries seen commonly in patients with complete pulmonary atresia.

In patients with TOF, there are varying factors in the right ventricular outflow tract to the pulmonary vasculature that may cause a range of disease severity. Obstruction may range from pulmonary stenosis (infundibular, valvular, or in the main pulmonary artery) to complete pulmonary artery atresia. Depending on the degree of obstruction, varying amounts of systemic venous blood will be shunted across the nonrestrictive VSD into the aorta. This will result in cyanosis of the neonate.

Our patient displayed signs of cyanosis within the first 24 hours of life. In general, clinical findings at birth vary with the severity of pulmonary stenosis. When the ductus arteriosus closes shortly after birth in a child with complete

TABLE 11-1

Common Cyanotic Congenital Cardiac Lesions

Lesion	Examination findings	ECG findings	CXR findings
Tetralogy of Fallot • Large VSD • RV tract outflow Obstruction • RVH • Overriding aorta	• Loud systolic ejection murmur at LSB • Loud single S_2 • ± Thrill • Tet spells: as RVOT obstruction increases, increased shunting across VSD increases intensity of murmur and cyanosis	• RAD and RVH	• Boot-shaped heart • Normal heart size • Decreased pulmonary vascular markings
Transposition of the great vessels	• Extreme cyanosis • S_2 single and load • ± murmur → seen if VSD or PS	• RAD and RVH • Upright T wave in V_1	• "Egg on a string" with cardiomegaly • May have increased pulmonary vascular markings
Total anomalous pulmonary venous return • Pulmonary veins drain into RA or other location beside LA. Must have ASD or PDA for survival	• Hyperactive RV impulse • S_2 fixed and widely split • 3/6 SEM at LUSB • Mid-diastolic rumble at LLSB	• RAD • RVH • May see right atrial enlargement	• Cardiomegaly • Increased pulmonary markings • "Snowman in a snowstorm": usually seen after 4 months of age
Tricuspid atresia • Absent tricuspid valve and small RV and PA • Must have ASD, PDA, or VSD for survival Other (<1% frequency) • Pulmonary atresia • Truncus arteriosus • Ebstein anomaly • Double outlet right ventricle	• Single S_2 • Harsh systolic regurgitation murmur at LLSB if VSD	• Superior QRS axis • Right atrial enlargement, and LVH	• Normal or slightly enlarged heart • May have boot-shaped heart

Adapted from Gajewski, R. Chapter 6: Cardiology. In: The Harriet Lane Handbook. *17th ed. Robertson J, and Shilkofski N, eds. Elsevier Mosby; 2005.*

ASD, atrial septal defect; CXR, chest x-ray; ECG, electrocardiogram; LA, left auricle; LLSB, left lower sternal border; LSB, lower sternal border; LUSB, left upper sternal border; LVH, left ventricular hypertrophy; PA, pulmonary artery; PDA, posterior descending artery; PS, pulmonary stenosis; RA, right auricle; RAD, reactive airway disease; RV, right ventricular; RVH, right ventricular hypertrophy; RVOT, right ventricular outflow tract; VSD, ventricular septal defect.

atresia, cyanosis will result from the dramatic decrease in pulmonary blood flow and thus an acute substantial increase in right-to-left shunting. This is often the first presentation of cardiac disease in the infant, also called a hypercyanotic episode, or a "Tet spell." The cyanosis associated with these spells is often severe and hyperpnea is often present, which is thought to be in response to the acute hypoxia and a secondary metabolic acidosis. These episodes can occur spontaneously or after early morning feedings or prolonged crying.

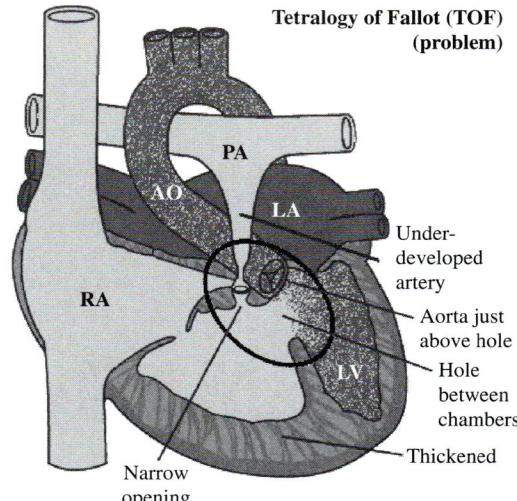

**Tetralogy of Fallot (TOF)
(problem)**

Under-developed artery

Aorta just above hole

Hole between chambers

Thickened

Narrow opening

Figure 11-2 Tetralogy of Fallot.

Whereas a witnessed Tet spell would obviously warrant a further workup of a child for a cardiac defect, there are several children with only moderate pulmonary outflow obstruction who may not present acutely at birth. Physical examination findings in these children can include a prominent right ventricular impulse on palpation, a normal S_1 and a single S_2 (with absent pulmonic component), and a harsh crescendo–decrescendo systolic ejection murmur heard best along the left midsternal border, with radiation to the back. As the degree of obstruction increases, and in complete pulmonary atresia, the murmur may be less obvious because of decreased flow across the obstruction.

After a swift but thorough physical examination, further workup for a cyanotic infant would include an ABG, a CXR, an ECG and an echocardiogram. An ABG on 100% oxygen may help delineate cardiac disease from other sources of cyanosis in an infant. Infants with TOF and restricted pulmonary flow will have a PaO_2 of around 50 on 100% FiO_2. If cyanosis is caused by respiratory or neurological causes, PaO_2 will be well greater than 150. A chest roentgenogram in the neonate with tetralogy will show a normal-sized heart with decreased vascular markings in the lung fields (see Fig. 11-1). Because the right ventricular outflow tract and main pulmonary artery segments are hypoplastic, there will be a characteristic concavity in the upper left margin of the heart shadow, thus resulting in a "boot-shaped" heart. Although an ECG is not essential in the diagnosis of tetralogy, there are several subtle abnormalities that may be noted (see Fig. 11-3). Right axis deviation and right ventricular hypertrophy may be seen, although this may be viewed as normal findings in neonates where there is a physiologic prominence of the right ventricle.

Echocardiography is the diagnostic test of choice for diagnosis of TOF (see Fig. 11-4). Findings include a dilated aortic root over a large VSD. Varying degrees of right ventricular outflow obstruction will be seen ranging from pulmonary valve stenosis to complete atresia. Hypoplasia and narrowing of the main and branch pulmonary arteries will also be seen. Finally, abnormal coursing coronary arteries may be seen on echocardiogram. These are important to find, as it may alter choice for location of right ventricular outflow patch. Cardiac catheterization may also be

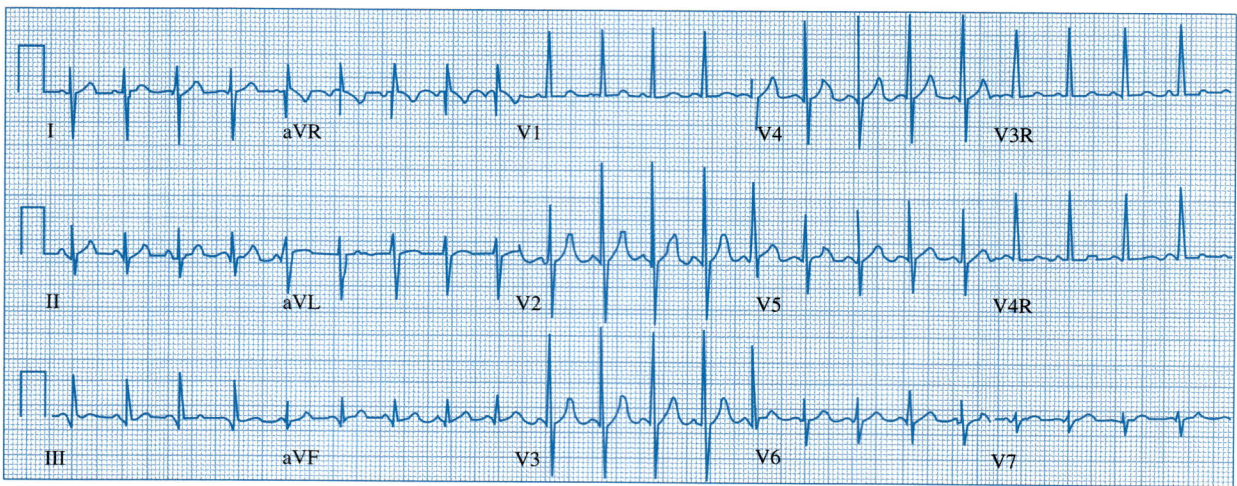

Figure 11-3 ECG with right ventricular hypertrophy. ECG, electrocardiogram.

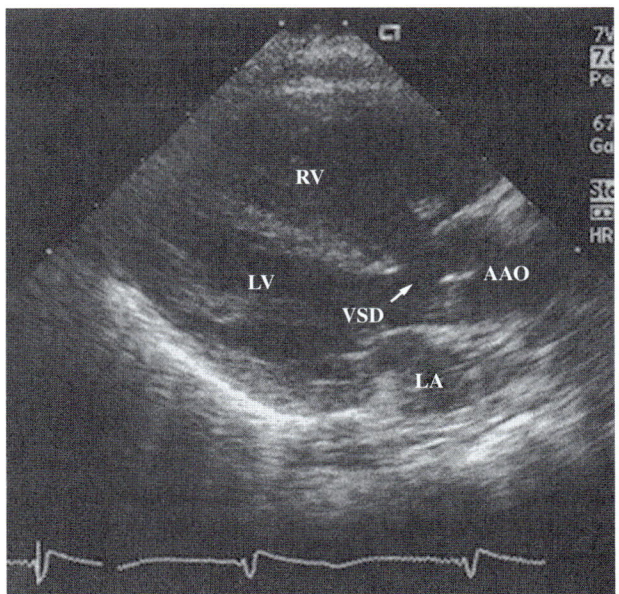

Figure 11-4 Echocardiogram. Parasternal two-dimensional long axis showing VSD.
AAO, ascending aorta; LA, left atrium; LV, left ventricle; RV, right ventricle; VSD, ventricular septal defect.

preformed to obtain additional morphologic and physiologic information that may not be seen on echocardiogram.

After the diagnosis of TOF, the ultimate goal is correction of the anatomical defect so as to relieve right ventricular obstruction and revert to normal four-chambered circulation. While surgery will provide definitive treatment, it is important to review medical interventions that should be carried out prior to surgical repair as well as those that may be required acutely for hypercyanotic episodes.

In neonates with cyanotic spells and instability or shock-like picture soon after birth, prompt initiation of prostaglandin E1 is essential. This will allow the ductus arteriosus to remain open and allow pulmonary blood flow. After initial stabilization, echocardiography and other diagnostic studies stated above should be performed to determine degree of right ventricular outflow obstruction and degree of hypoplasia and stenosis of pulmonary vasculature. Only children who have ductal dependent pulmonary blood flow must be continued on Prostin until palliative or corrective surgical repair is possible. In most infants with TOF, however, there will be some right ventricular outflow, and pulmonary blood flow will not be solely ductal dependent. These children may be followed without early surgical intervention; however, education of caregivers for recognition of hypercyanotic spells is essential.

Treatment for a Tet spell is directed at lowering limitation of pulmonary blood flow and increasing systemic vascular resistance, so as to minimize right-to-left shunting of unoxygenated blood. Table 11-2 reviews different treatment options for these hypercyanotic spells. While these options may provide short-term relief for these episodes, episodes

TABLE 11-2

Treatment Options for "Tet Spells"

Treatment	Rationale
Oxygen	Reduces hypoxemia (limited value)
Calm child, encourage knee-to-chest position	Decreases venous return and increases systemic resistance
Propranolol	Negative inotropic effect on infundibular myocardium, improves pulmonary blood flow
Morphine	Decreases venous return, depresses respiratory center, relaxes infundibulum.
Phenylephrine	Increases systemic vascular resistance
Methoxamine	Increases systemic vascular resistance
Sodium bicarbonate	Reduces metabolic acidosis
Correct anemia	Increases delivery of oxygen to tissues
Correct pathologic tachyarrhythmias	May abort hypoxic spell
Infuse glucose	Avoids hypoglycemia from increased utilization and depletion of glycogen stores

Adapted from Gajewski, R. Chapter 6: Cardiology. In: The Harriet Lane Handbook. 17th ed. Robertson J, and Shilkofski N, eds. Elsevier Mosby 2005.

that are increasingly frequent or cause hemodynamic instability indicate the need for more immediate management. Surgical intervention may be either palliative or corrective, and will depend on age and size of the patient as well as cardiac anatomy. Palliative procedures are often reserved for those patients in whom intracardiac (corrective) repair is contraindicated because of prematurity, small size, hypoplastic pulmonary arteries, or coronary artery anatomy. The concept of palliative repair involves constructing a connection between the aorta or right ventricle and the pulmonary arteries. This can either comprise of a prosthetic Gore-Tex shunt between the ascending aorta and the pulmonary arteries (modified Blalock-Taussig shunt,), or a valved outflow patch from the right ventricle to the main pulmonary artery. In these cases, the VSD is left open, so as to not allow unrestricted pulmonary blood flow. Performing these palliative procedures initially allows for growth of the infant as well as further development and growth of the hypoplastic pulmonary arteries prior to future corrective repair. If the child has aortopulmonary collaterals, these may also be unifocalized to supply an additional aortic to pulmonary conduit.

Complete intracardiac repair of TOF is usually done within the first year of life, but can be performed in infants as young as 3 months of age. The repair consists of patch closure of the VSD and revision of the right ventricular outflow tract. This is done by repairing the pulmonary valve and resecting the infundibular muscle and augmenting the right ventricular outflow tract with a transannular patch. This will allow unobstructed flow from the right ventricle out to the pulmonary arteries. If palliative repair was done initially, full repair involves takedown of the previously placed shunts.

Surgical repair of TOF is a fairly common procedure with low mortality rates ranging between 0% and 3%, depending on institution. Postoperative complications that may occur include pulmonary regurgitation, residual right ventricular outflow obstruction, and cardiac arrhythmias including ventricular tachycardia and atrioventricular (AV) block. Long-term survival in children after complete repair is excellent with rates of 80% to 90% at three to four decades from time of repair.

In summary, TOF is one of the most common cyanotic heart lesions encountered in the neonatal period. It involves a constellation of symptoms with wide anatomic variations leading to a range of presenting symptoms. Early and thorough evaluation of the cyanotic infant will allow diagnosis of the lesion and influence timing of repair. With proper medical and surgical intervention, TOF is a correctible congenital heart lesion, which can be repaired to allow children to live a relatively normal life.

Selected References

1. Gajewski, R. Chapter 6 Cardiology. In: *The Harriet Lane Handbook*. 17th ed. Robertson J, and Shilkofski N eds. Elsevier Mosby; 2005.
2. Bernstein, D. Chapter 423: Cyanotic Congenital Heart Lesions: lesions associated with decreased pulmonary blood flow. In: *Nelson Textbook of Pediatrics. 17th Ed*. Berhman R, Kleigman R, and Jenson H, eds. Saunders Elsevier. 2004.

35-Year-Old Male with Neck Pain

C
12

CASE PRESENTATION

A 35-year-old healthy white man presents to the clinic with neck pain and fatigue which he has noticed for several weeks. A few weeks prior to presentation, he was at the beach with his children (ages 2 and 5), and he noticed onset of neck and shoulder pain. The pain was moderate, 6 to 7 out of 10 at its worst. He felt that his neck was stiff, but he did not have limited range of motion. Over the prior few weeks, the pain had been intermittent, coming and going gradually. The pain is improved with ibuprofen and not worsened by anything. There are no consistent aggravating factors. He has also noticed that since the onset of the pain he has had decreased exercise tolerance. He has been an avid jogger, but he has not been able to make his usual 3 to 5 mi/day for the past few weeks. He was not short of breath and did not have chest pain. He did not have headache, vision changes, or photophobia. He did not have fever, chills, sweats, or weight loss. He denied any injury to his neck. He denied bleeding problems, skin rash, tick exposure, and focal weakness.

Physical Examination

The patient was healthy appearing and comfortable, appearing stated age. Vital signs: temperature 36°C, pulse 58 beats/min, respiratory rate 16 breaths/min, blood pressure 120/78 mm Hg, with room air oxygen saturation of 100%. Head, eyes, ears, nose, and throat: pupils equally round and reactive, extraocular muscles intact, good dentition. Neck: supple with no lymphadenopathy, no bruit, and no jugular venous distension. Tenderness elicited over trapezius muscles bilaterally. Diffusely enlarged thyroid is appreciated, with no nodules. Cardiovascular: bradycardic with regular rhythm, with no murmurs or gallops. Normal S_1, S_2. Lungs: clear bilaterally. Abdomen: soft, nontender, normal bowel sounds, no hepatosplenomegaly. Extremities: no edema or tenderness. The remainder of the examination was unremarkable.

Laboratory Studies

Chemistry 10 normal, white blood cells 5.6, hemoglobin 14.6, hematocrit 45. Mean corpuscular volume 80. Platelets 235. Thyroid-stimulating hormone (TSH) 54.5, T4 0.1, free T3 normal.

Case Resolution

The patient was diagnosed with primary hypothyroidism, and he was started on levothyroxine 100 mcg po qd from the clinic. He had subsequent complete resolution of the neck pain and fatigue. His dose of levothyroxine was eventually titrated up to 150 mcg daily.

Question

What is the most likely explanation of the patient's hypothyroidism?

Answer

In this patient's case, the most likely cause is primary hypothyroidism from chronic autoimmune (Hashimoto) thyroiditis causing neck pain, prominent thyroid, and fatigue.

Discussion

Primary hypothyroidism is a common and important cause of morbidity, which can be diagnosed and treated from a primary care setting in many cases. The prevalence varies by study but is estimated to be 5% to 15% of women and 1% to 5% of men. It is more common in women, becomes more frequent with age, and is more common in whites and Mexican Americans than in blacks.[1] Family history of thyroid disease and other autoimmune diseases is a good indicator of risk for a patient to develop hypothyroidism.[2]

There are several varieties of hypothyroidism, including primary hypothyroidism from thyroiditis, iatrogenic or environmental hypothyroidism, and hypothyroidism secondary to pituitary or hypothalamic dysfunction.

Primary hypothyroidism is the most common cause of hypothyroidism in United States and Europe. It is usually caused by chronic autoimmune thyroiditis. Hashimoto disease refers to the goitrous thyroid form, and there is also an atrophic thyroid form. Primary hypothyroidism is thought to be an autoimmune process, in which helper (CD4) T cells become activated, stimulating autoreactive B cells to be recruited into the thyroid and to secrete thyroid autoantibodies. The primary targets are thyroglobulin, the thyroid microsomal antigen (thyroid peroxidase), and the thyrotropin receptor. Levels of these antibodies can be measured in the serum. The activated helper T cells also recruit killer (CD8) T cells to the thyroid. The direct killing by these cells is thought to be the main method of tissue destruction and the resulting hypothyroidism, although the auto-antibodies may have some pathogenic role.[3]

Because many tissues in the body have thyroid hormone receptors, patients can present with a wide variety of symptoms, as shown in Table 12-1, which makes clinical diagnosis difficult. Most symptoms result from generalized slowing of metabolic processes or accumulation of matrix substances. All patients with overt, symptomatic hypothyroidism are recommended for treatment, which is detailed below. Asymptomatic patients with TSH levels

TABLE 12-1

Symptoms and Signs of Hypothyroidism

Mechanism	Symptoms	Signs	Laboratory findings
Slowing of metabolic processes	Fatigue and weakness Cold intolerance Dyspnea on exertion Weight gain Cognitive dysfunction Mental retardation (infant) Constipation Growth failure	Slow movement and slow speech Delayed relaxation of tendon reflexes Carpal tunnel syndrome Bradycardia Carotenemia	
Accumulation of matrix substances	Dry skin Hoarseness Edema	Coarse skin Puffy facies and loss of eyebrows Periorbital edema Enlargement of the tongue Myxedema	
Others	Decreased hearing Myalgia and paresthesia Depression Menorrhagia Arthralgia Pubertal delay	Diastolic hypertension Pleural and pericardial effusions Ascites Galactorrhea	Hyponatremia Increased creatinine Hyperlipidemia

greater than 10 are also recommended for treatment. Asymptomatic patients with an abnormal TSH less than 10 are classified as subclinical hypothyroidism and do not require immediate treatment, but the patient should have follow-up in 6 months for reevaluation of symptoms and recheck of laboratory abnormalities. Risk stratification can be accomplished in these patients with subclinical hypothyroidism by measuring levels of thyroid antibodies, as a strongly positive result correlates with risk for progression. Those older than 45 years and especially men are also more likely to progress to overt hypothyroidism.

There have been several studies to determine whether routine screening would be useful for this condition which is so common and easily diagnosed by laboratory testing. However, no benefit has been shown for treating early, subclinical hypothyroidism in general, so this has not been widely undertaken. The only exception to this is prenatal care screening, as aggressive treatment in pregnant women can be justified.[2,3,4]

During pregnancy, physiologic changes in thyroid function occur which should not be misinterpreted as pathological. Beta-human chorionic gonadotropin (β-hCG) has a weak thyroid-stimulating effect and causes small increases in free T4, total T4, and total T3 levels, with a proportionate compensatory decrease in TSH level. This correlates with the level of β-hCG rise during the first trimester and levels off over the second and third trimesters. Women on thyroid replacement therapy before pregnancy may require an increase in dosage during pregnancy because of this physiology. This benign condition must be differentiated from true thyroid disorders, which also may be seen in pregnancy. These need treatment in order to ensure a good pregnancy outcome. Untreated hypothyroidism during pregnancy is associated with gestational hypertension, low birth weight, and spontaneous abortion. Within 1 year following delivery, about 5% to 10% of women may exhibit postpartum autoimmune thyroid dysfunction, which results in permanent hypothyroidism in about 25% to 30% of cases.[5]

Primary hypothyroidism occasionally can be transient, not requiring continuous thyroxine supplementation, but trials of medication should be followed closely with TSH checks every 6 weeks.

There are several common environmental and iatrogenic causes of hypothyroidism, and thorough medical history taking is the key to their diagnosis. The most common cause of hypothyroidism worldwide is iodine deficiency (defined as <100 mcg/day). This is uncommon in countries where iodized salt is used. Iodine inhibits biosynthesis and release of thyroid hormone; it does not seem to have any effect on thyroid autoimmunity. Interestingly, iodine oversupplementation, including use of medications like amiodarone which is 35% iodine by weight, seems to augment thyroid autoantibody production in those who are susceptible and thus can induce a chronic autoimmune thyroiditis.[3] Thyroidectomy, radioiodine treatment, and external radiation therapy (2500 rad or more) are well-known causes of hypothyroidism, although many patients who undergo subtotal thyroidectomy may retain some thyroid function and not require replacement therapy. The same is true for patients with Graves who have received iodine 131, although more of these patients do progress to true hypothyroidism.[7] There are a number of medications which are implicated, shown in Fig. 12-1.

Central hypothyroidism is secondary to either TSH or thyrotropin-releasing hormone (TRH) deficiency and is much less common than primary, environmental, and iatrogenic hypothyroidism. Less than 1% of patients with hypothyroidism have one of these forms of central hypothyroidism. Although the mechanisms of the types of central hypothyroidism are different, they are usually grouped together for initial diagnostic purposes.

Patients with central hypothyroidism have low or normal serum TSH concentrations (but inappropriately low in the presence of low-serum T4 and T3 concentrations). Causes of secondary (TSH deficiency) hypothyroidism include pituitary tumor; postpartum pituitary necrosis (Sheehan syndrome); trauma; hypophysitis; nonpituitary tumors such as craniopharyngiomas, infiltrative diseases, and inactivating mutations in the gene for either TSH or the TSH receptor. TSH deficiency may be isolated, but more often it occurs in association with other pituitary hormone deficiencies.

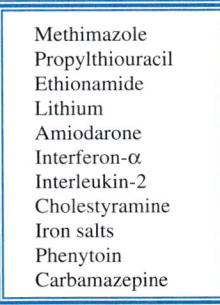

Methimazole
Propylthiouracil
Ethionamide
Lithium
Amiodarone
Interferon-α
Interleukin-2
Cholestyramine
Iron salts
Phenytoin
Carbamazepine

Figure 12-1 Medications which can cause hypothyroidism.[3,6]

TABLE 12-2

Diagnostic Testing for Hypothyroidism

	Primary hypothyroidism	Subclinical hypothyroidism	Central hypothyroidism
Serum TSH	High (>10)	High (usually <10)	Low (can also be normal or slightly high)
Serum free T4	Low	Normal	Low
Serum T3	Normal or low	Normal	Normal or low

TSH, thyroid-stimulating hormone.

Tertiary (TRH deficiency) hypothyroidism can be caused by any disorder that damages the hypothalamus or interferes with hypothalamic–pituitary portal blood flow, thereby preventing delivery of TRH to the pituitary. It can also be caused by mutations in the gene for the TRH receptor. Like TSH deficiency, TRH deficiency can be isolated or occur in combination with other hormonal deficiencies. Hypothalamic damage results from tumors, trauma, radiation therapy, or infiltrative diseases.[8]

The diagnostic biochemical tests TSH, free T4, and T3 should be ordered in patients with symptoms, and an interpretation of the results is discussed in Table 12-2. The presence of antithyroid antibodies can be commercially assessed and can be useful for risk stratification, but it is not necessary for diagnosis of primary hypothyroidism. If secondary or tertiary hypothyroidism is suspected, other pituitary or hypothalamic function tests can also be ordered, although the two cannot be distinguished by biochemical tests. Any patient with findings suggestive of central hypothyroidism should undergo magnetic resonance imaging (MRI) of the hypothalamus and pituitary.

The first step in treating hypothyroidism is, if necessary, to discontinue potentially causative medications and correct iodine deficiency. Then, initiate medical replacement therapy if still indicated. The staple of medical treatment for hypothyroidism of any description is thyroxine (T4) replacement with levothyroxine. Levothyroxine can be dosed according to weight initially. A full replacement dosage is 1.6 mcg/kg body weight, which is usually about 75 to 100 mcg/day for women and 100 to 150 mcg/day for men. Elderly patients have a much lower starting dose, usually around 12.5 to 25 mcg/day. The most important part is that the dose be titrated based on serial TSH measurements, drawn every 6 to 8 weeks, until a normal TSH is accomplished.[9]

There have been a number of studies which looked at T3 replacement with liothyronine to determine whether this gives added benefit. No advantage has been shown for combination therapy, and adverse effects (palpitations, irritability, nervousness, dizziness, and tremor) were more frequent.[10]

Key Points

- Most common type of hypothyroidism worldwide: iodine deficiency
- Most common type of hypothyroidism in countries with iodized salt: primary hypothyroidism from chronic autoimmune thyroiditis
- Symptoms: can be anything related to slowing of metabolic processes or accumulation of matrix substances
- Initial diagnostic testing: serum TSH, free T4, T3
- Treatment: levothyroxine, initially weight-based dosing, then dose titrated according to TSH levels

References

1. Hollowell JG, Staehling NW, Flanders WD, et al. Serum TSH, T5, and thyroid antibodies in the United States population (1988 to 1994): National Health and Nutrition Examination Survey (NHANES III). *J Clin Endocrinol Metab.* 2002;87:489.
2. Surks MI, Ortiz E, Daniels GH, et al. Subclinical thyroid disease: scientific review and guidelines for diagnosis and management. *JAMA.* 2004 Jan 14;291(2):228–238.
3. Dayan CM, Daniels GH. Chronic autoimmune thyroiditis. *N Engl J Med.* 1996;335:99.
4. Bach-Huynh TC, Jonklaas J. Thyroid medications during pregnancy. *Ther Drug Monit.* 2006 Jun;28(3):431–441.
5. Karabinas CD, Tolis GJ. Thyroid disorders and pregnancy. *J Obstet Gynecol.* 1998 Nov;181:509–515.

6. Ross D. Disorders that cause hypothyroidism. In: Rose, BD (ed). *UpToDate*. Waltham, MA, 2007. Version 15.3. Sept 2007.

7. Franklyn JA, Daykin J, Drolc Z, et al. Long-term follow-up of treatment of thyrotoxicosis by three different methods. *Clin Endocrinol (Oxf)*. 1991 Jan;34(1):71–76.

8. Samuels MH, Ridgeway EC. Central hypothyroidism. *Endocrinol Metab Clin North Am*. 1992 Dec;21(4):903–919.

9. Mandel SJ, Brent GA, Larsen PR. Levothyroxine therapy in patients with thyroid disease. *Ann Intern Med*. 1993 Sep 15;1191:492–502.

10. Escobar-Morreale H, et al. Treatment of hypothyroidism with combinations of levothyroxine plus liothyronine. *J Clin Endocrinol Metab*. 2005 Aug 15;90(8);4946–4954.

11. Surks MI. Clinical manifestations of hypothyroidism. In: Rose, BD (ed), *UpToDate*. Waltham, MA, 2007. Version 15.3. Aug 2007.

2-Day-Old with Lethargy and Hypothermia

CASE PRESENTATION

The patient was a 2-day-old female, born by normal spontaneous vaginal delivery to a mother who tested positive for group B streptococci during pregnancy. Membranes were ruptured for 15 hours, and the mother was treated with three doses of penicillin prior to delivery. The infant was at 50th percentile for weight, length, and head circumference. She was the second child of her parents, and her brother was healthy. On the second day of life, the mother became concerned that her daughter did not breastfeed well and "wasn't acting right." The infant became hard to arouse, hypotonic, and tachypneic. Septic workup and antibiotics were initiated.

Physical Examination

Vital signs: temperature 36°C, pulse 163 beats/min, respiratory rate 80 breaths/min, and blood pressure 66/30 mm Hg. The child was lethargic and responsive only to pain. The anterior fontanel was soft and flat. Facial features were not dysmorphic. The heart had a regular rate and rhythm with no murmurs. She was tachypneic, and lungs sounds were clear and equal. Abdomen was soft, nontender, nondistended, with normally active bowel sounds. No hepatosplenomegaly was appreciated. Muscle tone was decreased. Capillary refill was 3 seconds. The remainder of her examination was normal.

K	3.5 mmol/L	3.7–5.9 mmol/L
Cl	112 mmol/L	98–107 mmol/L
CO_2	8 mmol/L	21–30 mmol/L
BUN	21 mg/dL	2–19 mg/dL
Creatinine	0.9 mg/dL	0.6–1.1 mg/dL
Glucose	70 mg/dL	65–199 mg/dL
Urine ketones	3+	negative
Ammonia	354 mmol/L	9–33 mmol/L

BUN, blood urea nitrogen; WBC, white blood cells.

Laboratory Tests

Test	Level	Range
pH	7.08	7.35–7.45
Pco_2	10 mm Hg	35–45 mm Hg
Po_2	136 mm Hg	80–110 mm Hg
HCO_3	3 mmol/L	22–27 mmol/L
WBC	16×10^9/L	6–17.5×10^9/L
Hemoglobin	40%	28%–42%
Platelets	448×10^9/L	150–440×10^9/L
Na	140 mmol/L	135–145 mmol/L

Question

How would you determine the underlying cause of this patient's decompensation?

Answer

Although sepsis is in first place on the list of the causes of decompensation of the newborn, it is important to think of inherited inborn errors of metabolism, particularly in a patient who has acidosis and hyperammonemia. Children who have metabolic disorders are often well at birth because the toxic intermediates are cleared by the placenta during the pregnancy. As the child moves into independent life, she will have a lowered calorie intake until oral feeding skills develop. Stored glycogen, fat, and body proteins are used for fuel while a feeding routine is established. A defect in energy metabolism may become apparent during the first few days of life. The initial laboratories in this case indicated severe ketoacidosis, and the physician checked an ammonia level which was elevated. Further testing to determine the diagnosis included an acylcarnitine profile, plasma amino acids, urine organic acids, and carnitine.

For this patient, metabolic testing results were available in 2 days and are shown in Table 13-1. These findings are consistent with propionic acidemia, which is caused by deficiency of propionyl-coenzyme A (CoA) carboxylase. Plasma amino acids (not shown) were normal except for increased glycine. To complete the diagnosis, one must also rule out a disorder affecting all carboxylases, such as biotinidase deficiency or multiple carboxylase deficiency. Both disorders are owing to the limited synthesis of the carboxylases' cofactor biotin. The absence of other elevated compounds on the plasma acylcarnitine profile and the urine organic acid study indicate that the other carboxylases are functioning normally.

TABLE 13-1

Metabolic Laboratory Testing

Test	Level	Range
Carnitine, total	17 nmol/mL	22–47 nmol/mL
Carnitine, free	2 nmol/mL	21–38 nmol/mL
Carnitine, acyl	15 nmol/mL	5–9 nmol/mL
Plasma acyl-carnitine profile		
Propionyl carnitine	9.63 nmol/mL	<0.75 nmol/mL
Acetylcarnitine	0.96 nmol/mL	2.0–15.7 nmol/mL
Urine organic acids (qualitative)	Elevated propionyl glycine, methyl citric acid, and ketones	Undetectable

Discussion

Organic acidemias, such as propionic acidemia, can be associated with secondary hyperammonemia, particularly in the newborn period. Hyperammonemia occurs when the function of the urea cycle (Fig 13-1) is disrupted, either

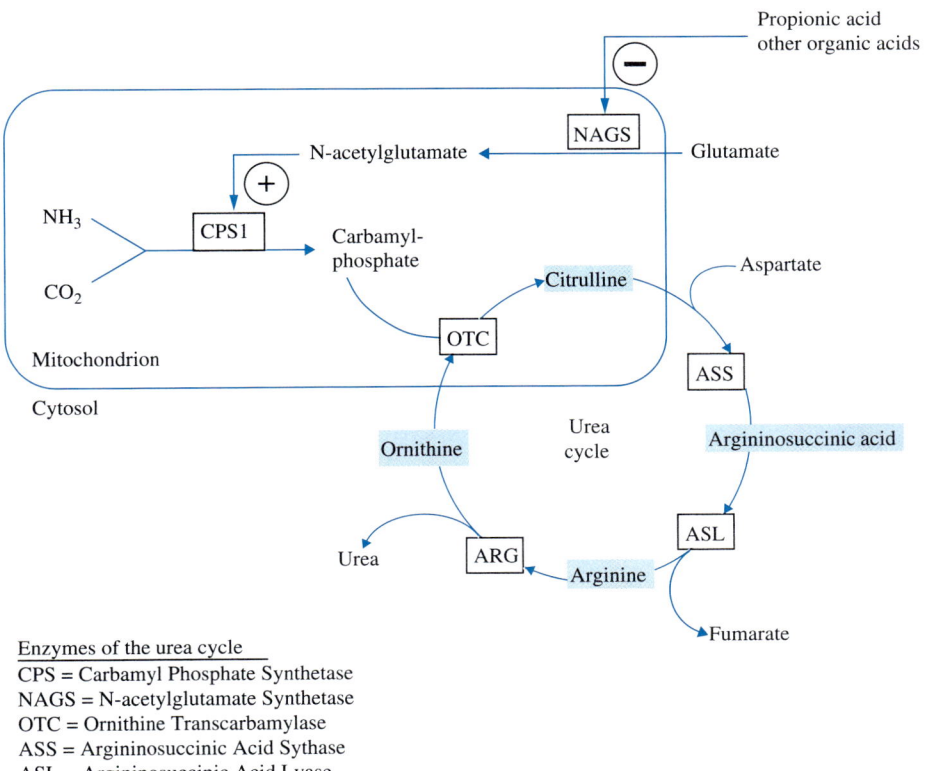

Enzymes of the urea cycle
CPS = Carbamyl Phosphate Synthetase
NAGS = N-acetylglutamate Synthetase
OTC = Ornithine Transcarbamylase
ASS = Argininosuccinic Acid Sythase
ASL = Argininosuccinic Acid Lyase
ARG = Arginase

Figure 13-1 The key enzymes involved with the urea cycle.

by *primary* deficiency of one of the urea cycle enzymes or by *secondary* deficiency because of inhibition of the enzyme *N*-acetylglutamate synthetase (NAGS) by organic acid metabolites (as in this case). NAGS is an obligate, positive activator of the first step of the urea cycle, carbamoyl phosphate synthetase (CPS).

When you are considering a metabolic disorder with hyperammonemia, the blood gas and the respiratory rate will help you determine whether you are observing a primary or secondary hyperammonemia.

- Primary hyperammonemia may cause respiratory alkalosis owing to the depressive effects of ammonia on the respiratory centers of the brainstem. The pH will be normal or mildly alkalotic. The child is not usually tachypneic.

- Secondary hyperammonemia because of organic acidemia is associated with primary metabolic acidosis with respiratory compensation. The pH will be acidotic, and the child will usually have tachypnea.

Treatment

General

Begin treatment of a child with a suspected metabolic disorder immediately, without waiting for confirmation of a diagnosis. Most of the diagnostic laboratories are performed at specialty centers and take several days for reports. You may be able to check the patient's newborn screen if the state screens for an expanded panel of metabolic disorders (see references for list).

Specific Therapy

Treatment of a patient with both acidosis and hyperammonemia requires the following steps: (1) Treat acidosis by increasing calorie input and halting catabolism, which is producing harmful compounds. (2) Decrease ammonia, either with dialysis or with drugs that scavenge ammonia and promote its excretion. (3) Replace HCO_3 conservatively, as it will correct as catabolism is halted. (4) Perform testing to determine the metabolic disorder and initiate specific diet therapy. (5) Provide any necessary supplements or medications for that condition.

1. Glucose is an excellent source of calories that is used by both body and brain tissues. Administer glucose at a physiologic rate for the patient. As the catabolic process is halted, the anion gap will improve as acid production is stopped and acids begin to clear.

2. Hyperammonemia is treated either with medications that remove ammonia groups as conjugates excreted in the urine, through dialysis, or with a combination of the two. A combination of both may be used in patients with severe hyperammonemia, for example, starting intravenous (IV) treatment medications while the dialysis equipment and lines are arranged. Ammonia-scavenging medications are sodium phenylacetate and sodium benzoate.

3. HCO_3 may be helpful to replace lost stores, but the correction of acidosis in organic acidurias is achieved by halting catabolism of body proteins and providing carbohydrate calories. You may also add IV lipid emulsion for increased calories under direction of a metabolic specialist.

4. When diagnosis is established, add an appropriate metabolic formula prepared by a metabolic nutritionist. The child's diet would be regulated to provide just enough of the "offending" amino acids, the ones the child cannot catabolize properly, to allow normal growth and development. In this case, the offending amino acids are valine, isoleucine, threonine, and methionine. Regular infant formula or breast milk is measured to provide the required amount of the offending amino acids. The remainder of the infant's formula is made of a chemically modified medical formula that is devoid of the offending amino acids. The prescription for the formula is modified as the child grows and as the plasma amino acid levels are monitored for appropriate levels of valine, isoleucine, methionine, and threonine.

5. Carnitine, a compound that is synthesized from lysine, is also used to treat patients with organic acidemias or other disorders that deplete carnitine. Either carnitine or CoA bind and transport acyl units from organic acid and fatty acid metabolism in the mitochondria and the cytosol. In a metabolic disorder, there may be an excess of acyl units in the mitochondria. These acyl units will bind to CoA and slow energy production. Carnitine can bind the excess acyl units, transport them out of the mitochondria, and

promote excretion of the bound units in the urine. Carnitine is produced by the body, but the requirement in organic acidemias often exceeds the body's synthetic capacity. Replacement carnitine is available in an IV form when the child is ill and in an oral form when the child is well. Patients with organic acidemias usually take supplemental carnitine daily because of increased urinary losses.

References

Deodato F, Boenzi S, Santorelli FM, et al. Methylmalonic and propionic aciduria. *Am J Med Genet C Semin Med Genet.* 2006; 142(2):104–112.

Nyhan WL, Barshop BA, Ozand PT. *Atlas of Metabolic Disease.* 2nd ed. London, UK: HodderArnold; 2005:8–17.

Seashore MR. The organic acidemias: an overview. www.geneclinics.org. Accessed August 14, 2006.

19-Month-Old Female with Ataxia and Wandering Eyes

CASE PRESENTATION

The patient is a 19-month-old Caucasian female who presented to her primary care physician with 6 weeks of progressive ataxia. According to her mother, the child had been well with normal growth and development up to this point. She began sitting at approximately 6 months of age, crawling at 9 months of age, and walking at 12 months of age. Six weeks ago, she noticed that her daughter would take a few steps and then stumble. The child's disability progressed to where she needed one hand held to assist in ambulation. At presentation, the patient is unable to walk independently. In addition to her gait, the mother has also noticed some "shakiness" and "jerkiness" of her torso. Given these abnormal movements, the child is unable to reach for objects, feed herself, or sit unassisted. The workup for this current illness this far has included a head computed tomography (CT) scan which showed sphenoid sinusitis. She subsequently completed a course of amoxicillin/clavulanate for the sinusitis. She was then referred to outpatient neurology. Magnetic resonance imaging (MRI) of the brain was performed at that time which was normal.

Past medical history is otherwise unremarkable. She was born by cesarean section at 40 weeks' gestation secondary to a delivery complicated by a nuchal cord. She is currently on no medications. She has had no surgeries. Family history is negative for cancers or neurologic disorders. Review of symptoms was otherwise negative including no reported fevers, chills, weight loss, nausea, vomiting, or abdominal pain.

Physical Examination

Patient was alert but anxious with periodic jerking of her upper extremities. Vital signs: temperature 36°C, pulse 120 beats/min, respiratory rate (RR) 24 breaths/min, blood pressure (BP) 105/53 mm Hg. Weight 11.08 kg, height 80.7 cm, head circumference 46 cm. Head, eyes, ears, nose, and throat (HEENT): head appeared normocephalic and atraumatic. Examination of the eyes showed jerky movements; pupils equal, round, reactive to light and accommodation (PERRLA). Neck: supple without lymphadenopathy. Cardiovascular (CV): regular rate and rhythm with no murmur/gallop/rub; S_1, S_2. Lungs: clear to auscultation bilaterally with a normal work of breathing. Abdomen: soft, nontender, normal bowel sounds; no hepatosplenomegaly. Extremities: no edema. Neurology: patient had 2+ patellar reflexes.

Strength was intact. She had ataxia of trunk, head, and extremities. No clonus. She was unable to ambulate without assistance.

Laboratory Studies/Imaging

Complete blood count showed white blood cells 6.7, hemoglobin 11.3, hematocrit 31, platelets 227, Na 140, K 4.1, Cl 107, HCO_3 20, blood urea nitrogen 16, creatinine 0.4, ionized calcium 4.6. Liver panel was within normal limits. Uric acid 5.9, albumin 4.5, lactate dehydrogenase 905. Cerebrospinal fluid was obtained and showed 4 red blood cells/high-powered field, 0 WBC, glucose 52, protein 29. Urine vanillylmandelic acid (VMA) 51.3 mg/g of creatinine (normal 0–15.5) and urine homovanillic acid (HVA) 83.8 mg/g of creatinine (normal 3–20).

CT scan of Chest/Abdomen/Pelvis

Calcifications were seen at the level of the right renal hilum with a small enhancing mass in the paraspinal position on the right. Abdominal MRI showed a normal liver and spleen. Adrenal glands were normal bilaterally. There was a soft tissue density at the level of the right hilum which extends behind and around the inferior vena cava (IVC). An iodine 123 metaiodobenzylguanidine (MIBG) scan performed in nuclear medicine was negative. Bone scan was negative. Skeletal survey and bone marrow biopsy was negative for metastasis. Excisional biopsy performed under general anesthesia showed a ganglioneuroblastoma.

Case Resolution

Given the patient's abnormal clinical examination and a CT scan of her abdomen showing a possible paracaval mass with calcifications, the patient underwent an excisional biopsy which confirmed a ganglioneuroblastoma. Following excisional biopsy, the patient received several courses of intravenous immunoglobulin (IVIG) with improvement of her opsoclonus–myoclonus. She was then placed on prednisone at 2 mg/kg/day which was slowly tapered over the course of 18 months. The patient had a slight relapse following a viral gastroenteritis at which time she received a course of rituximab. Her repeat CT scans have remained negative and her urine VMA and homomandelic acid (HMA) levels are within normal limits. She continues to have some ataxia but is ambulating independently. She had some developmental delays likely from the opsoclonus–myoclonus syndrome but is currently attending school and doing well while receiving physical, occupational, and speech therapy services.

Question

What elements of the history and physical examination findings suggest the diagnosis of neuroblastoma?

Answer

The child in the vignette was suffering from loss of milestones and had definitive signs of opsoclonus–myoclonus–ataxia (OMA). This is an autoimmune paraneoplastic syndrome as described and occurs in 1% to 3% of patients with neuroblastoma, and conversely up to 50% of patients with OMA will have an accompanying neuroblastoma. The characteristic symptoms as seen in this patient are rapid dancing eye movements, rhythmic jerking, and/or ataxia.

Discussion

Neuroblastomas rank as the most common extracranial solid tumor in children accounting for 8% to 10% of all pediatric cancers. Median age of diagnosis is 2 years of age with 90% appearing before 5 years of age. Neuroblastomas represent a collection of tumors that arise from the peripheral sympathetic ganglion cells and fall under the category of small, round blue cell neoplasms. Neuroblastomas are unique in their presentation since they reflect a spectrum of histopathologic characteristics and arise in various locations (Fig. 14.1).

Neuroblastomas usually present with diverse symptomatology based on the site of origin and extent of metastases. The most likely presentation involves detection of a firm, nontender, nodular abdominal mass palpable in the flank or midline and causing abdominal pain by history. Forty percent of neuroblastomas are found arising from the adrenal gland or retroperitoneal sympathetic ganglia. Thirty percent of remaining neuroblastomas originate from the cervical, thoracic, or pelvic ganglia. The table below compares the site of origin with the coexisting signs and symptoms (Table 14-1).

Neuroblastomas may also have accompanying paraneoplastic syndromes as described in the vignette above, such as OMA. As mentioned previously OMA occurs in 1% to 3% of patients with neuroblastoma, and conversely up to 50% of patients with OMA will have an accompanying neuroblastoma. The current mechanism is thought to be autoimmune driven based on the presence of plasma neural antigen autoantibodies and a documented clinical response to immunosuppressive therapy such as IVIG and steroids. About 70% to 80% of patients suffering from OMA will have permanent neurologic deficits including cognitive and motor delays with accompanying language deficits and behavioral problems.

Another neuroblastoma-associated paraneoplastic syndrome is intractable secretory diarrhea that results from the secretion of vasoactive intestinal peptide (VIP) by the tumor. VIP secretion can be most commonly found with ganglioneuroblastomas or ganglioneuromas. Removal of the tumor causes resolution of the diarrhea. Catecholamine release (ie,

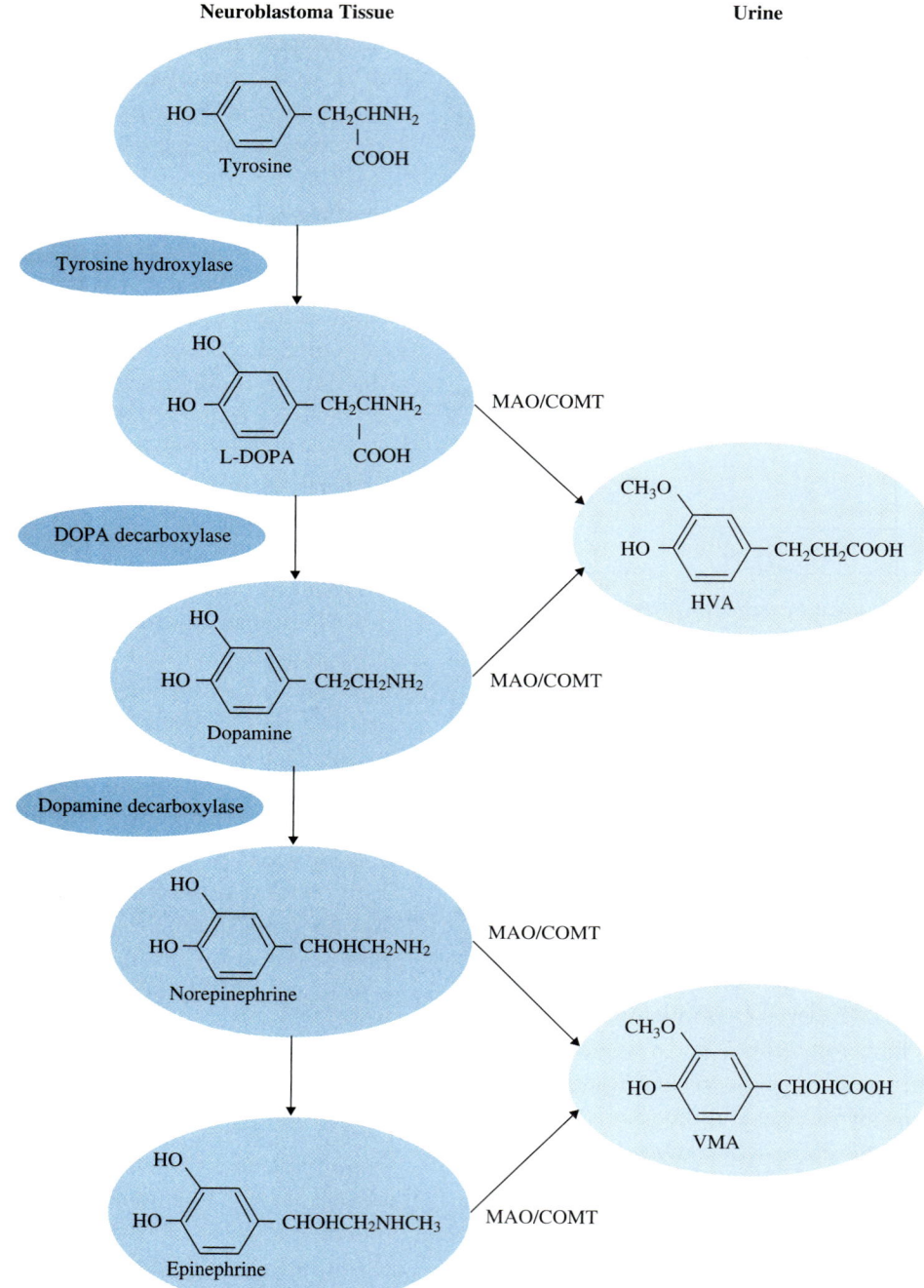

Figure 14-1 Catecholamine metabolism in neuroblastoma tissues leading to urinary metabolite VMA and HVA. COMT, catechol-O-methyltransferase; HVA, homovanillic acid; MAO, monoamine oxidase, VMA, vanillylmandelic acid.

epinephrine) from the tumor can also result in hypertension, tachycardia, flushing, or sweating. In general, neuroblastoma cells have dysregulated catecholamine metabolism whereby dopamine, HVA, and VMA build up in excess. Neuroblastomas often express enzymes involved in catecholamine metabolism including monoamine oxidase (MAO) and catechol-O-methyltransferase (COMT) that result in an abundance catecholamine of metabolites that can subsequently be quantified. Ninety-five percent of patients with neuroblastoma will have elevated levels of catecholamine metabolites, HVA, and VMA in the urine. The pathway of catecholamine metabolism is outlined in Figure 14-1.

TABLE 14-1

Tumor Origin and Coexisting Signs and Symptoms

Location	Signs and symptoms
Abdominal mass	Abdominal fullness or pain, palpable mass noted on routine well child check-up, constipation secondary to obstruction, edema secondary to venous compression, hepatomegaly
Thoracic tumors	Respiratory symptoms, stridor from tracheal deviation or narrowing, SVC syndrome from mechanical obstruction
Paravertebral tumors	Spinal cord compression resulting in pain, motor or sensory deficits, loss of bowel or bladder control
Cervical involvement	Horner syndrome (ptosis, miosis, anhidrosis) from high thoracic/cervical mass
Metastatic infiltration of marrow and bone	Anemia, pancytopenia, bone pain, fever, limp, bleeding, increased risk of infection
Metastasis to orbital bones	Periorbital ecchymoses ("raccoon eyes"), ptosis, proptosis
Metastasis to skin	Papules or subcutaneous nodules, one-third of congenital NB will have firm, nontender, bluish red skin lesions that show central blanching with halo of surrounding erythema when rubbed

NB, neuroblastoma; SVC, superior vena cava.

As demonstrated in the table above, neuroblastomas metastasize via both hematogenous and lymphatic routes. In children with localized disease, 35% will have regional lymph node involvement. Extension of lymph node infiltration outside of the location of the primary tumor represents disseminated disease. Hematogenous sites include bone, bone marrow, skin, and liver.

Early diagnosis of neuroblastomas can be made on prenatal ultrasounds; however, they are more commonly diagnosed by CT or MRI along with HVA or VMA elevation in the urine. To confirm the diagnosis, patients will undergo bone marrow aspiration and biopsy along with possible biopsy and resection of the primary tumor. Surveys for metastases are performed with bone films, bone scans, and/or I-MIBG scans. MIBG chemically resembles norepinephrine which can then be taken up by sympathetic nervous system tissues such as neuroblastomas. MIBG can then be labeled with radioactive iodine and detected using scintigraphy to determine the extension of the disease process.

Staging of neuroblastomas is based on the International Staging System (INSS) used to categorize the complexity of the primary neoplasm as well as metastatic dissemination. The INSS incorporates stages 1 to 4 with 4S representing a distinct category of tumors in children less than 1 year of age with a localized primary tumor and dissemination to the liver and skin. Stage 4S tumors often result in a favorable outcome with spontaneous resolution of the neuroblastoma requiring little to no intervention. Treatment plans of the other stages are then designed based on the age at diagnosis, INSS staging, presence of the proto-oncogene MYCN, Shimada histology, and DNA ploidy of the tumor. Based on the factors above, each patient will undergo a combination of surgery, chemotherapy, and radiation for treatment. In severe disease, bone marrow transplantation may be indicated.

As a result of the diversity in location and presentation, the differential diagnosis of neuroblastoma is broad. Other abdominal masses that can mimic neuroblastomas include Wilms tumor and other germ cell tumors. Differentiation from Wilms tumor can be made with the presence of calcifications which are typically absent in Wilms tumors. Signs of bone marrow and lymph node involvement can easily be confused with other leukemias and lymphomas. The bone marrow aspirate/biopsy aids in determining the underlying neoplastic process. With neuroblastomas, the marrow will show clusters of neuroblasts forming pseudorosettes while leukemias such as acute lymphoblastic leukemias (ALL) show diffuse involvement. Other tumors such as rhabdomyosarcoma, Ewing sarcoma, and other neoplasms with bone marrow infiltration should be considered. Patients presenting with signs resembling OMA should also undergo complete neurologic evaluation to rule out primary neurologic etiologies. Other causes of OMA include infections, toxins, and ingestions along with metabolic abnormalities.

Selected References

National Cancer Institute. *Neuroblastoma (PDQ): Treatment Health Professional Version.* Bethesda, MD: National Cancer Institute; www.cancer.gov. Last modified December 1, 2007.

Ater JL. Neuroblastoma. In: Behrman R, Kliegman R, Jenson H, eds. *Nelson Textbook of Pediatrics.* 17th ed. Philadelphia, PA: Saunders; 2004:1709–1710.

Brodeur GM, Maris JM. Neuroblastoma. In: Pizzo PA, Poplack DG, eds. *Principles and Practice of Pediatric Oncology.* 5th ed. Philadelphia, PA: Lippincott Wilkins & Wilkins; 2006: 933–970.

Silverman LB, Sallan SE. Acute lymphoblastic leukemia. In: Nathan D, Orkin S, Ginsburg D, et al, eds. *Hematology of Infancy and Childhood.* 6th ed. Philadelphia, PA: Saunders; 2003:1144, Vol. 2.

32-Year-Old Male with Worsening Dyspnea on Exertion

CASE PRESENTATION

A 32-year-old elementary school teacher established himself as a new patient with a local primary care physician. At that time, he complained of cough, mild wheezing that worsened at night, decreased appetite, and worsening fatigue of approximately 1 week's duration. Although he had no known history of asthma, he said he "used to wheeze a lot" as a child. He occasionally smoked cigarettes (no more than 15–20/week) and also smoked 3 cigars/day. His physical examination at that time was notable for wheezing and rhonchi audible in nearly all lung zones. He was diagnosed with a reactive airway disorder in exacerbation and given a 5-day course of azithromycin, a 1-week burst of prednisone (40 mg dose), and an albuterol inhaler. He was also encouraged to use over-the-counter cough medicine as needed. Although his symptoms seemed to improve over the next week, he returned to the same primary care physician roughly 1 month later because his original symptoms had worsened. He was now also complaining of orthopnea and nightly episodes of paroxysmal nocturnal dyspnea as well as a vague feeling of chest discomfort that came on with exertion. He was most distressed about his activity level. Six months previously he had been an avid basketball player, he now couldn't exercise at all because of easily "getting winded," and over the past 2 days had lacked the energy to go to work. Based on the patient's story and physical examination that day, the primary care physician sent the patient to our emergency department via emergency medical services (EMS).

Physical Examination

The patient was a young, athletic-looking man who was quite anxious and unable to lie down flat. Vital signs: temperature 36.9°C, pulse 107 beats/min and regular, blood pressure (BP) 154/83 mm Hg, and respiration rate (RR) 24 breaths/min with oxygen saturations of 96% to 98% on 2 L of oxygen via nasal cannula. His lung examination, performed after administration of nebulizers by EMS personnel, still demonstrated faint wheezing at his bilateral bases as well as fine end-inspiratory rales roughly one-third up each side. His work of breathing was mildly increased without grunting or retractions. His cardiac examination revealed a grade 4/6 decrescendo murmur heard throughout diastole that was equally loud throughout the precordium. An S_3 was present but jugular venous distention was not appreciable. He had no cyanosis, clubbing, or peripheral edema. His pulses were strong and equal throughout all four limbs. His neurological examination revealed no focal abnormalities. The remainder of his examination was unremarkable.

Laboratory Studies

Complete blood count, chemistry-10 panel, and erythrocyte sedimentation rate (ESR) were within normal ranges. His total creatine kinase (CK) was elevated at 490 U/L (reference range 70–185) but creatine kinase MB (CK-MB) and troponin T levels were not elevated. An electrocardiogram (ECG) signaled sinus tachycardia, normal electrical axis, normal intervals, left ventricular hypertrophy, left atrial enlargement, and concave upward ST-segment elevations of 1 mm in leads V_1 through V_3 consistent with early repolarization changes. A chest x-ray (Fig. 15-1) showed patchy parenchymal lung opacities in both lower

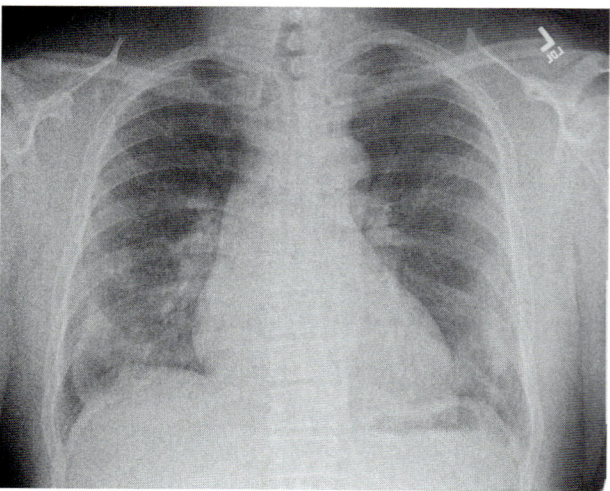

Figure 15-1 Chest x-ray (PA and lateral views) of this patient is consistent with pulmonary edema.
PA, posteroanterior.

and upper lobes bilaterally. The cardiac silhouette was mildly enlarged and the aorta was tortuous.

Case Resolution

This previously healthy 32-year-old man with new, uncompensated heart failure was admitted to the cardiology service where a transthoracic echocardiogram (TTE) was performed, revealing severe aortic valve regurgitation by color flow and continuous-wave Doppler examination. The TTE also showed mildly increased left ventricular wall thickness with normal chamber size and contraction; mild mitral valve regurgitation; normal right ventricular wall thickness, chamber size, and contraction; and no evidence of pericardial effusion. He eventually underwent aortic valve replacement.

Question

What inherited connective tissue disorders should be considered in a young individual presenting with aortic insufficiency?

Answer

In Marfan syndrome, abnormal production of the structural protein fibrillin can lead to abnormalities in the aortic valve leaflet and/or the aortic root. Ehlers-Danlos syndrome (in particular, type IV or vascular Ehlers-Danlos

syndrome) involves a deficiency in the production of type III collagen and subsequent compromise of the aortic root or ascending aorta.

Discussion

Echocardiography should be performed in all patients (young and old) with new-onset heart failure. The sensitivity and specificity of two-dimensional echocardiography for the diagnosis of heart failure (which has a broad differential diagnosis) approach 80% and 100%, respectively. An echocardiogram provides detailed information about ventricular size and function; regional wall motion abnormalities are compatible with ischemic cardiomyopathies from coronary artery disease. Pericardial thickening in constrictive pericarditis, abnormal myocardial texture in infiltrative cardiomyopathies, and abnormal right ventricular size and function in right-sided heart failure can be diagnosed by echocardiography as well. Echocardiography is especially important in assessing valvular integrity in heart failure and other disease states. In the case presented above, a TTE not only diagnosed severe aortic insufficiency as the cause of this young man's heart failure symptoms, but, as we shall discuss below, also provided an explanation for the valve's defect.

Aortic valve insufficiency results from leakage and backflow of blood that is ejected from the left ventricle into the ascending aorta back into the left ventricle. The variety of mechanisms contributing to aortic insufficiency can be divided into abnormalities of the aortic valve leaflets and pathologies of the proximal aortic root (Table 15-1).

TABLE 15-1

Major Causes of Aortic Regurgitation

Leaflet abnormalities	Aortic root or ascending aorta
Rheumatic fever	Systemic hypertension
Endocarditis	Aortitis (eg, syphilis)
Bicuspid aortic valve	Reiter syndrome
Trauma	Ankylosing spondylitis
Rheumatoid arthritis	Trauma
Myxomatous degeneration	Dissecting aneurysm
Marfan syndrome	Ehlers-Danlos syndrome
Fenfluramine–Phentermine	Inflammatory bowel disease

This patient's echocardiogram showed a trileaflet aortic valve with well-preserved mobility but a dilated aortic root measuring approximately 4.3 cm at the sinotubular junction as well as a dilated ascending aorta measuring approximately 5.4 cm above the sinotubular junction. A follow-up CT angiogram of the chest (Fig. 15-2) detailed aneurysmal dilatation of the proximal ascending thoracic aorta measuring approximately 5.5 cm without evidence of dissection. An ascending thoracic aortic aneurysm had led to severe aortic regurgitation and ensuing heart failure symptomatology in this young man.

Thoracic aortic aneurysms, less common than abdominal aortic aneurysms (6 cases/100,000 patient years compared to 15–37 cases/100,000 patient years), can be either fusiform (uniform in shape with symmetrical dilatation involving the entire circumference of the aortic wall) or saccular (more localized, appearing as an outpouching of only a portion of the aortic wall). A pseudoaneurysm (also termed false aneurysm) is a collection of blood and connective tissue outside the aortic wall, usually the result of a rupture (Fig. 15-3). Four general anatomic categories of thoracic aortic aneurysms exist, catalogued by the aneurysm's point of origin (Fig. 15-4), although some aneurysms involve more than one segment. Ascending aortic aneurysms arise from the aortic valve to brachiocephalic trunk and account for roughly 60% of thoracic aneurysms. Aortic arch aneurysms, present in 10% of cases, describe any thoracic aneurysm that involves the brachiocephalic

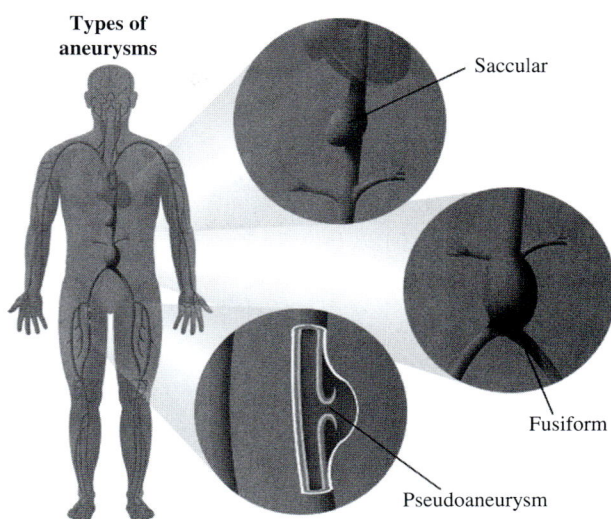

Figure 15-3 Descriptive terms used for thoracic aortic aneurysms. *Image taken from http://www.stanfordhospital.com/healthlib/greystone/ heartcenter/heartconditionsinadults/thoracicaorticaneurysm*

vessels. Descending aortic aneurysms, arising distal to the left subclavian artery, are seen in 40% of cases and thoracoabdominal aneurysms coexist in thoracic and abdominal aortic segments in approximately 10% of aortic aneurysms.

Thoracic aortic aneurysms occur two to four times more commonly in men than in women. Because it is degenerative, arteriosclerotic disease is the most common cause of thoracic aneurysms, typically seen in older populations. In addition to age-associated changes in collagen and elastin, smoking, hypertension, atherosclerosis, and bicuspid or unicuspid aortic valves are other factors contributing to the degeneration of the thoracic aorta's integrity. In younger patients, such as the one presented above, other etiologies for thoracic aneurysms must be sought. Inherited disorders of connective tissue such as Marfan syndrome and Ehlers-Danlos syndrome predispose to aneurysm formation, and as high as 42% of asymptomatic women with Turner syndrome have some form of aortic root dilatation owing to bicuspid aortic valves, coarctation of the aorta, and/or uncontrolled hypertension. Aortitis refers to a broad array of inflammatory and infectious disorders that can occasionally cause aortic aneurysm. These include giant cell arteritis, syphilitic aortitis, mycotic aneurysm (typically in the setting of bacterial endocarditis), Takayasu arteritis, rheumatoid and psoriatic arthritis, ankylosing spondylitis, Wegener granulomatosis, and Reiter syndrome. Finally, the familial thoracic aortic aneurysm syndrome describes the roughly 15% to 20% of patients with an aneurysm or dissection and a family history of this disorder independent of Marfan or

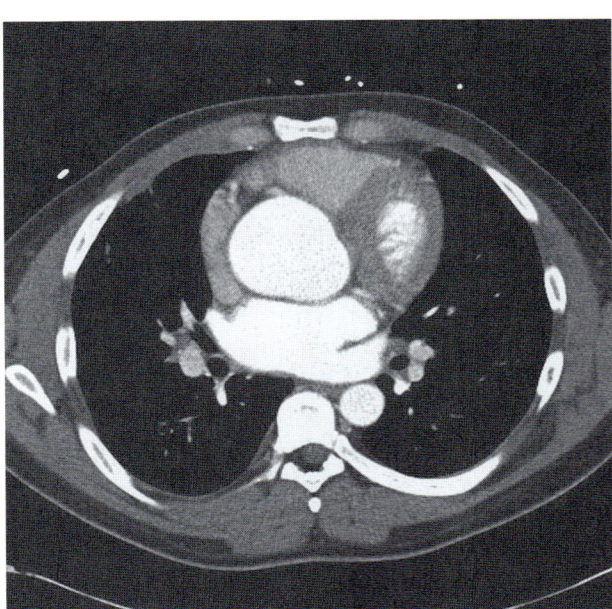

Figure 15-2 CT angiogram of the chest of this patient reveals an ascending thoracic aortic aneurysm. CT, computed tomography.

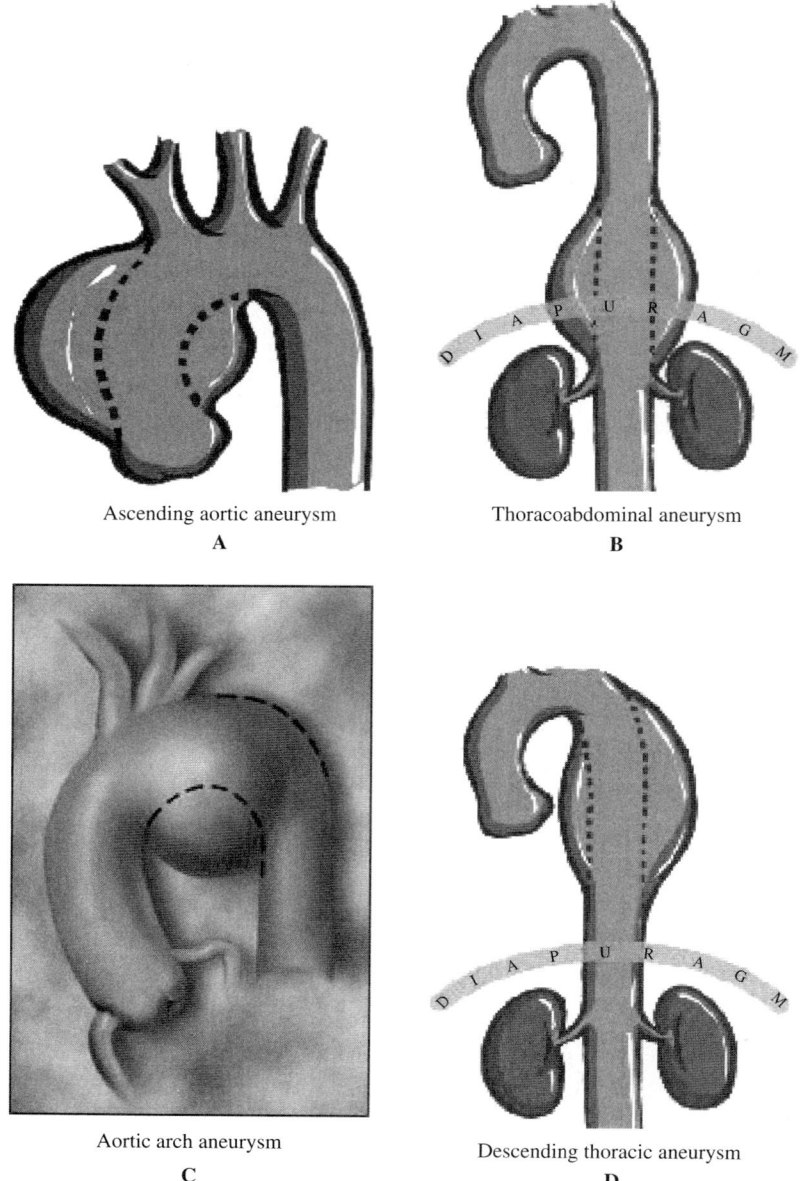

Ascending aortic aneurysm
A

Thoracoabdominal aneurysm
B

Aortic arch aneurysm
C

Descending thoracic aneurysm
D

Figure 15-4 Thoracic aortic aneurysm categories.

Images taken from http://www.slrctsurgery.com/Thoracic%20aortic%20aneurysms.htm and http://www.columbiasurgery.org/pat/aortic/ aneurysms.htm

Ehlers-Danlos syndrome; these patients present at significantly younger ages than do those with sporadic aneurysms. The patient presented above phenotypically displayed no evidence for a collagen vascular disease and an extensive serological workup was negative for many of the diseases categorized under aortitis. Pathological review of his surgically removed aortic valve and portion of his proximal aorta showed only degenerative disease. He was unaware of any familial history of aortic aneurysms or dissections.

Most patients with thoracic aortic aneurysms have no symptoms until their aneurysms begin to leak or expand. At that point, patients can present with chest, back, flank, or abdominal pain, depending on the aneurysm's location and attributed to compression or distortion of adjacent structures or vessels. Ascending aortic aneurysms can present with heart failure symptoms because of aortic regurgitation, as in the case presented above, and compression of a coronary artery can result in myocardial ischemia or infarction. If a thoracic aneurysm erodes into the mediastinum, compression of adjacent structures can lead to a myriad of symptoms, as seen with the left vagus or left recurrent laryngeal nerves (hoarseness), phrenic nerve (hemidiaphragm paralysis), tracheobronchial tree (wheezing, cough, hemoptysis, dyspnea), and esophagus (dysphagia). Dissections or leakages are the most serious, life-threatening complications of aneurysms and require immediate medical and surgical attention.

Imaging studies are required in the diagnosis of thoracic aortic aneurysms. A chest x-ray showing widening of the mediastinal silhouette, enlargement of the aortic knob, or displacement of the trachea from midline is often how asymptomatic aneurysms are detected. However, chest x-rays cannot distinguish an aneurysm from a tortuous aorta, and one series found plain film abnormalities detectable in only 61% (22 of 36) of patients presenting with acute-onset chest or back pain and found to have nondissecting thoracic aneurysms. Therefore, CT angiogram is the preferred test to detect a thoracic aortic aneurysm, determine its size, and define aortic and branch vessel anatomy. Magnetic resonance angiography can substitute for a CT angiogram, and actually is preferred for aneurysms involving the aortic root because CT images the root less well and is less accurate in sizing its diameter. Transthoracic echocardiography is of limited value in thoracic aortic disease because of nonconductance of the signal by lung air, but imaging within the mediastinum using transesophageal echocardiography can be useful when a coexistent dissection is suspected.

For most ascending thoracic aortic aneurysms, surgery is indicated at a diameter of more than or equal to 5.5 cm; this threshold can be raised to 6 cm or more among those with an increased operative risk, while ascending aortic repair is recommended when aneurysms reach only 5 cm (or even smaller diameters) for patients who are at increased risk of aortic dissection or rupture (eg, Marfan syndrome). The aneurysm is generally resected and replaced with a prosthetic Dacron tube graft of appropriate size. When the aneurysm involves the aortic root and is associated with significant aortic regurgitation, surgery typically involves a composite aortic repair (the Bentall procedure, used for the patient presented above) in which a tube graft with a prosthetic aortic valve is placed. Alternatively, when the aortic valve leaflets are structurally normal and the aortic regurgitation secondary to dilatation of the root is mild, a valve-sparing root replacement can be performed. Most descending thoracic aortic aneurysms are surgically repaired at an aortic diameter of more than or equal to 6 cm with either open resection and replacement with prosthetic graft or, alternatively, with a transluminally placed endovascular stent graft.

Selected References

1. Isselbacher EM. Thoracic and abdominal aortic aneurysms. *Circulation.* 2005;11(6):816–828.
2. Coady MA, Davies RR, Roberts M, et al. Familial patterns of thoracic aortic aneurysms. *Arch Surg.* 1999;134(4):361–367.
3. Erbel R, Schweizer P, Krebs W, et al. Sensitivity and specificity of two-dimensional echocardiography in detection of impaired left ventricular function. *Eur Heart J.* 1984;5(6):477–489.
4. Coselli JS, Conklin LD, LeMaire SA. Thoracoabdominal aortic aneurysm repair: review and update of current strategies. *Ann Thorac Surg.* 2002;74(5):S1881–S1884 (discussion S1892–S1898).

3-Year-Old Female with Tachypnea

CASE PRESENTATION

A 3-year-old female presented to our emergency room with a 2-week history of persistent fever and one witnessed seizure. The seizure occurred several hours prior to presentation and was felt to be consistent with a febrile seizure. Over the last 2 weeks, the child had seen multiple physicians at various urgent care centers and received varying treatments for her febrile illness. The patient has no significant past medical history and no history of prior seizures. No known exposure to tuberculosis (TB) or human immunodeficiency virus (HIV). She had no known sick contacts and no recent ingestion of undercooked meat. Recent travel: notable for travel to the New England area, no foreign travel. She was treated approximately 14 days prior to presentation for a urinary tract infection (UTI) with trimethoprim/sulfamethoxazole. She was also treated approximately 10 days prior to presentation with a 10-day course of azithromycin after findings of diffuse haziness on a chest x-ray (CXR) taken by her primary care physician (PCP). Her review of systems was significant only for the persistent fever and occasional increased work of breathing as noted by the parents. One such episode of "fast breathing" was associated with perioral cyanosis. The parents denied any change in activity level, oral intake, emesis, rashes, or swollen glands.

C 16

Physical Examination

Patient was slightly tachypneic, but in no apparent distress. Vital signs: temperature 36.8°C, pulse 127 beats/min, respiratory rate 40 breaths/min, blood pressure 130/94 mm Hg. Head, eyes, ears, nose, and throat (HEENT): normocephalic; atraumatic; tympanic membranes clear, shiny, and grey; bilaterally. Neck: supple, no lymphadenopathy. Cardiovascular (CV): regular rate and rhythm (RRR), no murmur. Normal S_1, S_2. Lungs: clear to auscultation bilaterally, tachypneic. No grunting, nasal flaring, or retractions. No use of accessory muscles. Abdomen: soft, nontender, nondistended; no hepatosplenomegaly. Neurology: cranial nerves (CN) II to XII appear intact. Normal strength and tone. Developmental history normal.

Laboratory Studies

White blood cells (WBC) 18.1, absolute neutrophil count (ANC) 12.7, absolute lymphocyte count (ALC) 4.4, absolute eosinophil count (AEC) 0, hematocrit (Hct) 40.1, platelets 428. Arterial blood gas (ABG) (from the outside hospital): 7.39/39.5/25/25/-1. Cerebrospinal fluid (CSF): red blood cells (RBC) 5, white blood cells (WBC) 6, glucose 45, protein 21, cultures negative. Urinalysis (U/A): unremarkable. C-reactive protein (CRP) 8.5. Chest radiograph and head CT are shown below in Fig. 16-1 and Fig. 16-2, respectively.

Case Resolution

The patient was initially treated with vancomycin, ceftriaxone, and erythromycin for presumed pneumonia. Her symptoms persisted for the next 6 days and she was then transferred to a tertiary care center for further workup and management. Owing to her history of new-onset seizure, a head CT was obtained (Fig. 16-2) and showed a left temporoparietal-enhancing mass. She was then placed on steroids, antituberculous medications, and antiepileptics. Blood and urine cultures from the initial hospital remained negative. Three serial gastric aspirates were negative for acid-fast bacillus

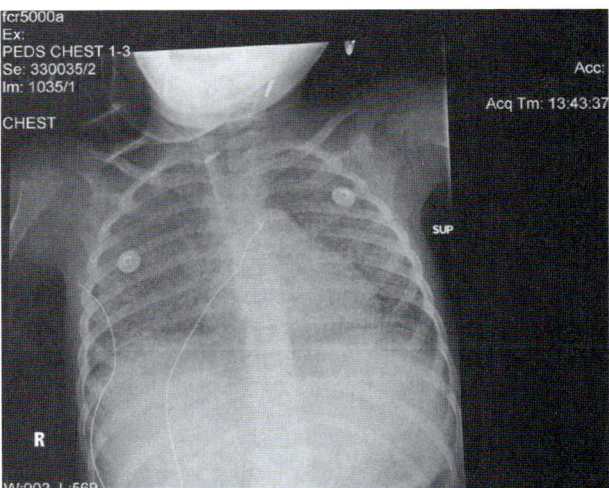

Figure 16-1 PA and lateral chest x-ray.

(AFB) and were culture negative. Stool cultures remained negative. Screen for parasites, fungi, and actinomyces was also negative. A screening immune workup was initiated and showed normal serum immunoglobulin levels, normal lymphocyte markers, and normal neutrophil function. HIV, rheumatoid factor, and ANA were all negative.

Question

Is there a single pathology causing her pulmonary symptoms and brain mass?

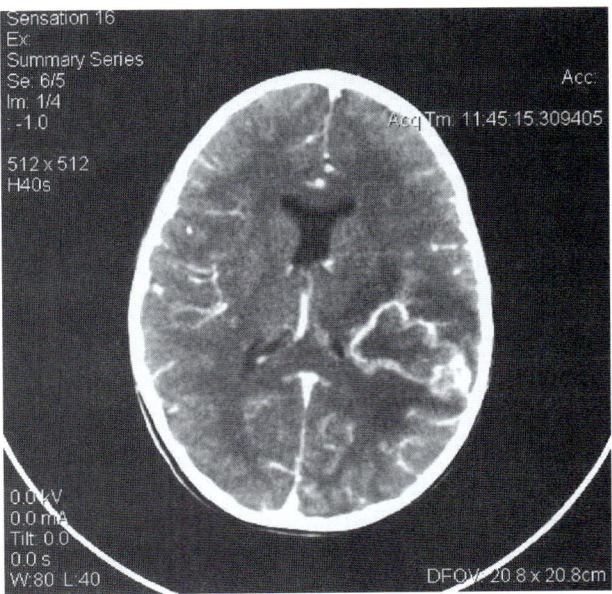

Figure 16-2 Contrast-enhanced head computed tomogram.

Answer

Primary TB can cause significant respiratory compromise and, especially in children, can cause tuberculoma formation. She underwent a bronchoscopy with bronchoalveolar lavage (BAL) that grew out *Mycobacterium tuberculosis* complex. Brain biopsy was also performed which also grew *M. tuberculosis*.

Discussion

TB is a common infection worldwide and can be seen by medical professionals who treat any age group. National surveillance and control methods have made infection with *M. tuberculosis* less common in the United States with each passing year. Despite progress in monitoring and treatment, TB still remains the most common infectious cause of death worldwide. For 2005, in the United States, the incidence of TB is 4.8 cases/100,000 population. This is a 3.8% decrease from the prior year. Unfortunately, multidrug-resistant TB is still on the rise and there is still a disparity between US-born and foreign-born persons as well as between Caucasians and racial/ethnic minorities[1].

TB is a serious illness, yet not a common one in the United States; therefore, a high index of suspicion is often necessary to diagnose TB. Obviously, not every patient with signs of a respiratory infection is going to have TB, and not need a TB screening or workup. Therefore, it is helpful if a physician is aware of populations that are at greater risk of TB infection and can raise their level of suspicion appropriately. There are a number of patient populations that are at increased risk for TB infection. Risk factors for TB include:

1. HIV-positive status
2. Immunosuppressive medications
3. Patients with cancer, most notably hematologic neoplasms
4. Homeless patients
5. IV drug users
6. Foreign-born patients
7. Low socioeconomic status
8. Inmates of prisons or jails

Possible TB infection can find a home on nearly any differential diagnosis list, in turn making it difficult to diagnose. Infection with *M. tuberculosis* commonly begins with inhalation of the bacteria into the lungs. After inhalation into the lungs, there are three common outcomes.

1. The host immune system effectively and immediately clears the infection.

2. Progressive or primary disease

3. Chronic or latent TB infection (LTBI), often leading to reactivation disease after many years

The clinical presentation of TB depends on what stage of the illness the patient presents in. The patient in this case presented with primary TB, and many pediatric patients do, and had the classic finding of persistent fever for 14 to 21 days. Other likely symptoms include chest pain or pleuritic pain. Less common, but possible, symptoms include cough, fatigue, pharyngitis, and arthralgias.

Reactivation of latent TB is more often seen in adults and adolescents and usually follows a more indolent course, presenting with the classic findings of persistent cough, weight loss, fatigue, fever, night sweats, and possible hemoptysis. Chest pain and dyspnea are sometimes seen as well. The cough of reactivation TB is often persistent and may or may not be productive of sputum.

The gold standard for diagnosis of TB is culture of *M. tuberculosis*. Tuberculin skin testing (TST) with purified protein derivative (PPD) is useful only for screening and is nondiagnostic. Skin tests should be read at 48 to 72 hours and a positive test depends on age and which, if any, risk factors are present (see Table 16-1). CXR may be used for screening in patients with a positive TST and is also useful in diagnosing pulmonary TB. While CXR findings vary widely depending on the stage of illness and immune status of the patient, typical findings often include hilar lymphadenopathy; involvement of a segment or lobe, possibly with atelectasis or infiltrate; pleural effusion; cavitary lesions; and miliary disease.[2] There are three common methods in use to obtain material for culture: induced/expectorated sputum, gastric aspirate, or bronchoscopy with BAL. Which method to utilize often depends on the clinical situation and age of the

---

TABLE 16-1

Definitions of Positive Tuberculin Skin Testing Results in Children and Adolescents

Induration ≥5 mm
    Children or adolescents in close contact with a known or suspected infectious case of TB
    Children or adolescents with suspected TB disease:
        Finding on chest radiograph consistent with active or previously active TB
        Clinical evidence of TB disease
    Children or adolescents who are immunosuppressed (eg, receiving immunosuppressive therapy or with immunosuppressive conditions [eg, HIV infection])
Induration ≥10 mm
    Children or adolescents at increased risk of disseminated disease:
        Those <4 years old
        Those with concomitant medical conditions (eg, Hodgkin disease, lymphoma, diabetes mellitus, chronic renal failure, or malnutrition)
    Children or adolescents with increased risk of exposure to cases of TB disease:
        Those born in a country with a high prevalence of TB cases
        Those who travel to a country with a high prevalence of TB cases
        Those with parents born in a country with a high prevalence of TB cases
        Those frequently exposed to adults with risk factors for TB disease (eg, adults who are HIV infected or homeless, users of illicit drugs, those who are incarcerated or institutionalized, or migrant farm workers)
Induration ≥15 mm
    Children ≥4 years old with no known risk factors

Adapted from American Academy of Pediatrics. Tuberculosis. In: Pickering L, ed. Red Book: 2000 Report of the Committee on Infectious Diseases. 25th ed. Elk Grove Village, IL: American Academy of Pediatrics; 2000:593–613.

patient. Sputum induction is generally the preferred method of sample collection. Induced sputum can be cultured for *Mycobacterium* and also stained for AFB. Gastric aspiration is more commonly used with pediatric patients who are unable to produce sputum on their own. Gastric contents are aspirated each morning prior to rising from bed or the first meal, in order to collect any sputum swallowed during the night. In general, gastric aspirates are less reliable than induced sputum samples when used for culture.[3] Gastric aspirates are also unsuitable for AFB staining, since it is possible to find nonpathogenic *Mycobacterium* species in the stomach. In this case, the second gastric aspirate grew *Mycobacterium gordonae*, one of the least pathogenic species of mycobacterium and likely part of her flora. Bronchoscopy with BAL is also an effective method and has been shown to be roughly equivalent to sputum induction.[4] A positive AFB stain is often sufficient to diagnose TB, but culture is both the gold standard and necessary to guide treatment.

Treatment of *M. tuberculosis* should always be guided by drug susceptibility and resistance of the isolated bacterium. Drug resistance has increased in both the United States and worldwide in the last few years, making multidrug-resistant TB a serious concern and in turn making culture with susceptibility data vital in order to treat the infection. Treatment itself varies based on whether the patient has active or latent TB. Latent TB in children is usually treated with isoniazid for 9 months. Treatment of active TB should always utilize a multidrug regimen and directly observed therapy (DOT). The purpose of DOT is to increase adherence to treatment and reduce relapse rates, treatment failures, and drug-resistance rates. There are a number of recommended treatment regimens, generally using three- or four-drug regimens. The most commonly used treatment regimens use a combination of ethambutol, isoniazid, pyrazinamide, and rifampin or rifapentine, with streptomycin utilized occasionally. The duration of treatment is usually for either 6 or 9 months.

In this case, TB was suspected based on CXR findings, but not definitively diagnosed until culture results showed *M. tuberculosis*. This patient was started on isoniazid, rifampin, pyrazinamide, and streptomycin. The local health department was notified and began an investigation into the source, although no source was found. The patient's brother was also found to have been exposed and started on therapy for latent TB.

Selected References

1. Centers for Disease Control and Prevention. Trends in tuberculosis—United States, 2005. *MMWR Morb Mortal Wkly Rep.* 2006;55:305–308.
2. American Academy of Pediatrics. Tuberculosis. In: Pickering L, ed. *Red Book: 2000 Report of the Committee on Infectious Diseases.* 25th ed. Elk Grove Village, IL: American Academy of Pediatrics; 2000:593–613.
3. Zar H, Hanslo D, Apolles P, et al. Induced sputum versus gastric lavage for microbiological confirmation of pulmonary tuberculosis in infants and young children: a prospective study. *Lancet.* 2005;365:130–134.
4. Conde M, Soares S, Mello F, et al. Comparison of sputum induction with fiberoptic bronchoscopy in the diagnosis of tuberculosis: experience at an acquired immune deficiency syndrome reference center in Rio de Janeiro, Brazil. *Am J Respir Crit Care Med.* 2000;162:2238–2240.

11-Year-Old Female with Fatigue and Icterus

CASE PRESENTATION

A previously healthy 11-year-old Caucasian female presented to her pediatrician with a 2-week history of light-headedness. She is found to have bilateral tympanic effusions and cervical lymphadenopathy on physical examination. She is started on a 1-week course of cefprozil and guaifenesin for treatment of presumed otitis media with resultant labyrinthitis. Her symptoms seem to improve. One week later, her mother notices that her daughter's sclera appear yellow and her abdomen seems distended. The patient returns to her pediatrician for evaluation. Her mother reports intermittent fever over the last several days. Upon further questioning, the patient reports increasing fatigue, poor appetite, and less, but dark urine output. Her review of systems is otherwise unremarkable. She has no known drug allergies and takes no regular medications. Her past medical history is also unremarkable. Her mother reports that she was the product of a full-term pregnancy that was without perinatal complications. She has had no surgeries and no hospitalizations.

Her family history is significant only for coronary artery disease on her father's side of the family. There is no history of liver problems of any kind. The patient has four siblings all of whom are healthy. She is in the sixth grade. She is active in sports and school activities. The family did not report any international travel or camping trips. The family dwelling uses city water.

Physical Examination

Vital signs: temperature 37°C, heart rate (HR) 100 beats/min, respiratory rate (RR) 20 breaths/min, blood pressure (BP) 90/70 mm Hg. Head, eyes, ears, nose, and throat (HEENT): normocephalic and atraumatic. Tympanic membranes (TMs) visualized b/l without effusions. Oropharynx is without erythema or exudate; Frenular jaundice; scleral icterus, pupils equal, round, reactive to light (PERRL), extraocular movement intact (EOMI); nasal mucosa is normal. Neck: No appreciable lymphadenopathy. Cardiovascular: regular rate and rhythm with grade 2 to 3/6 systolic ejection murmur at the left upper sternal border without radiation. Lungs: no increased work of breathing or respiratory distress, but decreased air movement on the right side with egophony and dullness to percussion approximately half way up the chest on the right side. Abdomen: abdominal distention with ascites. Spleen tip is palpable 3 to 4 cm below the costal margin. Liver is palpable 3 to 4 cm below the costal margin. Span of liver is 13 to 15 cm on percussion. Genitourinary: Tanner stage I. Extremities: 1+ pitting edema to the knees bilaterally. Neurologic: cranial nerves tested and intact. Muscle strength 5/5 in all extremities. Deep tendon reflexes (DTRs) 2+ in all extremities. Sensation normal. No cerebellar signs. No asterixis. Psychiatry: appropriate effect

Skin: jaundice; no rashes, lesions, or ecchymosis

Laboratory Studies/Imaging

Chemistries: Na 139, K 2.8, Cl 110, HCO_3 22, blood urea nitrogen (BUN) 18, creatinine (Cr) 0.9, total bilirubin 5.8, direct bilirubin 3.1, aspartate aminotransferase (AST) 151, alanine aminotransferase (ALT) 45, alkaline phosphatase (ALP) 99, gamma-glutamyltransferase (GGT) 202

Complete blood count (CBC): white blood cells (WBC) 4.8, hemoglobin (Hgb) 7.6, hematocrit (Hct) 21.7, platelets 118

Coagulation: prothrombin time (PT) 28.5, partial thromboplastin time (PTT) 53.4, international normalized ratio (INR) 2.7

Urinalysis (U/A): specific gravity 1.025, pH 5, protein 1+, bilirubin 1+

Ceruloplasmin 8

Chest x-ray (CXR): bilateral pleural effusions with the right greater than left

Abdominal ultrasound (U/S): marked splenomegaly, common bile duct is upper limits of normal at 5.1 mm. No intrahepatic ductal dilatation. Large right pleural and a moderate left pleural effusion, ascites.

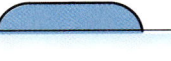

Case Resolution

The above patient underwent an orthotopic liver transplant and continues to do well.

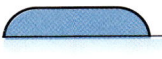

Question

How can the cause of this child's coagulopathy be discerned?

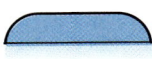

Answer

There are many potential causes of coagulopathy in this case. In the setting of anemia and low platelets, microangiopathic anemia or disseminated intravascular coagulation (DIC) must be considered. Review of the blood smear for evidence of hemolysis such as spherocytes or schistocytes is the first step in evaluation. Splenic sequestration could also explain the low platelets. Liver failure or disease leading to splenomegaly could explain the clinical scenario of thrombocytopenia and coagulopathy. A nutritional deficiency of vitamin K could also explain the coagulopathy. Selective testing of clotting factors will lead to the answer. This approach takes advantage of the diverse origin of clotting factors. Factor five is produced in the liver but is not

TABLE 17-1

Clotting Factor Patterns in Disease States

	Factor five	Factor seven	Factor eight
DIC	↓	↓	↓
Liver failure	↓	↓	↔
Nutritional deficiency	↔	↓	↔

DIC, disseminated intravascular coagulation.

vitamin K-dependent for gamma-carboxylation. Factor seven is also made in the liver and is vitamin K-dependent for gamma-carboxylation. Factor eight is synthesized in the vascular endothelium. DIC will consume all clotting factors. All factor levels will be depressed in this setting. Liver failure will lead to low levels of both factors: five and seven. Nutritional deficiency of vitamin K will lead to a low value of factor VII (see Table 17-1).

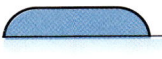

Discussion

This is an 11-year-old female with new-onset hepatosplenomegaly, jaundice, and fulminant hepatic failure with anemia and coagulopathy of liver disease. Differential diagnoses for her fulminant hepatic failure includes:

- Infectious etiology including
  - Hepatitis A, B, and C
  - Epstein-Barr virus
  - Cytomegalovirus
- Autoimmune hepatitis
- Wilson disease (WD)
- Alpha-1 antitrypsin deficiency
- Toxin ingestion (eg, acetaminophen)
- Vascular event (Budd-Chiari syndrome, ischemia)

The patient's age, fulminant liver failure with mild encephalopathy, low-alkaline phosphatase and ceruloplasmin on laboratory analysis, and a nonimmune hemolytic anemia were most consistent with WD.

The diagnosis was confirmed by liver biopsy which revealed a markedly elevated quantitative copper level as seen in Fig. 17-1.

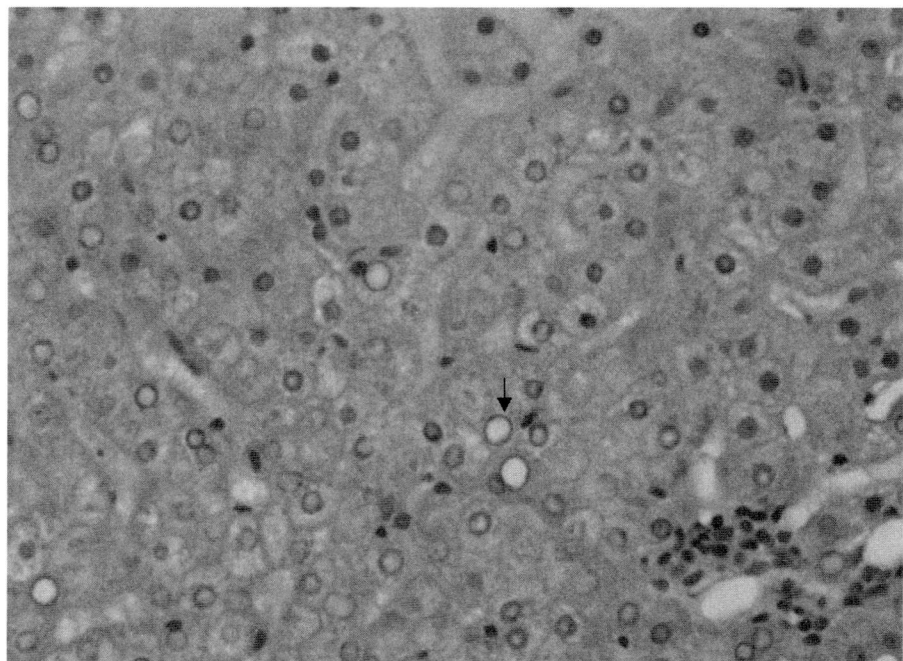

Figure 17-1 Liver biopsy revealing the glycogen depositions seen in Wilson disease.

Wilson Disease

WD, also known as hepatolenticular degeneration, is an inborn error of metabolism that is inherited in an autosomal recessive pattern. It is a disease of copper metabolism marked by the accumulation of toxic levels of copper in the liver, brain, and eyes. It has an incidence of 1 in 30,000 worldwide and a carrier rate 1 in 100.

The disease was first described by a British neurologist, Dr Samuel Alexander Kinnier Wilson, in 1912. The association with copper accumulation was later made by Dr J.N. Cumings in 1948.

The hallmarks of the disease are the presence of liver disease, neurologic symptoms, and Kayser-Fleischer corneal rings. The leading neurologic symptoms in WD are dysarthria, dyspraxia, ataxia, and Parkinson-like extrapyramidal signs. Changes in basal ganglia in the brain magnetic resonance image (MRI) are characteristic features of the disease.

Most patients with WD will present between the ages of 5 and 40 years, but the average median age at presentation of liver dysfunction is 10 to 15 years with neurologic presentations typically occurring later in the course of the disease.

The diagnosis should be considered in all patients with fulminant hepatic failure or unexplained liver disease, patients with liver disease who are less than 40 years old,

patients with viral-negative hepatitis, patients who are less than 40 years old with Parkinson-like symptoms, young individuals with behavioral changes without substance abuse, and in all patients who have first-degree relatives with WD.

WD is a relatively rare disease that has a spectrum of clinical presentations making the diagnosis rather challenging. Hepatitis with WD can be mild manifest as transaminitis, or more severe, with jaundice and elevated bilirubin levels. With severe hepatitis, hemolysis may occur as a consequence of the release stored copper from dying hepatocytes. Therefore, hemolysis in the setting of liver disease should raise the suspicion of WD.

Neurologic manifestations of WD mimic a movement disorder without affecting muscle strength or sensation and mimicking parkinsonism. Speech is the modality that is often affected early and manifests as slurred, hypokinetic speech with progression to frank dysarthria later in the disease. Tremor and dystonia occur frequently with the disease. Loss of coordination also occurs which manifests as difficulty with handwriting and abnormal gait.

The behavioral abnormalities that occur in WD are extremely diverse and include mood lability, difficulty with concentration, and even paranoia and hallucinations.

There is no gold standard for the diagnosis of WD and an accurate diagnosis requires a combination of clinical signs and symptoms in conjunction with biochemical tests.

Findings suggestive of the disease include:

- Presence of Kayser-Fleischer rings on slit lamp examination
- Elevated serum-free copper level (>25 µg/dL)
- Low-serum ceruloplasmin (<20 mg/dL)
- Elevated 24-hour urinary copper level (>100 µg)
- Elevated hepatic copper levels on biopsy (>250 µg/g dry weight) (10)

WD is secondary to a genetic defect on chromosome 13, in linkage with esterase D locus. The gene involved is *ATP7B* (shares homology with *ATP7A* which is involved in Menke disease, another disorder of copper metabolism) which encodes a gene for transmembrane copper-transporting adenosine triphosphate (ATPase), localized to the hepatocyte canalicular membrane. Although the disease mechanism is unclear, it is postulated that the liver is responsible for appropriate copper balance through the excretion of excess copper. Thus, the underlying defect may be secondary to defective secretion of copper into bile for elimination from the body as there is diminished export from the liver into the circulation. As copper accumulates in the liver, hepatic injury occurs presumably secondary to free radical generation as a consequence of the pro-oxidant properties of copper. Over time, progressive hepatocyte damage leads to hepatitis and then to cirrhosis. Once cirrhosis develops, copper leaks into the plasma and accumulates in other tissues producing the neurologic, hematologic, and nephrologic manifestations of the disease. The organ most sensitive to extrahepatic copper deposition is the brain where deposition in the basal ganglia leads to the movement disorder and neuropsychiatric manifestations of the disease. Early recognition and diagnosis of WD is paramount as it is an unusual genetic disease in that it is remarkably effectively treated.

References

1. Wilson SAK. Progressive lenticular degeneration: a familial nervous disease associated with cirrhosis of the liver. *Brain.* 1912;34:295–507.
2. Cumings JN. The copper and iron content of brain and liver in the normal and in hepato-lenticular degeneration. *Brain.* 1948;71:410–415.
3. Walshe JM. Penicillamine: a new oral therapy for Wilson's disease. *Am J Med.* 1956;21:487–495.
4. Kitzberger R, Madl C, Ferenci P. Wilson disease. *Metab Brain Dis.* 2005 Dec;20(4):295–302.
5. Brewer GJ. Behavioral abnormalities in Wilson's disease. *Adv Neurol.* 2005;96:262–274.
6. Ferenci P. Wilson's disease. *Clin Gastroenterol Hepatol.* 2005 Aug;3(8):726–733.
7. Brewer GJ, Askari FK. Wilson's disease: clinical management and therapy. *J Hepatol.* 2005;42(suppl 1):S13–S21.
8. Brewer GJ. Recognition, diagnosis, and management of Wilson's disease. *Proc Soc Exp Biol Med.* 2000 Jan;223(1):39–46.
9. Fink JK, Hedera P, Brewer GJ. Hepatolenticular degeneration (Wilson's disease). *Neurologist.* 1999;5:171–185.
10. Green G, Harris I, Lin G, et al. *The Washington Manual of Medical Therapeutics.* 31st ed. Philadelphia, PA: Lippincott Williams & Wilkins; 2004.
11. Frommer DJ. Defective biliary excretion of copper in Wilson's disease. *Gut.* 1974;15:125–129.
12. Gibbs K, Walshe JM. Biliary excretion of copper in Wilson's disease. *Lancet.* 1980;2:538–539.
13. Iyengar V, Brewer GJ, Dick RD, et al. Studies of cholecystokinin-stimulated biliary secretions reveal a high-molecular-weight, copper-binding substance in normal subjects that is absent in patients with Wilson's disease. *J Lab Clin Med.* 1988;111:267–274.
14. Harris ZL, Takahashi Y, Miyajima H, et al. Aceruloplasminemia: molecular characterization of this disorder of iron metabolism. *Proc Natl Acad Sci USA.* 1995;92:2539.
15. Wilson disease foundation. http://www.wilsonsdisease.org, accessed last February 20, 2008.

70-Year-Old Caucasian Female with Hypertension and Depression

CASE PRESENTATION

A 70-year-old Caucasian female with a past medical history of hypertension, hyperlipidemia, tobacco use, gastroesophageal reflux disease (GERD), and depression presented with loss of consciousness after reported complaints of headache, light-headedness, shortness of breath, and right arm tingling. The patient awoke confused and disoriented. At that time she was combative and unable to articulate her thoughts. Per the patient's husband and son, she had been behaving oddly for the past several weeks. She lost her job 2 weeks prior and since that time she had become increasingly agitated, depressed, and forgetful. On the morning of admission, the patient was eating at a diner and locked her keys in her car. Loss of consciousness occurred while awaiting help to open the car at the diner.

When she arrived at the outside hospital, she had an elevated blood pressure measured at 193/98 mm Hg and had an electrocardiogram (ECG) which demonstrated ST-segment elevation greater than 1 mm in leads V_2 through V_5, I, and aVL. The patient had worsening altered mental status with increasing combativeness, and required sedation and eventually she was intubated. She received a β-blocker for hypertension and was transferred to a tertiary care hospital for further management.

Physical Examination

The patient was sedated and intubated and appeared well-nourished. Vital signs: temperature 37.5°C, pulse 70 beats/min, blood pressure (BP) 105–130/65–85 mm Hg. The ventilator was set to a synchronous intermittent mandatory ventilation (SIMV) rate of 8 at an FIO_2 of 0.60. She was not breathing over the ventilator. Pupils were equal round and reactive to light. Her neck was supple and without jugular venous distention or thyromegaly. Heart rate and rhythm were regular with normal S_1 and S_2 and no auscultated S_3 or S_4. No murmur, gallop, or rub were present. The point of maximal intensity (PMI) was normal. Breath sounds were coarse with mild rales posteriorly in the bases. Abdominal examination was benign. Her lower extremities were not edematous and were warm. Examination was otherwise normal.

Laboratory Studies

Cardiac biomarkers revealed creatine kinase (CK) 2339, creatine kinase MB (CK-MB) 12.9, and troponin T 0.418. Pro–brain natriuretic peptide (pro–BNP) was 2224. Potassium was 3.5 and creatinine was normal at 0.7. Liver function tests were normal. Thyroid-stimulating hormone (TSH) was normal. Urine toxicology screening was positive for opiates, but otherwise negative and the patient had known exposure of opiates at the outside hospital for sedation. Complete blood count with white blood cells (WBC) 14.8, hemoglobin 14.2, hematocrit 41.9, and platelets 215.

ECG 1 pictured below (Fig. 18-1) was obtained at the time of presentation to the emergency department at the tertiary care center. It demonstrated sinus tachycardia with anteroseptal infarct pattern ST-segment elevations in precordial leads V_2 through V_4. Chest x-ray revealed an appropriately

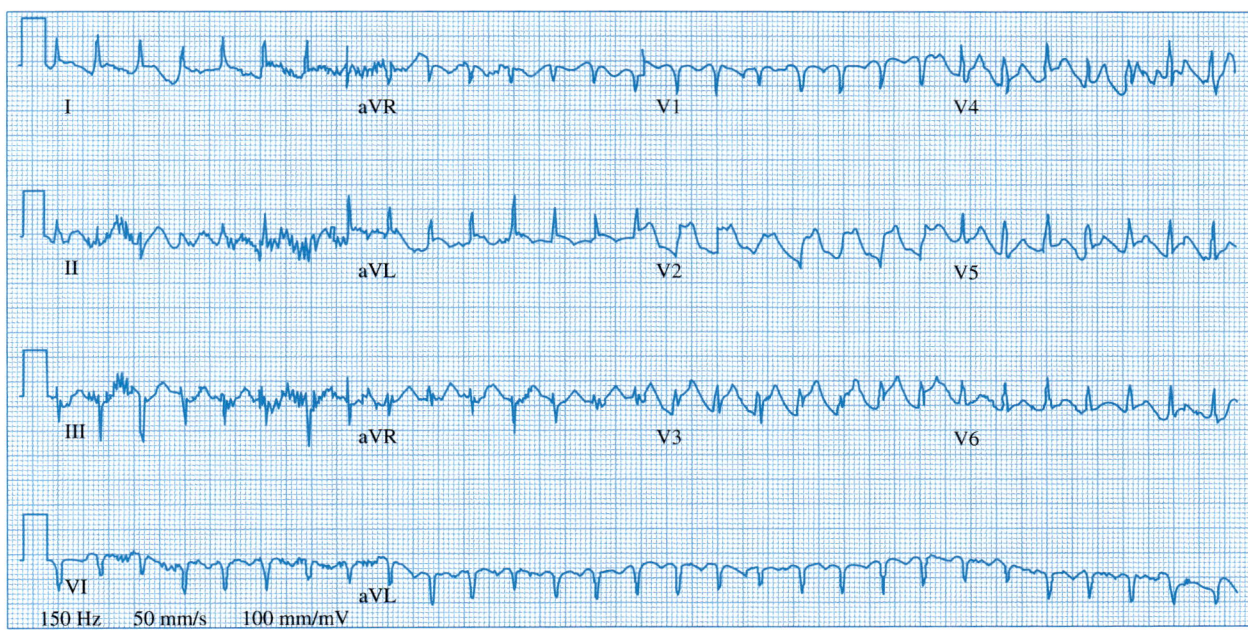

Figure 18-1 ECG 1 obtained at the time of presentation. ECG, electrocardiogram.

positioned endotracheal tube with focal areas of atelectasis or developing infiltrate in the perihilar region and left upper and left lower lung zones as well as perihilar vascular congestion.

Case Resolution

The patient received aspirin, β-blocker, and heparin and was taken emergently for coronary angiography, given the elevation of cardiac biomarkers and ST-segment elevations on her ECG. The patient had a left ventricular ejection fraction of 20% and had akinesis/ballooning of the apex of the left ventricle by left ventriculogram. However, angiography demonstrated no hemodynamically significant coronary artery disease. The patient was transferred to the cardiac intensive care unit for further management and started on a loop diuretic, angiotensin-converting enzyme (ACE) inhibitor, low-dose β-blocker, and continued on continuous heparin infusion overnight. Echocardiogram following cardiac catheterization is pictured below (Fig. 18-2) and demonstrates ballooning of the left ventricle at the apex, and sparing of the mid to basal septal, inferior and anterior left ventricular walls. Ejection fraction at that time was 35% to 40%. ECG 2 (Fig. 18-3) was obtained the morning following cardiac

catheterization and demonstrated normal sinus rhythm; left axis deviation; a slightly prolonged QT; inferior infarct pattern with abnormal Q waves in leads II, III, and aVF; and persistent ST-segment elevations in lateral and anterior leads. The patient was hospitalized for 5 days and was treated medically. She developed no complications during hospital admission and was discharged to home with follow-up to cardiology. Repeat echocardiogram 1 month after discharge revealed complete resolution of the left ventricular ballooning and wall motion

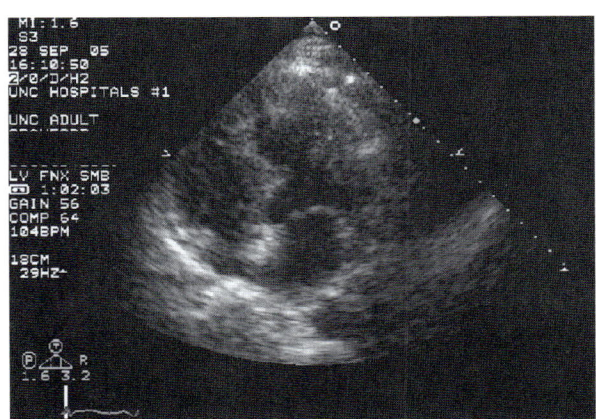

Figure 18-2 Echocardiogram from morning following presentation.

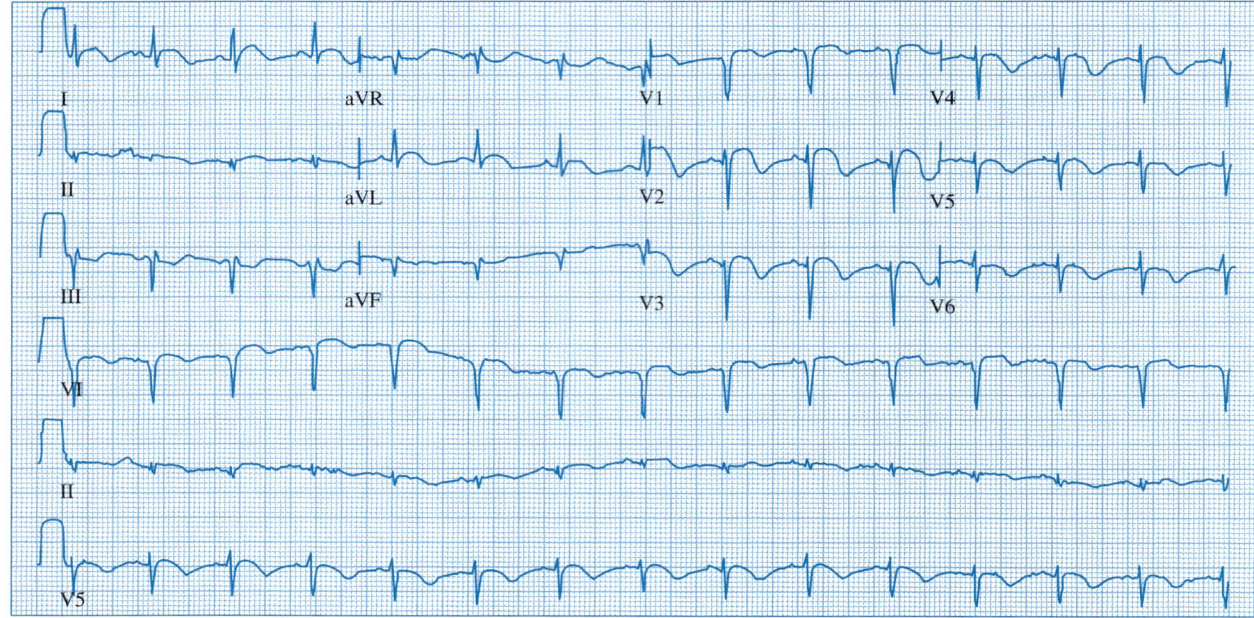

Figure 18-3 ECG 2 obtained morning following cardiac catheterization. ECG, electrocardiogram.

abnormality and the patient had a normal left ventricular ejection fraction.

Question

What can cause congestive heart failure without flow-limiting coronary artery disease?

Answer

There are many causes of congestive heart failure. In multiple, large cohort series, ischemic heart disease is the leading cause of heart failure accounting for 35% to 50% of cases of newly diagnosed heart failure. Hypertensive heart disease is usually the second most identifiable cause of heart failure followed by a wide variety of causes. A recent cohort study examined the etiology of heart failure in patients referred for evaluation after initially unexplained heart failure. In this cohort, the cause remained idiopathic in 50% of the patients (see Table 18-1). The pattern in the current patient of apical left ventricular dysfunction/ballooning without associated coronary artery atherosclerotic disease is characteristic of transient left ventricular apical ballooning, also known as stress-induced cardiomyopathy or Tako-Tsubo syndrome.

TABLE 18-1

Etiology of Heart Failure in a Cohort of Patients with Initially Unexplained Heart Failure Referred to Tertiary Care

Diagnosis	Prevalence (%)
Idiopathic	50
Myocarditis	9
Ischemic heart disease	7
Infiltrative myocardial disease	5
Peripartum cardiomyopathy	4
Cardiomyopathy caused by HIV	4
Cardiomyopathy caused by hypertension	4
Cardiomyopathy because of connective tissue disease	3
Cardiomyopathy owing to substance abuse (alcohol and cocaine)	3
Others	10

HIV, human immunodeficiency virus.

Discussion

This case, as with most cases of transient left ventricular apical ballooning (also known in the literature as Tako-Tsubo physiology or stress-induced cardiomyopathy), presented with symptoms consistent with an ST-segment elevation myocardial infarction. First recognized in the literature in 1991 with a series of case reports from Japan, the patients typically present after an emotional or physical stress-triggering event with symptoms such as chest pain, dyspnea, and ECG changes such as ST-segment elevations and T-wave inversions.[1] However, when coronary angiography is performed, there is no evidence of hemodynamically significant coronary atherosclerotic disease.

Many articles have addressed this new phenomenon since its recognition in the 1990s including reports from Japan, United States, and Europe. The clinical characteristics, prognosis, and treatment have been defined, but no etiology has been identified.

The clinical presentation classically associated with transient left ventricular apical ballooning includes onset of symptoms after an emotionally or physically stressful event such as the death of a spouse, bad financial news, or the exacerbation of a chronic disease such as an asthma.[2,3,4,5,6] In all case series, the condition afflicts women far more often than men. Symptoms at the time of onset include chest pain and dyspnea, but these are not universally present. The most common finding on ECG is ST-segment elevation which is typically present in the precordial leads. Many patients also have associated T-wave inversions present either at the time of presentation or at some point during hospitalization.[3,4,6] Cardiac biomarkers including CK, CK-MB specific to cardiac tissue, and troponin T or I often rise, but not to the degree observed in acute coronary syndrome (ACS). Additionally, in contrast to the slow rise and fall in cardiac biomarker levels recorded in ACS, the levels are often at their peak at the time of patient presentation.[3,4] As patients typically present with ECG changes mimicking ST-segment elevation myocardial infarction, they are taken for coronary angiography and presence of hemodynamically significant coronary artery atherosclerosis is excluded. Additionally, several studies have attempted to observe or induce coronary vasospasm during coronary angiography but have demonstrated that coronary vasospasm does not play a role in onset of symptoms.[2,5] Finally, cardiac imaging studies demonstrate left ventricular dilatation at the apex with associated akinesis and decreased left ventricular ejection fraction which do not correlate with a specific coronary artery territory.[5]

Disease prognosis is generally excellent. Complications include cardiogenic shock, left ventricular thrombus, and congestive heart failure. Other less commonly observed complications are arrhythmia (atrioventricular block, ventricular tachycardia or fibrillation, sinus bradycardia, paroxysmal atrial fibrillation), cerebral vascular accident, left ventricular rupture, and ventricular septal defect. Complications, however, are uncommon and patients generally return to cardiac function as prior to event within days to weeks,[3,4] with recurrence of disease being exceedingly rare.[3]

The etiology of transient left ventricular apical ballooning has been studied including the examination of myocardial biopsy, assessment of viral antibody titers at presentation and several weeks later, attempted induction of coronary vasospasm during a coronary angiogram, myocardial imaging to search for the presence of myocardial ischemia, and evaluation for the presence of pheochromocytomas or cardioexcitatory drugs such as cocaine.[2,3,6] None of these causes have been identified as the etiology of the disease. At this time, theories persist that catecholamine-mediated myocardial stunning may be the cause of pathology, as occurrence of the disease is frequently associated with emotionally or physically stressful events.[2,5,7] A recent study from United States measured plasma catecholamine levels in patients with transient left ventricular apical ballooning and compared them to patients diagnosed with Killip class III myocardial infarction. Plasma catecholamine levels among those patients with transient left ventricular apical ballooning were significantly increased compared to patients with myocardial infarction.[7] Further studies are needed to definitively identify a causal relationship.

Treatment of transient left ventricular apical ballooning includes ACE inhibition (afterload reduction/remodeling), diuretics, and beta-blockade (once euvolemically and hemodynamically stable). Intra-aortic balloon counterpulsation may be required in severe cases and is preferred over the use of pressors, given the implication of sympathetic hypersensitivity as demonstrated by elevated levels of plasma catecholamines.[7]

Patients do not require anticoagulation as with intracoronary thrombus unless left ventricular thrombus develops, caused by left ventricular wall motion abnormalities. Length of hospitalization is typically less than 1 week unless catastrophic complications occur. Patients generally return to their preadmission level of functioning rapidly.

Selected References

1. Dote K, Sato H, Tateishi H, et al. Myocardial stunning due to simultaneous multivessel coronary spasms: a review of 5 cases. *J Cardiol.* 1991;21(2):203–214.

2. Abe Y, Kondo M, Matsuoka R, et al. Assessment of clinical features in left ventricular apical ballooning. *J Am Coll Cardiol.* 2003;41(5):737–742.

3. Bybee K, Kara T, Prasad A, et al. Systematic review: transient left ventricular apical ballooning: a syndrome that mimics ST-segment elevation myocardial infarction. *Ann Int Med.* 2004;141(11):858–865.

4. Donahue D, Movahed M. Clinical characteristics, demographics and prognosis of transient left ventricular apical ballooning syndrome. *Heart Fail Rev.* 2005;10(4):311–316.

5. Skarkey S, Lesser J, Zenovich A, et al. Acute and reversible cardiomyopathy provoked by stress in women from the United States. *Circulation.* 2005;11(4):472–479.

6. Tsuchihashi K, Ueshima K, Uchida T, et al. Transient left ventricular apical ballooning without coronary artery stenosis: a novel heart syndrome mimicking acute myocardial infarction. *J Am Coll Cardiol.* 2001;38(1):11–18.

7. Wittstein I, Thiemann D, Lima J, et al. Neurohumoral features of myocardial stunning due to sudden emotional stress. *N Engl J Med.* 2005;352(6):539–548.

8. Felker GM, Thompson RE, Hare JM, et al. Underlying causes and long-term survival in patients with initially unexplained cardiomyopathy. *N Engl J Med.* 2000;342:1077–1084.

77-Year-Old Male with History of Nephrolithiasis, DVT, and Diverticulosis

CASE PRESENTATION

The patient is a 77-year-old man with past medical history of nephrolithiasis, deep vein thrombosis (DVT), and diverticulosis who presented to the Emergency Department (ED) of a large tertiary care medical center with well-localized, right-sided flank and leg pain of 4 days' duration. The pain was described as constant, dull, and aching in nature. The patient reported that at its most severe the pain was moderate, rated 4/10, but worsened with changes in position. The patient first noticed the discomfort after a long day of working on his tractor; he is the owner and manager of a 100-acre farm. He initially noticed mild pain in his right thigh on the evening of his tractor work. During the 24 hours prior to presentation, the pain worsened in severity and moved superiorly in location. He also reported improved symptoms with the application of a heating pad to the right leg. The patient denies cough, shortness of breath, and hemoptysis. The patient reports a distant history, greater than 30 years ago, of DVT secondary to an ipsilateral leg injury that occurred while he repaired irrigation pipes. The patient denies history of malignancy, coagulation disorder, surgery, and hip fracture.

Physical Examination

Patient was pleasant, in no distress, and appeared comfortable. Vital signs: temperature 37.6°C, blood pressure (BP) 142/69 mm Hg, pulse 83 beats/min, respiration rate (RR) 22 breaths/min; O_2 saturation 99% on room air (RA). Head, eyes, ears, nose, and throat (HEENT): atraumatic; normocephalic; pupils equal, round, reactive to light and accommodation (PEERLA); extraocular movement intact (EOMI). Neck: supple, no lymphadenopathy, no bruit, no jugular venous distension. Cardiovascular system (CVS): regular rate and rhythm (RRR); no murmurs, gallops, or rubs appreciated. S_1, S_2 normal. Chest: appears symmetric, nontender to palpation, breath sounds clear to auscultation bilaterally without wheezes rales or rhonchi. Abdomen: soft, nontender without organomegaly; normal active bowel sounds. Extremities: warm and well perfused; no edema, no erythema, no tenderness, no palpable cords; normal range of motion. The remainder of his examination was unremarkable.

Laboratory Studies

White blood cells (WBC) 10, hemoglobin/hematocrit (Hgb/Hct) 14/39, platelets (Plt) 198. Prothrombin time (PT) 12.1, international normalized ratio (INR) 1.1, partial prothrombin time (PTT) 36.5. Creatine kinase (CK) 90, creatine kinase-MB (CK-MB) 3.2, troponin (TRP) I <0.029. Aspartate aminotransferase (AST) 33, alanine aminotransferase (ALT) 43, total bilirubin (Tbilli) 0.7, alkaline phosphatase (AlkP) 56. Urine analysis: yellow, cloudy; specific gravity (SG) 1.025, leukocyte esterase (LE) negative. Nitrates: negative, red blood cells (RBC) <1, white blood cells (WBC) <1. Chest x-ray: no acute process, crisp borders of diaphragm and cardiac silhouette.

Peripheral vascular laboratory LE venous duplex scan:

Right leg: There is evidence of intraluminal obstruction in the femoral vein in the thigh. There are ultrasound (U/S) characteristics of an acute process. Intraluminal material appears to be poorly attached to the vessel wall.

Left leg: There is no evidence of deep venous obstruction.

Case Resolution

After the results of the lower extremity venous Doppler were positive for venous thrombus, the patient was immediately started on intravenous (IV) heparin and oral warfarin. Follow-up laboratory tests for congenital causes of hypercoagulable states were found to be negative.

Question

How long should a patient with recurrent DVT be on oral anticoagulation for the prevention of subsequent DVT/pulmonary embolism (PE)?

Answer

Current recommendations from the American College of Chest Physicians (ACCP) insist on a 3- to 6-month treatment for patients with initial presentation of idiopathic DVT. For recurrent DVT, however, oral anticoagulation should be extended indefinitely unless, of course, the patient acquires a contraindication for treatment (1).

Question

Are low-molecular-weight heparins contraindicated as DVT treatment in geriatric patients?

Answer

A randomized controlled trial with a study population of 100 consecutive patients with proximal deep vein thrombi ages greater than 75 years compared enoxaparin versus oral anticoagulation. This study found no statistically significant difference between rates of recurrent venous thromboembolism (VTE) major hemorrhage, and mortality (2).

Discussion

Lower extremity VTE is clinically classified according to the anatomic location of the vein in which they occur: either superficial or deep and either distal or proximal. Lower extremity veins that are both proximal to the knee and deep include the femoral, iliac, and popliteal veins. DVTs in these veins are of clinical importance because of their considerable risk of PE and subsequent death. Thrombi in veins that are either superficial or distal are of lesser clinical significance since they are associated with a much lower risk of embolization. Unless specified otherwise, in this discussion, DVT will refer to proximal deep vein thromboemboli.

In 1856, Virchow first identified three factors that predispose patients to the development of VTEs: venostasis, vascular injury, and hypercoagulability. Venostasis increases risk by slowing the clearance of clotting factors (3). Vascular injury deters the endothelial inhibition of coagulation and initiation of fibrinolysis. Hypercoagulability is secondary to factors that are either acquired or inherited. Acquired risk factors include age, trauma, neoplasm, pregnancy, estrogen use, and previous DVT. Inherited causes for a hypercoagulable state include factor V Leiden mutation, prothrombin gene mutation, antithrombin III deficiency, protein C deficiency, protein S deficiency, and antiphospholipid antibodies. The annual incidence of VTE is nearly 0.1%, and it increases with age to an annual rate of nearly 1% for patients older than 60 (4, 5).

The classic clinical presentation of DVT includes unilateral edema, warmth, erythema, tenderness, a palpable cord, superficial vein distention, limb cyanosis (*phlegmasia cerulea dolens*), or limb pallor (*phlegmasia alba dolens*). Calf pain is the most common complaint. A study comparing clinical evaluation versus objective testing for DVT found the sensitivities of pain, edema, and warmth to be 86%, 97%, and 72% respectively (6). It has been well-established that clinical findings of DVT are unreliable and cannot be depended upon for diagnoses. The majority of patients with findings that clinicians find suspicious do not actually have DVTs. Therefore, clinical suspicion should be followed with objective testing to confirm the diagnosis of DVT (7). Options for objective diagnosis include venous compression U/S, impendence plethysmography (IPG), and compression venography (CV). According to the American Thoracic Society, CV is the gold standard for DVT diagnosis and is both 100% sensitive and specific with a proficient technician (8). Venography, however, is invasive, expensive, requires IV contrast, and can be complicated by pain, phlebitis, and hypersensitivity reactions. Compression U/S is the method most commonly used in United States for the diagnosis of DVT. Duplex U/S combines Doppler flow detection and real-time sonography to provide information on both blood flow velocity and oxygen saturation. The sensitivity and specificity for U/S are both greater than 95%. This test is safe, noninvasive, inexpensive, portable, and has been studied extensively in clinical trials. IPG is another noninvasive diagnostic procedure used to diagnose DVTs. This procedure uses electrical impulses to detect resistance to venous flow and is more popular in European hospitals than in the United States.

Because of the risk of PE after DVT and low reliability of clinical suspicion alone to diagnose and risk stratify DVT, clinical prediction guidelines have been developed and validated by systematic review. One such group, the Wells criteria, was developed by P.S. Wells and others at the University of Ottawa and first described in *Lancet* 1995 as a means to estimate pretest probability and stratify for diagnostic testing and management (9). The criteria use patient medical history (cancer, immobilization, previous DVT), physical examination (edema, tenderness), and clinician impression of alternate diagnoses to classify patients as high, moderate, or low pretest probability (see Table 19-1) and recommend management accordingly (10). The original Wells criteria recommended a single negative U/S for patients with low probability was sufficient to rule out DVT (11). However, moderate- and high-risk patients with normal U/S were recommended follow-up U/S and CV respectively. The most recent recommendations for use of Wells criteria, a compilation of multiple studies published in the *Journal of American Medical Association* 2006, established that low pretest probability combined with a negative serum D-dimer has 95% sensitivity and is sufficient to rule out DVT without U/S (12).

Initial treatment should begin immediately after objective identification of a proximal vein clot. Less than 25% of untreated calf VTEs will eventually extend into proximal veins and this typically occurs within a week of diagnosis (13). If the thrombus is distal, immediate therapy is not necessary; still a follow-up study in 1 week is indicated to ensure the distal clot has not propagated to involve a deep proximal vein. The goal of DVT treatment is the prevention of PE by stabilizing the thrombus. Anticoagulation prevents extension of the clot and promotes thrombolysis. Options for initial therapy include IV unfractionated heparin versus subcutaneous low-molecular-weight heparin (UFH vs. LMWH). UFH is administered via an IV bolus and subsequently set at an infusion rate to maintain an activated partial thromboplastin time (aPTT) that is two times the control value. LMWH, formed by depolymerization of UFH, has been proven in multiple

TABLE 19-1

Wells Criteria Clinical Characteristics

Active cancer (treatment ongoing or within 6 months or palliative)	+1
Paralysis, paresis, or recent plaster immobilization of lower extremity	+1
Recently bedridden for >3 days or major surgery within 4 wks	+1
Localized tenderness along the distribution of the deep venous system	+1
Entire leg swelling	+1
Calf swelling by >3 cm when compared to the asymptomatic leg	+1
Pitting edema (greater in the symptomatic leg)	+1
Previous DVT documented	+1
Collateral superficial veins (nonvaricose)	+1
Alternative diagnosis (as likely or > that of DVT)	−2

In patients with symptoms in both legs, use the more symptomatic leg.

Sum Pretest Probability Score

High probability: ≥3 (85% prevalence of DVT)

Moderate probability: 1 or 2 (33% prevalence of DVT)

Low probability: ≤0 (5% prevalence of DVT)

Adapted from Anand SS, Wells PS, Hunt D, et al. Does this patient have deep vein thrombosis? JAMA. 1998;279(14): 1094–1099. Wells PS, Owen C, Doucette S, et al. Does this patient have deep vein thrombosis? JAMA. 2006;295(2): 199–207.

DVT, deep vein thrombosis.

trials to be as safe and efficacious and cost effective as UFH, since it can be administered in fixed doses, does not require laboratory monitoring, and allows outpatient management for stable patients. Oral anticoagulation with warfarin or subcutaneous LMWH is considered an acceptable long-term management of proximal DVT; however, warfarin remains standard therapy (3). If warfarin is chosen, it should be started as soon as possible and should overlap with initial therapy (UFH or LMWH) for 5 days to ensure that the patient's INR is therapeutic (range 2.0–3.0). For patients with a first occurrence of idiopathic DVT, anticoagulation should continue for at least 3 months, beyond which continuing anticoagulation should be balanced with risk of bleeding. If a patient has known recurrence of DVT, then anticoagulation should continue indefinitely.

For patients who have a contraindication to anticoagulation or who have failed therapy with recurrence while anticoagulated, an inferior vena cava filter should be placed.

Selected References

1. Geerts WH, Pineo GF, Heit JA, et al. Prevention of venous thromboembolism: the Seventh ACCP Conference on Antithrombotic and Thrombolytic Therapy. *Chest.* 2004;126:(suppl 3) 338S–400S.
2. Veiga F, Escriba A, Maluenda MP, et al. Low molecular weight heparin (enoxaparin) versus oral anticoagulant therapy (acenocoumarol) in the long-term treatment of deep venous thrombosis in the elderly: a randomized trial. *J Thromb Haemost.* 2000;84(4):559–564.
3. Bates SM, Ginsberg JS. Clinical practice: treatment of deep-vein thrombosis. *N Engl J Med.* 2004;351(3):268–277.
4. Nordstrom M, Lindblad B, Bergqvist D, et al. A prospective study of the incidence of deep-vein thrombosis within a defined urban population. *J Intern Med.* 1992;232(2):155–160.
5. Silverstein MD, Heit JA, Mohr DN, et al. Trends in the incidence of deep vein thrombosis and pulmonary embolism: a 25-year population-based study. *Arch Intern Med.* 1998;158(6):585–593.
6. Sandler DA, Martin JF, Duncan JS, et al. Diagnosis of deep-vein thrombosis: comparison of clinical evaluation, ultrasound, plethysmography, and venoscan with x-ray venogram. *Lancet.* 1984;2(8405):716–719.
7. Creager MA, Dzau VJ. Vascular diseases of the extremities. In: DL Kasper, et al, eds. *Harrison's Principles of Internal Medicine.* 16th ed. New York, NY: McGraw-Hill; 2005:1486–1494, Vol. 2.
8. Tapson VF, Carroll BA, Davidson BL, et al. The diagnostic approach to acute venous thromboembolism: clinical practice guideline: American Thoracic Society. *Am J Respir Crit Care Med.* 1999;160(3):1043–1066.
9. Wells PS, Hirsh J, Anderson DR, et al. Accuracy of clinical assessment of deep-vein thrombosis. *Lancet.* 1995;345(8961):1326–1330.
10. Anand SS, Wells PS, Hunt D, et al. Does this patient have deep vein thrombosis? *JAMA.* 1998;279(14):1094–1099.
11. Wells PS, Anderson DR, Bormanis J, et al. Value of assessment of pretest probability of deep-vein thrombosis in clinical management. *Lancet.* 1997;350(9094):1795–1798.
12. Wells PS, Owen C, Doucette S, et al. Does this patient have deep vein thrombosis? *JAMA.* 2006;295(2):199–207.
13. Lagerstedt CI, Olsson CG, Fagher BO, et al. Need for long-term anticoagulant treatment in symptomatic calf-vein thrombosis. *Lancet.* 1985;2(8454):515–518.

4-Year-Old Male with History of Sickle Cell Disease

CASE DESCRIPTION

A 4-year-old African American male with a history of sickle cell disease presented with a 3-day history of fever and cough. The patient's father also reports that for the past 2 days his son has had difficulty speaking and has been acting very "lethargic." The child initially presented to an outside emergency department, where he was reported to be unresponsive to voice, somnolent, and unable to use the right side of his body. He was fluid resuscitated at the outside facility and sent for admission to the pediatric intensive care unit. No other past medical, social, or family history is available.

Physical Examination

The patient was somnolent, responsive only to pain, and tachypneic with shallow breaths. Vital signs: temperature 36.1°C, pulse 140 beats/min, blood pressure 88/50 mm Hg, respiratory rate 45 breaths/min. Oxygen saturation of 100% on 100% O_2 via a non–rebreather face mask. The patient was in moderate respiratory distress with bilateral retractions and nasal flaring. His lung fields were clear except for crackles diffusely throughout the right lung fields. His cardiovascular examination revealed tachycardia and a grade 2/6 systolic ejection murmur heard best at the left sternal border. His abdominal examination revealed hepatomegaly to the level of the umbilicus, and a nonpalpable spleen. He did not move his extremities on his right side. The remainder of his physical examination was normal.

Laboratory Studies

A summary of the patient's laboratory studies include a complete blood count with white blood cells 4.8 with an absolute neutrophil count of 3.2, hemoglobin 4.1, and platelets 386. Reticulocyte count was 9.1%. Approximately 80% of the child's hemoglobin was of the sickled type. Arterial blood gas (ABG) was consistent with impending respiratory failure. Chemistries included Na 144, K 4.3, Cl 114, HCO_3 19, blood urea nitrogen 66, and creatinine 1.7. Serum transaminases included aspartate aminotransferase 68 and alanine aminotransferase 28. Blood, urine, and bronchial lavage cultures were drawn. Chest x-ray (CXR) is shown below in Fig. 20-1. Brain magnetic resonance image (MRI) is also shown below in Fig. 20-2.

Case Resolution

The patient was intubated immediately upon arrival both to protect his airway and support his impending hypoxemic respiratory failure. He was treated for acute chest syndrome with oxygen and empiric antibiotics. A large pleural effusion was drained via a chest tube. He underwent emergent exchange transfusion as well on the day of admission as treatment for his apparent cerebrovascular accident (CVA). Blood and pleural fluid cultures ultimately revealed *Streptococcus pneumoniae* as the causative organism for sepsis and antibiotics were tailored accordingly. The child eventually recovered almost full function of the right side of his body with preservation of his cognitive activity as well.

Question

Besides pain crisis, what potential life-threatening emergencies are faced by those with sickle cell disease?

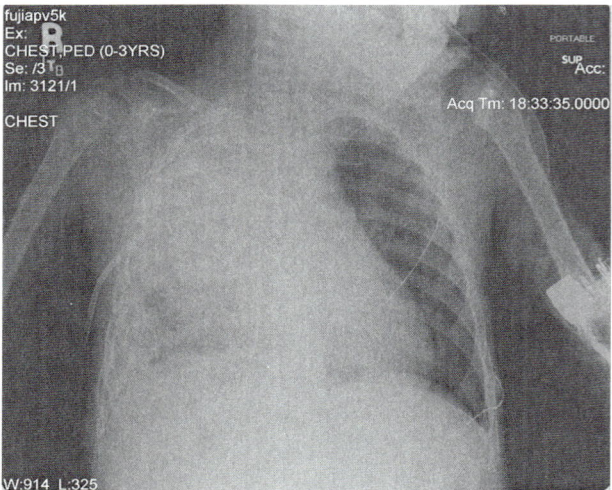

Figure 20-1 PA and lateral radiographs of the chest showing acute chest syndrome. Notice the left lower lobe infiltrate. PA, posteroanterior.

Answer

Life-threatening emergencies in patients with sickle cell disease include acute chest syndrome, CVAs/transient ischemic attack (TIA), fulminant bacterial sepsis, aplastic crisis, myocardial infarction, and splenic sequestration. Prompt recognition of these clinical entities should lead to appropriate and often time lifesaving therapy.

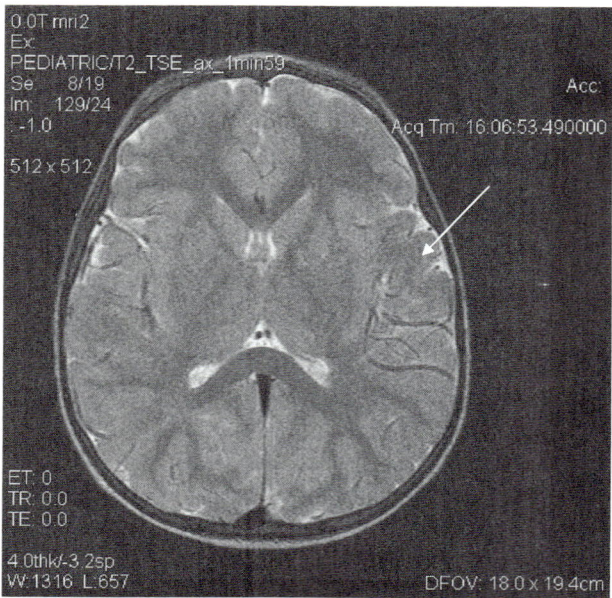

Figure 20-2 T2-weighted axial image demonstrating watershed hypoperfusion and prominent collateral circulation (arrow).

Discussion

Sickle cell anemia is an autosomal recessive disorder that results when a single base substitution in the beta-globin gene chain results in a valine being substituted for glutamine on the sixth amino acid position. It has been recognized as a disease state for centuries in areas of the world where malaria is endemic. Individuals who are heterozygotes (sickle cell trait) for the disease are at a selective advantage owing to increased resistance to infection from *Plasmodium falciparum*, the causative agent in malaria. It occurs mainly in individuals of sub-Saharan African descent for this reason, and also in individuals of Mediterranean, Hispanic, and Indian descent. In fact, sickle cell anemia is the most common autosomal recessive disorder in African Americans, with an incidence of 1 in 625 live births.

In individuals affected with sickle cell disease, hemoglobin forms highly ordered polymers under conditions of hypoxia that causes the red cells to distort into a rigid, crystal-like rod, the so-called "sickled" cell. Because of the distortion of the shape of the pathologic cells, erythrocytes in patient with sickle cell disease have a shorter life span, resulting in a chronic hemolytic anemia. These inflexible and brittle red cells also occlude the microvasculature which slows blood flow and results in further hypoxia as well as tissue ischemia and infarction with distinct sequelae in various organs, such as the CVA seen in the patient described above.

Early identification after birth of individuals with sickle cell anemia has been shown to significantly decrease morbidity and mortality with timely institution of comprehensive medical care. Thus, screening programs for sickle cell disease have been mandated for infants born in the United States. In newborns with the disease, quantitative hemoglobin electrophoresis reveals predominantly fetal hemoglobin (Hb F) with a small amount of sickle hemoglobin (Hb S) and no normal hemoglobin (Hb A). Other hemoglobinopathies are also routinely diagnosed via this method (Table 20-1).

Individuals with sickle cell disease rarely exhibit symptoms in the first few months of life. Anemia and other manifestations result when fetal hemoglobin is replaced with Hb S at 4 to 6 months of age. Common manifestations of anemia in infancy can include pallor, jaundice, splenomegaly, and a systolic ejection murmur.

The hallmark of sickle cell disease is severe acute pain episodes, which represent the most common reason for hospitalization for individuals with this disease. Vaso-occlusion

TABLE 20-1

Electrophoretic Patterns in Common Hemoglobinopathies

Condition	Hgb A	Hgb S	Hgb C	Hgb F	Hgb A2
Normal	95–98*	0	0	<1	<3.5
Beta-thalassemia minor	90–95	0	0	1–3	>3.5
Sickle cell trait	50–60	35–45†	0	<2	<3.5
Sickle-beta (+) thalassemia	5–30	65–90	0	2–10	>3.5
Sickle-beta (0) thalassemia	0	80–92	0	2–15	>3.5
Sickle-Hgb C disease	0	45–50	45–50	1–8	<3.5
Homozygous sickle cell disease	0	85–95	0	2–15	<3.5

Hgb, hemoglobin.

*Numbers indicate the percent of total hemoglobin for an untransfused adult patient. Ranges are approximate and may vary depending upon the particular laboratory and method of determination.

†Percent Hgb S can be as low as 21% in patients with sickle cell trait in conjunction with alpha-thalassemia.

within the bone marrow vasculature leads to bone infarction and release of inflammatory mediators that cause pain. Though not fatal themselves, repeated hospitalizations for acute pain episodes are associated with a higher mortality. Morbidity is high, however, in that episodes are unpredictable and greatly affect an individual's ability to function. Acute pain often occurs spontaneously, but can occur after infection, dehydration, stress, fatigue, menstruation, changes in temperature, or exposure to high altitudes. The pain is often described as "bone pain," and commonly involves the lower back, chest, femoral shafts and hip joints, ribs, knees, abdomen, and head. Pain tends to recur in a limited number of sites in individual patients. In infants, pain episodes often involve the hands, feet, fingers, and toes. This discrete entity is referred to as dactylitis, and is often the first clinical manifestation in an infant with sickle cell disease. Priapism is another discrete painful episode of prolonged erection that occurs in boys between 5 and 13 years of age and is caused by sickling in the sinusoids of the penis. It can result in loss of sexual function. The management of acute pain crises includes outpatient therapy with oral pain medications, and failing that, inpatient therapy with parenteral analgesics and other adjuvants such as oxygen and antibiotics, if indicated.

Among those more life-threatening clinical entities that affect patients with sickle cell disease, acute chest syndrome is the second most common cause of hospitalization in children with sickle cell disease and the leading cause of death. The etiology of acute chest syndrome is unknown, but recent clinical studies reveal that infectious agents, such as *Chlamydia pneumoniae, Mycoplasma pneumoniae, Staphylococcus aureus,* and *S. pneumoniae,* as well as pulmonary fat emboli are causative in the majority of cases. Symptoms at presentation are age dependent, but in young children include wheezing, cough, and fever. Fever, new pulmonary infiltrate on chest radiograph (Fig. 20-1), as well as hypoxemia must be present to make the diagnosis. The cornerstone of treatment for acute chest syndrome includes administration of oxygen, respiratory therapy in the form of nebulized albuterol, and administration of empiric antibiotics. Blood transfusion or exchange transfusion is indicated for progressive hypoxemia, respiratory failure, and worsening anemia.

Acute splenic sequestration is unique to young children with sickle cell anemia. Because of occlusion of splenic blood vessels, large amounts of blood pools in the spleen acutely which may lead to hypovolemic shock and subsequent death. Large studies support a fatality rate of approximately 10% after the first event. Symptoms include splenic enlargement, an acute drop in the child's hemoglobin, and subsequent shock. The mainstay of treatment is blood transfusion. Survivors face a recurrence risk of approximately 50%, and mortality increases to 20% with the second episode. Experts recommend splenectomy after the first episode of acute splenic sequestration crisis for this reason. Prevention of this potentially fatal event is also undertaken with parent education in the examination of their child's spleen and instruction to seek medical attention promptly if splenic enlargement develops.

Individuals with sickle cell anemia develop functional asplenia over time as a consequence of sickling, infarction, and consequent fibrosis within the spleen. This process, known as autoinfarction, is the reason that 95% of children have a nonpalpable spleen by the age of 5. Autoinfarction is also responsible for placing the child with sickle cell disease at a higher risk for overwhelming sepsis since the spleen can no longer effectively filter encapsulated bacteria such as *S. pneumoniae*. For this reason, fever in a child with sickle cell anemia represents a clinical emergency. Approximately one-quarter of children with sickle cell disease who develop bacteremia will die if not properly treated. Thus, management of fever in these children involves administration of empiric antibiotics until blood culture results are confirmed negative. Administration of daily oral penicillin for prophylaxis starting at the age of 2 months until the child reaches at least 3 years of age; transition to twice weekly penicillin until age 5 has been shown in several landmark studies to greatly decrease the incidence of bacteremia with *S. pneumoniae*. Administration of routine childhood vaccinations, including those against *S. pneumoniae* and *Haemophilus influenzae* type B, hepatitis B, and influenza virus, is also essential in minimizing a child's risk of infection.

Children with sickle cell disease are at risk for stroke secondary to occlusion of large cerebral vessels. Just as in the patient in the case, children present with mental status changes, seizures, and/or focal paresis or paralysis. Management is exchange transfusion, subsequent rehabilitation, and chronic transfusion therapy in order to prevent recurrent stroke. Children at high risk for stroke identified with routine transcranial Doppler study are also placed on chronic transfusion therapy in order to prevent stroke and its subsequent cognitive and physical deficits.

In conclusion, sickle cell anemia is a disease with significant morbidity and sometimes mortality in affected children. A comprehensive approach to therapy must include early diagnosis, parental and patient education, preventative care including complete vaccination, antibiotic prophylaxis, and careful medical attention when emergencies arise.

Selected References

Dees D. Guidelines for the management of the acute painful crisis in sickle cell disease. *Br J Hematol*. 2003;120:744–752.

Gill FM, Sleeper LA, Weiner SJ, et al. Clinical events in the first decade in a cohort of infants with sickle cell disease. *Blood*. 1995;86(2):776–783.

Powell RW, Levine GL, Yang Y, et al. Acute splenic sequestration crisis in sickle cell disease: early detection and treatment. *J Pediatr Surg*. 1992;27(2):215–219.

Quinn K, Vichinsky E. In: *Nelson Textbook of Pediatrics*. 17th ed. Philadelphia, PA: Saunders; 2003. Chapter 454.

Shafer FE, Lorey F, Cunningham GC, et al. Newborn screening for sickle cell disease: 4 years of experience from California's newborn screening. *J Pediatr Hematol Oncol*. 1996;18(1):36–41.

Vichinsky EP, Neumayr LD, Earles AN, et al. Causes and outcomes of the acute chest syndrome in sickle cell disease. *NEJM*. 2003;342(25):1855–1865.

Vichinsky EP, Styles LA, Colangelo LH, et al. Acute chest syndrome in sickle cell disease: clinical presentation and course. *Blood*. 1997;89(5):1787–1792.

West DC, Andrada E, Azari R, et al. Predictors of bacteremia in febrile children with sickle cell disease. *J Pediatr Hematol Oncol*. 2002;24(4):279–283.

Yaster M, Kost-Byerley S, Maxwell LG. The management of pain in sickle cell disease. *Pediatr Clin North Am*. 2000;47(3):699–710.

1-Year-Old Female with Lymphadenopathy and Fever

CASE PRESENTATION

A 1-year-old female presented to the pediatric emergency department for evaluation of a "lump" on her neck. Her parents first noticed a grape-sized mass 3 days prior to presentation. She had been seen as an outpatient and was being treated with oral antibiotics. The lump continued to grow, exceeding the size of a golf ball. She developed fever to 103°C, was increasingly fussy, and had a poor appetite. She had no upper respiratory infection (URI) symptoms and her review of systems was otherwise negative. She had never traveled out of United States, had never had contact with any travelers or incarcerated persons, and did not attend day care. There were no pets at home.

Physical Examination

She was febrile to 38.7°C. Respiratory rate was 28 beats/min. Her pulse was 118 beats/min. The examination was remarkable for dry mucous membranes; mild tachycardia; and a large, well-demarcated mass on the left anterior neck. The mass was firm and very tender to palpation with no obvious fluctuance. There was no lymphadenopathy in the axillary or inguinal areas. The remainder of the physical examination was unremarkable.

Laboratory Studies

A complete blood count (CBC) was obtained, with white blood cell (WBC) count of 21.6, an absolute neutrophil count of 14.7, and a 2+ left shift. C-reactive protein was elevated at 8.6. Platelets were slightly elevated at 493. The remainder of the CBC and peripheral smear were unremarkable. A computed tomography (CT) scan of the neck demonstrated a single 4 cm × 3 cm mass in the left anterior cervical region with a central area of enhancement (see Fig. 21-1). Magnetic resonance imaging (MRI) was performed the following day to further characterize the mass (see Fig. 21-2).

Question

What is the most likely etiology of this neck mass?

Answer

The differential diagnosis of a neck mass in a child is broad. Malignant conditions such as lymphoma, sarcoma, and histiocytosis may present as unilateral neck masses possibly with fevers, as seen in this case. Congenital causes such as branchial cleft cysts or thyroglossal duct cysts will present in a similar location as the patient in this case. Given the leukocytosis, fever, and appearance on imaging, cervical lymphadenitis is most likely.

Discussion

Cervical lymphadenitis is a common pediatric illness, most often seen in children between 1 and 6 years of age. It is caused by acute or chronic inflammation of a cervical lymph node (not to be confused with lymphadenopathy, a reactive process of the lymph node). The epidemiology varies by the child's age, geographic location,

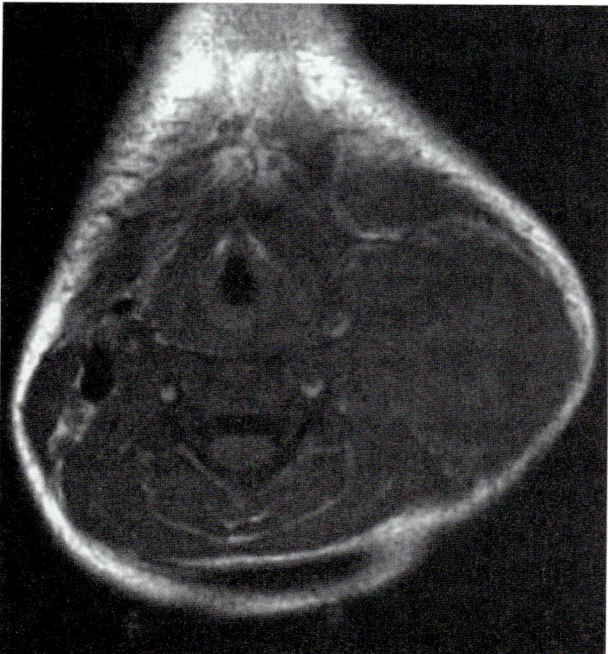

Figure 21-1 CT demonstrated 4 cm × 3 cm mass in the anterior cervical region with questionable ring enhancement in the center of the mass.
CT, computed tomography.

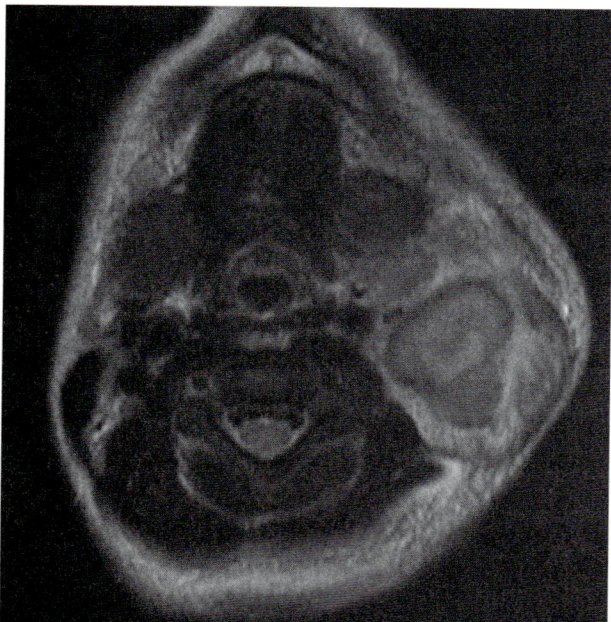

Figure 21-2 MRI demonstrating a poorly marginated mass with diffuse stranding of the subcutaneous fat and several areas of centrally located low density suggesting necrosis. The mass enhances strongly with gadolinium.
MRI, magnetic resonance imaging.

and socioeconomic status; these are all markers for infectious exposure. The history frequently reveals a preceding upper respiratory infection, sore throat, or earache. Cervical lymphadenitis most commonly occurs in submandibular nodes, followed by upper cervical nodes, submental notes, occipital nodes, and lower cervical nodes. Infected cervical nodes are usually between 1 and 6 cm in diameter, and approximately one-quarter to one-third become fluctuant.

Surgical intervention is required when abscess formation occurs. The rate of suppuration requiring drainage in children with lymphadenitis varies greatly in the literature, depending on the inclusion criteria of the study. A retrospective cohort study involving all inpatients at a pediatric tertiary care hospital examined the factors predictive of surgical drainage and reported a 21% rate of surgical intervention. Their findings also suggest that surgical intervention was more likely in children who were symptomatic more than 48 hours prior to admission and who were under a year of age.

Staphylococcus aureus and *Streptococcus pyogenes* are the causative agents in 65% to 89% of cases of acute cervical lymphadenitis across multiple studies. In neonates, the most common organisms responsible for acute cervical lymphadenitis are group B streptococcus and *S. aureus.* Chronic and subchronic cervical lymphadenitis is more frequently caused by *Bartonella henselae*, mycobacteria, or toxoplasmosis. Atypical mycobacteria can be the cause of cervical lymphadenitis without the classic mycobacterial tuberculosis risk factors. Therapy for lymphadenitis caused by mycobacterial disease often involves excisional biopsy. Placement of skin test for mycobacteria is often advocated at the time of initiation of antibiotics in the setting of lymphadenitis. A plethora of organisms is responsible for the remainder of cases (see Table 21-1). A careful history and physical examination provides clues to identifying atypical organisms. Periodontal disease may contribute to infection with anaerobic organisms, a tick bite could suggest tularemia, and a pustular lesion may be the visible evidence of an inoculation site for *Nocardia asteroides,* actinomycosis, sporotrichosis, plague, or cutaneous diphtheria. A scratch from a kitten is the classic history for *B. henselae.* Hepatomegaly, splenomegaly, and diffuse lymphadenopathy should prompt consideration of a generalized process or systemic illness. Physical location of the mass also helps to narrow the differential diagnosis, as common congenital masses have characteristic locations. Midline congenital masses include thyroglossal duct cysts, epidermoid

TABLE 21-1

Causes of Pediatric Lymphadenitis

Infectious causes	
Bacteria	**Viruses**
Staphylococcus aureus	Cytomegalovirus
Streptococcus pyogenes (group A)	Ebstein-Barr
Streptococcus agalactiae (group B)	Herpes simplex
Bacillus anthracis	Human herpesvirus 6
Corynebacterium diphtheriae	Varicella-zoster
Bartonella henselae	Adenovirus
Haemophilus influenzae	Human immunodeficiency virus
Serratia marcescens	Influenza
Acinetobacter species	Measles
Escherichia coli	Mumps
Proteus species	Parainfluenza
Pseudomonas aeruginosa	Respiratory syncytial virus
Salmonella typhi	Rubella
Shigella species	Coxsackieviruses
Brucella species	Rhinoviruses
Francisella tularensis	
Yersinia pestis	
Yersinia enterocolitica	
Yersinia pseudotuberculosis	Mycobacteria and actinomycetes
	Actinomyces israelii
Anaerobic organisms	Mycobacterium tuberculosis
(Peptostreptococcus species, Bacteroides species)	Mycobacterium avium-intracellulare
	Mycobacterium scrofulaceum
	Nocardia asteroides
Noninfectious causes	
Neoplasia	Histiocytosis
Collagen vascular disease (lupus, JRA)	Sarcoidosis
Kawasaki disease	Kikuchi disease
Immunologic deficiencies (chronic granulomatous disease, hyper-IgE syndrome, leukocyte adhesion deficiency)	

Adapted from Peters TR, Edwards KM. Cervical lymphadenopathy and adenitis. Pediatr Rev. 2000 Dec;21(12):399–405.
IgE, immunoglobulin E; JRA, juvenile rheumatoid arthritis.

cysts, lipomas, and thyroid tumors. Rarely, a lymph node may be found in the midline. Branchial cleft cysts are located on the anterior border of the sternocleidomastoid. Cystic hygromas may be found posterior to the sternocleidomastoid. Malignancies are most likely to be found posterior to the sternocleidomastoid or both anterior and posterior. The exception to this is the rare midline thyroid tumor.

Although serious sequelae of cervical adenitis (jugular vein thrombosis, septic emboli, mediastinal abscess, pericarditis) have been described in the literature, they are exceedingly rare and most children recover without complication. Since this child failed outpatient therapy, she was admitted to the pediatric inpatient unit and started on intravenous Unasyn. She had no clinical response after 24 hours, so vancomycin was added. The initial CT was suggestive of lymphadenitis, but rhabdomyosarcoma could not be excluded. To further confirm the diagnosis, an MRI was performed and the child also underwent a needle aspiration. Needle aspiration confirmed the MRI impression of cervical lymphadenitis. She improved rapidly on vancomycin, with normalization of her WBC by hospital day 5. She was discharged home on oral clindamycin and had complete resolution of her mass.

Selected References

Feigen RD, Cherry JD, eds. *Textbook of Pediatric Infectious Diseases.* 3rd ed. Philadelphia, PA: WB Saunders; 1992.

Luu TM, Chevalier I, Gauthier M, et al. Acute adenitis in children: clinical course and factors predictive of surgical drainage. *J Paediatr Child Health.* 2005;41:273–277.

Martinez-Aguilar G, Hammerman WA, Mason EO Jr, et al. Clindamycin treatment of invasive infections caused by community-acquired, methicillin-resistant and methicillin-susceptible *Staphylococcus aureus* in children. *Pediatr Infect Dis J.* 2003 Jul;22(7):593–598.

Peters TR, Edwards KM. Cervical lymphadenopathy and adenitis. *Pediatr Rev.* 2000 Dec;21(12):399–405.

31-Year-Old Female with Pica, Alopecia, and Hirsutism

CASE PRESENTATION

A 31-year-old female presented to urgent care with a complaint of ongoing hair loss from the top of her head and at her temples as well as worsening fatigue. She stated that she had infrequent (6–7/year) but very heavy periods lasting at least 7 days in duration. These had worsened over the prior 2 years as she continued to gain weight. She noted an increase in body hair, especially on the chest and face, though states that as long as she can remember it has "just kept on growing." Review of systems was positive for pica, with ice eating. The patient furthermore revealed recent polydipsia, polyphagia, and polyuria. She had previously been diagnosed with iron deficiency anemia but did not take her iron because of constipation. Other past medical history included hypertension that was untreated.

Physical Examination

The patient was a well-appearing, obese African American female, in no distress. Blood pressure was 155/92 mm Hg, pulse 95 beats/min, respiratory rate 18 beats/min, weight 203 lb, height 5 ft 6 in. The patient had pale mucus membranes of the mouth and conjunctival pallor. There was thinning of the hair of both temples and at the top of her head. Terminal hair development was seen at the upper lip, chin, and sideburns. The patient's abdomen was obese, but soft and nontender with normal bowel sounds. Dark hair was seen in the periumbilical area and along the linea alba. Pelvic examination was negative for masses, and there was no cervical or adnexal tenderness. The remainder of the examination was unremarkable.

Laboratory Studies

A complete blood count revealed white blood cells 9.1, hematocrit 26.1, mean corpuscular volume 59, platelets 316, iron 9 mg/dL, transferrin 329 mg/dL, percent saturation 2, ferritin 4 mg/mL. Thyroid-stimulating hormone (TSH) 2.12, hemoglobin A1c 7.8%. Chemistries all within normal limits with the exception of a fasting blood sugar of 130. Urine pregnancy test is negative.

Case Resolution

The patient was started on oral iron replacement therapy with subsequent improvement in her hematocrit as well as iron indices. She had improved energy. Given her elevated fasting glucose and hemoglobin A1c as well as characteristic symptoms, she was given a diagnosis of diabetes and started on metformin. After initiating this medication, she lost 15 lb. She felt some improvement in her menorrhagia, and a decrease in facial hair growth. Subsequent hemoglobin A1c was 5.2. She still continued to have menstrual irregularity, however, and was started on a combined estrogen/progestin oral contraceptive. Serum prolactin and insulin-like growth factor-1 (IGF-1) levels were within normal limits. The 24-hour urine examination for free cortisol was within normal limits.

Question

The constellation of signs and symptoms seen in this patient are likely representative of which clinical syndrome?

Answer

This patient presented with menstrual irregularity, alopecia, hirsutism, obesity, and diabetes. This aggregation of findings is characteristic of polycystic ovarian syndrome (PCOS).

Discussion

PCOS is comprised of an array of signs and symptoms that may vary or evolve over time. An important point is that it is a syndrome, a phenotype with significant heterogeneity of presentation. Diagnosis is based on the presence of menstrual irregularity and signs of androgen excess. PCOS is one of the most common endocrinopathies in women, with several studies suggesting a prevalence of 4.7% to 8.0%. When clinical manifestations are overt and fully expressed, this syndrome is easily identified. More often than not, however, the presentation of PCOS is more subtle and the diagnosis more challenging.

Though controversy persists regarding the diagnosis of PCOS, the National Institutes of Health (NIH) criteria remains the most utilized guideline. According to the NIH consensus, PCOS is diagnosed when there is each of the following:

- Menstrual irregularity because of oligo- or anovulation
- Evidence of hyperandrogenism, either clinical or biochemical
- Exclusion of other causes of hyperandrogenism and menstrual irregularity

It should be noted that documentation of polycystic ovaries by imaging is not included in these criteria. A more recent diagnostic tool (the Rotterdam criteria) does consider ultrasonographic evidence of polycystic ovaries in identification of the syndrome. Ultrasonographic criteria include the finding of at least 12 small (2–9 mm) follicles in each ovary and/or increased ovarian volume of greater than 10 mL. A transvaginal approach should be used when imaging the ovaries. These findings are fairly sensitive and specific for polycystic ovaries, but often loosely interpreted, and therefore, in the opinion of some experts, too difficult to apply diagnostically. In addition, the Rotterdam criteria only stipulate that either menstrual irregularity or evidence of hyperandrogenism be present when polycystic ovaries are documented. This would apply the diagnosis of PCOS to a broader segment of the population as compared with the NIH criteria, and the validity of this diagnostic labeling remains in some question.

The Rotterdam criteria are summarized as follows and require two out of three plus the exclusion of other etiologies:

- Oligo- and/or anovulation
- Clinical and/or biochemical signs of hyperandrogenism
- Polycystic ovaries
- Exclusion of other etiologies (congenital adrenal hyperplasia [CAH], androgen-secreting tumors, Cushing syndrome)

PCOS is a complex disorder of apparent polygenic etiology. The pathogenesis is complex and not fully understood; however, there appears to be intrinsic abnormality in the hypothalamic–pituitary–ovarian axis. Affected women appear to have an increased luteinizing hormone (LH) pulse frequency, most likely because of both accelerated hypothalamic gonadotropin-releasing hormone (GnRH) secretion and a lowered suppressive influence of estradiol and progesterone. Low-circulating progesterone levels also result in increased GnRH. LH regulates androgen production in ovarian theca cells. These cells increase production of androgens and more efficiently convert androgenic precursors to testosterone, likely because of both increased stimulation by LH and ovarian hyperresponsiveness to gonadotrophic stimulation.

It is also thought that the characteristic hyperinsulinism seen in PCOS plays a role in the pathogenesis of the syndrome. Insulin is believed to act synergistically with LH to increase production of androgens within theca cells. At the same time, increased insulin levels inhibit synthesis of sex hormone-binding globulin (SHBG), increasing the proportion of biologically active, unbound free testosterone.

The oligo- or anovulation of PCOS usually presents as oligo- or amenorrhea. Decreased ovulation leads to a deficiency of progesterone secretion. In some women, continuous estrogenic stimulation of the endometrium leads to anovulatory breakthrough bleeding or dysfunctional uterine bleeding that can be very frequent or heavy (Table 22-1). The menstrual irregularities may start around the time of puberty. In some women, however, the onset of menstrual abnormalities is associated with weight gain. Decreased ovulatory events result in fertility problems for many women with PCOS. Continuous unopposed estrogenic stimulation of the endometrium increases the incidence of endometrial hyperplasia and may increase the risk of endometrial carcinoma.

TABLE 22-1

Some Characteristics of Menstruation and Other Disorders Associated with PCOS

Type of menses	Prevalence
*Oligomenorrhea	64%
*Amenorrhea	16%
*Normal menses	16%
*Polymenorrhea	4%
Other signs, symptoms, or conditions	
*Hirsutism	70%
*Acanthosis nigricans	2%
*Acne	11%
Diabetes	10% by fourth decade
Impaired glucose tolerance	30%–40%
Obesity	30%–75%
Obstructive sleep apnea	Unknown but 30× increase risk
Endometrial, breast, and ovarian cancer	Unknown
Hypertension	Unknown
Infertility	Unknown

Data marked with * are from a series of 240 women with the polycystic ovarian syndrome.

From Carmina E, Lobo RA. Hirsutism, alopecia, and acne. In: Becker KL, Rebar RW, eds. Principles and Practice of Endocrinology and Metabolism. *Lippincott Williams & Wilkins: Philadelphia, PA; 2001:998–1005. Other data in tables adapted from that reviewed in Ehrmann D. Polycystic ovary syndrome.* N Engl J Med. *2005;352:1223–1236.*

PCOS, polycystic ovarian syndrome.

Hyperandrogenism is most often manifest by hirsutism, acne, and male pattern baldness. Hirsutism refers to the development of thick "terminal" hairs in the region of the upper lip, chin, areolae, and linea alba. The degree of hirsutism depends highly on the sensitivity of the hair follicle to androgenic stimulation, and therefore does not correlate well with the measured androgen level. In approximately 50% of women with mild to moderate hirsutism, this manifestation is idiopathic, occurring in the absence of excess androgen. Hirsutism in the presence of hyperandrogenism is most commonly caused by PCOS. Other, infrequent, causes of androgen excess include nonclassic CAH owing to 21-hydroxylase deficiency, androgenic medications, Cushing syndrome, hyperprolactinemia, acromegaly, and thyroid disease. The latter four conditions, Cushing's syndrome, hyperprolactinemia, acromegaly, and thyroid disease, usually present with symptoms other than hirsutism. Screening for nonclassic CAH by measuring serum 17-hydroxyprogesterone levels can usually be limited to high-risk women of Ashkenazi Jewish descent because of its rarity in other populations. The rapid development of hirsutism, or the presence of overt symptoms of virilization such as deepened voice, increased muscle mass, and clitoromegaly, is less suggestive of simply PCOS and should prompt a search for a virilizing tumor.

Otherwise, laboratory testing in the evaluation of PCOS is variable (Table 22-2), and typically guided by history and physical examination. In the setting of oligomenorrhea or amenorrhea, serum human chorionic gonadotropin (hCG) should be sent to assess to rule out pregnancy. Measurements of serum prolactin, TSH, and follicle-stimulating hormone (FSH) should also be considered to rule out hypothyroidism or ovarian failure. Moderate to severe hirsutism and other signs of hyperandrogenism may be evaluated with measurement of serum testosterone, and if available, serum free testosterone. If there is concern for virilizing tumor, dehydroepiandrosterone sulfate (DHEA-S) should also be sent to assess for adrenal source.

TABLE 22-2

Conditions That Are in the Differential Diagnosis of PCOS That Should be Excluded Before the Diagnosis of PCOS Can Be Assigned

Conditions to rule out	Mimics PCOS how?	How to tell apart from PCOS	
		History/physical examination	Tests to run
Nonclassic congenital adrenal hyperplasia	Increased androgens	Family history, newborn screening or ethnic heritage suggestive (see text)	AM level of 17-hydroxyprogesterone
Cushing syndrome/disease	Menstrual problems + Increased androgens	Stigmata of hypercortisolism including refractory hypertension, "buffalo hump," moon facies striae, peripheral wasting	24-hour collection of urine for free cortisol, additional workup needed if elevated
Prolactin-secreting tumor	Menstrual problems	Often history of galactorrhea	Elevated serum prolactin or pituitary mass on MRI
Androgen-secreting tumor (adrenal or ovarian in origin)	Menstrual problems + Increased androgens	Difficult but may have rapid onset of virilization including clitorimegaly, rapid acquisition of alopecia	Serum androgen levels (testosterone, androstenedione, dehydroepiandrosterone sulfate)
Hypothyroidism	Menstrual problems	Other historical or examination features of hypothyroidism including constipation, fatigue, goiter, history of thyroiditis, other endocrinopathies	Serum TSH and serum free thyroxine level
Uterine cancer/uterine abnormality Iatrogenic causes	Menstrual problems Variable	Possible abnormal pelvic examination History of exposure to androgens, phenytoin, valproate, minoxidil, etc	Ultrasound of uterus N/A
Miscellaneous including ovarian failure (OF), simple obesity (SO), acromegaly (AM)	Variable	Signs of early menopause (OF), obesity in history (SO), coarse features, and prognathism (AM)	Low estrogen, high follicle-stimulating hormone (OF), N/A (SO), elevated serum IGF-1 (AM)

Menstrual problems may include dysfunctional uterine bleeding, oligomenorrhea, or amenorrhea. Increased androgen may include hirsutism, deepened voice, male pattern alopecia, clitorimegaly.

Adapted with some minor additions from Ehrmann D. Polycystic ovary syndrome. NEJM. *2005;352:1223–1236.*

MRI, magnetic resonance imaging; PCOS, polycystic ovarian syndrome.

High levels of testosterone (>200 ng/dL) and DHEA-S (>700 mcg/dL) increase the likelihood of underlying neoplasm. Routine measurements of serum LH levels are not recommended owing to unclear clinical implications.

Other clinical manifestations of PCOS include obesity, impaired glucose tolerance and type 2 diabetes, hypertension and vascular endothelial dysfunction, dyslipidemia, and obstructive sleep apnea (Table 22-1). Once the diagnosis of PCOS is made, close attention must be paid to the identification and treatment of each of these conditions. It is estimated that approximately 50% of women with PCOS are obese. The cause of this is unclear. Insulin resistance and impaired glucose tolerance of PCOS, however, appear independent of obesity, although the combination of obesity and PCOS does seem to have a synergistic adverse influence on glucose tolerance. The degree of impaired vascular endothelial function and hypertension, as well as obstructive sleep apnea, also appears independent of obesity. Also, persons with PCOS may have an increased risk of certain cancers (endometrial, breast, and ovarian) because of prolonged anovulation and other hormonal disruption.

Treatment of PCOS should focus on alleviating the cutaneous manifestations of hyperandrogenism, managing the menstrual abnormalities, and improving glucose tolerance. Simple weight loss should be included in every treatment regimen as weight loss improves insulin sensitivity and may lead to less anovulatory menstrual cycles. Combined estrogen–progestin oral contraceptives remain a mainstay of treatment. The estrogen component suppresses LH, resulting in decreased theca cell androgen production. At the same time, it enhances the production of SHBG, therefore limiting the proportion of free testosterone. Estradiol is typically combined with a nonandrogenic progestin such as norgestimate or desogestrel. The progestin component inhibits endometrial proliferation. Spironolactone has antiandrogenic effects that appear to act synergistically with oral contraceptives. Drospirenone, a spironolactone analog, has been combined with ethinyl estradiol and has proven effective in the treatment of PCOS.

Metformin is also a very effective medication in the treatment of PCOS. By inhibiting the production of hepatic glucose, metformin lowers insulin concentrations and reduces androgen production within theca cells. Metformin also appears to have direct inhibitory effects on ovarian steroid production. Some of the positive effects of metformin may be associated with the weight loss typically seen early in the course of treatment with this medication. In the absence of any pharmacologic therapy, weight loss alone in women with PCOS has been associated with decreased androgen levels, improved ovulatory function, and improved glucose tolerance. Thiazolidinediones are also effective at lowering insulin and androgen levels, but are associated with weight gain and are less commonly used owing to an unclear safety profile in pregnancy. Glucocorticoids such as prednisone and dexamethasone can also be used to treat severe androgen excess but should be used for only a limited time because of their diabetogenic effects. Other medications that have been used to treat PCOS and its symptoms include finasteride for hirsutism and clomiphene citrate for the induction of ovulation. A recent randomized trial of 626 infertile women with PCOS randomized patients to one of three study groups receiving metformin, clomiphene citrate, or both and examined live birth rates in each cohort. In the study, the live birth rate was 7.2% (15 of 208) in the metformin group, 22.5% (47 of 209 subjects) in the clomiphene group, and 26.8% (56 of 209) in the combination therapy group, indicating that clomiphene alone or in combination with metformin was best to treat infertility in PCOS. It should be noted that there was higher multiple birth rate.

The patient in the above case displayed characteristic adrenergic features of PCOS. She had menstrual irregularity characterized by menorrhagia, presumably secondary anovulatory dysfunctional uterine bleeding. She had characteristic clinical manifestations of PCOS including obesity, diabetes, and hypertension. Symptoms were insidious enough that they did not prompt aggressive evaluation for a virilizing neoplasm. History and physical examination did not point to an alternative explanation for androgenic excess. Thyroid function was normal. Additionally, her symptoms improved with the initiation of metformin and modest weight reduction. At this point, she was started on a combined oral contraceptive. A fasting lipid panel should be checked. A comprehensive approach should be taken to the outpatient management of her PCOS.

Selected References

Carmina E, Lobo RA. Hirsutism, alopecia, and acne. In: Becker KL, Rebar RW, eds. *Principles and Practice of Endocrinology and Metabolism.* Lippincott Williams & Wilkins; Philadelphia, PA: 2001:998–1005.

Dunaif A, Segal KR, Futterweit W, et al. Profound peripheral insulin resistance, independent of obesity, in polycystic ovary syndrome. *Diabetes.* 1989;38(9):1165–1174.

Ehrmann D. Polycystic ovary syndrome. *NEJM.* 2005;352:1223–1236.

Legro RS, Barnhart HX, Schlaff WD, et al. Cooperative Multicenter Reproductive Medicine Network. Clomiphene, metformin, or both for infertility in the polycystic ovary syndrome. *N Engl J Med.* 2007 Feb 8;356(6):551–566.

Rebar R. Disorders of menstruation, ovulation, and sexual dysfunction. In: Becker KL, et al, eds. *Principles and Practice of Endocrinology and Metabolism.* Lippincott Williams & Wilkins; Philadelphia, PA: 2001:956–960.

Norman RJ, Masters L, Milner CR, et al. The Rotterdam ESHRE/ASRM-Sponsored PCOS Consensus Workshop Group. Revised 2003 consensus on diagnostic criteria and long-term health risks related to polycystic ovary syndrome (PCOS). *Hum Reprod.* 2004;19(1):41–47.

Rosenfield R. Hirsutism. *NEJM.* 2005;353:2578–2588.

Dostou JM. Hisuitism. In: Runge M, Greganti A, eds. *Netter's Internal Medicine.* Teterboro, NJ: Icon Learning Systems; 2003:208–212.

2-Day-Old Male with Respiratory Distress

CASE PRESENTATION

A 2339-g infant was born at 36 weeks to a 21-year-old mother after an uncomplicated pregnancy and vaginal delivery. The mother's history was unremarkable, with negative pre-natal laboratory tests. A murmur was noted in the initial newborn period. The infant was active, pink, with bilateral symmetric femoral pulses, and a normal capillary refill time. A grade 2/6 systolic murmur, heard best at the left lower sternal border, persisted on day of life 2, and a pulse oximetry was performed revealing a saturation of 92% on room air. This was confirmed on repeat measurement. The rest of the examination remained unchanged, with clear lung fields and a liver edge palpable just below the costal margin. A chest x-ray was obtained (Fig. 23-1) demonstrating cardiomegaly and increased pulmonary vascularity.

Question

What is the most likely cause of this infant's hypoxia?

Answer

Congenital cardiac lesions that present with a soft murmur and minimal cyanosis in the immediate newborn period include truncus arterious (TA) and Ebstein anomaly. Tetralogy of Fallot may present with profound cyanosis or intermittent cyanosis, depending on the degree of pulmonary stenosis. Hypoplastic left heart syndrome may present with cyanosis in the immediate neonatal period or at several days of life as the ductus arterious closes. Total anomalous pulmonary venous return is highly variable in presentation with severe cyanosis to no cyanosis depending on the degree of obstruction of the pulmonary vessels. In this child's case, her murmur and mild hypoxia were caused by TA. The diagnosis was confirmed by echocardiogram. This infant had a common arterial trunk overriding a large subarterial ventricular septal defect (VSD) with mild truncal stenosis. The truncal valve was tricuspid with mild valvular insufficiency. A main pulmonary artery segment was identified arising from the truncus and bifurcating into left and right pulmonary arteries, defining her heart lesion as TA, type I.

Discussion

TA is a rare congenital cyanotic heart lesion consisting of a single arterial trunk arising from the right ventricle that supplies the pulmonary, systemic, and coronary circulation (Fig. 23-2). A VSD is always present, as well as a truncal valve that may have two to six cusps. TA is further defined into four types by the position of the pulmonary artery. The main pulmonary artery arises from the lateral side of the truncus and divides into the left and right pulmonary arteries in type I. Types II and III have no main pulmonary trunk and the left and right pulmonary arteries arise from either the posterior aspect of the truncus (type II) or the lateral aspect of the truncus (type III). Type IV has no connection between the heart and pulmonary arteries; instead the pulmonary blood flow is supplied from aortopulmonary collateral arteries that arise from the aorta. TA has an estimated incidence of 0.8/10,000 live births, accounting for 1% of congenital heart disease.

Conotruncal defects are frequently associated with 22q11.2 deletion syndrome, also known as DiGeorge syndrome and velocardiofacial syndrome. The incidence is estimated at approximate 1/3000 to 1/6000 live births. The most common phenotypic abnormalities associated with 22q11.2 deletion syndrome are thymus and parathyroid hypoplasia, cardiac anomalies, cleft lip and palate, velopharyngeal

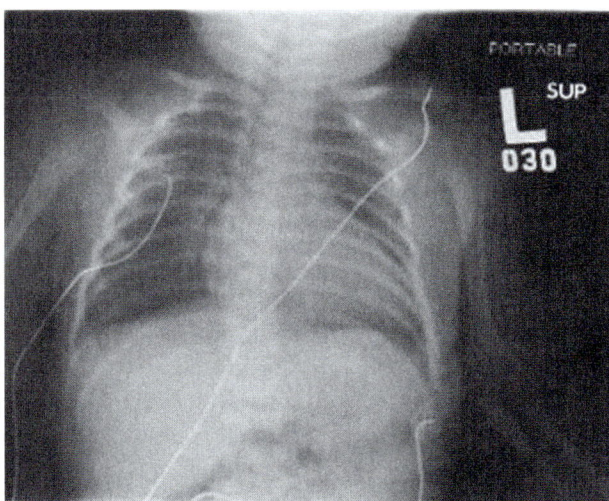

Figure 23-1 Chest radiograph demonstrating cardiomegaly and increased pulmonary vasculature.

insufficiency, and characteristic facial features. Population studies suggest that 22q11.2 deletion syndrome contribute to 1/5 cases of TA. Therefore fluorescence in situ hybridization (FISH) screening for 22q11.2 deletion is recommended for children diagnosed with a conotruncal heart defect such as TA.

Clinical manifestations of TA are dependent on the patient's age and are directly related to pulmonary vascular resistance. In the immediate neonatal period, when pulmonary vascular resistance is high, the infant may exhibit only minimal cyanosis (Table 23-1). As pulmonary vascular resistance falls, pulmonary blood flow increases and older infants manifest signs of congestive heart failure. A complex murmur may be auscultated with a loud, single second heart sound; a systolic ejection murmur over the left sternal border, occasionally accompanied by a thrill; an early systolic click; and an apical mid-diastolic rumble caused by increased flow across the mitral valve, and if truncal valve insufficiency is present, a high-pitched early diastolic decrescendo murmur. Older children develop pulmonary vascular restrictive disease resulting in decreased pulmonary blood flow and progressive cyanosis accompanied by polycythemia and clubbing.

The differential diagnosis of cyanosis in the newborn period is broad and includes hypoventilation (sedation, central nervous system injuries, neuromuscular disorders, seizures), structural and infectious respiratory causes (upper and lower airway), cardiac right-to-left shunting (cyanotic congenital heart disease, persistent pulmonary hypertension of the newborn), and methemoglobinemia. This can be narrowed quickly with an appropriate series of studies.

Hyperoxia Test

The hyperoxia test is used to help distinguish between pulmonary and cardiac disease in a cyanotic newborn. In infants with congenital heart disease, breathing 100% oxygen will generally not increase arterial PaO_2 above 150 mm Hg. An arterial PaO_2 greater than 150 mm Hg suggests a pulmonary cause for cyanosis but does not exclude all forms of congenital heart disease.

Chest X-Ray

A chest x-ray may help differentiate between cardiac and pulmonary disease. In cardiac disease, the cardiac shadow and degree of pulmonary vasculature and pulmonary blood flow may be helpful. Chest x-ray findings in TA are variable, but include cardiac enlargement with prominence of both ventricles and increased pulmonary vasculature and pulmonary edema after the first week of life.

Electrocardiogram

Electrocardiogram findings in TA are limited to right, left, or combined ventricular hypertrophy.

Echocardiogram

An echocardiogram is a definitive noninvasive test to evaluate cardiac structure. Echocardiogram provides the

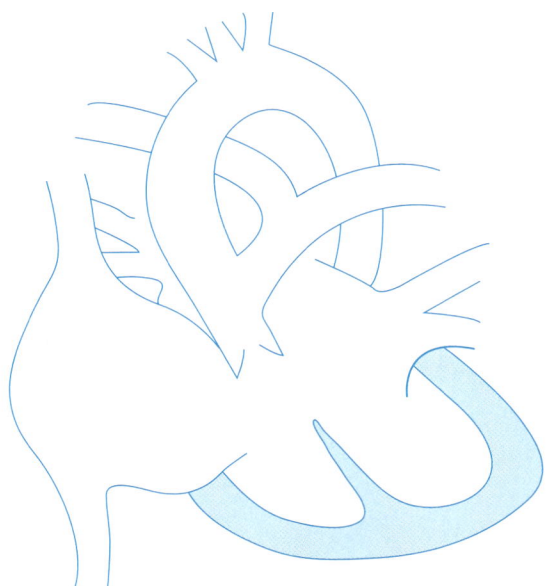

Figure 23-2 Type I truncus arteriosus.

TABLE 23-1

Physical and Diagnostic Findings in Cyanotic Congenital Heart Disease

Heart lesion	Examination findings	Electrocardiogram	Chest x-ray
Truncus arteriosus	A loud, single second heart sound and a systolic ejection murmur over the left sternal border	Ventricular hypertrophy: right, left, or combined	Cardiac enlargement with prominence of both ventricles, and increased pulmonary vasculature and pulmonary edema after the first week of life
Transposition of the great arteries	Cyanosis and tachypnea are most often present If large VSD, cyanosis may be subtle with delayed onset. Second sound is usually single, loud No murmur or soft systolic murmur at the midleft sternal border	Normal neonatal pattern	Mild cardiomegaly Narrow mediastinum "Egg on a string" sign
Tricuspid atresia	Cyanosis evident at birth Increased left ventricular impulse Holosystolic murmur left sternal border Single second heart sound	Left axis deviation Left ventricular hypertrophy Biphasic P waves	Decreased pulmonary vasculature
Tetralogy of Fallot	Cyanosis may be absent to severe Substernal right ventricular impulse Loud, harsh murmur at left sternal border, may be preceded by click Second heart sound single or soft	Right axis deviation Right ventricular hypertrophy Dominant R-wave precordial leads P wave tall and peaked	"Boot" or "wooden shoe" shaped heart Concavity of left heart border in region of main pulmonary artery Right ventricular hypertrophy Decreased pulmonary vasculature
Total anomalous pulmonary venous return	Cyanosis may be absent to severe Murmur may be absent or systolic murmur over LSB with gallop rhythm	Right ventricular hypertrophy	"Snowman" sign: large supracardiac shadow (masked by thymus in infants) Cardiomegaly Prominent main pulmonary artery and right ventricle Increased pulmonary vasculature
Hypoplastic left heart	Cyanosis and hypoperfusion with weak or absent pulses (may develop after 48 hours of life) Palpable right ventricular parasternal lift Nondescript systolic murmur	Initial: R ventricular dominance P Poor voltage Later: right ventricular hypertrophy Prominent P waves	Variable in first days of life Cardiomegaly Increased pulmonary vasculature
Ebstein anomaly	Cyanosis highly variable Quiet precordium Holosystolic murmur radiating over left anterior chest Gallop common Multiple clicks left lower sternal border Diastolic murmur left sternal border	Right bundle branch block with increased right precordial voltage Normal or tall/broad P waves Prolonged PR interval Wolfe-Parkinson-White (delta wave or SVT) may be present	Heart size varies from normal to enlarged and box shaped Vascular markings may be increased or decreased

(Continued)

TABLE 23-1

Physical and Diagnostic Findings in Cyanotic Congenital Heart Disease (*Continued*)

Heart lesion	Examination findings	Electrocardiogram	Chest x-ray
Critical pulmonic stenosis	Cyanosis only with critical stenosis Loud, harsh systolic murmur over pulmonic area, radiating over precordium, lung fields, neck, and back Parasternal right ventricular lift Elevation of venous pressure	Right ventricular hypertrophy Tall, spiked P waves	Cardiac enlargement Prominence of right ventricle and atrium

LSB, left sternal border; SVT, supraventricular tachycardia; VSD, ventricular septal defect.

diagnosis, revealing a truncal artery overriding a VSD. An interrupted aortic arch can be associated with TA.

Cardiac catheterization/Angiography

Cardiac catheterization is invasive, but provides additional information about the structure of the heart, including the origin of coronary arteries. In TA, catheterization demonstrates left-to-right shunting at the ventricular level with right-to-left shunting into the truncus. Systolic pressures are similar across the right and left ventricles and the truncus.

The initial treatment of any infant with suspected cyanotic congenital heart disease should be the initiation of prostaglandin infusion (Table 23-1). A significant side effect of prostaglandin infusion is respiratory depression or apnea; therefore, an experienced physician should be present and prepared to intubate and provide respiratory support.

Without correction, many infants die within the first year of life. Survival depends on the degree of pulmonary circulation and the consequences of obstructive pulmonary vascular disease. Prior to the development of techniques for surgical repair, survival was infrequent and associated with significant disability. Surgical correction consists of closure of the VSD, division of the pulmonary arteries from the truncus, and placement of a conduit to connect the right ventricle and pulmonary arteries. This surgical correction has a 3% to 5% mortality rate in the immediate postoperative period with long-term survival rates 71% to 85% at 10 years. Reoperation is frequently necessary to replace conduit material as a child grows, with reoperation rates greater than 50% and a median time of 5 years to reoperation.

Once a child has developed obstructive pulmonary vascular disease, corrective repair is no longer possible and heart–lung transplantation becomes the only surgical option.

Selected References

1. Bernstein D. In: Behrman Re, Kliegman Rm, Jenson Hb, eds. *Nelson Textbook of Pediatrics*. 17th ed. Philadelphia, PA: Saunders; 2004. Chap. 418.
2. Botto LD, May K, Fernhoff PM, et al. A population-based study of the 22q11.2 deletion: phenotype, incidence, and contribution to major birth defects in the population. *Pediatrics*. 2003 Jul;112(1 Pt 1):101–107.
3. Canfield MA, Honein, MA, Yuskiv N, et al. National estimates and race/ethnic-specific variation of selected birth defects in the United States, 1999–2001. *Birth Defects Res A*. 2006;76: 747–756.
4. Koppel RI, Druschel CM, Carter T, et al. Effectiveness of pulse oximetry screening for congenital heart disease in asymptomatic newborns. *Pediatrics*. 2003 Mar;111(3):451–455.
5. Marcelletti C, McGoon DC, Mair DD. The natural history of truncus arteriosus. *Circulation*. 1976 Jul;54(1):108–111.
6. Monro JL, Alexiou C, Salmon AP, et al. Reoperations and survival after primary repair of congenital heart defects in children. *J Thorac Cardiovasc Surg*. 2003 Aug;126(2):511–520.
7. Perez E, Sullivan KE. Chromosome 22q11.2 deletion syndrome (DiGeorge and velocardiofacial syndromes). *Curr Opin Pediatr.* 2002 Dec;14(6):678–683.
8. Rajasinghe HA, McElhinney DB, Reddy VM, et al. Long-term follow-up of truncus arteriosus repaired in infancy: a twenty-year experience. *J Thorac Cardiovasc Surg*. 1997 May;113(5): 869–878; discussion 878–879.
9. Thompson LD, McElhinney DB, Reddy M, et al. Neonatal repair of truncus arteriosus: continuing improvement in outcomes. *Ann Thorac Surg*. 2001 Aug;72(2):391–395.

38-Year-Old Female with Hand Swelling

CASE PRESENTATION

A 38-year-old Caucasian woman with no past medical history presented to urgent care complaining of stiffness. She noticed it when she woke up 5 days ago. The stiffness seemed to be located mostly in her hands, but she also described a whole body stiffness associated with fatigue. She had limited range of motion in her hands as well as overall difficulty moving around. The pain was worse in the morning, and improved somewhat with moving around for 30 to 60 minutes. She denied fevers and chills. She had no past rheumatologic conditions; no rashes; and no history of exposures, tick bites, or diarrhea. She initially denied having any sick contacts, but upon specific questioning, did remember a neighbor's child having "slapped cheek" disease about a month ago. The patient is a married mother of three who lives on a horse ranch. She is not on any medicines and has no known drug allergies.

Physical Examination

Well-appearing woman, moving stiffly, vital signs: temperature 36.6, respiratory rate of 15 breaths/min., blood pressure 113/62 mm Hg, pulse 90 beats/min. Head, eyes, ears, nose, and throat pupils equal, round, reactive to light. Oropharynx clear, no ulcerations. Tympanic membranes normal. Pulmonary: clear to auscultation bilaterally, no wheezes. Cardiovascular: regular rate and rhythm. No murmurs. Abdomen: soft, nontender, nondistended. No hepatosplenomegaly. Skin: no rashes. Musculoskeletal: mildly tender; symmetrical swelling of the wrists, hands, digits, feet, and toes. She has severely limited flexion and mildly limited extension of the distal interphalangeal (DIP), proximal interphalangeal (PIP), and metacarpophalangeal (MCP) joints of her hands. Flexion and extension is also limited at the carpal–metacarpal joints and all metatarsophalangeal (MTP) joints. No erythema or synovial thickening can be appreciated. Large and more proximal joints appear normal, but have mildly decreased range of motion.

Laboratory Studies

Electrolytes within normal limits. Erythrocyte sedimentation rate (ESR) 21. C-reactive protein (CRP) <0.5. White blood cells 5.3, hemoglobin 11.1, hematocrit 33.1, mean corpuscular volume 88, platelets 187. Reticulocytes 2.8%. Iron studies, B$_{12}$, folate within normal limits. Antinuclear antibody test (ANA) negative, rheumatoid factor negative. Parvovirus immunoglobulin G 5.64 (<0.90 = negative, 0.90–1.10 = equivocal, >1.10 = positive). Parvovirus IgM 20.40 (<0.90 = negative, 0.90–1.10 = equivocal, >1.10 = positive).

Case Resolution

The patient was felt to be suffering from acute parvovirus–associated polyarthritis. This is a self-limited, benign condition. Patient was reassured and recommended to take nonsteroidal anti-inflammatory drugs (NSAIDs) for pain. Within several weeks, all symptoms had resolved and she had resumed her normal activities.

Question

What aspects of this presentation are most helpful to narrow down the differential diagnosis?

TABLE 24-1

Differential Diagnosis for Acute Polyarticular Arthritis

Infectious arthritis:

Parvovirus B19, enterovirus, adenovirus, EBV, Coxsackie virus, CMV, rubella, mumps, hepatitis B, varicella-zoster virus, HIV, *Neisseria gonorrhoeae*, *Staphylococcus aureus*, gram-negative bacilli, *Borrelia burgdorferi*, *Mycobacterium tuberculosis*, fungi

Postinfectious (reactive) arthritis:

N. gonorrhoeae, bacterial endocarditis, campylobacter, chlamydia, salmonella, shigella, yersinia, *Tropheryma whippelii*, group A streptococci

Crystal induced:

Gout, pseudogout, hydroxyapatite

Spondylarthritides:

Ankylosing spondylitis, psoriatic arthritis, inflammatory bowel disease

Systemic rheumatic disease:

Rheumatoid arthritis, systemic lupus erythematosus, polymyositis/dermatomyositis, juvenile rheumatoid arthritis, scleroderma, Sjögren syndrome, Behçet syndrome, polymyalgia rheumatica, Wegener granulomatosis, giant cell arteritis

Endocrine disorders:

Hyperparathyroidism, hyperthyroidism, hypothyroidism

Malignancy:

Metastatic cancer, multiple myeloma

Other:

Osteoarthritis, hypermobility syndromes, sarcoidosis, fibromyalgia, osteomalacia, Sweet syndrome, serum sickness

Adapted from Mies RA, Francis ML. Diagnostic approach to polyarticular joint pain. Am Fam Physician. 2003;68:1151–1160.
CMV, cytomegalovirus; EBV, Epstein-Barr virus; HIV, human immunodeficiency virus.

Answer

The differential diagnosis for adults presenting with acute polyarticular arthritis is broad (see Table 24-1). Although there are many different approaches to this complaint, five aspects of the history and physical examination can help narrow the list of possible etiologies. These are chronology of symptoms, associated inflammation, distribution of joint pain, associated symptoms, and demographics.[1] Although none are extremely sensitive or specific, together they provide clues which help lead the practitioner in the right direction.

Discussion

Chronology describes both the onset of symptoms and the disease course. Acute onset of symptoms, like for the patient in the presentation, are more likely to lead to viral, crystal, or reactive arthritis than rheumatoid arthritis (RA) or systemic lupus erythematosus (SLE), which tends to be insidious in onset.[1] Following the course of the disease can provide other clues to the diagnosis. Many causes of acute-onset arthritis also resolve spontaneously and do not recur. Arthritis that resolves completely but then does

recur makes a crystal-associated arthritis, such as gout, more likely.[1] Several etiologies can cause migratory arthritis which is inflammation of a few joints, which improves over the course of a several days, but then different joints become involved. Gonococcal arthritis, rheumatic fever, sarcoidosis, SLE, Lyme disease, bacterial endocarditis, and Whipple disease all cause migratory arthritis.[1]

Joint pain is classified as arthritis when it is associated with signs of inflammation, such as erythema, warmth, and swelling. Joint pain in the absence of inflammation is termed arthralgia. Severe inflammation causes prolonged morning stiffness as well as systemic side effects such as fatigue, fever, and potential weight loss.[1] The physical examination of the joints should systematically evaluate every peripheral joint as well as the spine.[2] Signs of inflammation, range of motion, and crepitus should all be noted. Infections, gout, RA, SLE, and reactive arthritis are all associated with inflammation.

The distribution of joint pain can be very helpful in differentiating the etiology of polyarthritis (Table 24-2). Osteoarthritis (OA) tends to involve the DIP and PIP, whereas RA typically involves the PIP and MCP joints. Lyme disease rarely affects the hands. OA rarely affects the elbows, wrists, and ankles. RA, SLE, polymyalgia rheumatica, and viral arthritides all cause fairly symmetric joint involvement.

TABLE 24-2

Etiology of Polyarthritis According to Patterns

Symmetric arthritides	SLE, RA, scleroderma
Arthritides associated with dactylitis	Ankylosing spondylitis, Reiter syndrome, psoriatic arthritis
Arthritides associated with sacroiliitis	Ankylosing spondylitis, IBD, psoriatic arthritis
Arthritis affecting the DIP joint	Osteoarthritis (Heberden nodes), psoriatic arthritis
Arthritis affecting the PIP joint	Osteoarthritis (Bouchard nodes), rheumatoid arthritis, SLE, scleroderma
Arthritis affecting the MCP joint	RA, SLE, scleroderma, hemachromatosis

DIP, distal interphalangeal; IBD, inflammatory bowel disease; MCP, metacarpophalangeal; PIP, proximal interphalangeal; RA, rheumatoid arthritis; SLE, systemic lupus erythematous.

Reactive arthritis, gout, and psoriatic arthritis tend to have asymmetric involvement. Spondyloarthropathies, such as ankylosing spondylitis, psoriatic arthritis, inflammatory bowel disease–associated arthropathy, and reactive arthritis are much more likely to have axial involvement.[3]

Extra-articular manifestations are varied as virtually any organ system can be involved in the different etiologies of polyarthritis.[1] SLE is associated with malar rash, oral ulcers, and serositis. RA can cause subcutaneous nodules. Parvovirus has a very distinctive rash in children, but may only cause a lacy rash or no rash at all in adults. Ankylosing spondylitis is associated with iritis and tendonitis. Psoriatic arthritis is obviously associated with psoriasis, but also with dactylitis and onychodystrophy.

Several aspects of patient demographics can be helpful. Women are much more likely to develop RA and SLE; however, after the age of 50, the gender difference is less significant. Women are also more likely to have joint involvement with parvovirus infections. Younger people are more likely to be diagnosed with rheumatic fever, SLE, RA, reactive arthritis, and spondyloarthropathies. Older people are more likely to develop OA, polymyalgia rheumatica, and giant cell arteritis. Sarcoidosis and SLE are more common in black people. White people are more likely to have polymyalgia rheumatica and Wegener granulomatosis.

Based on the history and physical examination of the patient in this case, a preliminary diagnosis was made for parvovirus B19–associated polyarthritis. The diagnosis was confirmed with the elevated IgM antibody titers.

Parvovirus B19, named for the plate and position on which it was incidentally discovered, belongs to a family of capsid viruses characterized by their small size. Infection is common worldwide, with about half of all adolescents and 80% to 90% of elderly adults having specific antibodies.[5]

The virus is spread by respiratory droplets, with infection rates among household contacts being very high. Most cases of parvovirus infection are asymptomatic, with the clinical presentation of symptomatic patients being variable depending on age and gender.

Parvovirus B19 infections during childhood cause erythema infectiosum (EI), a syndrome associated with a characteristic erythematosus rash predominantly on the cheeks; hence the common name, slapped cheek disease. The rash may recur with exposure to sunlight, heat, or exercise. The disease is also called fifth disease, as it was the fifth common childhood exanthem described (first was measles, then scarlet fever, rubella, Duke disease, which probably does not exist as a separate entity, EI, and finally roseola). EI is associated with fever and nonspecific symptoms early. This is the viremic stage. The cutaneous eruption occurs about 2 weeks later, with the appearance of antiviral antibodies. The rash is likely caused by deposition of immune complexes in the skin.

In adults, particularly middle-aged women, parvovirus can cause significant arthropathy, associated with arthralgia and inflammatory arthritis. As noted above, the disease is typically symmetric and occurs usually in the hands. Ankles, knees, and wrists can be involved. Symptoms typically resolve over the course of a few weeks. Joint destruction does not occur. Like the rash, the etiology of the arthritis is thought to be because of immune complex deposition.

In patients with a high demand for erythropoiesis, such as hereditary spherocytosis and sickle cell disease, parvovirus B19 can be lethal. The virus has extreme tropism for human erythroid progenitor cells. Even in normal volunteers exposed to the virus, reticulocyte counts fall to 0. At-risk patients can develop an aplastic crisis potentially associated with profound anemia, congestive heart failure, cerebrovascular accidents, and acute splenic sequestration. Viremia is present during the crisis. Red cell production resumes with the development of specific antibodies, conferring a lifelong protective immunity.

Immunocompromised patients, such as congenital immune deficiency, HIV/AIDS, or transplant recipients on immunosuppressive therapy, are at risk for persistent parvovirus infection. Antibodies are absent, so these patients do not develop EI or arthritis. Effective treatment options in these cases, include intravenous immunoglobulins. Response is prompt, with a decline in viremia; however, relapses are possible. A side effect of treatment can be EI or arthritis as immune complexes are now present.

Infection with parvovirus B19 during pregnancy can cause hydrops fetalis because of transplacental transfer of the virus. Particularly during the second trimester, the virus can infect the fetal liver and inhibit erythrocyte production, leading to profound anemia and congestive heart failure. The risk of transplacental transfer is approximately 30%. The risk of fetal loss is 5% to 9%.

Although the vast majority of parvovirus infections are benign and self-limited, the rare, but severe, reactions can be devastating. A recombinant vaccine consisting of empty capsids elicited neutralizing antibodies in phase 1 trials[6]. Unfortunately, like many therapies, commercial interests will likely dictate further development and distribution.

Selected References

1. Mies RA, Francis ML. Diagnostic approach to polyarticular joint pain. *Am Fam Physician.* 2003;68:1151–1160.
2. McCarty DJ. Differential diagnosis of arthritis: analysis of signs and symptoms. In: Keepman WJ, Moreland LW, eds. *Arthritis & Allied Conditions.* Philadelphia, PA: Lippincott Williams & Wilkins; 2005:37–49, Chapter 2. (Accessed online at Books@Ovid)
3. El-Gabalawy HS, Duray P, Goldbach-Masky R. Evaluating patients with arthritis of recent onset: studies in pathogenesis and prognosis. *JAMA.* 2000;284:2368–2373.
4. Young NC, Brown KE. Parvovirus B19. *N Engl J Med.* 2004;350:586–597.
5. Kelly HA, Siebert D, Hammond R, et al. The age-specific prevalence of human parvovirus immunity in Victoria, Australia, compared with other parts of the world. *Epidemiol Infect.* 2000;124:449–457.
6. Ballou WR, Reed JL, Noble W, et al. Safety and immunogenicity of a recombinant parvovirus B19 vaccine formulated with MF59C.1. *J Infect Dis.* 2003;187:675–678.

horizontally (community acquired). In general, late-onset disease has a less fulminant course than early-onset disease and manifests as bacteremia (45%–60%), meningitis (25%–35%), or focal infections (20%). Focal infections include osteomyelitis, septic arthritis, pneumonia, urinary tract infections, and skin or soft tissue infections.

The incidence of early-onset GBS disease has decreased sharply since the widespread implementation of intrapartum chemoprophylaxis, declining by as much as 80%. The rate of 1.7/1000 live births from 2004 represents a significant decrease from the prechemoprophylaxis era rate of 9.34/1000 live births in 1993. The rate of late-onset disease has remained stable from 1999 to 2004 at a rate of 0.35/1000 live births. The current guidelines recommend a culture-based approach to screening at 35 to 37 weeks' gestation. Women with documented GBS bacteriuria or a history of previous infants with GBS disease do not require screening as they should receive intrapartum antibiotic therapy. Women testing positive during this third trimester screening are treated with penicillin at rupture of membranes or onset of labor. If culture results are not available at the onset of labor, a risk-based approach is used. Risk factors include gestation less than 37 weeks, membrane rupture greater than 18 hours, or intrapartum fever.

As a result of intrapartum antibiotics, most cases of invasive GBS are now seen in adults. Group B streptococcus infections in pregnant and parturient women may manifest as urinary tract infection, bacteremia, endometritis, rate of 8% to 15%. Cases of GBS disease are seen less frequently in older children; however, the overall case fatality rate is higher at 9%.

Ampicillin plus an aminoglycoside are the antibiotics of choice for suspected invasive GBS infection in a newborn. This provides broad antibiotic coverage while the organism is identified, along with synergistic bactericidal activity against GBS. Antibiotic choice can be narrowed to penicillin G, once GBS has been positively identified and the patient is clinically improving. Treatment regimens vary from 10 days for uncomplicated bacteremia to several weeks for osteomyelitis, endocarditis, or ventriculitis.

Selected References

1. Todd J. *Nelson Textbook of Pediatrics.* 17th ed. Philadelphia, PA: Saunders; 2004. Chapter 169.
2. Committee on Infectious Diseases. In: Pickering LK, Baker CJ, Long SS, McMillan JA, eds. *Red Book: 2006 Report of the Committee of Infectious Diseases.* 27th ed. Elk Grove, IL: American Academy of Pediatrics; 2006.
3. ACOG Committee Opinion. Prevention of early-onset group B streptococcal disease in newborns. *Obstet Gynecol.* 2002;100:1405–1412.
4. Centers for Disease Control and Prevention. Early-onset and late-onset neonatal group B streptococcal disease: United States, 1996–2004. *MMWR Morb Mortal Wkly Rep.* 2005;54:502–505.
5. Schrag SJ, Zywicki S, Farley MM, et al. Group B streptococcal disease in the ear of intrapartum antibiotic prophylaxis. *N Engl J Med.* 2000 Jan 6;342(1):15–20.

34-Week Twins with Difficulty Feeding

CASE PRESENTATION

A set of 34-week twins was admitted to the neonatal intensive care unit (ICU) for temperature instability and difficulty feeding. After a 3-week convalescent period, they were feeding well, gaining weight, and approaching discharge. Baby A suddenly refused to feed and her nurse noted a mottled appearance to her skin.

Physical Examination

On examination, she was responsive, but her extremities were cool and her skin was pale and mottled. Laboratory studies were obtained including complete blood count and urine cultures, (see next), and an intravenous line (IV) was placed. Because of an elevated C-reactive protein (CRP), she was started on antibiotics. Shortly thereafter, she became apneic and was intubated. A lumbar puncture revealed purulent cerebrospinal fluid (CSF). Blood culture

Question

Which organism is the most likely to cause meningitis and sepsis in a 3-week-old premature infant?

Discussion

Group B streptococci (GBS) are gram-positive cocci com-

15-Month-Old Females with Tonic–Clonic Seizure

CASE PRESENTATION

A 15-month-old female presented to the emergency department (ED) by private car after a brief generalized tonic–clonic seizure at home. She had been sent home from day care that morning with fever. Her parents reported several days of upper airway congestion and intermittent cough. After waking up from her nap, she was active and playful. Her mother heard a strange sound and found her on the floor with jerking movements of her arms and legs. The TV was on at home and the mother estimates the episode lasted no more than a commercial break. The child had no significant past medical history; however, her parents both had a history of febrile seizures as children. They described normal growth and development for this child. On arrival to the ED, she had a temperature of 41°C and was somewhat fussy, with a normal physical examination. After receiving acetaminophen and ibuprofen, her repeat temperature was 38°C and she had returned to her energetic, playful baseline. Neither laboratory studies nor imaging was performed.

A second 15-month-old female presented to the ED by ambulance after onset of generalized tonic–clonic seizure at home. By her mother's estimation, the seizure activity had been ongoing for about 40 minutes prior to arrival at the hospital. The child received rectal diazepam in route plus Ativan and fosphenytoin in the emergency room with resulting cessation of her seizure activity. She has a past medical history significant for asthma and no contributory family history.

Physical Examination

The second child described above had a 2-day history of fever to 39°C and upper respiratory infection symptoms. Her complete blood count was reassuring with white blood cells (WBC) 11.4 and normal differential, hemoglobin 12.6, and platelets 293. Her electrolytes were within normal limits with the exception of low sodium at 133. Her serum glucose was 108. Urine was obtained with a specific gravity of 1.023, a pH of 5.5, negative urinalysis, negative Gram stain, and negative urine drug screen. Cerebrospinal fluid (CSF) was obtained with glucose 63, protein 14, 1 RBC and 1 WBC; Gram stain was negative for bacteria. Computed tomography (CT) of the head was negative. Rapid antigen testing for influenza A was positive.

Question

What are the risk factors for the development of a first febrile seizure and do these two cases have risk factors for recurrent febrile seizures?

Answer

A family history of febrile seizures is a risk factor for a first febrile seizure and recurrent febrile seizures. Previous observational studies have suggested several risk factors for a first febrile seizure: neonatal discharge after more than 28 days of life, delayed development, child care attendance, low serum sodium, and very high fever. Several historical features are associated with recurrent febrile seizure:

first febrile seizure at a young age, family history of afebrile seizures, short duration of fever, and a relatively low fever at the time of initial seizure.

Discussion

Febrile seizures are the most common type of seizure disorder in childhood and occur in 2% to 5% of young children. After the first episode of febrile seizure, approximately 30% to 35% of children have a recurrence of seizure. The risk of developing epilepsy after a febrile seizure is less than 5%, although certain risk factors (Table 26-1) associated with the seizure may indicate increased risk for the later development of epilepsy. Most febrile seizures occur between 9 months and 5 years of age with a peak age of onset between 14 and 18 months. By definition, febrile seizures must occur in the context of a febrile illness. The seizure may occur after several days of fever or may be the presenting sign of illness. Otitis media and viral syndromes (particularly roseola) are most frequently identified as the etiology of fever leading to febrile seizures. A positive family history of febrile seizures can be found in 25% to 40% of children presenting with febrile seizure. Population-based studies have found no association between febrile seizures and later impairment of cognitive function or neurologic deficits.

Febrile seizures can be classified as "simple" or "complex." A simple febrile seizure consists of generalized tonic–clonic movements lasting less than 10 minutes and resolving spontaneously. They must not have any focal features and the child should quickly return to his or her baseline status without any further seizure activity. Complex febrile seizures are characterized by a focal onset, a focal feature during the seizure or postictal period, duration greater than 10 minutes, or recurrence within 24 hours.

The initial evaluation should be directed toward identifying the etiology of the fever. A new-onset seizure may signal a serious underlying infection such as sepsis or meningitis or may be entirely related to the fever itself. Other causes of seizure include toxins, drug exposures, and electrolyte disturbances. The evaluation should be tailored to the symptoms of the child, with no laboratory studies or imaging routinely recommended. The American Academy of Pediatrics guidelines for the evaluation and treatment of febrile seizure recommend the strong consideration of a lumbar puncture in children younger than 12 months of age recognizing that the classic signs of meningitis may be absent or subtle in young children. Neuroimaging should be considered in children with focal seizures, underlying neurological conditions (including neurocutaneous disorders and micro-/macrocephaly), or a persistent postictal neurologic defect.

Treatment of febrile seizure is primarily directed at treating the underlying cause of the fever. Antipyretics are used for fever control. Phenobarbital has been shown to be effective in preventing recurrent seizure. It is not routinely used as phenobarbital is associated with short-term memory dysfunction, disrupted concentration, and changes in behavior. Valproic acid is also effective but is associated with hepatotoxicity, bone marrow suppression, and pancreatitis. As febrile seizures are self-limited with no long-term sequelae; the risks of anticonvulsant therapy outweigh the benefits. Parents are often advised to give antipyretics at the first sign of fever; however, this has not been shown to reduce the risk of febrile seizure during an acute illness. The use of intermittent diazepam during febrile illnesses has been shown to be effective; however, studies have demonstrated relatively low rates of compliance and significant rates of side effects. Practically, education and reassurance of the parents are the mainstays of treatment.

TABLE 26-1

Risk Factors for Later Development of Epilepsy

Atypical features of seizure

Atypical postictal period

Family history of epilepsy

Initial febrile seizure before 9 months of age

Delayed developmental milestones

Preexisting neurological disorder

Selected References

1. Johnson M. In: Behrman, Kleigman, Jenson, eds. *Nelson Textbook of Pediatrics*. 17th ed. Philadelphia, PA: Saunders; 2004. Chapter 586.
2. Waruiru C, Appleton R. Febrile seizures: an update. *Arch Dis Child.* 2004;89:751–756.
3. Duffner PK, Baumann RJ. A synopsis of the American Academy of Pediatrics' Practice parameters on the evaluation and treatment of children with febrile seizures. *Pediatr Rev.* 1999;20(8):285–287.
4. Baumann RJ. Technical report: treatment of the child with simple febrile seizures. *Pediatrics.* 1999;103(6):e86.
5. Rosman NP, Colton T, Labazzo J, et al. A controlled trial of diazepam administered during febrile illnesses to prevent recurrence of febrile seizures. *N Eng J Med.* 1993;329(2):79–84.

25-Year-Old Male with Recurrent Aseptic Meningitis

CASE PRESENTATION

A 25-year-old African American male with a past medical history of hypertension, childhood asthma, and three bouts of "seizures secondary to viral meningitis" diagnosed by an outside hospital over the previous 2 years presented to the floor of a major university medical center from an outside hospital for further evaluation of recurrent headaches over the past 4 days. The headaches are predominantly frontal in location and are described as a "sharp, throbbing pain." The pain radiates to the occiput and has been present at "all times" over the past 4 days. It is particularly worse after experiencing nausea and is relieved only minimally by nonsteroidal anti-inflammatory drugs (NSAIDs) and acetaminophen (APAP). Associated symptoms include subjective fevers, chills, night sweats, and photophobia. He also reports a possible "seizure-like" episode and recent "memory problems." These memory issues are manifested as short-term memory loss, which has been persistent for the past 1 year. He has a penile lesion that has been present for the past 2 days and a sore on his anus that has been slowly healing over the past 3 weeks. Also significant in his review of system is a 2-week history of "pain in his mouth." His medications at this time only include a calcium channel blocker for his hypertension and an occasional APAP or an over-the-counter NSAID for his headache. While he denies any intravenous (IV) drug and alcohol use, he does admit to a remote history of smoking marijuana and cigarettes.

Physical Examination

Vital signs: temperature 36.8°C, blood pressure 145/65 mm Hg, heart rate 82 beats/min, respiration rate 14 breaths/min. Oxygen saturation was 98% on room air. Patient was awake; alert; and oriented to person, place, and time. On oropharyngeal examination, patient had a rounded ulceration approximately 1.1 cm in diameter that had a white necrotic-appearing base. The remainder of his head, eyes, ears, nose, and throat examination, including a funduscopic examination, was unremarkable. His neck was supple, without lymphadenopathy.

His neck was supple, with no signs of meningismus. His cardiovascular, pulmonary, and abdominal examinations were unremarkable. There was a maculopapular rash in his suprapubic region and a genitourinary examination that was notable for a superficial ulceration seen on the scrotum near the base of his penis. There was no discharge, but it was quite painful with palpation. There was also a perianal lesion that was approximately 1 cm in diameter, indurated and notable for clear discharge. His neurological examination was notable for normal cranial nerve examination, no deficits in either strength or motor function. Patient had normal cerebellar function.

Laboratory Studies

Initial laboratories obtained were notable for serum Na 141, K 5.7, Cl 101, HCO_3 28, blood urea nitrogen 28, creatinine 0.7, and glucose 138. Complete blood count revealed white blood cells 9.4 (with absolute neutrophil count of 8.0, absolute lymphocyte 0.9, absolute monocyte 0.3, and absolute eosinophils 0.0), hematocrit 45.1. Blood and urine cultures were unremarkable. Human immunodeficiency virus (HIV) test was negative as was a purified protein derivative skin testing. Cerebrospinal fluid (CSF) from a lumbar puncture revealed a pleocytosis with low/normal glucose and high protein with bacterial, cryptococcal antigen; VDRL, rapid plasma reagin (RPR), and acid-fast bacillus (AFB), herpes simplex virus (HSV) polymerase chain reaction (PCR) and enterovirus PCR were all negative.

Diagnostic Imaging

Noncontrast head computed tomography (CT) as well as brain magnetic resonance imaging (MRI) were unremarkable.

Case Resolution

The differential diagnosis for unremitting headaches and recurrent aseptic meningitis was extensive and included aseptic meningitis secondary to HSV. The patient was initially placed on broad-spectrum antibiotics until bacterial meningitis was ruled out. His antibiotic coverage was then narrowed to acyclovir until results of the HSV PCR from the CSF came back negative. Despite spiking the temperature to 39.7°C on the night of admission, patient's serum and CSF serologies for viral and bacterial etiologies were negative. The patient was continued on antibiotics for 48 hours after his initial temperature spike. These antibiotics were subsequently discontinued as an infectious workup to this point was unremarkable. It was then decided to obtain a biopsy of the penile lesion. Results of the biopsy were negative for RPR and HSV, but were significant for a process consistent with necrotizing vasculitis. While the erythrocyte sedimentation rate (ESR) was elevated at 65, antinuclear antibody test (ANA), double-stranded DNA, rheumatoid factor (RF), proteinase 3-enzyme-linked immunosorbent assay (PR3-ELISA), and myeloperoxidase-ELISA (MPO-ELISA) serologies were all negative.

Question

Is there a unifying diagnosis for this patient's aseptic meningitis and mucosal ulcerations?

Answer

The differential diagnosis of aseptic meningitis is very broad (Table 27-1). However, the recurrent aseptic meningitis in

TABLE 27-1

Common Causes of Aseptic Meningitis

Viral	Echoviruses
	Coxsackieviruses types A and B
	Herpes simplex type 2 (Mollaret, recurrent)
	Human immunodeficiency virus
	Lymphocytic choriomeningitis virus
	Arboviruses
	Mumps
	Poliovirus
Bacterial	Parameningeal bacterial infection (epidural, subdural abscess)
	Partially treated bacterial meningitis
	Leptospira species
	Borrelia burgdorferi (Lyme disease)
	Mycobacterium tuberculosis
	Bacterial endocarditis
Drugs	Ibuprofen
	Trimethoprim – sulfamethoxazole
	Other NSAIDs
Cancer	Lymphoma
	Leukemia
	Metastatic carcinomas and adenocarcinomas
Autoimmune	Sarcoid
	Behçet disease
	Systemic lupus erythematosus

NSAID, nonsteroidal anti-inflammatory drugs.

combination with associated oral and genital lesions (Table 27-2) suggests a diagnosis of Behçet disease (BD). BD is considered a chronic, multisystem inflammatory vasculitis that is often clinically recognized by recurrent oral and genital ulcerations, uveitis, and erythema nodosum (Table 27-3). The disease is relapsing in nature, with an undulating course of unpredictable exacerbations and remissions. The size of vessels affected vary, as does the type and localization. Treatment is often empiric and directed to the individual and his/her manifestations.

Discussion

The cause of BD has not been fully elucidated. However, the most likely theory centers on the idea of BD as

TABLE 27-2

Diseases Associated with Genital Ulcers

Herpes simplex virus
Syphilis
Chancroid
Lymphogranuloma venereum
Granuloma inguinale
Behçet disease

the result of an autoimmune reaction triggered by certain infectious or environmental agents in a genetically predisposed individual. Suggested infectious etiologies include *Streptococcus sanguis* while immunopathogenic features of BD consist of increased T- and B-cell responses to heat–shock proteins (HSP), increased neutrophil and monocyte activity, and alterations in cytokine levels.

Cases of this multisystem inflammatory vasculitis have been reported from around the world. However, it is more prevalent in countries along the ancient Silk Road, which includes the regions within the Far East (Japan, Korea, etc), the Middle East (Iran, Iraq, Israel, Saudi Arabia, etc), and countries around the Mediterranean Sea (Egypt, Greece, Italy, Turkey, etc). This geographic distribution, in combination of its association with HLA-B5 haplotype as well as the familial aggregation of some affected individuals, supports the idea of a genetic component to BD.

The mean set of onset of BD is 20 to 35 years. The prevalence is higher in men than women, with a male to female ratio of 3:2. It is also more severe and associated with a worse prognosis in young men.

TABLE 27-3

Diagnostic Criteria of Behçet Disease

Major:

Recurrent oral aphthae (at least 3×/year)
+
Minor:

Any *two* of the following:
1. Recurrent genital lesions
2. Eye lesions (uveitis, retinal vasculitis)
3. Skin lesions (eg, nodosum, pseudofolliculitis)
4. Positive pathergy

In 1990, the International Study Group for Behçet disease proposed the following diagnostic criteria: recurrent oral aphthae (defined as occurring at least three times a year) plus any two of the following: recurrent genital ulcerations, positive pathergy, eye lesions (uveitis, retinal vasculitis), skin lesions (erythema nodosum, pseudofolliculitis).

Oral ulcerations are the first manifestation of BD in approximately 87% of patients. The most common sites include the tongue, lips, buccal mucosa, gums, and soft palate. They are either single or multiple in number and are very painful. These oral aphthae are herpetiform in nature and are usually rounded with a white or yellow necrotic base. They are termed as "minor if they are less than 1 cm in size, major if they are greater than 1 cm." These oral lesions usually occur about three times a year and may last anywhere from 1 to 3 weeks.

Genital ulcerations are usually larger, deeper, more painful, and last longer than oral lesions. They rarely occur at the onset of BD. The incidence of genital lesions approaches 75% of patients. They are characterized by a fibrin-covered base. For males, genital ulcers typically involve the scrotum and less frequently on the shaft of the penis and inguinal areas. In females, the most common site of involvement is the labia, but can also include the vagina, as well as the cervix and perianal areas. Scarring is associated with these lesions.

The pathergy reaction is a nonspecific hyperactivity/hypersensitivity reaction induced by an intradermal needle stick. It is performed by puncturing the forearm skin with a 20- or 22-guage sterile needle. A positive test occurs if an erythematous, sterile papule greater than 2 mm diameter develops 24 to 48 hours later. The test reflects polymorphonuclear leukocyte (PMN) infiltration. It is positive in approximately 40% of patients.

Ocular manifestations are the most worrisome complication of BD. The incidence reaches 43% to 65% of patients and usually occurs approximately 3 years after initial symptoms. Again, both the venous and arterial systems can be affected. Involvement usually occurs with anterior uveitis with hypopyon formation or posterior uveitis with retinal involvement. The relapsing nature of BD and ocular manifestations usually resolve after a period of weeks, but can lead to blindness within 5 years if not treated.

The neurological manifestations, as in the patient above, have a prevalence of about 5% to 30%. It can either affect the parenchyma or the vascular system within the central nervous system (CNS). Neurological symptoms usually present after systemic symptoms. Manifestations include meningoencephalitis, cranial nerve palsies, hemiplegia, or peripheral nerve involvement. Imaging studies, such as

MRI, can reveal the multifocal nature of the disease and lesions that are 4 to 10 mm in size. Interestingly, BD does not affect periventricular regions. Neuropathology usually reflects demyelination with vasculitis, multifocal necrosis, and perivascular cuffing with lymphocytes or PMNs.

There are a few controlled studies of the management of the BD. Moreover, the assessment of efficacy of therapy is limited by the natural waxing and waning of the disease. Thus, treatment for BD is largely symptomatic and empirical. It is usually tailored to the clinical manifestations of each patient. Hence, mucocutaneous manifestations of BD may be treated with topical anesthetics, topical glucocorticoids, oral colchicines, dapsone, and/or topical sucralfate. More severe ulceration may require systemic steroids, thalidomide, or immunosuppressive agents. Ocular lesions can be treated with topical mydriatics, glucocorticoids, and/or other systemic immunosuppressive agents. Significant ocular, neurologic, and vascular manifestations may require both steroids as well as other immunosuppressive agents. Prednisone at 1 mg/kg/day for 1 month is a recommended starting dose for steroid therapy; however, pulse therapy with IV methylprednisolone may be used for life-threatening disease.

BD runs a chronic course that is characterized by unpredictable exacerbations and remissions. It is thought that BD may become less severe after approximately 20 years. Increased severity is noted to be increased amongst the young, male, and Middle Eastern or Far Eastern patients. Mortality is approximately 9.8% amongst BD patients. This comes largely from CNS, ocular, and large vessel arterial/venous involvement. Mucocutaneous and ocular disease is typically worst during the early years of BD. For those patients who develop CNS and large vessel disease, these manifestations typically occur later during the course of the disease.

Selected References

1. Al-Otaibi L. Behcet's disease: a review. *J Dent Res.* 2005;84(3): 209–222.
2. Haghighi A, Pourmand R, Nikseresht AR. Neuro-Behcet disease: a review. *Neurologist.* March 2005;11(2):80–89.
3. Onder M. The multiple faces of Behcet's diease and its aetiological factors. *J Eur Acad Dermatol Venereol.* 2001;15:126–136.
4. http://vasculitis.med.jhu.edu/typesof/behcets

3-Day-Old Female Infant with a Murmur

CASE PRESENTATION

The patient is a 3-day-old Caucasian female infant born at 36 weeks to a 22-year-old gravida 1, para 1 with blood type A+, with otherwise normal prenatal laboratory tests. The infant was born via normal spontaneous vaginal delivery after preterm labor, complicated by premature and prolonged rupture of membranes. The maternal prenatal course was uncomplicated and the mother had normal screening ultrasounds at 8 and 20 weeks' gestation. Birth weight was 2339 g and Apgar scores were 8 and 9 at 1 and 5 minutes, respectively. The patient was transferred to the newborn nursery without immediate postnatal complications. She was observed only during the first 24 hours of life, but was noted on day of life 2 to have increased work of breathing with breast feedings and baseline tachypnea. Subsequently, during the second routine newborn examination, the patient was noted to have a murmur that prompted further evaluation. There was no family history of congenital heart disease (CHD) nor were there early childhood deaths in the family. Parents were both without illnesses.

Physical Examination

Patient is a small-for-gestational-age infant, in mild respiratory distress. Vital signs: temperature 37°C, pulse 158 beats/min, blood pressure 80/55 mm Hg, respiratory rate 50 breaths/min, SaO_2 98% on room air. Head, eyes, ears, nose, and throat: normocephalic; atraumatic; anterior fontanelle was open, soft, and flat; mild micrognathia; and low-set ears. Cardiovascular examination: grade 3/6 systolic ejection murmur (see Table 28-1 for grading murmurs), low pitched and blowing, best heard at left lower sternal border with radiation to the axilla; the patient had a hyperdynamic precordium, but otherwise normal S_1 and S_2 heart sounds were audible. Upper and lower extremity pulses equal and 1+, with greater than 3-second capillary refill. Pulmonary examination showed tachypnea but symmetric chest raise bilaterally, lungs clear, no retractions, or increased work of breathing. Abdomen was soft, nondistended, normal active bowel sounds, liver palpable 1 cm below costal margin. Skin examination was warm and well perfused, no rashes or lesions. Infant was moving all extremities, no hip clicks, no cyanosis or edema. Neurological examination was normal grossly with normal tone, normal root, normal suck.

Laboratory Studies

Initial arterial blood gas showed pH 7.5/PCO_2 41/PaO_2 94. Chemistries revealed Na 134, K 2.8, glucose 101, ionized calcium 3.8, hemoglobin 10 g/dL. Two-dimensional echocardiogram showed normal atrial sidedness and atrioventricular (AV) connections, but a common arterial trunk overriding a large subaortic ventricular septal defect (VSD), mild truncal insufficiency, and stenosis. A main pulmonary artery segment bifurcating into left and right pulmonary arteries was noted, consistent with truncus arteriosus type I, with right ventricular hypertrophy (RVH) and patent ductus arteriosus (PDA).

Chest x-ray: Cardiomegaly with increased pulmonary vascularity.

Electrocardiogram (ECG): RVH, but otherwise normal for age with normal intervals.

Case Resolution

After truncus arteriosus was documented on echocardiography, the patient was transferred from the newborn nursery to the pediatric intensive care unit (PICU) and

TABLE 28-1

Classification of Murmurs Based on Intensity and the Presence or Absence of a Palpable Thrill on Physical Examination

Grade of murmur	Intensity	Thrill or no thrill
1	Barely audible	NO Thrill
2	Soft but easily audible	NO Thrill
3	Loudest sound in the chest	NO Thrill
4	Loudest sound in the chest	Thrill
5	Loud, stethoscope barely on the chest	Thrill
6 (rare)	Audible, stethoscope off chest	Thrill

Adapted from Park, Myung. The Pediatric Cardiology Handbook. *3rd ed. Philadelphia PA: Mosby Inc; 2003.*

started on an intravenous prostaglandin infusion to maintain patency of the ductus arteriosus, to allow mixing of systemic oxygenated blood flow. She was managed with supportive care in the PICU for weight gain in anticipation of surgical repair. On day of life 10, she developed worsening feeding intolerance and respiratory distress and was taken to the operating room for repair. The patient's intraoperative course was unremarkable. However, postoperatively, the infant developed junctional ectopic tachycardia and cardiac failure. The patient went on to survive and was transferred to the cardiac stepdown unit 14 days after surgery.

Question

What is the incidence of murmur and CHD in the newborn population? What abnormalities on this patient's physical examination prompted further evaluation and when is further diagnostic evaluation warranted?

Answer

The incidence of CHD is less than 1% of all live births; however, up to 90% (average 50%–70%) of infants in the newborn period up to 6 months of age will have a murmur on physical examination. There are a few things noted on this patient's physical examination that prompted further evaluation, including a systolic ejection murmur, diminished pulses, and decreased capillary refill, as well as the facial anomalies including the noted micrognathia and

low-set ears which are often associated with CHD. Although it is difficult to define the character of a neonatal murmur on routine neonatal examination, it is important never to miss a diastolic, continuous, or greater than grade 3/6 murmur which is generally associated with structural heart disease and requires echocardiographic evaluation. Also it is important to listen for abnormalities of the second heart sound which is most commonly associated with structural heart disease.

Discussion

The prevalence of CHD is approximately 6 cases/1000 live births, but most cases are asymptomatic at birth because of some persistence of fetal circulation. Because there is a spectrum of severity of CHD in newborns, the newborn clinical examination is integral in identifying patients with CHD. By performing serial newborn examinations and watching for specific signs and symptoms of heart disease in the newborn period, those infants with life-threatening anomalies requiring intervention are identified. See Table 28-2 for quick reference of most common murmurs found on physical examination of the newborn and young infant and the associated CHD.

It is well documented that detecting congenital or structural heart disease in the neonatal period is quite difficult. A prospective study in England evaluated 7204 newborn infants born between 1995 and 1996 and concluded that only 44% of cardiac malformations are found with routine neonatal evaluation, defined as abnormal physical examination, namely, cyanosis or murmur. However in

TABLE 28-2

Murmurs in the Neonatal Period and Recommended Evaluation

Murmur	Post natal age audible	Anatomic abnormality	Evaluation	Refer to cardiology (yes or no)	Treatment or intervention
Soft 1–2/6 systolic ejection murmur (SEM) at LUSB with radiation to back and axilla	Birth–6 months	Peripheral pulmonic stenosis (**PPS**): benign murmur due to branch pulmonary artery hypoplasia	No further evaluation necessary, follow clinically	No or yes if louder at > 6 months	None (disappears with age)
Continuous "machine like," 2-4/6 SEM	dol 1–2 but can persist in premature infants	Patent ductus arteriosis (**PDA**): persistent fetal circulation with connection between aorta and pulmonary artery	CXR, ECHO	Yes	Close clinical monitoring for closure or surgical closure if symptomatic
Grade 3/6 SEM if small and grade 1–2/6 if large	2–6 weeks	Ventricular septal defect (**VSD**): most common, can present with heart failure, lesion is large with large L to R shunt	CXR, ECG, ECHO	Yes	Small: likely to close spontaneously (70–80% by 2 yr), large requires operative closure
Grade 1–3/6 SEM best heard at the left back	1–6 weeks	Coarctation of the aorta (**COA**): narrowing of aorta usually at the ductus arteriosis	CXR (rib notching), ECG, ECHO, examine LE pulses	Yes	Surgical repair of aortic narrowing
Grade 2–5/6 SEM at RUSB	Newborn	Aortic valve stenosis (**AS**): subvalvar, valvar, or supravalvar obstruction, often associated with bicuspid aortic valve	ECHO	Yes	Balloon opening of valve area or surgical replacement of valve
Grade 2–5/6 SEM at LUSB, sometimes continuous at back	Newborn	Pulmonary valve stenosis (**PS**): valvular, subvalvular, or supravalvular obstruction, usually with Tetralogy of Fallot (**TOF**) or Noonan syndrome	ECHO	Yes	Prostaglandin E2 immediately, long-term management with balloon valvuloplasty or surgical repair
Grade 2–4/6 systolic ejection murmur at LMSB Loud S2	Newborn – 1 month	Tetralogy of Fallot (**TOF**): RVOT obstruction, VSD, overriding aorta, RV hypertrophy (remember murmur is RVOT obstruction not VSD)	ECHO, CXR	Yes	Prostaglandin E2 immediately if PS (cyanosis), long-term staged or one-time complete repair

(*Continued*)

TABLE 28-2

Murmurs in the Neonatal Period and Recommended Evaluation (*Continued*)

Murmur	Post natal age audible	Anatomic abnormality	Evaluation	Refer to cardiology (yes or no)	Treatment or intervention
Grade 2–3/6 SEM, diastolic rumble. Sometimes no murmur present	Newborn (if venous obstruction present)	Total anomalous pulmonary venous return (**TAPVR**): pulmonary veins drain to RA or tributaries instead of LA	ECHO, CXR (snowman sign)	Yes	Prostaglandin E2 immediately, long-term surgical repair
Grade 2–4/6 SEM at LUSB + high pitched diastolic murmur	Newborn	Truncus arteriosis (**TA**): single vessel for pulmonary and systemic circulation, always VSD (murmur), 4 types	ECHO	Yes	Inotropic support with digoxin and afterload reduction with diuretics
Grade 3–4/6 holosystolic murmur at LLSB, thrill and dynamic precordium	Newborn – 3 months	Atrioventricular septal defect (**AVSD**): endocardial cushion defect, ASD with VSD, Most common in Down syndrome	ECHO, CXR (cardiomegaly)	Yes	Inotropic support with digoxin and afterload reduction with diuretics
Grade 2–3/6 SEM if VSD present, no murmur with loud S2 if no VSD	Newborn – 6 weeks	Transpoistion of the great arteries (**TGA**): aorta from RV and pulmonary artery from LV, requires PDA or VSD for mixing	ECHO, CXR (egg-shaped heart, narrow mediastinum)	Yes	Prostaglandin E2 immediately, if no VSD then atrial septostomy (Rashkind procedure)

this study, if a murmur is present on examination, there is a 54% chance that the patient has structural heart disease and should be referred for further evaluation and diagnosis. These data were further supported by a large study of 20,000 infants whose sole abnormal physical examination finding was a murmur. In this cohort, 86% were found to have structural heart lesions on echocardiogram, thus supporting the idea that if a murmur is noted on physical examination during the neonatal period, further evaluation is warranted.

Luckily, the patient mentioned above was found to have a murmur on physical examination and referred for further evaluation and immediate therapy. However, this is not always the case and it should make clinicians more aware of physical examination findings that are consistent with CHD. A retrospective study looking at children born with CHD in England between 1987 and 1994 noted that only 45% were diagnosed during the first routine neonatal examination, one-third were diagnosed by abnormal physical examination findings at 6 weeks, and all were diagnosed by 3 months. However, owing to the fact that more than 50% were discharged from the hospital without detection of disease and final diagnosis did not occur until 3 months of age suggests that a thorough cardiac examination and further evaluation of murmurs should be part of the routine neonatal physical examination likely through a year of age.

It is important to understand the limitations of physical examination when it comes to the definitive diagnosis of structural heart disease, solely based on a murmur. Further evaluation is required with imaging in most cases of neonatal murmurs. Currently the gold standard for evaluation of a child with a murmur is an echocardiogram. Classical teaching has taught that chest x-ray and ECG are also helpful in the diagnosis of CHD, but recent literature would suggest otherwise. A study of asymptomatic infants with a murmur who were evaluated by chest radiograph showed little predictive value in identifying the presence or absence of heart disease. Similarly, a study looking at a parallel population who were evaluated by ECG noted no significant difference in the detection of heart disease, and often times the study was misleading. However, once a structural lesion is identified on echocardiogram, an ECG can be helpful in further defining the disease.

In summary, the cardiac examination in a newborn infant is imperative for the identification of structural heart disease. A murmur noted on examination in the newborn period is more likely to be indicative of CHD than that found in an older child. It is also important to continue thorough cardiac examination during the first 6 months of life because of life-threatening lesions that may present after hospital discharge. In most cases, detection of a murmur in the neonatal period should prompt referral to a pediatric cardiologist where an echocardiogram can be completed and a definitive diagnosis obtained.

Selected References

1. Ainsworth S, Wyllie J, Wren C. Prevalence and clinical significance of cardiac murmurs in neonates. *Arch Dis Child Fetal Neonatal Ed.* 1999;80:F34–F45.
2. Wren C, Richmond S, Donaldson L. Presentation of congenial heart disease in infancy: implications for routine examination. *Arch Dis Child Fetal Neonatal Ed.* 1999;80:F49–F53.
3. Birkeback NH, Hansen LK, Elle B, et al. Chest roentgenogram in the evaluation of heart defects in asymptomatic infants and children with a cardiac murmur: reproducibility and accuracy. *Pediatrics.* 1999;103(2):E15.
4. Poddar B, Basu S. Approach to a child with a heart murmur. *Indian J Pediatr.* 2004;71(1):63–66.
5. Danford DA, Gumbiner CH, Martin AB, et al. Effects of electrocardiography and chest radiograph on the accuracy of preliminary diagnosis of common congenital cardiac defects. *Pediatr Cardiol.* 2000;2(4):334–340.
6. Park MK. *The Pediatric Cardiology Handbook.* 3rd ed. Philidelphia, PA: Mosby Inc; 2003.
7. Rein AJ, Omokhodion SI, Nira A. Significance of a cardiac murmur as the sole clinical sign in the newborn. *Clin Pediatr (Phila).* 2000 September;39(9):511–520.
8. Frommelt M. Differential diagnosis and approach to a heart murmur in term infants. *Pediatr Clin N Am.* 2004;51:1023–1032.
9. Altman CA. Suspected heart disease in the newborn: criteria for referral. www.uptodateonline.com. Accessed August 2006.

3-Year-Old Male with Presumed Viral Upper Respiratory Infection

CASE PRESENTATION

A 3-year-old male presented to his primary care physician with the chief complaint of fever, congestion, rhinorrhea, and cough. Rapid influenza and streptococcal tests performed in the office were negative. He was sent home with symptomatic care for presumed viral upper respiratory infection (URI). He returned to his primary medical doctor's office 2 days later with nonbilious, nonbloody vomiting; persistent fever (T_{max} 41°C); and poor oral intake. His parents denied any history of diarrhea or rash. He was sent to the emergency room for evaluation, found to have a right lower lobe infiltrate chest x-ray, and was admitted for intravenous (IV) ceftriaxone and rehydration. The day following admission he developed coffee-ground emesis, epistaxis, tea-colored urine, pallor, tachycardia, and periorbital edema. His past medical history is significant for Marfan syndrome and autism with severe speech delay. The patient's sister had also been sick with fever and URI symptoms. The following examination and laboratory information is from his hospital day 1.

Physical Examination

The patient was a toxic-appearing male, tachypneic and moaning. Vital signs: temperature 38°C, pulse 152 beats/min, respiratory rate 42 breaths/min, blood pressure (BP) 95/63 mm Hg, saturations 95% on room air. Head, eyes, ears, nose, and throat examination revealed dried blood in the right nares. Neck revealed no rigidity, but patient moaned on attempted passive motion. Cardiovascular examination revealed tachycardia and a hyperdynamic precordium with grade 2/6 systolic ejection murmur. The right lung field had markedly decreased air movement with crackles at the base. He had mild intercostal retractions, but no flaring or grunting. Abdominal examination was unremarkable. Examination of the extremities revealed scattered petechiae over the dorsum of both feet with generalized mottling and delayed capillary refill of 4 to 5 seconds. Neurological examination was nonfocal but difficult, given the patient's underlying nonverbal status.

Laboratory Studies

Complete blood count (CBC) showed white blood cells (WBC) 11.5, hemoglobin 9.4, hematocrit (Hct) 27.4, platelets (plt) 9. Chemistries showed Na 129, K 3.9, Cl 106, HCO_3 14, blood urea nitrogen (BUN) 59, creatinine (Cr) 1.4. Lactate dehydrogenase was three times the upper limit of normal. Direct Coombs test was normal. Chest x-ray (CXR): right-sided mobile effusion and right lower lobe infiltrate (Fig. 29-1). Blood culture were drawn. Repeat laboratory tests 6 hours later were significant for Hgb 6.8, Hct 19, BUN 74, and Cr 1.8.

Case Resolution

Blood cultures on admission were positive for *Streptococcus pneumoniae,* with intermediate resistance to penicillin and sensitivity to ceftriaxone. The patient was transferred to an

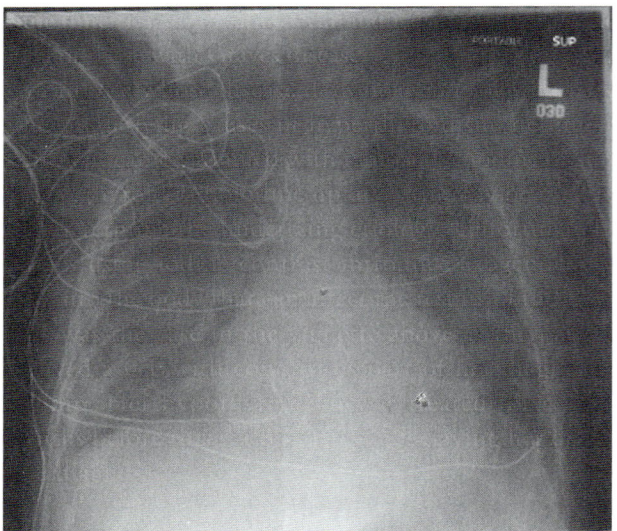

Figure 29-1 Anterioposterior CXR showing an infiltrate in the right lower lobe and an pleural effusion.

intensive care setting where he was resuscitated with 60 mL/kg of normal saline, transfused platelets, and red blood cells (RBCs); started on vancomycin and IV proton pump inhibitor. He had a 15-second episode of generalized tonic–clonic activity and was loaded with fosphenytoin. Head computed tomography was negative. Echocardiogram revealed no vegetations. The following morning he developed oliguria and hypertension. Urinalysis revealed 3+ blood, 2+ protein, hyaline and muddy brown casts suggestive of acute tubular necrosis. His Cr rose to 3.0 and he had a persistent metabolic acidosis necessitating transfer to a tertiary care center for dialysis. Peripheral blood smear revealed schistocytes, and his working diagnosis was *Streptococcus pneumoniae*–associated hemolytic uremic syndrome (SP–HUS), pneumococcal pneumonia, and presumed meningitis. Initially he required dialysis daily for 3 days, transitioned to 3 × /week dialysis for 1 week, and subsequently had return of his renal function. He did require several blood transfusions for ongoing hemolysis and multiple antihypertensive medications. Additionally he required chest tube placement for pleural effusion associated with his pneumonia. Pleural fluid was sterile. A lumbar puncture (LP) was never performed owing to his thrombocytopenia and he was treated for 21 days with vancomycin and ceftriaxone for presumed meningitis. He was discharged home on hospital day 24 on furosimide, atenolol, and lisinopril to control his BP.

Question

How frequently is *S. pneumoniae* associated with HUS and what is the prognosis?

Answer

HUS is classified as typical (D+) or atypical (D−). Ninety percent of cases of HUS are typical, associated with infectious colitis. The remaining 10% are because of a variety of causes including drugs, chronic illnesses, and other organisms. *Streptococcus pneumoniae* is one of the more recognized causes of atypical HUS. The true incidence is unknown.

Discussion

HUS is the most common cause of acute renal failure in infants and young children. HUS is characterized by the triad of hemolytic anemia, thrombocytopenia, and acute renal failure. In most instances, HUS is associated with infectious colitis, namely, because of *Escherichia coli* 0157:H7, and is referred to as D+ HUS. Other causes of D+ HUS include shigella and salmonella. The atypical, or D−, form of HUS is less common in childhood. Etiologies implicated in D− HUS include certain drugs, especially chemotherapeutics; underlying medical conditions, including systemic lupus erythematous, cancer, bone marrow transplant; and other infectious agents, including streptococcal pneumoniae, Epstein-Barr virus, coxsackievirus, and influenza.

The pathogenesis of *E. coli*–associated HUS is caused by Shiga toxin production by the bacteria, which causes endothelial injury and a release of mediators which lead to thrombus formation. Endothelial injury in the glomerular capillaries accounts for the nephropathy. Additionally, circulating RBCs are deformed and injured by traveling in occluding vessels (causing characteristic schistocytes), get picked up and destroyed by the reticuloendothelial system, and cause anemia. The pathogenesis of SP–HUS has been theorized to be mediated by neuraminidase produced by the bacteria. This neuraminidase has been proposed to expose a usually hidden T-cell antigen on the surface of RBCs causing an antibody–antigen-mediated activation and ensuing injury.

Laboratory data supporting a diagnosis of HUS include normochromic normocytic anemia, elevated reticulocyte count, thrombocytopenia, blood smear with schistocytes or helmet cells, normal coagulation profile, negative direct Coombs test, elevated lactate dehydrogenase, and decreased haptoglobin. There are varying degrees of renal involvement which may manifest as uremia and/or electrolyte abnormalities.

Renal involvement in HUS is varied. Clinical features range from normal urine output with minimal hematuria and proteinuria to severe renal failure/anuria requiring dialysis. Progression to end-stage renal disease (ESRD) has been documented. Hypertension is common, occurring in 50% of children with HUS.

It is generally known that the prognosis for D+ HUS is better than for D− HUS. D− HUS comes with an increased risk for ESRD, chronic renal failure, hypertension, and recurrence. A 2002 *Pediatrics* article by Brandt et al compared clinical outcomes of 12 patients with SP–HUS with 17 patients with *E. coli*–associated HUS. Their findings supported the generally held belief of worse outcomes for D− HUS, citing increased need for dialysis, longer hospital stay, and greater number of RBC transfusions. The chart below summarizes the results of the study.

Treatment for D+ and D− HUS is largely supportive and consists of fluid/electrolyte management, dialysis, if indicated, and control of hypertension to prevent encephalopathy and congestive heart failure. RBC transfusion may be required depending on the degree of ongoing hemolysis. Platelet transfusion is controversial and generally required only pre-procedure or for active bleeding. There is some thought that platelet transfusion may contribute to ongoing microthrombus formation.

In summary, HUS is a common cause of acute renal failure in children. Although less common, SP–HUS is a recognized entity. While treatment of HUS is the same regardless of the cause, the prognosis for D− HUS is generally worse.

	Dialysis	Hospital days	Days of oliguria	Number of RBC transfusions	ESRD
D+ HUS	59%	16	5.9	2	5%
SP– HUS	75%	33	13.2	8	17%

ESRD, end-stage renal failure; HUS, hemolytic uremic syndrome; RBC, red blood cells; SP−HUS, *Streptococcus pneumoniae–associated hemolytic uremic syndrome.*

Adapted from Brandt J, Wong C, Mihm S, et al. Invasive pneumococcal disease and hemolytic uremic syndrome. Pediatrics. *2002;110:371–376.*

Selected References

1. American Academy of Pediatrics. Pneumococcal infections. In: Pickering LK, ed. *Red Book: 2006 Report of the Committee on Infectious Disease.* 27th ed. Elk Grove Village, IL: American Academy of Pediatrics; 2006:525–537.
2. Brandt J, Wong C, Mihm S, et al. Invasive pneumococcal disease and hemolytic uremic syndrome. *Pediatrics.* 2002;110:371–376.
3. Durbin WJ. Pneumococcal infections. *Pediatrics Rev.* 2005;22:418–424.
4. Corrigan JJ, Boineau FG. Hemolytic-Uremic syndrome. *Pediatrics Rev.* 2001;22:365–369.
5. Cochran JB, Panzarino VM, Maes LY, et al. Pneumococcal-induced T-antigen activation in hemolytic uremic syndrome and anemia. *Pediatr Nephrol.* 2004;19:317–321.
6. Siegler R, Oakes R. Hemolytic uremic syndrome: pathogenesis, treatment, and outcome. *Curr Opin Pediatr.* 2005;17:200–204.

36-Year-Old Male with New Bilateral Lower Extremity Edema

CASE PRESENTATION

A 36-year-old African American male presents to the urgent care clinic Saturday morning complaining of swelling in his lower extremities. He first noted the swelling upon waking 5 days prior and has never had it before. He denies associated pain, skin changes, trauma or insect/tick bites, and has no relevant surgical history. He reports occasional dyspnea with prolonged exertion, but denies any episodic shortness of breath while at rest or performing his daily activities. He denies orthopnea and paroxysmal nocturnal dyspnea, but states that he snores, and that his wife occasionally has to nudge him from sleep when, as she describes, he stops breathing. He denies hematuria, dysuria, urinary hesitancy, and incontinence. He has two to three episodes of nocturia most nights, and reports some foaming in his urine. He does not have a personal physician, and last sought medical attention 1 year ago for a kidney stone which he passed without incident. He has had no recent illnesses, including respiratory infections, and denies any other past medical history. He rarely drinks during the week, but often has 4 to 8 beers on Friday and Saturday nights, and has done so since he was a teenager. He smokes 5 to 10 cigarettes per day for the past 20 years but denies any history of intravenous drug use. He has several tattoos from various tattoo parlors he trusts. He has been married 3 years, and been monogamous with the same woman for 10 years preceding their marriage. He takes no medications on a regular basis, but uses ibuprofen occasionally for knee pain after playing basketball. His family history is notable for breast cancer in his mother, alcoholism in his father, and diabetes amongst several of his 15 brothers and sisters.

Physical Examination

The patient is a well-appearing, obese male, sitting comfortably in a clinic chair, his feet propped on an adjacent chair. Vital signs: temperature 37°C, pulse 75 beats/min, blood pressure 144/92 mm Hg, respiratory rate 14 breaths/min; body mass index (BMI) 40. His sclerae are nonicteric, his neck supple, and thyroid symmetric. His cardiac examination reveals a normal S_1, S_2; a regular rate and rhythm; without murmurs, gallops, or rubs. His right-sided jugular vein is barely detectable 2 in above his sternal notch. The lung fields are clear bilaterally. His abdomen is obese, protuberant, but soft, nontender, without palpable organomegaly or masses, or detectable shifting dullness. There is no hepatojugular reflux. He has 2+ pitting edema from his feet to his mid pretibial regions bilaterally, without local skin changes. He has strong palpable pulses in all extremities.

Laboratory Studies

Initial laboratory values obtained include Na 139, K 3.8, Cl 111, HCO_3 25, blood urea nitrogen (BUN) 17, creatinine 1.9, glucose 96. Thyroid-stimulating hormone (TSH) was 1.82. Glycohemoglobin (HgbA1C) was 5.9.

A routine urinalysis showed a specific gravity of 1.010, pH 6.5, leukocyte esterase negative, nitrite negative, protein 3+, glucose negative, blood 1+.

Urine microscopy revealed occasional oval fat bodies with multiple hyaline casts and rare fine granular casts.

No white blood cells (WBCs) or red blood cells (RBCs). No cellular casts.

Case Resolution

With what appeared to be nephrotic syndrome of unknown etiology in the setting of significant renal insufficiency, a nephrology consultant was called to see the patient in the urgent care center. They noted the above findings on urine microscopy and requested a more detailed serologic evaluation to gain insight into the origin of the patient's condition. The patient was discharged to home later that afternoon. His final laboratory results were as follows:

Albumin 2.2, total protein 4.9, human immunodeficiency virus enzyme-linked immunosorbent assay (HIV ELISA) negative, hepatitis B panel negative, hepatitis C antibody negative, rapid plasma reagin (RPR) negative, antineutrophil cytoplasmic antibody (ANCA) negative, C3/C4 = within normal limits, myeloperoxidase (MPO), and proteinase 3-ANCA (PR3-ANCA) negative, antinuclear antibody test (ANA) negative, serum protein electrophoresis (SPEP) and urine protein electrophoresis (UPEP) without monoclonal protein, urine protein/creatinine ratio = 6.17, total cholesterol 329, low-density lipoproteins (LDL) 219, triglycerides 319.

One week later, with no clear etiology for the patient's condition, a renal biopsy was performed. Examination of the tissue by light microscope revealed multiple glomeruli with segmental sclerotic lesions. Immunofluorescence was notable for the absence of immunoglobulin deposits. Electron microscopy was notable for broad visceral epithelial (podocyte) foot process effacement and the absence of any immune complex deposits.

Question

What causes of nephrotic syndrome should be considered in this patient prior to biopsy and what is his final diagnosis considering all available information?

Answer

Conditions causing nephrotic syndrome defined as massive proteinuria, hypoalbuminemia, hyperlipidemia, and edema may be considered in two categories. The first is primary renal diseases, conditions that mainly affect the kidney. Examples include glomerular nephropathies. The second category includes secondary systemic diseases, those whose effects are seen throughout multiple organ systems. Examples include diabetes, amyloidosis, and systemic lupus erythematosus (SLE). Though this division is somewhat artificial and not a systemic disease, it does not rule out the need for a detailed renal evaluation, it may be helpful in constructing a focused differential diagnosis. In this case, there was no evidence of a systemic disease process.

Consideration of a patient's age and race can further focus the differential diagnosis (Table 30-1). This is well illustrated

TABLE 30-1

Age-Related Differences in Causes of Unexplained Nephrotic Syndrome in White and Black Adults: Top Four Diagnoses Ranked by Relative Frequency

Rank	White patients <45	White patients ≥45	Black patients <45	Black patients ≥45
1	Membranous nephropathy	Membranous nephropathy	FSGS	FSGS
2	Minimal-change nephropathy	Minimal-change nephropathy/ FSGS@	Membranous nephropathy	Membranous nephropathy
3	FSGS	Amyloid	Minimal-change nephropathy	Minimal-change nephropathy
4	IgA nephropathy	IgA nephropathy	IgA Nephropathy	Amyloid

FSGC, focal segmental glomerulosclerosis.

Table modified from M. Haas et. al. Changing etiologies of unexplained adult nephrotic syndrome: a comparison of renal biopsy findings from 1976–1979 and 1995–1997. Am. J Kidney Dis. 1997 Nov;30(5):621–31.

in a retrospective review of biopsies from patients with nephrotic syndrome, but without an identified responsible systemic disease. For instance, biopsies from patients with diabetes, the most common cause of nephrotic syndrome, lupus, hepatitis B, and hepatitis C, were excluded. In this review, amyloidosis, a rare condition in young adults, was the fourth most common cause of idiopathic nephrotic syndrome in those older than 45 years of age. It should therefore be considered in any older adult presenting with heavy proteinuria. Also of note, the most common cause of idiopathic nephrotic syndrome in white adults of all ages was membranous nephropathy. Meanwhile, in black adults, focal segmental glomerulosclerosis (FSGS) was most common.

Applying the population data above to the presented case, the most common causes of idiopathic nephrotic syndrome in young African American adults is FSGS, membranous nephropathy, and minimal change nephropathy. The absence of sizeable immune complex deposits by electron microscopy eliminates membranous nephropathy from the differential. The finding of segmental sclerosis on light microscopy eliminates minimal change disease, a condition defined by normal-appearing glomeruli on light microscopy, but foot process effacement by electron microscope. The findings of segmental sclerosis by light microscopy and podocyte foot process effacement by electron microscopy, in the context of the clinical presentation, are most consistent with FSGS. The next important step is to determine whether this is primary or secondary disease.

Discussion

FSGS describes the common pathologic finding of partial glomerular consolidation/sclerosis in a limited number of glomeruli, and may result from any number of disease processes. Multiple overlapping classification systems exist in an attempt to organize causal processes and define effective treatments. One such system, increasingly seen in the literature, defines five distinct histologic patterns of FSGS: collapsing, tip, perihilar, cellular, and FSGS not otherwise specified, attempting to link each with clinical characteristics of disease. However, as the clinical utility of this system is evolving, arguably the most basic and essential categorical distinction for clinical management is that of secondary versus primary FSGS, as this determination is critical to defining a treatment plan. Table 30-2 illustrates overlap in several categorizations.

TABLE 30-2

Classification of Focal Segmental Glomerulosclerosis (FSGS) into Primary or Secondary Varieties with Associated Conditions

Primary (idiopathic) FSGS
Typical (not otherwise specified) FSGS
Glomerular tip lesion variant of FSGS
Collapsing glomerulopathy variant of FSGS
Perihilar variant of FSGS
Familial FSGS – with no discernable mutation (see below in Secondary FSGS)

Secondary (with associated causes) FSGS and known associations
With advanced HIV disease (typically collapsing variant)
With IV drug abuse
With glomerulomegaly (usually perihilar variant) seen in
- Morbid obesity
- Sickle cell disease
- Cyanotic congenital heart disease
- Hypoxic pulmonary disease
Reduced renal mass seen in
- Unilateral renal agenesis
- Oligomeganephronia
- Reflux-interstitial nephritis
- Postfocal cortical necrosis
- Post nephrectomy
Drug toxicity
- Pamidronate (typically collapsing)
- Lithium
Specific familial mutations described
- α-actinin-4 mutations (autosomal dominant)
- Podocin mutations (autosomal recessive)
- Nephrin mutations (autosomal recessive)

Secondary FSGS describes the above pattern of glomerular scarring in the context of a strongly associated exposure including HIV, heroin, or pamidronate or a clinical condition including vasculitis, SLE, hypertension, or morbid obesity. Though the precise pathogenesis is dependent upon the causal condition or exposure, and in most cases, is incompletely understood, two distinct, but often overlapping, pathways have been described.

In the first, an independent systemic process, such as vasculitis or SLE, causes local injury which, in the healing phase, results in focal sclerosis. As an example, in the case of SLE, complexes of antigen and immunoglobulin deposit within the layers of the glomeruli. This stimulates local inflammation, cytokine release, and ultimately, scarring. Patients may continue to have stable levels of proteinuria long after the initial injury has occurred and the causal process is controlled. In the second, often overlapping, process, glomeruli undergo a transition to hypertrophy and hyperfiltration, either as a compensatory adaptation to nephron loss, as in the setting of renal agenesis or hypertensive nephrosclerosis, or as the result of renal vasodilatation, as in the setting of obesity and diabetic nephropathy. The associated hemodynamic changes lead to intraglomerular hypertension, transcapillary passage of macromolecules, and ultimately segmental sclerosis. It is thought that the hemodynamic modulating effects of angiotensin-converting enzyme inhibitors (ACE-Is) and angiotensin receptor blockers (ARBs) may temporize this destructive physiology.

In comparison to secondary FSGS, primary FSGS (also known as idiopathic FSGS) has no identifiable cause. One commonly sighted investigation identified the presence of a circulating "permeability factor" in patients with FSGS, and suggested this factor may be responsible, in part, for the high rate of FSGS recurrence in transplanted kidneys. It is this rationale that supports the use of plasmapheresis after renal transplant in FSGS patients in an attempt to prevent recurrence, though this has proven to be of limited value. As FSGS is a common pathologic outcome of various heterogeneous processes, there is unlikely a single cause for what is currently labeled primary/idiopathic disease.

For example, recent investigations suggest an increasing role for genetic mutations, viruses and viral infections, and dysregulated cytokine expression. Genetic mutations including mutations in the *ACTN4* gene, encoding α-actinin-4, have been associated with an autosomal dominant form of FSGS, though, technically, familial forms of FSGS would not be considered idiopathic. Parvovirus B19 is commonly present in patients with FSGS, and cytokines such as transforming growth factor-β1 have been implicated in the pathogenesis of FSGS.

Clinical presentation, past medical history, and laboratory evaluation can be helpful in distinguishing primary from secondary disease. Primary FSGS typically presents as the acute onset of nephrotic syndrome, compared to secondary FSGS which has a more indolent course and rarely is associated with hypoalbuminemia or edema. The presence of known risk factors for proteinuria or strong family history of kidney disease should raise suspicion for secondary disease, but does not rule out the possibility of primary FSGS. For example, hypertension, obesity, and obstructive sleep apnea (OSA) are widely prevalent in the American population and commonly associated with proteinuria. However, they are rarely associated with nephrotic syndrome, so that a patient presenting with these conditions and high levels of proteinuria, edema, and hypoalbuminemia may suffer from primary FSGS or another glomerular disease.

Examination of kidney tissue is mandatory to make a diagnosis of FSGS, or any other glomerulonephropathy, and is often helpful in distinguishing primary from secondary forms. For example, a collapsing pattern of glomerular injury and tubuloreticular inclusions by light microscopy in a patient with HIV is consistent with a unique form of HIV nephropathy, ruling out primary/idiopathic disease. Meanwhile other patterns may be more subtle. Foot process effacement identified by electron microscopy (EM) is generally diffuse in primary disease, while it is more concentrated around areas of sclerosis in secondary disease. Further, EM and immunofluorescence may reveal the presence of immune complexes and other such findings associated with a secondary process, such as vasculitis or SLE.

The clinical course of secondary FSGS is largely determined by the causal process. Treatment focuses on modifying risk factors for nephron loss and hyperfiltration. For example, blood sugar and blood pressure should be tightly controlled in those with diabetes and/or hypertension. Blood pressure targets for patients with chronic kidney disease vary for the general population, with goal systolic and diastolic pressures <130/<80 mm Hg. Obese patients should be encouraged to lose weight through appropriate diet and physical activities. Angiotensin converting enzyme inhibitors (ACE-Is) and angiotensin receptor blockers (ARBs), ACE are both proven effective in reducing proteinuria and slowing the progression of some proteinuric kidney diseases, although they are not specifically proven in secondary or primary FSGS. They are often used, independent of their blood pressure lowering effects, to treat patients with secondary FSGS.

There is great variability in the clinical course of primary FSGS, further supporting multiple etiologies. Risk factors for progression to end-stage renal disease include massive proteinuria, elevated serum creatinine at the time of diagnosis, interstitial fibrosis on biopsy, and a lack of response to initial therapy.

Treatment of primary FSGS typically includes immune suppression in combination with secondary risk factor modification, as well as ACE-Is and/or ARBs, as above.

While a detailed discussion of treatment is beyond the scope of this discussion, it is important to note that the decision to use immune suppression and selection of an appropriate immune modulating agent should take into consideration patients' risk factors for disease progression, the potential for response to treatment, as well as the risks of treatment. For example, one may consider avoiding immune suppression in patients with normal renal function and subnephrotic proteinuria, as they will likely have an indolent disease course and may be one of the few who experience spontaneous remission. One may also consider avoiding immune suppression in patients with advanced renal failure and diffuse fibrosis on biopsy, as they have little hope for recovery of renal function. Steroids, arguably the first line of treatment for patients with idiopathic FSGS, may be avoided or used in lower doses in combination with a second immune-modulating agent in patients with uncontrolled diabetes. Alternative medications include cyclosporine and mycophenolate mofetil. Given the heterogeneity of this disease, rapidly evolving treatment strategies, and the toxicity associated with therapy, patients with FSGS should be managed by a nephrologist.

The patient presented above had several risk factors for secondary FSGS, including morbid obesity and sleep apnea, both associated with hyperfiltration, as well as modest hypertension, associated with nephron loss. However, his presentation included the acute onset of nephrotic syndrome; his pathology demonstrating diffuse foot process effacement; and his age and race associated with a high prevalence of primary FSGS, are all consistent with primary disease, the final diagnosis.

The initial treatment plan for this patient included aggressive risk factor modifications including weight loss, blood pressure control, referral for OSA treatment, and use of an ACE-I under close observation, along with a diuretic for his edema, and a 3-hydroxy-3-methylglutaryl coenzyme A reductase inhibitor (statins) for his hyperlipidemia. Steroids were avoided initially given the patient's morbid obesity and a strong family history of diabetes. Further, not presented above, alternative immune suppression was delayed given multiple missed appointments and the risks of unmonitored immune suppression. Low-dose steroids, perhaps in combination with cyclosporine, may be considered in the future if the benefits are judged to outweigh the risks.

Selected References

Appel GB, Cattran DC. Treatment of primary focal glomerulosclerosis. In: Rose BD, ed. Waltham, MA: *UpToDate;* 2007.

Falk R, Jennette JC, Nachman P. Primary glomerular disease. In: Brenner BM, et al, eds. *Brenner & Rector's The Kidney.* 7th ed. Philadelphia, PA: Saunders; 2004:Chapter 28.

D'Agati VD, Fogo AB, Bruijn JA, et al. Pathologic classification of focal segmental glomerulosclerosis: a working proposal. *Am J Kidney Dis.* 2004;43:368.

Haas M, Meehan SM, Karrison TG, et al. Changing etiologies of unexplained adult nephrotic syndrome: a comparison of renal biopsy findings from 1976–1979 and 1995–1997. *Am J Kidney Dis.* 1997 November;30(5):621–631.

Kambham N, Markowitz GS, Valeri AM, et al. Obesity-related glomerulopathy: an emerging epidemic. *Kidney Int.* 2001; 59:1498.

Kaplan JM, Kim HS, North KN, et al. Mutations in ACTN4, encoding alpha-actinin-4, cause familial focal segmental glomerulosclerosis. *Nat Genet.* 2000;24:251.

Praga M, Morales E, Herrero JC, et al. Absence of hypoalbuminemia despite massive proteinuria in focal segmental glomerulosclerosis secondary to hyperfiltration. *Am J Kidney Dis.* 1999;33:52.

Rennke HG, Klein PS. Pathogenesis and significance of nonprimary focal and segmental glomerulosclerosis. *Am J Kidney Dis.* 1989;13:443.

Rose B. Pathogenesis and diagnosis of focal glomerulosclerosis. In: Rose BD, ed. Waltham, MA: *UpToDate;* 2007.

Savin VJ, Sharma R, Sharma M, et al. Circulating factor associated with increased glomerular permeability to albumin in recurrent focal segmental glomerulosclerosis. *N Engl J Med.* 1996;334: 878–883.

Tanawattanacharoen S, Falk RJ, Jennette JC, et al. Parvovirus B19 DNA in kidney tissue of patients with focal segmental glomerulosclerosis. *Am J Kidney Dis.* 2000;35:1166–1174.

5-Year-Old Male with Fever and Conjunctivitis

C
31

CASE PRESENTATION

A 5-year-old Caucasian male with no significant past medical history presented with the chief complaint of fever for the last 6 days. The fever has been recorded at home as high as 40°C. There is temporary relief of fever from administration of acetaminophen. He has had decreased oral intake since his illness began, but his mother denies any other symptoms, including cough, sore throat, emesis, diarrhea, and rash. He has no known sick contacts. He has felt tired and ill since the fever began; most of his time has been spent lying in bed. Prior to this illness, he was very active and energetic in all of his kindergarten activities. His immunizations are up-to-date, and there have been no concerns about his overall growth or development. Family history is noncontributory; he lives with his parents, two older siblings, and a pet dog. He is not exposed to cigarette smoke at home.

Physical Examination

Patient appears ill, and is quiet and somewhat listless during the examination. Vital signs: temperature 39°C, blood pressure 97/44 mm Hg, heart rate 137 beats/min, respiration rate 28 breaths/min, SpO_2 99%. Head, eyes, ears, nose, and throat: normocephalic/atraumatic, bilateral injection of the bulbar conjunctivae with sparing of the limbus, no discharge from the eyes, no nasal discharge, tympanic membranes are grey and mobile bilaterally, buccal mucosa is dry, tongue is very erythematous with numerous raised bright red papillae. Neck: supple, normal carotid pulses. Lymph nodes: multiple enlarged lymph nodes in the submandibular and cervical areas bilaterally; all nodes are nontender and mobile, and all measure between 0.5 and 2.0 cm in diameter. Cardiovascular: regular rate and rhythm, no murmurs, rubs, or gallops, normal S_1 and S_2, radial and dorsalis pedis pulses are 2+ and equal bilaterally. Pulmonary: clear to auscultation bilaterally, no wheezes or rales. Abdomen: soft, nontender, nondistended, liver edge palpable 2 cm below costal margin, no splenomegaly. Extremities: no clubbing, cyanosis, or edema. Skin: no rash, no skin changes in hands or feet.

Laboratory Studies

White blood cells 19.2 (polymorphonuclear leukocytes [PMNs] 88%), hemoglobin 11.7, hematocrit 34, platelets (plt) 277; chemistries normal; aspartate aminotransferase 133, alanine aminotransferase 142, total bilirubin 1.1, alkaline phosphatase 119, total protein 7.0, albumin 4.1; erythrocyte sedimentation rate (ESR) 44, C-reactive protein (CRP) 8.7; urinalysis (U/A) significant for 13 WBC, 0 red blood cells (RBC), + leukocyte esterase (LE), negative nitrite. Chest x-ray was normal.

Case Resolution

The patient was admitted for observation and intravenous (IV) hydration. The day following admission, he developed a diffuse rash over his trunk and extremities, characterized by fine, erythematous papules. On the morning of the next day, he was found to have erythematous and mildly edematous palms. He was treated for his condition, and his symptoms improved over the next 5 days. He was discharged from the hospital after resolution of his fever on hospital day 8.

Question

What is the appropriate treatment for this patient's condition?

Answer

The child described in the case scenario has Kawasaki disease and should be treated with intravenous immunoglobulin (IVIG) and high-dose aspirin. The patient should have an echocardiogram performed as well to evaluate for the presence of coronary artery pathology.

Discussion

Kawasaki disease (KD) is an acute, generally self-limited vasculitis that occurs primarily in infants and young children. The disease was first described by Dr. Tomisaku Kawasaki as the mucocutaneous lymph node syndrome in 1967 after he studied a series of cases that appeared in Japan. Although KD is much more common in Japan than elsewhere in the world, with an annual incidence of greater than 100 cases/100,000 children younger than 5 years old, the disease has been described in endemic and epidemic forms throughout the world. In comparison, the incidence rate in the United States in 1997 and 2000 was 17 cases/100,000 children younger than 5 years old. Despite this disparity in incidence, KD is the leading cause of acquired heart disease in children in United States.

The diagnosis of classic KD requires the presence of fever for at least 5 days and at least four of the following: bilateral nonpurulent conjunctival injection, erythema or edema of hands or feet, rash, changes in the lips or oral cavity (cracked lips, strawberry tongue), and cervical lymphadenopathy (at least one node >1.5 cm in diameter) (Table 31-1). Incomplete presentations of KD, also called atypical KD, can occur and are more common in infants than young children. Although those children with incomplete presentations of KD do not fulfill all of the classic clinical criteria, they are still at significant risk for developing coronary artery pathology. The diagnosis should be suspected in any infant with fever lasting longer than 7 days with no known cause. Evaluation of the coronary arteries with an echocardiogram and other laboratory values should be considered in order to diagnose incomplete presentations of KD. Fewer than four of the diagnostic criteria are

TABLE 31-1

Diagnostic Criteria for Kawasaki Disease

Fever for at least 5 days, plus at least four of the following:

Extremity changes: erythema and/or painful induration of palms or soles of feet in acute phase, cracking and peeling of skin on hands and feet occurs in subacute phase

Rash: usually diffuse, maculopapular eruption developing around day 5 of illness; may also be urticarial, scarlatiniform, or resemble erythema multiforme

Bilateral conjunctival injection: usually affects bulbar conjunctivae, exudate is absent, painless

Changes in lips and oral cavity: erythema, cracking, peeling of lips; strawberry tongue; diffuse erythema of oral mucosae

Cervical lymphadenopathy: usually unilateral, at least one lymph node >1.5 cm in diameter; nonfluctuant, firm, usually nontender

Adapted from Burns JC, Glode MP. Kawasaki syndrome. Lancet. *2004;364;533–544.*

necessary for diagnosis, if coronary artery disease is found by echocardiography. A recent consensus statement endorsed by the American Academy of Pediatrics (AAP) and American Heart Association (AHA) is of particular utility in using echocardiography and accessory laboratory data to guide therapy in the incomplete presentation of KD.

The systemic arteritis seen in KD can affect blood vessels throughout the body. Virtually all autopsy specimens show involvement of the muscular coronary arteries, although aneurysms have been demonstrated in specimens of other extraparenchymal arteries, such as the celiac, mesenteric, femoral, iliac, renal, axillary, and brachial arteries. Of course, involvement of the coronary arteries leads to the most significant adverse outcomes, including coronary aneurysms and resulting myocardial infarction or sudden death. Other common clinical and laboratory features of KD seen in the patient described above include leukocytosis (with neutrophilia), elevated erythrocyte sedimentation rate and CRP, sterile pyuria, hepatomegaly, and elevated serum transaminases (Table 31-2). As mentioned above, additional findings may also include or be related to inflammation of other medium-sized arteries, arthritis/arthralgia, diarrhea, vomiting, abdominal pain, gallbladder hydrops, aseptic meningitis, urethritis, and a desquamating rash in the groin.

TABLE 31-2

Laboratory Abnormalities in Acute Kawasaki Disease

Laboratory abnormality Patients	%
C-reactive protein	~ 80%
CSF pleocytosis	~35%
γ-Glutamyl transferase >37 U/L	~65%
Alanine aminotransferase > 50 U/L	~30%
Platelet count >45 × 10⁹/L	~40%
WBC count >15 × 10⁹/L	~40%
Anemia (hemoglobin <2 SD below mean for age)	~40%
Erythrocyte sedimentation rate > 60 mm/h	~60%

CSF, cerebrospinal fluid; SD, standard deviation; WBC, white blood cells.

Adapted from Burns JC, Mason WH, Glode MP, and the Kawasaki Disease Multicenter Study Group. Clinical and epidemiological characteristics of patients referred for evaluation of possible Kawasaki disease. J Pediatr. 1991;118:680–686. Burns JC, Glode MP. Kawasaki syndrome. Lancet. 2004;364;533–544.

Untreated, 15% to 25% of patients with KD will develop coronary artery aneurysms; treatment during the acute phase of the illness reduces this risk to less than 5%. The mainstay of treatment is aspirin and IVIG. IVIG, when administered alone or in combination with aspirin, has consistently been shown to reduce the incidence of coronary artery abnormalities in patients with KD. It is typically administered as one dose of 2 g/kg and it appears most effective if given in the first 5 to 7 days of the illness, but it is still effective if given in the first 10 days of illness. A second dose of IVIG is sometimes used for patients who fail to respond to the first treatment, but the effectiveness of multiple doses of IVIG is not well established. Aspirin is initially administered at doses of 80 to 100 mg/kg/day. Variability exists on the length of high-dose aspirin treatment. Many clinicians decrease the aspirin dose to 3 to 5 mg/kg/day when fever has abated for more than 48 to 72 hours while others treat until day 14 of the illness and more than 48 to 72 hours of absent fever. Although aspirin does not have an effect on the development of coronary artery aneurysms, it is felt to have important antithrombotic and anti-inflammatory effects. Low-dose aspirin is generally continued for 6 to

8 weeks after the onset of illness, until no evidence of coronary pathology is demonstrated on follow-up echocardiography. For those patients with coronary artery pathology, aspirin use may be indefinite and may be combined with such agents as dipyridamole, clopidogrel, and in some cases, warfarin. The role of steroids in the treatment of KD is unclear. Several small studies have shown some benefit from including steroids in initial treatment regimens. In 2007, a larger placebo-controlled trial demonstrated no added benefit of adding corticosteroids to IVIG therapy. Other agents being studied for treatment of refractory cases of KD include pentoxifylline, infliximab, abciximab, and cyclophosphamide.

Patients who are unfortunate to develop coronary pathology are a special subgroup and warrant close follow-up and distinct clinical management (Table 31-3). Based on the number, size, and complexity of lesions, there are distinct recommendations with regards to therapy, restrictions on activity, follow-up surveillance, and the need for invasive testing. For those patients who convalesce without the development of detectable coronary artery pathology, long-term follow-up is recommended, although long-term outcome data are not yet available as to the significance of the risk increase for the development of significant coronary artery disease in the future.

The underlying cause of the systemic inflammatory response seen in the vasculature of the patients with KD is unknown, although several theories exist. These range from a superantigen-mediated systemic immune activation to a ubiquitous pathogen (or pathogens) that has tissue tropism to vascular beds. Perhaps genetic factors such as cytokine gene, chemokine gene, matrix metalloproteinase gene, or TOLL receptor gene polymorphisms make certain persons, families, or populations more susceptible to the syndrome which may simply manifest in a common final pathway that is clinically expressed as KD. What is known is that multiple nonspecific inflammatory and immune-mediated perturbations have been described in patients suffering from KD including elevations in serum levels of proinflammatory cytokines, widespread activation and expansion of specific receptor families of T cells, and activation of affected endothelial beds. Studies of affected arterial tissue consistently demonstrate evidence of endothelial swelling, subendothelial edema with an influx of neutrophils early in the inflammatory cascade with later transition to mononuclear cells, T cells, and plasma cells. Later there is destruction of the elastic intima and possibly fibrosis and healing. Elegant studies in the arterial tissues of autopsy

TABLE 31-3

Risk Stratification and Recommendations for Treatment, Activity Restrictions, Recommended Follow-Up Tests (Invasive and Noninvasive)

Risk level	Pharmacological therapy	Physical activity	Follow-up testing	Invasive testing
I: no coronary artery changes at any stage of illness	None beyond aspirin first 6–8 weeks	None beyond the first 6–8 weeks	Cardiovascular risk assessment and counseling at 5-year intervals	None
II: transient coronary artery ectasia that disappears within 6–8 weeks	None beyond aspirin first 6–8 weeks	None beyond the first 6–8 weeks	Cardiovascular risk assessment and counseling at between 3- and 5-year intervals	None
III: 1 small–medium coronary artery aneurysm/major coronary artery	Low-dose aspirin at least until aneurysm regression noted	<11 years old: none beyond the first 6–8 weeks, 11–20 years old: activity guided by stress test, perfusion scan performed biennially, contact sports discouraged for those taking antiplatelet agents	Annual cardiology follow-up with echocardiogram, ECG, CV risk assessment and counseling. Biennial stress test, evaluation of myocardial perfusion scan	Angiography only if noninvasive tests suggest ischemia
IV: > or = 1 large or giant coronary artery aneurysm, multiple or complex aneurysm in same artery without obstruction	Long-term antiplatelet therapy and warfarin therapy, combined in cases of giant aneurysm	Contact or high-impact sports should be avoided because of risk of bleeding, activity guided by stress test, perfusion scan performed biannually	Biannual cardiology follow-up with echocardiogram, ECG, annual stress test, evaluation of myocardial perfusion scan	Angiography at 6–12 months or sooner if indicated, repeated only if noninvasive tests, clinical scenario suggests ischemia
V: coronary artery obstruction	Long-term low-dose aspirin, warfarin or LMWH if giant aneurysms persist	Contact or high-impact sports should be avoided because of risk of bleeding, activity guided by stress test, perfusion scan performed biannually	Biannual cardiology follow-up with echocardiogram, ECG, annual stress test, evaluation of myocardial perfusion scan	Angiography recommended to address therapeutic options

CV, cardiovascular; ECG, electrocardiogram; LMWH, low-molecular-weight heparin.

Adapted from Newburger JW, Takahashi M, Gerber M, et al. Diagnosis, treatment, and long-term management of Kawasaki disease: a statement for health professionals from the committee on rheumatic fever, endocarditis, and Kawasaki disease: Council on Cardiovascular Disease in the Young, American Heart Association. Pediatrics. *2004;114:1708–1733.*

cases have revealed the evidence of oligoclonally expanded IgA-producing plasma cells in the walls of damaged arteries, suggesting very strongly of an antigen-driven response, perhaps to a mucosally derived ubiquitous pathogen. Studies using reverse genetics have shown that when the genes for these specific IgA molecules are expressed *ex vivo,* the resultant antibodies cross-react to a number of specimens derived from different KD patient but does not control. Despite these compelling findings, the search for the elusive universal KD antigen has produced nothing but a long list of pathogens that do not appear to cause the disease.

Selected References

Newburger JW, Takahashi M, Burns JC, et al. Treatment of Kawasaki syndrome with intravenous gamma globulin. *N Engl J Med.* 1986;315:341–347.

Burns JC, Mason WH, Glode MP, and the Kawasaki Disease Multicenter Study Group. Clinical and epidemiological characteristics of patients referred for evaluation of possible Kawasaki disease. *J Pediatr.* 1991;118:680–686.

Newburger JW, Takahashi M, Beiser AS, et al. Diagnosis, treatment, and long-term management of Kawasaki disease. *Circulation.* 2004;110:2747–2771.

Newburger JW, Takahashi M, Gerber M, et al. Diagnosis, treatment, and long-term management of Kawasaki disease: a statement for health professionals from the committee on rheumatic fever, endocarditis, and Kawasaki disease: Council on Cardiovascular Disease in the Young, American Heart Association. *Pediatrics.* 2004;114:1708–1733.

Durongpisitkul K, Gururaj VJ, Park JM, et al. The prevention of coronary artery aneurysm in Kawasaki disease: a meta-analysis on the efficacy of aspirin and immunoglobulin treatment. *Pediatrics.* 1995;96:1057–1061.

Holman RC, Curns AT, Belay ED, et al. Kawasaki syndrome hospitalizations in the United States, 1997 and 2000. *Pediatrics.* 2003;112:495–501.

Newburger JW, Sleeper LA, McCrindle BW, et al. Randomized trial of pulsed corticosteroid therapy for primary treatment of Kawasaki disease. *N Engl J Med.* 2007;356:663–675.

Burns JC, Glode MP. Kawasaki syndrome. *Lancet.* 2004;364;533–544.

Rowley AH, Baker SC, Shulman ST, et al. Detection of antigen in bronchial epithelium and macrophages in acute Kawasaki disease by use of synthetic antibody. *J Infect Dis.* 2004;190:856–865.

Rowley AH, Shulman ST, Mask CA, et al. IgA plasma cell infiltration of proximal respiratory tract, pancreas, kidney, and coronary artery in acute Kawasaki disease. *J Infect Dis.* 2000;182:1183–1191.

Rowley AH, Shulman ST, Mask CA, et al. Oligoclonal IgA response in the vascular wall in acute Kawasaki disease. *J Immunol.* 2001 January 15;166(2):1334–1343.

1-Year-Old with Linear Growth Failure for 3 Months

C
32

CASE PRESENTATION

A 1-year-old Caucasian male was admitted to the pediatric hospital ward for the investigation of linear growth failure for 3 months. Both his weight and head circumference were following the 45th percentile growth curve for his age, while his height had fallen to below the 10th percentile. He had also been troubled by recurrent sinusitis and was treated with amoxicillin/clavulanate and azithromycin but showed no improvement. His parents denied any other prolonged illness, fevers, lethargy, or unexplained pain. They also denied respiratory distress, cough, abdominal pain, skin rashes, or changes in urination. He was taking a regular diet of varied table foods, but was still supplementing with 20 kcal/oz infant formula twice daily. He had recently been transitioned to whole cow's milk and took no more than two 8 oz glasses per day. The parents described him as "a good eater." He had no episodes of vomiting, and he passed well-formed stools once daily. Per his primary pediatrician, he was developing normally and meeting all motor, cognitive, and social milestones.

This child was the product of an uneventful pregnancy and a spontaneous vaginal delivery. The neonatal period was uncomplicated. He had not been previously hospitalized and had not undergone any surgery other than a routine circumcision. He did not have any allergies and was not taking any medications. Family history was negative for serious disease, and he did not have any siblings.

Physical Examination

The patient appeared well, and there was no sign of distress. He was well hydrated, chubby, and playful. His vital signs were unremarkable. Length was 73.5 cm (10th percentile), weight 22 lb, 13 oz (35th percentile), and head circumference 47.2 cm (45th percentile).

His skin was slightly pale without any notable lesions. Pupils were equal and reactive, with normal extraocular movements and positive red reflexes bilaterally. Head, eyes, ears, nose, and throat examination was normal, but for mild clear rhinorrhea. The chest was clear to auscultation and the cardiac examination was within normal limits. The abdomen was markedly protuberant with a liver edge felt approximately 6 cm below the right costal margin and extending across the midline. The spleen was also palpable 3 cm below the left costal margin. The abdomen was otherwise soft, nontender, and without any palpable masses. The genitourinary examination was normal, and extremities exhibited full ranges of motion without deformity. Finally, the neurologic examination showed normal strength, tone, reflexes, and balance.

From a developmental perspective, he was cruising and had developed a pincer grasp. He spoke one to two words and had positive stranger anxiety.

Laboratory Studies

A complete blood count (CBC) revealed white blood cells 9900, hemoglobin 12, platelet count 553,000, neutrophils 60%, lymphocytes 30%, and a normal peripheral blood smear. Laboratory studies into the marked hepatomegaly showed aspartate aminotransferase 240, alanine aminotransferase 265, gamma-glutamyltransferase 244, albumin 4.1, alkaline phosphatase 240, lactate dehydrogenase 313, and total bilirubin 0.3 with a direct value of less than 0.1. Coagulation studies and fibrinogen were within normal limits. Ammonia levels were normal. Creatine kinase (CK) was not elevated.

Uric acid was elevated at 8.3 with the normal range being up to 5.5. A venous blood gas revealed pH of 7.4 and serum bicarbonate 19. Also, lactate was elevated at 65 mg/dL with normal being up to 19.8 mg/dL. Screenings for hepatitis viruses, cytomegalovirus (CMV), Epstein-Barr virus (EBV), and human immunodeficiency virus (HIV) were negative. Urine homovanillic acid (HVA) and vanillylmandelic acid (VMA) levels were unremarkable. A sweat chloride test was also normal. Serologies for celiac sprue were negative. Alpha-1 antitrypsin level was normal.

Endocrine laboratory tests consisting of thyroid studies, cortisol, insulin, and growth hormone levels were normal. Lipid profile revealed cholesterol 117 mg/dL, triglycerides 707 mg/dL, and high-density lipoproteins (HDL) 32 mg/dL. Plasma amino acids, urine organic acids, pyruvate, and free fatty acids were within normal values. Both stool and urine were negative for reducing substances. Finally, electrolytes were normal, but for an initial blood glucose of 37 mg/dL. A subsequent fasting blood sugar value obtained 2 hours after a meal was 55 mg/dL.

Radiological Tests

An abdominal ultrasound showed a much enlarged, homogenous, echogenic liver and a somewhat hypoechoic and slightly enlarged spleen. There was no evidence of discrete liver masses or biliary tract disease, and blood flow in all hepatic vessels was normal.

Case Resolution

With hepatomegaly, fasting hypoglycemia, hyperuricemia, hypertriglyceridemia, high lactate, and failure of linear growth, glycogen storage disease (GSD) was at the top of the differential diagnosis. On further investigation, the parents stated the child often had a voracious appetite after napping and occasionally was diaphoretic upon waking in the morning. They denied any seizure activity. Further investigation into family history revealed a paternal great-grandfather and a paternal great-aunt who had some form of hypoglycemia that was diet controlled. A glucagon stimulation test produced very high lactate values with steady glucose levels in the low–normal range.

Blood samples were sent for genetic analysis of known mutations causing GSD. These results showed the patient was a compound heterozygote for GSD. A liver biopsy was not performed.

Question

Which subtype of GSD is this child most likely to have?

Answer

The child in this case most likely suffers from GSD types Ia, IIIb, or VI. With a normal CK, it is unlikely that he has types II, IIIa, IV, V, or VII which often affect skeletal or cardiac muscle. Without neutropenia, type Ib can also be eliminated. Types IIIb and VI usually have only mild elevations in triglycerides and uric acid. Normal CK, greatly elevated triglycerides, high uric acid, and large rise in lactate with glucagon stimulation all suggest GSD type Ia.

Discussion

GSDs, or glycogenoses, are a diverse group of metabolic disorders which affect the body's ability to mobilize glycogen stores in times of fasting. With more than 10 distinct subtypes of GSD, a myriad of body tissues and organs can be involved in the disease process causing numerous different symptoms (Table 32-1). GSD is often subdivided into hepatic glycogenoses, which primarily affect the liver's ability to store and retrieve glucose, and the muscle glycogenoses, which affect usage of glycogen in skeletal and cardiac muscle. With an overall incidence of 1/100,000 live births, GSD I, III, and VI are the most prevalent subtypes, accounting for approximately 75% of diagnosed cases. Most of the glycogenoses are inherited through an autosomal recessive pattern; however, GSD IX is exclusively X-linked recessive.

Clinical presentations of hepatic GSD can range from linear growth failure to profound metabolic acidosis, but 80% of patients develop some degree of hypoglycemia by 1 year of age. This often comes to attention when a child successfully sleeps through the night and does not awake for feedings. Presenting symptoms consist of diaphoresis, tremor, confusion, lethargy, voracious appetite, or even seizures. In muscle GSD, the primary symptoms are usually

TABLE 32-1

Classification of GSD

Abbreviation	Eponym	Enzyme defect	Clinical features
GSD 0		Glycogen synthase	Early-onset hypoglycemia, ketosis, and postprandial lactic acidosis without any hepatomegaly
GSD Ia	von Gierke disease	Glucose-6-phosphatase	Marked hepatomegaly, hypoglycemia, lactic acidosis, hyperuricemia, failure to thrive
GSD Ib, c, d		Hepatic transporters of glucose-6-phosphate, phosphate, or glucose	Marked hepatomegaly, hypoglycemia, lactic acidosis, hyperuricemia, failure to thrive, neutropenia, recurrent pyogenic infections
GSD II	Pompe disease	Acid maltase glucosidase	Hypertrophic cardiomyopathy, severe muscle weakness, early death
GSD IIIa, b	Forbes or Cori disease	Glycogen debrancher enzyme	Marked hepatomegaly, variable hypoglycemia, ketosis, evidence of hepatocellular dysfunction, variable myopathy, variable cardiomyopathy
GSD IV	Andersen disease	Glycogen branching enzyme	Severe early-onset cirrhosis
GSD V	McArdle disease	Muscle phosphorylase	Muscle cramps, exercise intolerance, episodic rhabdomyolysis, and myoglobinuria
GSD VI	Hers disease	Hepatic phosphorylase	Moderate hepatomegaly, fasting hypoglycemia
GSD VII	Tarui disease	Muscle phosphofructokinase	Early-onset muscle cramps, exercise intolerance, episodic rhabdomyolysis and myoglobinuria, hyperbilirubinemia, reticulocytosis
GSD VIII		Phosphorylase beta-kinase	Variable from fatal early-onset cardiomyopathy to asymptomatic hepatomegaly. Most cases inherited as autosomal recessive disorder; *some cases X-linked recessive*
GSD IX		Phosphoglycerate kinase	Hemolytic anemia, mental retardation. Myopathy, myoglobinuria, and exercise intolerance are inconsistent. *Inheritance X-linked recessive*
GSD X		Phosphoglycerate mutase	Exercise intolerance, cramps, myoglobinuria
GSD XI		Lactate dehydrogenase	Exercise intolerance, cramps, myoglobinuria

GSD, glycogen storage disease.
Adapted from Clarke JTR, Feigenbaum AJS. Metabolic genetics. In: Friedman J, Laxer RM, Gerstle T, et al, eds. Atlas of Pediatrics. Philadelphia, PA: Current Medicine; 2005.

cramping, rhabdomyolysis, and muscle weakness, but these can be mild and even have their initial presentation well into adulthood. For those forms affecting the cardiac muscle, patients can present with signs of congestive heart failure from hypertrophic cardiomyopathy. CK levels will usually be elevated in the muscle glycogenoses, while a normal CK level typically points to one of the hepatic glycogenoses (Table 32-2).

In GSD Ia, there is a defect in the glucose-6-phosphatase gene which normally cleaves glucose-6-phosphate to

organic glucose and transports it out of the endoplasmic reticulum (Fig. 32-1). This defect leads to marked hypoglycemia with hepatic production of lactic acid when fasting. Other laboratory findings include mild to moderate transaminase elevation, ketosis, hyperuricemia, and hyperlipidemia. Blood samples are often lipemic to the naked eye with triglyceride levels being strikingly elevated. Physical examination findings can include hepatomegaly, protuberant abdomen, cushingoid facial appearance, short stature, cutaneous xanthomas, gouty tophi, spider angiomas,

TABLE 32-2

Hepatic and Skeletal Muscle Involvement with the Various Types of GSD

Hepatic GSD	Muscle GSD
Type I	Type II
Type IIIb	Type IIIa
Type VI	Type IV
Type IX	Type V
Type 0	Type VII

GSD, glycogen storage disease.

delayed motor development, and even epistaxis because of platelet dysfunction, secondary to the acidemia.

If there is a history of recurrent pulmonary, oral, or skin infections, GSD Ib should be suspected as this could be a sign of associated neutropenia. Of note, the neutropenia may present as constant agranulocytosis or be missed completely as it appears in a more cyclical pattern. Often,

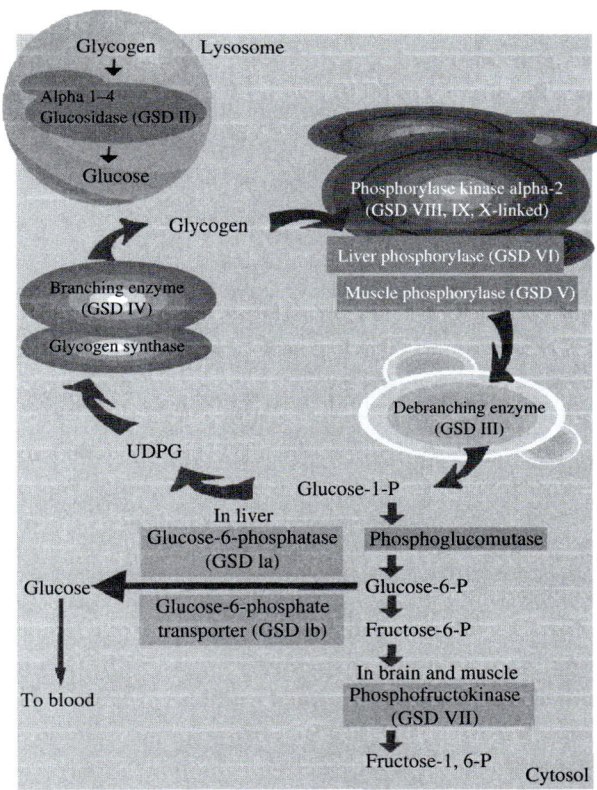

Figure 32-1 A summary of the enzymatic reactions involved in glycogenolysis, and the points of enzyme mutation in the various glycogenoses.

an inflammatory-like bowel disease can develop with this neutropenia. Otherwise, GSD Ib has the same metabolic derangements as its Ia counterpart, and the neutropenia can be treated with granulocyte colony-stimulating factor (G-CSF).

In GSD IIIb, which largely affects the liver, the glycogen debranching enzyme is affected, and this allows for some glucose mobilization through glycogenolysis of outer branch glycogen stores. Thus, there is clinical variability in the degree of hypoglycemia experienced by patients. Children can still present with severe hypoglycemia and growth failure as in GSD I; however, lactate and uric acid levels are often normal or only slightly elevated. In GSD IIIa, skeletal muscle is also involved, but the cramping and weakness usually does not present until the third decade of life. Overall, GSD III has a better prognosis than GSD I, with most symptoms improving by adulthood.

With GSD VI, the defect is in glycogen phosphorylase, and the clinical course is usually benign. Children can present with hypoglycemia but it is often mild and asymptomatic unless there has been a very prolonged fasting period. The children can also have hepatomegaly and mild growth delay, but unlike GSD I, there is no lactic or metabolic acidosis. By puberty, most patients have no sign of hepatomegaly, and their growth normalizes without intervention.

In children with suspected GSD, initial screening laboratory tests should consist of a venous blood gas with lactate, glucose, uric acid level, serum ketones, and a lipid panel. One should also obtain a CBC with differential, hepatic transaminases, albumin, coagulation studies, and a CK level. If possible, these laboratory tests should be drawn when the patient is fasting. The constellation of hypoglycemia, lactic acidemia, hyperlipidemia, and hyperuricemia are specific enough for a presumptive GSD diagnosis, pending genetic confirmation.

Radiographic imaging should include a hepatic ultrasound and cardiac echocardiography to assess overall cardiac function. A glucagon stimulation test can also be helpful as it will show a marked elevation of lactate with relatively steady glucose levels in GSD I. While this will help solidify the diagnosis of GSD I, it may not be as helpful in GSD III or VI, as there is seldom such a dramatic response (Table 32-3). In the past, hepatic or muscle biopsy was the gold standard for GSD diagnosis, but now genetic testing of the blood is preferred. Through mutation analysis and enzyme activity assays, GSD can be confirmed without invasive tissues biopsies.

TABLE 32-3

Metabolic Responses to Various Stimuli in GSD

Type	While hypoglycemic			Response to oral glucose		Response to glucagon (4 h after meal)	
	Triglyceride	Uric acid	Lactate	Glucose	Lactate	Glucose	Lactate
GSD I	↑↑↑	↑↑	↑↑↑	↑	↓↓	0	↑↑↑
GSD III	↑	N	N	↑	↑	0	0
GSD VI	↑	N	N	↑	↑	↑	0

GSD, glycogen storage disease.

↑ mild increase, ↑↑ moderate increase, ↑↑↑ marked increase, N normal, 0 no change, ↓↓ moderate decrease

Adapted from Wolfsdorf J, Weinstein D. Glycogen storage diseases. Rev Endocr Metab Disord. *2003;4:95–102.*

To avoid hypoglycemia and its associated symptoms, children are placed on a scheduled diet of uncooked corn starch. This corn starch acts as a reservoir of readily available glucose between meals and prevents hypoglycemia with resulting lactic acid production in the fasting state. Fructose, sucrose, and galactose are also completely eliminated from the diet as these have been proven to worsen lactic acidemia. Otherwise, children can partake in a regular diet.

In GSD I, children commonly develop numerous long-term complications and thus require close monitoring throughout their lives. The mechanisms of these sequelae are not readily apparent; however, experts believe they stem from a combination of direct glycogen deposition into tissues and chronic acidemia. Ninety percent of patients will develop hepatic adenomas by the second decade of life, and they require hepatic ultrasounds every 6 months with serum alpha-fetoprotein levels to monitor these lesions for malignant transformation, hemorrhage, or other complications. Renal function must also be monitored as these children can suffer proximal and distal tubular dysfunction as well as uric acid nephrolithiasis that can lead to renal failure. Urine alkalinization and citrate supplementation can prevent some of the renal complications. Many children will have a degree of developmental delay, and this is usually a direct result of severe hypoglycemia on brain development. With their hyperlipidemia, patients are at risk for pancreatitis and cholelithiasis; however, they do not suffer from cardiac complications owing to their altered lipid profiles. Yearly bone density scans are also needed to monitor for osteopenia, which results from the chronic acidemia. Other long-term effects are systemic hypertension, pulmonary hypertension, gout, bleeding disorders, anemia, growth restriction, and truncal obesity. Yearly monitoring for these issues is also recommended through corresponding tests.

Selected References

1. Wolfsdorf J, Weinstein D. Glycogen storage diseases. *Rev Endocr Metab Disord.* 2003;4:95–102.
2. Moses S. Historical highlights and unsolved problems in glycogen storage disease type I. *Eur J Pediatr.* 2002;161:S2–S9.
3. Rake JP, Visser G, Labrune P, et al. Glycogen storage disease type I: diagnosis, management, clinical course and outcome. Results of the European Study on Glycogen Storage Disease Type I (ESGSD I). *Eur J Pediatr.* 2002;161:S20–S34.
4. Rake JP, Visser G, Labrune P, et al. Guidelines for management of glycogen storage disease type I: European Study on Glycogen Storage Disease Type I. *Eur J Pediatr.* 2002;161:S112–S119.
5. Bodamer OA, Feillet F, Lane RE, et al. Utilization of cornstarch in glycogen storage disease type Ia. *Eur J Gastroenterol Hepatol.* 2002 November; 14(11):1251–1256.
6. Veiga-da-Cunha M, Gerin I, van Schaftingen E. How many forms of glycogen storage disease type I? *Eur J Pediatr.* 2000 May;159(5):314–8.
7. Clarke JTR, Feigenbaum AJS. Metabolic genetics. In: Friedman J, Laxer RM, Gerstle T, et al, eds. *Atlas of Pediatrics.* Philadelphia, PA: Current Medicine; 2005.
8. Amato AA. Sweet success—a treatment for McArdle's disease. N. Eng. J. Med. 2003;349:2481–2482.

25-Year-Old Woman with Headaches and Visual Changes × 3 Months

CASE PRESENTATION

A 25-year-old female began having headaches for the past month. She began to experience these headaches shortly after a miscarriage. She described the pain as mostly located in front of her head, occasionally also in the occipital region. She said the pain waxes and wanes, but is always present. They would occasionally be so severe that she would be unable to perform at work and would lie down in a darkened room. In the emergency department, she was given ibuprofen which did not help. She was also tried on Imitrex, which provided minimal relief, but the headache always remained. She was then given intravenous narcotics, which did alleviate the pain, but made her too sleepy. About a week and a half after the headache started, she started getting a "darkening" of her vision. This has progressed to the point now where she has difficulty walking downstairs. She stopped driving secondary to her vision, and lost her job. She says that her whole visual field is affected, with a global darkening and slightly blurring. For the past several weeks, she also reports some right jaw numbness, and associated drooling that has been intermittent. There is no associated jaw pain.

Physical Examination

Vital signs: temperature 37.2°C, blood pressure 140/80 mm Hg, pulse 80 beats/min, respiratory rate 18 breaths/min, pain 3/10, and body mass index (BMI) 47.9. She is an obese black woman in no apparent distress. The eye examination showed pupils equal round and reactive to light and her funduscopic examination revealed papilledema. Extraocular movements are intact. Her visual fields were intact, although she had decreased visual acuity. Her neurologic examination demonstrated that she was alert and oriented to person, place, and self. Cranial nerves II through XII are intact, with the exception of decreased sensation in the distribution of the third branch of cranial nerve V on the right side. Reflexes are difficult to elicit, but her toes are down going.

Laboratory Studies

Her original laboratory work was all within normal limits, including a full chemistry panel, complete blood count,

and coagulation studies. Computed tomography (CT) of her head revealed no acute findings. A lumbar puncture was performed and she had an elevated opening pressure at 48, but otherwise normal cell count and chemistry.

Case Resolution

The patient was admitted to neurology and treated with a therapeutic lumbar puncture with removal of 20 ml of cerebrospinal fluid and Diamox. She went on to have a shunt placed and an optic nerve fenestration. After these procedures, she regained vision in her right eye and her vision in her left eye stabilized.

Question

What about this patient should make you do further testing to investigate the etiology of her headache, and why should pseudotumor cerebri be at the top of your differential?

Answer

This patient had both focal neurologic symptoms and papilledema on examination. The key to diagnosing pseudotumor cerebri is a high level of suspicion. Her age, obesity, and papilledema all are very suggestive of pseudotumor cerebri. The lumbar puncture was confirmatory with the elevated opening pressure, normal cell counts, normal chemistry, and negative culture. Pseudotumor cerebri cannot be diagnosed unless the cerebral spinal fluid is found to be normal. The treatment of choice for pseudotumor cerebri includes everything from medication to ventriculoperitoneal shunt placement and optic nerve fenestration. Often neurology and neurosurgery specialists need to be involved with care.

Discussion

Significant morbidity is associated with headaches. In 1993, there were 150 million lost work days because of headaches. It is estimated that there are almost 400,000 lost school days each year. Ninety percent of all headaches fall into a benign category with migraine, tension-type headache, and cluster headaches being the primary diagnoses. Population-based studies reveal that 38% of the United States population experience tension-type headaches annually and 10% experience migraine headaches. Cluster headaches are estimated to have a prevalence of less than 1%. A study from United Kingdom revealed that 85% of patients seeking medical care for a headache were diagnosed with migraine-type headaches. While tension-type headaches are most prevalent in the population, migraine headaches are most prevalent in those who seek medical attention.

Migraine is derived from the word "hemicrania" which is Greek in origin. This was described originally by Galen in 200 AD as a pain syndrome affecting half the head. It is associated with huge costs as employers estimate $13 billion in lost revenue annually. The direct medical costs easily exceed $1 billion annually. The highest prevalence of this disease is among Caucasians. The prevalence decreases as income increases. The prevalence is estimated to be equal among boys and girls at approximately 4% until puberty. At puberty, migraine frequency increases more in girls than in boys with a peak incidence occurring in the fourth and fifth decade among both sexes. The pathophysiology of migraines is complex. The initiating event in the development of a migraine is neuronal activation and propagation. The spread of this neuronal activation throughout the cortices leads to the release of inflammatory mediators. It is these neuropeptides which stimulate nociception in the meningeal and dural vessels. The neurovascular changes in particular in the trigeminal system lead to the sensation of a migraine headache.

The manifestations of a migraine headache generally fall into a recognizable pattern. However, the true prevalence of premonitory symptoms varies widely from 20% to 60%. The "aura" of a migraine headache which may be visual, sensory, motor, language, or brain stem usually signals the onset of headache within 60 minutes. Eighty-five percent of migraine headaches can be described as unilateral, gradual in onset, and throbbing. Headaches may be bilateral and may become generalized after a unilateral start. The typical patient wants to lie down in a dark, quiet room and just be still. There are many symptoms associated with migraine headaches. They will last 4 to 72 hours and afterward patients describe being tired or washed out, irritable, and listless.

The drugs of choice to treat acute migraine attacks act at various subclasses of serotonin receptors. Serotonergic receptors located throughout the brain and along intracranial blood vessels have an inhibitory effect. Stimulation of these receptors will reduce protein extravasation and vasoconstriction. Triptan and ergot medications are felt to be the first line of therapy for aborting severe attacks and less severe attacks, unresponsive to nonsteroidal analgesics. Uncontrolled hypertension and coronary artery disease are contraindications for these medications. Prochlorperazine and metoclopramide have also been shown to have efficacy for acute therapy of migraines. For people with poor response to acute therapy, contraindication to acute therapy, migraine that interferes with function despite acute therapy, more than two headaches per week, prophylactic therapy should be initiated. Beta-blockers and calcium channel blockers have been well studied and used for many years, but many other drugs have been shown to be effective in well-done trials: amitriptyline, fluoxetine, divalproex sodium, sodium valproate, topiramate, botulinum toxin A.

Tension-type headaches are likely the most common form of headache syndrome. Patients will typically describe these headaches as being a pressure or tightness around the head which waxes and wanes in intensity. There is an overlap of symptoms with migraine headaches in some patients. This overlap predicts the future development of migraine headaches. Psychosocial factors are very common with tension-type headaches. Electromyogram (EMG) studies do not support the theory of muscle contraction and vasoconstriction. Given the overlap of symptoms with migraines, the unstable serotonergic neurotransmission associated with tension-type headaches, and the clinical response of tension-type headaches to triptan medications, migraine and tension-type headaches may represent a continuum. Nonsteroidal drugs are the treatment of choice for tension-type headaches. Antidepressants and biobehavioral techniques are effective for prophylaxis.

Deciding when a headache is an emergency and when to use neuroimaging are common and difficult issues for primary care physicians. The danger signs for a complaint of a headache are listed in Table 33-1. Several professional associations agree on three reasons to obtain neuroimaging: recent significant change in the pattern, frequency or severity of headaches, progressive worsening despite appropriate therapy, and focal neurological signs or symptoms. No conclusive data exist on the relative sensitivity of magnetic resonance imaging or CT scan.

TABLE 33-1

Danger Signs

Sudden-onset or severe rapidly crescendo headache
Absence of similar headache in the past
Worsening pattern
Focal neurological symptoms
Delirium
New headache: especially if age is <5 or >50

Selected References

Clinch R. Evaluation of acute headaches in adults. *Am Fam Physician.* 2001 February 15;63(4):685–692.

Silberstein S. Migraine. *Lancet.* 2004:363:381–91.

Mulleners W, Chronicle E. Anticonvulsant drugs for migraine prophylaxis. *Cochrane Database Syst Rev.* 2004;(3):CD003226.

Freitag FG. Drugs for migraines. Treat Guidel Med Lett. 2004; 2(25):63–66.

14-Year-Old Female with Dyspnea and Exercise Intolerance

CASE PRESENTATION

A 14-year-old female presented to her primary care pediatrician with the concern of progressive exercise intolerance. For the last 2 weeks at color guard practice, she was becoming increasingly fatigued with her usual level of exertion. When the patient initially began having difficulty keeping up in practice, she attributed it to symptoms of upper respiratory infection (URI). Her URI symptoms resolved, but she continued to have trouble in practice. She now has not participated in practice for the last few days as she feels like she cannot catch her breath once she starts performing the routines. Her mother has noticed that she is now "breathless" during activities of daily living. The patient pauses during climbing the stairs at the house. The previous day, she could not keep up with the family walking from the parking lot into church. The patient reports that her cough and congestion resolved 1 week ago. She feels somewhat short of breath even at rest and has tightness in her chest that worsens during activity. The patient complains of chest pain with inspiration even at rest. She denies fever, abdominal pain, vomiting, or diarrhea and also denies muscles aches or joint pain. The patient's past medical history is significant for overweight, but she has had no major illnesses, surgeries, or hospitalizations. The patient is sexually active. She uses an oral contraceptive which was started 4 months prior. The patient takes no other medicines with the exception of a daily multivitamin. She denies tobacco, alcohol, or illicit drug use. The patient was adopted as a young child after her mother was incarcerated and her father died suddenly at age 27 of a presumed myocardial infarction. On the day of presentation, the primary care physician obtained a chest radiograph which was read as normal and an electrocardiogram (ECG) that had nonspecific T-wave changes. The ECG was faxed to a pediatric cardiologist who requested the patient be seen in clinic later in the week for evaluation and an exercise stress test. The cardiologist also recommended obtaining a fasting lipid profile and screening for type 2 diabetes. Later in the week, the family presented to the pediatric cardiologist with requested screening laboratory tests all within normal limits. The patient initiated the exercise stress test and after about 5 minutes became very short of breath and complained of severe chest pain to the technician shortly before collapsing on the treadmill. She was then admitted to the intensive care unit at a tertiary care medical center.

Physical Examination

Patient was tachypneic and very anxious appearing. Vital signs: temperature 37.5°C, heart rate (HR) 155 beats/min, respiration rate (RR) 55 breaths/min, blood pressure 88/65 mm Hg. Oxygen saturation 98% on 100% nonrebreather. Weight 80 kg, body mass index (BMI) 28. Head, eyes, ears, nose, and throat: normocephalic, atraumatic, pupils equal, round, reactive to light. Neck: supple, no lymphadenopathy, no jugular venous distension. Cardiovascular examination (CV): tachycardic. No murmurs, gallops, rubs. No pain on palpation of the chest. Lungs: clear bilaterally, but patient taking shallow breaths, complaining of inspiratory pain. Abdomen: soft, nontender/nondistended, normoactive bowel sounds. Extremities: no edema or tenderness. The remainder of the examination was deferred.

Laboratory Studies

Arterial blood gas (ABG) on 100% non-rebreather. pH: 7.3, P_{CO_2} 50, P_{O_2} 95, HCO_3: 22, base balance -3.6, oxygen saturation 96%, Na 137, K 4.3, glucose 122, ionized calcium 4.0, hemoglobin 11.6, lactate 3.2. Creatine kinase 155, creatine kinase-MB 7.2, troponin T 0.34, D-dimer 537. Serum HCG: negative ECG and chest computed tomography (CT) results are shown in Fig. 34-1 and Fig. 34-2 respectively.

Case Resolution

The patient was started on intravenous heparin. She had a transthoracic echocardiogram that demonstrated right ventricular (RV) dysfunction and elevated pulmonary pressures.

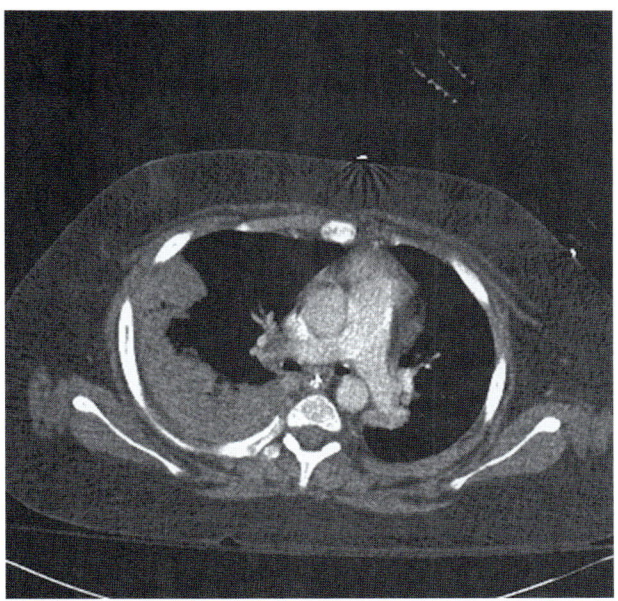

Figure 34-2 Chest CT. Note the filling defect in the region of the right pulmonary artery corresponding to a large pulmonary thromboembolus. This image also shows the peripheral area of lung infarction.
CT, computed tomography.

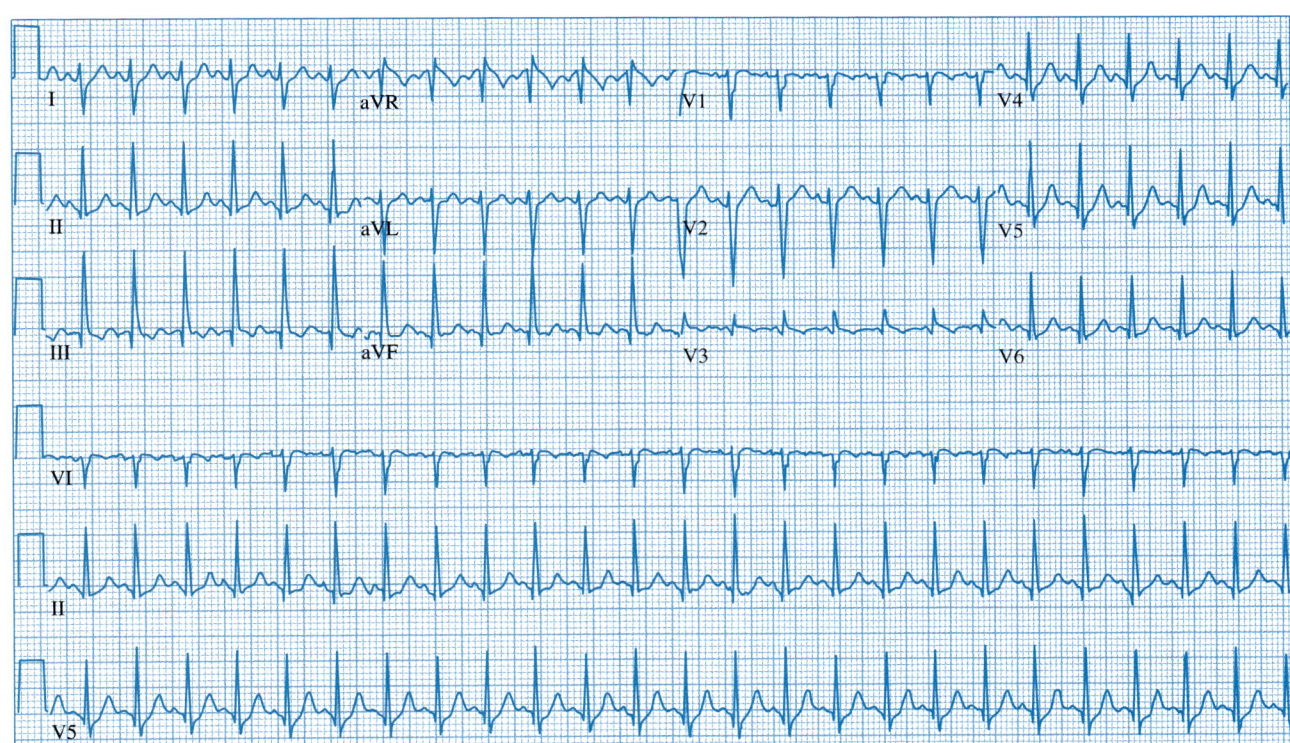

Figure 34-1 12-lead ECG reveals sinus tachycardia, mild right ventricular hypertrophy, and minor ST abnormalities. The classic finding of S1Q3T3 was not seen in this case.
ECG, electrocardiogram.

Lower extremity Doppler ultrasound did not demonstrate deep vein thrombosis (DVT). Owing to increasing cardiorespiratory compromise, the patient underwent thrombolysis which was without complication. During her hospital stay, the patient had a negative evaluation for hereditary thrombophilia, but test results were compromised as they were performed after anticoagulation was initiated. The patient was referred to a hematology clinic for further testing as an outpatient and was discharged home on low-molecular-weight heparin. In addition, the patient was counseled as she could no longer use hormonal contraception.

Question

What is the most likely explanation of the patient's progressive dyspnea and exercise intolerance and syncopal event during exercise stress testing?

Answer

Because of the history of antecedent URI and progressive dyspnea with exercise intolerance, cardiomyopathy secondary to viral illness was the initial concern of the primary care physician. However, the patient's collapse was caused by massive pulmonary embolism (PE). It is thought that the patient may have been experiencing small subsegmental pulmonary emboli during the symptomatic period before presentation to health care. The use of oral contraceptives may be the causative factor of the PE in this case, but concern for inherited thrombophilia state remains because of the sudden death of the patient's otherwise healthy father in his twenties. See Table 34-1 for risks associated with various genetic factors and the interaction with hormonal oral contraceptives.

Discussion

PE is a rare event in children with an estimated incidence of around 1 PE per 100,000 children per year. In contrast, the estimated annual incidence of PE in adults is around 120 events per 100,000 persons. Mortality in children with PE is around 2% for death directly attributable to PE, but all-cause mortality in the 2 years following PE is 16%. All-cause 2-year mortality in adults is also 16%. Morbidity caused by PE, such as recurrent thrombosis and post-thrombotic syndrome, is around 10%. Recurrent thromboembolism in

TABLE 34-1

Risks and Incidence of a First Episode of Venous Thrombosis

Condition/Risk factor(s)	Relative risk	Incidence, percent/year
Normal	1	0.008
Hyperhomocysteinemia (MTHFR 677T mutation)	2.5	0.02
	1	–
Prothrombin gene mutation	2.8	0.02
Oral contraceptives	4	0.03
Factor V Leiden (heterozygous)	7	0.06
Oral contraceptives + heterozygous factor V Leiden	35	0.29
Factor V Leiden (homozygous)	80	0.5–1.0

Adult patients only. Adapted from Leiden Thrombophilia Study

children occurs in around 8% of cases, but in adults, the recurrence rate is close to 20%. The decreased recurrence rate of thromboembolism is thought to be because of the more transient nature of predisposing factors in children as compared to adults. In general, children are at less risk for PE because of decreased prevalence of risk factors such as malignancy, heart disease, overweight, and chronic illness. However, the decreased incidence of PE in children has also been attributed to a reduced capacity to generate thrombin, increased thrombin inhibition by alpha-2 macroglobulin, and enhanced antithrombotic capacity of the vessel wall. It is not known whether the increasing prevalence of overweight among children with associated conditions such as hypertension and type 2 diabetes will increase the incidence of PE in children.

Study of PE in children is limited by the rarity of the disorder. However, multicenter studies and registries have allowed for the definition of underlying conditions that increase the risk for the development of a DVT and PE. Several studies have found that there is a bimodal peak in incidence for children less than 1 year of age and children in their teenage years. PE in children is most often associated with having a central venous catheter or significant systemic illnesses such as cancer or congenital heart disease. Nearly all neonates with PE have a history of a central venous catheter. Three-quarters of all children who develop thrombosis have several risk factors. For example, children with chronic illness often have a central venous catheter for receipt of needed medication, such as chemotherapy or intravenous antibiotics, thus compounding their risk for PE. Use of oral contraceptives is also an identified risk factor, but is less common than the previously mentioned risk factors. Adolescent women who use oral contraceptives do not appear to be at more or less risk than adult women who use hormonal contraception. A more complete list of predisposing conditions for DVT/PE in children can be found in Table 34-2.

Identifying both adults and children with PE remains enigmatic. Studies of PE in children have found that nearly all children presenting with PE have symptoms such as chest pain or tachypnea. However, the relative nonspecific nature of these symptoms may hamper identification of affected patients. Symptomatic children with relevant risk factors such as chronic illness or a central venous catheter should receive prompt evaluation to exclude the diagnosis of PE. Unfortunately the sensitivity and specificity of screening tests used to identify PE in adults have not been adequately studied in children. Chest x-ray and ECG may

be abnormal in PE but rarely provide data that are useful in confirming or excluding the diagnosis. Plasma D-dimer is produced by the breakdown of cross-linked fibrin in a clot and should be elevated in the setting of PE. Normal plasma D-dimer levels are used as a screening test to exclude adult patients with PE if they are relatively low risk. However, in a child deemed to be high risk for PE, a negative D-dimer should not preclude further evaluation. The gold standard for PE is angiography, but the invasive nature of this test prompts consideration of less-invasive initial testing prior to undertaking angiography. An example of a positive angiography for PE can be found in Fig. 34-3. Computed tomography angiography (CTA) is a sensitive test for identifying larger thrombi and is emerging as the first test of choice especially in patients presenting to the emergency room. This may be an especially good test in children as it is of short duration and can be interpreted even if children cannot cooperate fully with instructions. Ventilation-perfusion scanning and magnetic resonance imaging (MRI) angiography have also been used to identify PE in children.

One of the ways PE can be confirmed is through identification of a DVT, in the setting of symptoms compatible with PE. In adults, nearly two-thirds of DVTs are found in the lower extremity, while in children, nearly two-thirds of

TABLE 34-2

Underlying Conditions Resulting in Thrombosis for 405 Children with DVT/PE

Predisposing factor	% of cohort
Central venous catheter	60
Cancer/Bone marrow transplant	25
Cardiac disease	19
Surgery	15
Infection	12
MVA/Trauma	10
Others	8
Hormonal contraception	4
Spontaneous	3
Overweight	2
Hereditary thrombophilia	2
Systemic lupus erythematosus	1.5

DVT/PE, deep vein thrombosis/pulmonary embolism; MVA, moving vehicle accident.
Adapted from Monagle P. Outcome of pediatric thromboembolic disease: a report from the Canadian childhood thrombophilia registry. Pediatr Res. 2000;47(6):763–766.

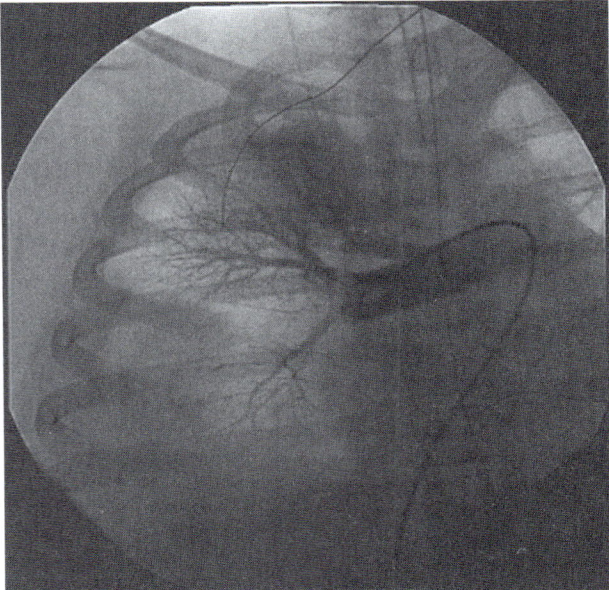

Figure 34-3 This arteriogram demonstrates evidence of pulmonary thromboembolus in the lower right lung. Note the paucity of vessel markings in the lower right branch pulmonary artery as compared to the upper branch pulmonary artery.

DVTs are found in the upper extremity. This complicates diagnosis as duplex ultrasonography used to identify DVT relies on compressibility of veins to exclude DVT. Upper extremity vessels are often not compressible because of the bony thorax. A recent study in children found ultrasonography to have a sensitivity of 20% for identification of intrathoracic thrombus. Venography is more sensitive than ultrasound for identification of an upper extremity DVT and is currently the recommended diagnostic test. However, venography should be combined with ultrasound to evaluate for jugular venous thrombosis as the sensitivity for this vessel is low with only venography. Currently CT- and MRI-based evaluations for DVTs are being tested but have not been shown to be superior.

Management of PE in children is generally equivalent to that of adults. Initial cardiorespiratory stabilization should be followed by anticoagulation. Intravenous heparin is often the initial choice, but low-molecular-weight heparin is gaining favor even in the initial management. Low-molecular-weight heparin does not require a continuous infusion, and confers less risk of bleeding, osteopenia, and heparin-induced thrombocytopenia. Low-molecular-weight heparin or warfarin may be used for anticoagulation in the 3 to 6 months following PE. Children with hereditary thrombophilia may require longer treatment. Children with significant cardiorespiratory compromise, who do not demonstrate improvement with initiation of anticoagulation, may require thrombolysis. Tissue plasminogen activator (TPA) is the most commonly used thrombolytic, but hemorrhagic complications from its use can be fatal. It is generally administered concomitantly with fresh frozen plasma in the effort to decrease complications. Of note, thrombolytic therapy with TPA may be less effective in infants and children owing to decreased plasminogen levels which is the active substrate for TPA. Because of the risk of a fatal complication and the possibility of decreased efficacy, the use of thrombolytics in children remains controversial.

Although there are differences in opinion regarding treatment of PE, there is much more debate how to treat DVT in children that has not yet resulted in PE. Generally, a DVT is identified in a child with a central venous catheter. Symptoms from the DVT can include loss of catheter patency, swelling, pain, or discoloration of the affected limb. Removal of the catheter may resolve the symptoms and prevent complications. In these children, the addition of anticoagulation, generally with low-molecular-weight heparin, can result in reduction of symptoms and may decrease the incidence of post-thrombotic syndrome.

Post-thrombotic syndrome results from damage to venous valves in deep vessels and manifests as pain, swelling, limb discoloration, and even ulceration. Some DVTs in children are identified incidentally during a study for other reasons or as part of a screening program. In children with identified DVT, catheter removal is recommended, but may not be possible in a child with chronic illness with limited intravascular access options. The role of anticoagulation to prevent PE in children with known DVTs caused by a central venous catheter is unclear. Children with central venous catheter-related DVTs are at increased risk for PE, but the risk has not been quantified nor has the efficacy of anticoagulation in prevention of PE been studied. Catheter-related DVT also increases the risk of bacterial colonization of the catheter and bacteremia secondary to catheter infection. There is a great need for further study of management of catheter-related DVT to determine if PE and infectious complications can be prevented.

In summary, this case describes a less common underlying etiology of PE in children, but highlights the need to consider this diagnosis in children presenting with chest pain and shortness of breath. The index of suspicion should be especially high in symptomatic children with chronic illness or a central venous catheter. There is a significant need for more information about the best way to diagnose, treat, and prevent PE in children to decrease morbidity and mortality associated with this condition.

Selected References

1. Andrew M, Cairney B, DeSai D. Venous thromboembolic complications (VTE) in children: first analysis of the Canadian registry of VTE. *Blood.* 1994;5:1251–1257.
2. Babyn PS, Gahunia HK, Massicotte P. Pulmonary thromboembolism in children. *Pediatr Radiol.* 2005;35:258–274.
3. Chan AK, Deveber G, Monagle P, et al. Venous thrombosis in children. *J Thromb Haemost.* 2003;1:1443–1455.
4. Johnson AS, Bolte RG. Pulmonary embolism in the pediatric patient. *Pediatr Emerg Care.* 2004;20(8):555–560.
5. Journeycake JM, Buchanan GR. Thrombotic complications of central venous catheters in children. *Curr Opin Hematol.* 2003;10:369–374.
6. Monagle P. Outcome of pediatric thromboembolic disease: a report from the Canadian childhood thrombophilia registry. *Pediatr Res.* 2000;47(6):763–766.
7. Stein PD, Kayali F, Olson RE. Incidence of venous thromboembolism in infants and children: data from the National Hospital Discharge Survey. *J Pediatr.* 2000;145(4):563–565.
8. Koster T, Rosendaal FR, de Ronde H, et al. Venous thrombosis due to poor anticoagulant response to activated protein C: Leiden thrombophilia study. *Lancet.* 1993;342:1503.

5-Year-Old Male with Syncope

CASE PRESENTATION

A 5-year-old Hispanic male presented to the emergency room via ambulance after a brief episode "passing out" just prior to emergency medical services' arrival. His mother stated that he woke up that morning very irritable, sweating, complaining of nonspecific pain, and suddenly became unresponsive. He had no history of ingestion. No fever, vomiting, diarrhea, or seizure activity per the mother. The patient's only remarkable past medical history was mild, intermittent asthma and sinusitis. His current medications included budesonide, albuterol, ceftibuten, and an over-the-counter cough medicine. Upon arrival to the emergency department (ED), he was found to have a fingerstick glucose of 40, rectal temperature of 35°C, but was responsive to stimulation. After warm intravenous fluids and oral glucose bolus, he was more interactive, asking for food, with a rectal temperature of 37°C and fingerstick glucose of 149. He was subsequently admitting to the pediatric floor for observation.

Physical Examination

Patient was a nontoxic appearing, well-developed, well-nourished child who is drowsy but responsive and in no apparent distress. Vital signs: temperature 35°C (repeat rectal), blood pressure 111/54 mm Hg, pulse 101 beats/min, respiration 18 breaths/min, oxygen saturation of 99% on room air, and weight 22.7 kg. Head, eyes, ears, nose, and throat: normocephalic, atraumatic, pupils equal, round, reactive to light, extraocular movement intact, tacky mucous membranes, scant clear rhinorrhea, unremarkable tympanic membranes and oropharynx. Neck: supple, no lymphadenopathy or thyromegaly. Cardiovascular: regular rate and rhythm no murmurs, gallops, rubs, good pulses, 2- to 3-second capillary refill. Lungs: clear to auscultation, no wheezing or retractions noted. Abdomen: soft, nontender, normoactive bowel sounds; no hepatosplenomegaly. Extremities: no cyanosis, clubbing, edema. Skin: diaphoretic, pallor, but no rash or lesions. Neurology: spontaneous eye opening with stimulation, drowsy but oriented. The remainder of the examination was unremarkable.

Laboratory Studies

Na 138, K 3.4, Cl 105, CO_2 17, blood urea nitrogen 14, creatinine (Cr) 0.6, glucose 43, venous blood gas pH 7.27, PCO_2 40, PO_2 35, HCO_3 19, white blood cells 11.9, hematocrit 42%, platelets 300, aspartate aminotransferase 49, alanine aminotransferase 24, total protein 23, albumin 4.2, urinalysis specific gravity 1.025, pH 5, large ketones, no protein, negative leukocyte esterase, negative nitrite, acetaminophen level < 10, salicylate level < 4, ammonia level 28, urine toxicology screen negative, thyroid-stimulating hormone 0.56, head computed tomography (CT) negative. Insulin level pending.

Case Resolution

After stabilization and a long-requested meal of crackers and juice in the ED, the patient was more interactive and very playful with the staff on the pediatric floor. A Spanish interpreter was called to obtain the complete history from the patient's mother. This interview revealed that the patient and his mother had been in a van traveling from New York to North Carolina with multiple family members. Because of time constraints, they were unable to make frequent stops for snacks and meals. Subsequently, the patient's last meal was around 5 PM the previous night, resulting in a fasting period of about 12 to 14 hours. During hospitalization, frequent fingerstick glucose checks were all normal and he was sent home in good condition. Days later, his insulin level sent from the ED came back normal.

Question

What is the most likely explanation of the patient's clinically significant and symptomatic hypoglycemia?

Answer

In an otherwise healthy child of this age with a prolonged fasting period and ketonuria, idiopathic ketotic hypoglycemia (IKH) is the most likely diagnosis. Also high on the differential would be toxins or medication ingestions such as oral hypoglycemic agents, insulin, salicylates, or alcohol. Hepatic and metabolic causes of hypoglycemia are ruled out with the absence of hepatomegaly or increased transaminases. Table 35-1 shows the differential diagnosis of hypoglycemia in infants and children.

Discussion

Hypoglycemia is defined as whole blood glucose less than 50 mg/dL in full-term infants or less than 60 mg/dL in a child or adult. However, like the child in the above case, severe symptoms may not occur until the blood glucose drops near 40 mg/dL. Older children with hypoglycemia may exhibit the classic symptoms of hypoglycemia seen in adults such as sweating, palpitations, hunger, lethargy, and headache; however, younger children and infants may present with subtle findings that can easily be overlooked. Neonates with hypoglycemia usually present with cyanosis, hypothermia, apnea, hypotonia, poor feeding, or seizures. As a result, it is not uncommon for children with episodic hypoglycemia to be misdiagnosed with epilepsy. Another common diagnostic pitfall occurs in children who present with a sudden deterioration in psychobehavioral functioning such

TABLE 35-1

Classification of Hypoglycemia in Infants and Children

Neonatal transient hypoglycemia
Prematurity
SGA
Normal newborn
Transient hyperinsulinism
Discordant twin
Birth asphyxia
Infant of diabetic mother

Neonatal, infantile, or childhood persistent hypoglycemia
Hyperinsulinism
Panhypopituitarism
Growth hormone deficiency
ACTH deficiency
Addison disease
Glycogen storage diseases
Galactosemia
Hereditary fructose intolerance
Fatty acid oxidation disorders

Other etiologies
Ketotic hypoglycemia
Ingestions
  Salicylates
  Alcohol
  Oral hypoglycemia agents
  Insulin
  Propranolol
  Ackee fruit (unripe)
  Vacor (rat poison)
  TMP-sulfa (w/ renal failure)
Liver disease
  Reye syndrome
  Hepatitis
  Cirrhosis
  Hepatoma
Amino acid and organic acid disorders
Systemic disorders
  Sepsis
  Malnutrition
  Malabsorption
  Renal failure
  Diarrhea

(Continued)

TABLE 35-1

Classification of Hypoglycemia in Infants and Children (*Continued*)

Shock
Burns
Nissen fundoplication
Falciparum malaria

ACTH, adrenocorticotropic; SGA, small for gestational age; TMP-sulfa, trimethoprim and sulfamethoxazole.

TABLE 35-2

Demographics of the Hypoglycemic Presentation of IKH

Average age	30.8 months
Sex	68% male
Race	75% Caucasian
Weight percentile for age	70% < 25th percentile
Average blood glucose	34 mg/dL
Symptom constellation	lethargy, seizure, vomiting, coma
Intercurrent illness	46%
Median time of presentation	7:56 AM

IKH, idiopathic ketotic hypoglycemia.
Adapted from Daly LP, Osterhoudt KC, Weinzimer SA. Presenting features of idiopathic ketotic hypoglycemia. J Emerg Med. 2003;25(1):39–43.

as behavior changes and inattention, mistakenly leading to a diagnosis of attention deficit disorder.

IKH is the most common cause of hypoglycemia among previously healthy children older than 6 months of age. It is defined as periodic episodes of hypoglycemia associated with ketonuria in an otherwise healthy child. Typically these episodes occur with a concurrent illness (such as a viral upper respiratory infection or gastroenteritis) or any other condition that leads to prolonged fasting. The classic history usually involves a child who eats poorly or completely skips dinner and then is difficult to arouse in the morning. If prompt medical treatment is delayed, they quickly progress to seizures or comatose by midmorning.

It is important to consider the age at presentation when considering the diagnosis of IKH. It rarely occurs before the age of 18 months and remits by the age of 8 to 9 years of age. In a recent case series of children presenting in an ED setting with the diagnosis of IKH, the mean age of presentation was 30.8 months. Table 35-2 shows the demographics of children in the study that presented to the ED with IKH.

Many investigations into the etiology of IKH have revealed several possible pathophysiologic explanations including disturbances in gluconeogenesis, glycolysis, brain glucose utilization, and impaired response to insulin in fasting states. However, the leading hypothesis into the pathogenesis is that children with IKH have a substrate deficiency attributed to lean body mass. Studies of children with IKH show that compared to age-matched controls they are frequently smaller and have decreased levels of plasma alanine levels. Alanine, produced in muscle, is a major precursor in gluconeogenesis. This theory may also explain why the condition remits with age and concurrent

increased muscle mass, therefore, providing more substrate for endogenous glucose production.

In the acute setting, treatment of IKH usually requires a bolus of a 25% dextrose and water solution, 2 to 4 mL/kg, then maintenance fluids with D10W, and electrolytes. If the child is unable to tolerate oral fluids or the hypoglycemia does not resolve after treatment, they should be admitted to the hospital. In the outpatient setting, prevention efforts should focus on frequent meals and snacks consisting of high-protein, high-carbohydrates foods. During intercurrent illness, parents should be instructed to give sugar-containing fluids and test the child's urine for ketones. Parent education should also include the signs and symptoms of hypoglycemia and reiterate the importance of prompt medical attention when the child exhibits these symptoms.

In summary, IKH is the most common cause of hypoglycemia in nondiabetic children. It usually presents in the morning hours after a history of fasting for 10 to 16 hours with ketones in the urine. Early and accurate diagnosis can prevent unnecessary testing and avoid future hypoglycemic episodes that can lead to complications such as developmental delay and recurrent seizures. Additional causes of hypoglycemia in children should be excluded in any child presenting with hypoglycemia less than 18 months of age, has a possible history of ingestion, or evaluation reveals hepatomegaly or elevated transaminases.

Selected References

1. Crain EF, Gershel JC. Endocrine emergencies: hypoglycemia. In: *Clinical Manual of Emergency Pediatrics*. 4th ed. Philadelphia, PA: McGraw-Hill Publishing; Sept 2002:chap 7.

2. Daly LP, Osterhoudt KC, Weinzimer SA. Presenting features of idiopathic ketotic hypoglycemia. *J Emerg Med*. 2003;25(1): 39–43.

3. Sperling MA. Hypoglycemia. In: Behrman RE, Kliegman RM, Jenson HB, eds. *Nelson's Textbook of Pediatrics*. 17th ed. Philadelphia, PA: Saunders, Elsevier Science; 2000:Chap 81.

39-Year-Old Female with Progressive Dyspnea on Exertion and Leg Edema

CASE PRESENTATION

A 39-year-old African American female presented to the hospital in early spring with a several-day history of nausea, vomiting, cough, shortness of breath, dyspnea on exertion, and edema. She attributed her gastrointestinal symptoms to sequelae from a cholecystectomy she had undergone 9 months prior. Although she tolerated the surgery well, she had suffered waxing and waning nausea and vomiting since that time and had been admitted to the hospital several times because of dehydration. The shortness of breath was new, however, and was accompanied by paroxysmal nocturnal dyspnea and intermittent chest pain. On further review of systems, she endorsed significant weight loss over the past several months, dysphagia, and frequent bowel movements.

The patient's past medical history is significant for diabetes mellitus and hypertension. The patient also reports having been diagnosed with possible cardiomegaly after a routine chest x-ray (CXR) 2 years prior, but could not provide further details. She worked in a textile factory. She denied tobacco use or illicit drug use. She did not have any recent travel. She did not think anyone in her family had premature heart disease or other heart problems. She had no children.

Physical Examination

On examination, she was moderately obese, afebrile, tachycardic. Vital signs: temperature 36°C, heart rate 134 beats/min, hypertension with initial blood pressure 171/112 mm Hg, respiration rate 24 breaths/min, and her oxygen saturation was 93% on room air. Her neck examination was remarkable for a soft, diffusely enlarged thyroid gland without discrete nodules. She did not have exophthalmos. She had diminished breath sounds at both bases and was noted to have bilateral 1+ edema of lower extremities. In addition to her tachycardia, she was noted to have an S_3 on heart examination. She had normoactive bowel sounds and no organomegaly, but was mildly tender to palpation in the epigastric area. Her reflexes were not checked on initial examination.

Laboratory Studies/Imaging

The patient's chest radiograph showed small bilateral effusions and an enlarged cardiac silhouette. Her electrocardiogram (ECG) (Fig. 36-1) showed sinus tachycardia with premature ventricular contractions and evidence of both left ventricular hypertrophy as well as left atrial enlargement. Serial cardiac enzymes were negative. A urine drug screen was negative. A pulmonary embolism (PE)-protocol computed tomography (CT) was negative for pulmonary embolus, but did show cardiomegaly with evidence of congestive heart failure. Her thyroid-stimulating hormone (TSH) was <0.01 μIU/mL and both her free triiodothyronine (T_3) and free thyroxine (T_4) levels were markedly elevated. A transthoracic echocardiogram done during admission showed dilated cardiomyopathy with an ejection fraction of 10% to 15%.

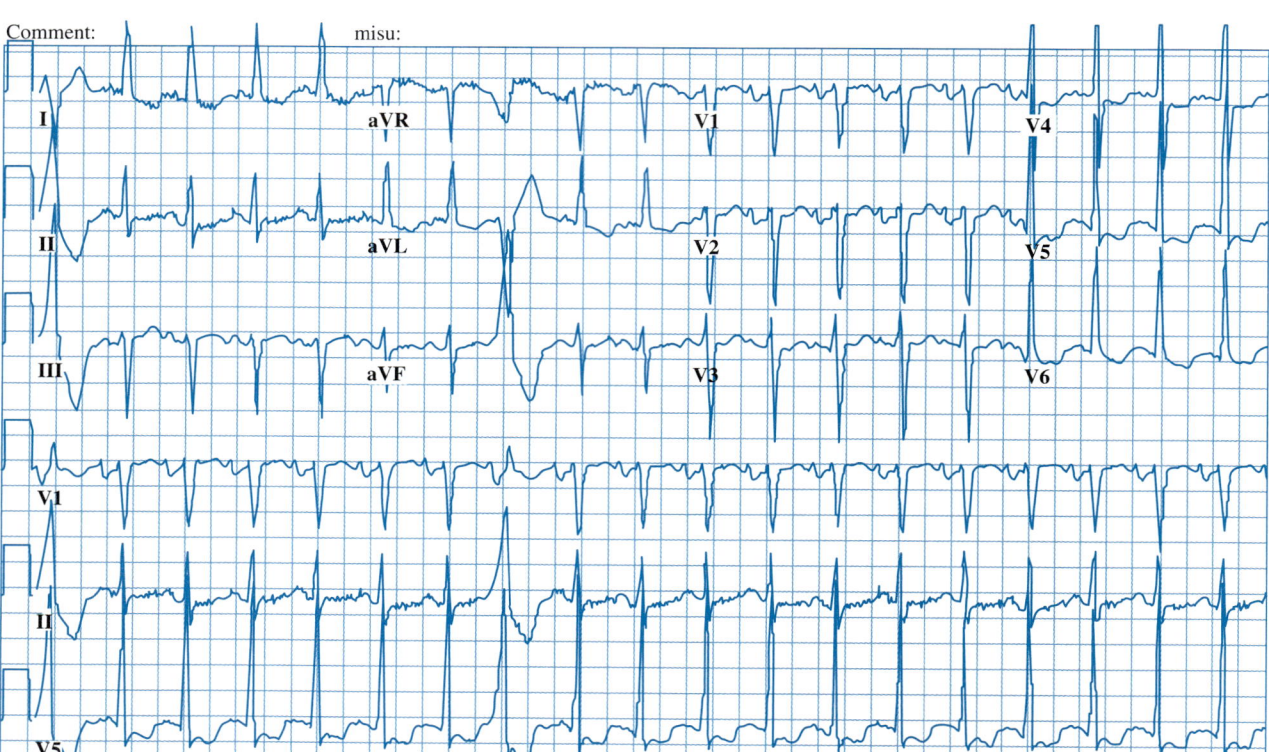

Figure 36-1 ECG from the patient described in vignette above showed sinus tachycardia with premature ventricular contractions and evidence of both left ventricular hypertrophy as well as left atrial enlargement. Subsequent two-dimensional echocardiogram showed dilated cardiomyopathy with an ejection fraction of 10%–15%. ECG, electrocardiogram.

Upon further direct questioning of the patient, she recalled being told several months prior that she had a "thyroid problem," but she had not undergone treatment.

Case Resolution

In the hospital, she was started on atenolol 50 mg/day and propylthiouracil (PTU). She was also given lisinopril and furosemide for afterload reduction and treatment of her newly diagnosed heart failure. Her nausea, vomiting, and dysphagia improved with the initiation of treatment for hyperthyroidism. As an outpatient, she was started on methimazole, and plans were made for her to undergo radioiodine uptake scan 2 to 3 months after her last contrasted study, which in this case was the PE-protocol CT scan.

Question

Based on the information presented in the case, what is the most likely cause of the patient's cardiomyopathy and clinical heart failure?

Answer

Given the patient's presentation, the most likely cause is long-standing hyperthyroidism, and her cardiomyopathy is secondary to her previously untreated thyroid disease and possibly to untreated hypertension.

Discussion

Hyperthyroidism occurs in about 2% of women and 0.2% of men. Graves disease is the most common cause of hyperthyroidism, but other causes range from Hashimoto thyroiditis to pituitary tumors that secrete TSH. The patient described in the vignette above had several complaints and physical examination findings consistent with hyperthyroidism including weight loss, dysphagia, frequent bowel movements, nausea and vomiting, tachycardia, and thyromegaly. Other classic signs and symptoms include heat intolerance, sweating, lid lag, exophthalmos (classically in Grave's disease) irregular menses, tremor, and anxiety.

Hyperthyroidism affects the cardiovascular system by increasing the heart rate, cardiac contractility, cardiac output, diastolic relaxation rate, and myocardial oxygen consumption and by reducing systemic vascular resistance and diastolic pressure (Table 36-1). This probably occurs via the binding of T_3 to cardiac myocyte nuclear receptors that influence cardiac gene expression and therefore protein synthesis. Part of the increased contractility and cardiac hypertrophy attributed to hyperthyroidism can be explained by the increased protein synthesis. Proteins such as cardiac actin and myosin heavy chain subunits are expressed at a higher level in the setting of hyperthyroidism. Moreover, expression of the calcium adenosine triphosphatase (ATPase) in the sarcoplasmic reticulum is increased in hyperthyroidism leading to more rapid diastolic relaxation compared to the euthyroid state. Other channels are affected directly without gene transcription and protein expression such as the sarcolemmal Na1 channel, the inward-rectifying K1 channel, voltage-activated potassium channels, and the aforementioned calcium ATPases. T_3 also has other extranuclear effects on the heart as well as effects on the sympathoadrenal system. T_3 may also influence the density of beta-adrenergic receptors on myocytes, increase the density of beta-receptor–coupled G proteins that stimulate the myocytes when beta-agonists bind the receptor, and lead to decreases in regulatory phosphodiesterase enzymes. Together these mechanisms likely produce many of the overall changes in contractility, cardiac output, and systemic vascular resistance described above.

The clinical manifestations of hyperthyroidism include palpitations, tachycardia, systolic hypertension with a widened pulse pressure, and varying degrees of exercise impairment. Two to twenty percent of patients with hyperthyroidism will experience atrial fibrillation; though it is important to keep in mind that less than 1% of new-onset atrial fibrillation is caused by overt hyperthyroidism and that sinus tachycardia is the most common arrhythmia seen in hyperthyroidism. On examination, a Means-Lerman "scratch" may be appreciated on auscultation; this is a raspy midsystolic murmur at the left sternal border and is attributed to the rubbing together of the pericardium and the pleura.

Heart failure owing to hyperthyroidism can occur, particularly in elderly patients with atrial fibrillation or in patients with severe, untreated hyperthyroidism. Prolonged high cardiac output, increased myocardial oxygen demand, impaired diastolic filling, and rapid left ventricular rate all contribute to the development of heart failure. These patients have poor cardiac contractility, low cardiac output, a third heart sound, and pulmonary congestion as our patient did, all the result of rate-related heart failure. Most commonly, hyperthyroidism exacerbates underlying heart disease. As described in the vignette above, this patient had been diagnosed with cardiomegaly in the past, which was probably related to untreated hypertension; the patient described likely had some degree of underlying hypertensive heart disease. There was not any definite evidence of ischemic heart disease in this patient, though a catheterization was not done.

Initial treatment in treating hyperthyroidism in general is aimed at lowering the heart rate using beta-blockers, usually propranolol, but other beta-blockers may be used including atenolol. Propranolol has one advantage over other less lipid-soluble agents in that it has the ability to inhibit conversion of T_4 to T_3 in peripheral tissues. Antithyroid drugs, known as thionamides, can also be used acutely, and include PTU or methimazole. These drugs decrease thyroid hormone synthesis. PTU has the additional mechanism of inhibiting the conversion of T_4 to metabolically active T_3 in peripheral tissues. This effect on peripheral conversion may make PTU a better presurgical therapeutic option. Moreover, because methimazole is associated with aplasia cutis in a developing fetus, PTU is more favorable in pregnancy. These medicines are typically started along with a beta-blocker and are continued for

TABLE 36-1

Cardiovascular Parameters that Change in the Hyperthyroid State

Increased with respect to euthyroid state	Decreased with respect to euthyroid state
Cardiac output	Diastolic blood pressure
Cardiac inotropy	Systemic vascular resistance
Cardiac chronotropy (HR)	Isovolumetric relaxation time
Ejection fraction	Diastolic blood pressure
Peripheral and cardiac oxygen consumption	Diastolic relaxation time
Pulse pressure	
Pulmonary artery systolic pressure	

HR, heart rate.
Adapted from data reviewed in multiple sources.

some time. The thionamides can induce remission in up to 60% of those with Graves disease.

In those whose disease does not remit or who have other underlying causes of hyperthyroidism, definitive treatment can be attained with radioactive iodine or surgery. A thyroid radioiodine uptake scan may be used to help determine the underlying etiology. Unfortunately, studies using iodine contrast introduce exogenous iodine into the body that can affect the results of the scan. This was the case in the vignette above as the patient received a CT with contrast as part of her diagnostic workup. Her hypothyroidism was treated for several months before this study was done, delaying her definitive diagnosis.

Selected References

1. Kahaly GJ, Dillmann WH. Thyroid hormone action in the heart. *Endocr Rev.* 2005;26:704–728.
2. Dillmann WH. Cellular action of thyroid hormone on the heart. *Thyroid.* 2002;12:447.
3. Klein I, Ojamaa K. Thyroid hormone and the cardiovascular system. *N Engl J Med.* 2001;344:501–509.
4. Davis PJ, Davis FB. Nongenomic actions of thyroid hormone on the heart. *Thyroid.* 2002;12:459.
5. Lozano HF, Sharma CN. Reversible pulmonary hypertension, tricuspid regurgitation and right-sided heart failure associated with hyperthyroidism: case report and review of the literature. *Cardiol Rev.* 2004 November–December;12(6):299–305.
6. Ventrella S, Klein I. Beta-adrenergic receptor blocking drugs in the management of hyperthyroidism. *Endocrinologist.* 1994;4:391.
7. Pearce EN. Diagnosis and management of thyrotoxicosis. *BMJ.* 2006;332:1369–1373.

10-Day-Old Female Infant with Persistent Jaundice

CASE PRESENTATION

The patient is a 3314-g product of a 38$\frac{1}{7}$ weeks' gestation to a 27-year-old gravida 1, para 1-0-0-1 (G2, P1-0-0-1) Jehovah's Witness Hispanic female with no significant past medical history, no pregnancy complications, with prenatal laboratory tests remarkable for A positive blood. Baby was B positive. Antibody screen negative, group B streptococcus (GBS) negative, gonococcus (GC)/chlamydia negative, hepatitis B negative, human immunodeficiency virus (HIV) negative, rapid plasma reagin (RPR) nonreactive, and rubella nonimmune (the mother did receive her rubella immunization prior to discharge). Baby was delivered via repeat routine C-section with Apgar scores of 9 and 9. Baby was very ruddy at delivery and a complete blood count (CBC) revealed hematocrit of 49.7. This did improve slightly during her hospitalization, but she remains with a slightly reddish hue.

The baby continued to have significant weight loss of approximately 14% with the development of jaundice. Her bilirubin peaked at 16.9 at 84 hours of life with continued weight loss and poor feeding; therefore, single phototherapy was instituted for 24 hours and bilirubin improved to 13.3. The parents continued to supplement her feeding and pumped breast milk with a syringe, feeding 30 to 40 cc of pumped breast milk every 2 hours plus putting the baby to breast.

The mother had hesitation that the baby may suffocate with breastfeeding and was somewhat hesitant to have her latch well, but the infant continued to remain jaundiced. There was no family history of infantile jaundice or hereditary anemia.

C

37

Physical Examination

Vital signs: temperature 37°C, weight 2.9 kg, heart rate 120 beats/min, oxygen saturation 100% on room air.

General: ruddy-appearing infant in no acute distress.

Head, eyes, ears, nose, and throat: anterior fontanelle open/soft/flat, bilateral red reflex present, extraocular movement intact, icteric sclera; mucus membranes moist

Cardiovascular: regular rate and rhythm, N1, S_1, S_2, no murmur; 2+ femoral pulses bilaterally

Pulmonary: clear to auscultation bilaterally, no wheeze

Abdomen: soft, nontender/nondistended, normoactive bowel sounds; no hepatosplenomegaly

Extremities: negative Ortolani and Barlow signs

Laboratory Studies

Newborn screening results on day of life 4 revealed thyroid-stimulating hormone (TSH) 566.2 and T_4 6.3. Diagnosis was confirmed on repeat laboratory tests and thyroxine therapy was initiated.

RPR was nonreactive. CBC: white blood cell count 17.4, hemoglobin 16.6, hematocrit 49.7, and platelets 261. Her blood type is B positive.

Question

What kind of jaundice does this infant have?

Answer

Unconjugated hyperbilirubinemia which may be physiologic jaundice, but in this case was attributed to congenital hypothyroidism.

Discussion

Jaundice is a common problem in the neonatal period. Up to 60% of term newborns will have clinical jaundice during the first week of life without any underlying pathology. Physiologic jaundice carries the small, but present, risk of bilirubin encephalopathy and kernicterus, as the newborn brain is uniquely susceptible to unconjugated bilirubin. Therefore a systematic approach to diagnosis, therapy, and follow-up of newborns is critical.

Most neonates experience physiologic jaundice with unconjugated hyperbilirubinemia. They produce twice the amount of bilirubin as adults do because of relative polycythemia and the rapid turnover of red blood cells; they have immature pathways for bilirubin conjugation and have increased enterohepatic circulation. See Table 37-1. Physiologic jaundice follows a typical pattern, with peak bilirubin at 3 to 4 days of life, rarely above 12 mg/dL in infants, without any risk factors and resolution by 10 to 14 days of life. Prematurity, a family history of jaundice, ABO incompatibility, as well as, cephalohematoma or other birth trauma, and delayed passage of meconium are risk factors that contribute to an exaggerated physiologic jaundice with bilirubin that may be as high as 17 mg/dL.

Breastfeeding may contribute to an exaggerated physiologic jaundice because of the initial relative caloric deprivation and dehydration with delayed meconium passage. Breast-fed infants are three to six times more likely to develop moderate or severe physiologic jaundice as compared to bottle-fed infants. Increased frequency of feedings helps improve the infant's hydration as well as stimulates milk production.

Late-onset *breast milk jaundice* usually occurs later with bilirubin peaking between day 6 and 14 of life. It usually resolves by 2 weeks of life, but may remain elevated for 1 to 3 months. Up to one-third of breast-fed infants are affected, but despite the high total bilirubin levels of 12 to 20 mg/dL, levels are not pathologic. The exact mechanism of breast milk jaundice is poorly understood; however, substances in the maternal milk may inhibit bilirubin metabolism. To confirm the diagnosis, breast feeding may be stopped for 48 hours and bilirubin levels should fall rapidly. Once the diagnosis is confirmed, breast feeding should be resumed.

All other forms of jaundice are considered pathologic jaundice. Pathologic jaundice may be unconjugated or conjugated. We will focus on unconjugated hyperbilirubinemia, as conjugated hyperbilirubinemia is beyond the scope of this discussion. Further workup is needed in any infant who has jaundice within the first 12 to 24 hours of life, whose total serum bilirubin (TSB) is greater than the 95th percentile or is rapidly increasing. Hemolytic disease, metabolic and endocrine disorders, gastrointestinal and hepatic disorders (Table 37-2), and infections may manifest as jaundice and require further evaluation (see Table 37-3).

The evaluation of jaundice always includes the measurement of fractionated bilirubin level (see Table 37-4 for recommended evaluation of neonatal jaundice). Jaundice that occurs early, within the first 24 hour of life, or late, more than 2 weeks old, is often pathologic and should be considered so, until proven otherwise. In the first 24 hours of life, pathologic jaundice is often attributed to hemolytic disease: ABO incompatibility or Rh erythroblastosis fetalis; occult hemorrhage; or infection including sepsis, rubella, or toxoplasmosis. Rh erythroblastosis fetalis occurs much less frequently now given the increased use of Rh immunoglobulin. ABO hemolytic disease often presents within the first 24 hours of life with rapidly increasing bilirubin concentration. The diagnostic criteria of ABO

TABLE 37-1

Risk Factors for the Development of Severe Hyperbilirubinemia

- Elevated predischarge from the newborn nursery bilirubin level
- Jaundice visible in the first 24 hours
- East Asian race
- Significant bruising
- Sibling that required phototherapy

TABLE 37-2

Most Frequent Causes of Liver Disease in Neonates and Infants

Cholestatic disorders

- Biliary atresia
- Choledochal cyst
- Paucity of intrahepatic bile ducts (eg, Alagille syndrome)
- Progressive familial intrahepatic cholestasis syndromes (Byler disease and syndrome)
- Benign recurrent intrahepatic cholestasis
- Caroli disease and syndrome
- Inspissated bile (s/p hemolytic disease)
- Cholelithiasis

Idiopathic neonatal hepatitis and mimickers

- Cystic fibrosis
- Alpha-1-antitrypsin deficiency
- Hypopituitarism/hypothyroidism
- Neonatal iron storage disease

Viral hepatitis or other infectious diseases in the neonate

- Cytomegalovirus
- Herpes simplex virus/herpes zoster virus/human herpes virus 6
- Epstein-Barr virus
- Parvovirus B19
- Rubella
- Reovirus, type 3
- Adenovirus
- Enterovirus
- Bacterial sepsis/urinary tract infection
- Syphilis
- Tuberculosis
- Toxoplasmosis

Metabolic disease

- Disorders of peroxisomal function (Zellweger syndrome)
- Disorders of bile acid metabolism
- Disorders of urea cycle (arginase deficiency)
- Disorders of amino acid metabolism (tyrosinemia)
- Disorders of lipid metabolism (Niemann-Pick type C/Gaucher/Wolman)
- Disorders of carbohydrate metabolism (galactosemia, fructosemia, type IV glycogen storage disease)

Toxic/pharmacologic injury (eg, acetaminophen, total parenteral nutrition, hypervitaminosis A)

Tumors (intra- and extrahepatic)

TABLE 37-3

Causes of Indirect Hyperbilirubinemia in the Neonate

Increased production or bilirubin load on the liver

- Immune mediated: Rh, ABO
- Hereditary spherocytes, G6PD deficiency
- Sepsis
- Polycythemia: infant of a diabetic mother
- Hematoma

Decreased clearance

- Prematurity
- Hypothyroidism
- Galactosemia
- Increased enterohepatic recirculation of bilirubin
- Intestinal obstruction

hemolytic disease are outlined in Table 37-5. G6PD deficiency must also be considered, especially in African American infants, as it is present in 11% to 13% of African American infants and males as the *G6PD* gene on the X chromosome. Infants with G6PD deficiency have increased red blood cells (RBC) turnover, but unlikely hemolysis, and impaired ability to conjugate bilirubin. Thirty percent of infants with kernicterus have been found to have G6PD deficiency.

Metabolic and endocrine disorders should be considered in patients with persistent or atypical jaundice. As in the infant in this case, congenital hypothyroidism can cause jaundice. Congenital hypothyroidism occurs in

TABLE 37-4

Usual Evaluation for Neonatal Jaundice

- Total serum bilirubin
- Conjugated fraction of bilirubin
- Blood type
- Coombs test
- Complete blood count
- Urinalysis and urine culture
- Sepsis evaluation if suspected

TABLE 37-5

Diagnostic Criteria for ABO Hemolytic Disease

Jaundice within 24 hours of birth

and

Mother with blood type O

and

Infant with blood type A or B

and

Direct Coombs test positive

or

Direct Coombs test negative with homozygous Gilbert syndrome

and

Microspherocytes on peripheral blood smear

TABLE 37-6

Common Signs and Symptoms of Congenital Hypothyroidism

Findings during the first 2 postnatal weeks
- Prolonged neonatal jaundice
- Edema of the eyelids, hands, and feet
- Gestation >42 weeks
- Birth weight >4 kg
- Poor feeding
- Hypothermia
- Protuberant abdomen
- Large anterior and posterior fontanelle

Findings beyond 1 month of age
- Darkened and mottled skin
- Stressful, frequent, and labored breathing
- Failure to gain weight, poor sucking ability
- Decreased stool frequency
- Decreased activity and lethargy

Findings after 3 months
- Umbilical hernia
- Infrequent and hard stools
- Dry skin with carotenemia
- Macroglossia
- Generalized swelling or myxedema
- Hoarse cry

1/3500 to 4000 newborns in areas where there is normal iodine nutrition and more often when there is iodine deficiency. Most cases are sporadic, and girls are affected twice as often as boys. It is also more common in Hispanic girls. Familial forms are much rarer with girls and boys equally affected as it is autosomal recessive. The cause of sporadic congenital hypothyroidism is unknown. Often congenital hypothyroidism is diagnosed on newborn screen; however, it may sometimes be missed and awareness of clinical signs as outlined in Table 37-6 is important to make the diagnosis. Therapy with thyroxine should be initiated as soon as serum TSH and free T_4 are obtained without waiting for laboratory results. Free T_4 is the test of choice as it is the biologically active hormone and total T_4 is influenced by protein binding and may provide false-positive or negative results. Normal intellectual and neurological development and linear growth is expected for infants treated appropriately beginning during their first few weeks of postnatal life.

The American Academy of Pediatrics (AAP) has developed clinical guidelines for managing jaundice in infants older than 35 weeks' gestation. After determining risk factors for jaundice and measurement of bilirubin, tables published by the AAP can be used to determine the risk of developing clinically significant jaundice and to guide follow-up. Traditional teaching has used the degree of yellowing of the skin with blanching to diagnose jaundice; however, given that a 2 to 3 mg/dL difference in bilirubin level may represent 50% versus 95% risk of critically high bilirubin levels, some experts recommend screening all infants with a bilirubin level at hospital discharge.

Treatment of physiologic jaundice often times is supported only with increased frequency of feedings. However for infants with exaggerated physiologic jaundice, phototherapy and, if needed, exchange transfusion is used. Blue wavelengths used in phototherapy alter unconjugated bilirubin in the skin to a much less toxic water-soluble photo isomer that can be excreted in the urine and bile without conjugation. Conjugated hyperbilirubinemia is the only contraindication to phototherapy as it may cause a discoloration of the skin, called bronze baby syndrome. With intensive phototherapy, bilirubin levels should decrease 1 to 2 mg/dL within 4 to 6 hours, and 30% to 40% in the first 24 hours. Phototherapy can usually be discontinued when levels are less than 15 mg/dL. If levels remain elevated despite intensive phototherapy, exchange transfusion should be considered. Exchange transfusion should be considered in the setting of hemolytic disease, severe anemia, rapidly increasing total bilirubin (>1 mg/dL/h in <6 hours), and if phototherapy fails to correct the hyperbilirubinemia. Intravenous immunoglobulin (IVIG) may be considered in infants with isoimmune hemolytic disease as it has been shown to significantly decrease the need for exchange transfusion.

Selected References

Foley TP. Hypothyroidism. *Pediatr Rev.* 2004;25:94–99.

Maisels MJ. Neonatal jaundice. *Pediatr Rev.* 2006;27:443–454.

Maisels MJ, Baltz RD, Bhutani V, et al. Management of hyperbilirubinemia in the newborn infant 35 or more weeks of gestation. *Pediatrics.* 2004;114:297–316.

Porter ML, Dennis BL. Hyperbilirubinemia in the term newborn. *Am Fam Physician.* 2002;65:599–606.

4-Year-Old Female with Abdominal Pain and Swelling

CASE PRESENTATION

A previously healthy 4-year-old female presented to her primary care physician with complaint of 3 weeks of abdominal pain. It has been primarily intermittent, but has worsened over the last 4 days. Her abdominal pain was described as diffuse and worse while lying flat. The pain would occasionally awaken her at night. At times she localized it more to the right side. She appeared to her parents to be short of breath when she laid flat. She had no fever or emesis. There was a single episode of diarrhea 2 days prior, but there was no blood in her bowel movements or urine. She had a markedly decreased appetite for 4 days, but good fluid intake. Her parents recall that she has had a history of complaining "seatbelts have been too tight" when they actually have not, and refusing to wear pants that do not have an elastic waistline, for the last couple of months. She has been increasingly fussy over the last 4 days. Review of systems included polydipsia (but no polyuria), back pain, and a several days of upper airway congestion and a productive cough. Past medical history was notable only for a C-section delivery for failure to progress. Social history was significant in that she lived with both parents, who were nonsmokers. She had no known sick contacts. Her mother worked as a researcher. Family history was significant for multiple family members with cancers (Hodgkin, melanoma, esophageal, thyroid, multiple ovarian cancers) and autoimmune diseases (systemic lupus erythematosus, rheumatoid arthritis, Type I diabetes).

Physical Examination

In general, she was uncomfortable appearing with intermittent tachypnea. Vital signs: temperature 36.3°C, pulse 137 beats/min, respiratory rate 32 breaths/min, blood pressure 117/90 mm Hg. Height 104 cm, weight 18.3 kg, SaO_2 is 96% on room air. Head, eyes, ears, nose, and throat examination was normal. Pupils were equal with no aniridia. She had markedly decreased breath sounds in the right base in mid lung fields, but no rhonchi or wheezing. Heart beat was regular with no murmurs. She had a prominently distended abdomen with prominent veins extending into chest region, tenderness to palpation along midline and right side. No discrete mass or organomegaly was detected. Genitourinary, lymph node, skin, and neurologic examinations were normal.

Laboratory Studies

Chemistries revealed Na 140, K 4.6, HCO_3 17, glucose 74, blood urea nitrogen 6, creatinine (Cr) 0.7, Ca 9.4. Liver function tests included an aspartate aminotransferase of 190, alanine aminotransferase 24, albumin 3.3, total protein 6.2, alkaline phosphatase 111, and bilirubin 1. C-reactive protein was 11.3, lactate dehydrogenase (LDH) was more than 11,000, and uric acid was 936 while lactate was 4.7. Complete blood count showed white blood cell (WBC) 14, hematocrit 33, and platelets 579 with a left shift on differential. Urinalysis showed 1+ ketones, a specific gravity of 1.030, and 1+ protein.

Chest x-ray (CXR) showed right-sided pleural effusion with a smaller left pleural effusion but no infiltrates (Fig. 38-1). Abdominal ultrasound showed ascites and a

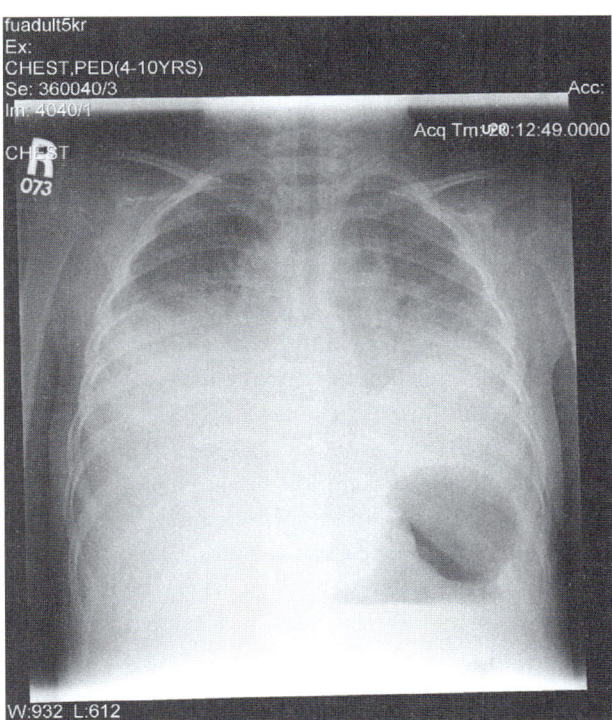

Figure 38-1 Chest x-ray at presentation. Bilateral pleural effusions are present.

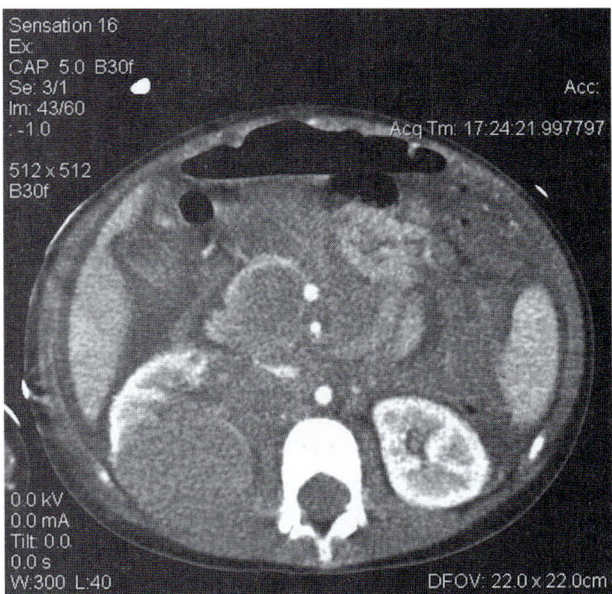

Figure 38-2 Abdominal CT. Lower pole of the right kidney is largely replaced by a mass. This appears to invade surrounding tissue as well as anteriorly displace the pancreas and bowel.

4-cm, posterior right renal mass. The liver had no apparent masses.

Case Resolution

The patient was transferred to our institution for further evaluation. She had a computed tomography (CT) of the chest (Fig. 38-2), abdomen, and pelvis, which showed a 6.7 cm × 4 cm right renal mass with retroperitoneal invasion encasing the retroperitoneal vasculature as well as displacement of the pancreas anteriorly. There was an additional mass in the right lower quadrant likely adjacent to a large bowel loop. Ascites and bilateral pleural effusions with adjacent atelectasis were also present. Thoracentesis showed chylous fluid. Biopsy of the renal mass revealed Burkitt lymphoma.

Question

Should tumor lysis syndrome be considered in this patient? If so, how should it be managed?

Answer

Originally described as acute uric acid nephropathy, tumor lysis syndrome is an oncologic emergency. Based on this child's tumor burden, tumor type, and laboratory results, tumor lysis syndrome should be considered. Tumor lysis syndrome most often follows combination chemotherapy. It can also occur following steroid treatment and has been reported prior to initiation of therapy. The risk of tumor lysis syndrome is highest with poorly differentiated lymphomas (such as Burkitt lymphoma), acute lymphoblastic leukemia, and acute myelogenous leukemia. In a cohort series of patients with high-grade non-Hodgkin lymphoma, 6% of patients developed tumor lysis syndrome. The syndrome is defined by the development of acute renal failure in the presence of hyperuricemia with or without hyperphosphatemia.

In addition to the elevation of uric acid and serum phosphate, associated laboratory findings include elevated lactate dehydrogenase, hyperkalemia, and hypocalcemia. Hypovolemia, elevated pretreatment uric acid, and poor baseline renal function predispose to the development of tumor lysis syndrome. Elevated pretreatment levels of LDH (as in this patient) are predictive of azotemia, hyperuricemia, and hyperphosphatemia following therapy. Prevention of the syndrome is through aggressive intravenous hydration. Allopurinol, a xanthine oxidase inhibitor, and recombinant uricase are also used to prevent or blunt the hyperuricemia. Urinary alkalinization is controversial, but commonly used. Alkaline urine promotes the conversion of uric acid to a more soluble urate salt. This reduces the likelihood of uric acid precipitation in the renal tubules.

Discussion

Abdominal masses in children are the most common presenting sign of malignancy, and they deserve careful evaluation with imaging (ultrasound or CT if possible). The most common abdominal tumors in children are Wilms tumor and neuroblastoma. Other considerations in the differential diagnosis of abdominal masses in children depending on the clinical scenario include trauma, intussusception, hernias, teratoma, benign tumors, lymphoma, choledochal cysts, hepatoblastoma, and abscess.

The diagnosis of Burkitt lymphoma is based on the classic "starry sky" appearance on biopsy (Fig. 38-3). This consists of small, noncleaved lymphoblasts with fewer large, clear histiocytes. The genetics of Burkitt lymphoma is very well researched. The most common chromosomal

translocation unites the c-myc proto-oncogene on chromosome 8 with the IgM heavy chain locus on chromosome 14, which is activated in B cells. Burkitt lymphoma is also associated with translocations of chromosome 8 with chromosomes 22 and 2, which code for other light and heavy chain loci. p53 mutations are also common, as are duplications of 1q and trisomy 7.

The presentation of Burkitt lymphoma is variable, regardless of whether the disease is seen in Africa or the West. Sixty percent of African children present with jaw tumors. However, abdominal tumors are the most common presentation in the West. These may include renal, ovarian, retroperitoneal, liver, or spleen masses. CNS presentation is not uncommon, though usually this is localized to the spinal cord. Other locations include the thyroid, salivary gland, long bones, bone marrow, penis, breast, heart, and skin. Marrow involvement is present in approximately 40%. "Burkitt leukemia" is also seen, which presents with bone marrow and nodal involvement with hepatosplenomegaly, but no discrete masses. The characteristics of endemic (equatorial Africa) and sporadic (western) Burkitt lymphoma are further delineated in Table 38-1.

There is also a strong association between Burkitt lymphoma and the Epstein-Barr virus. It is associated with 90% to 95% of African Burkitt and 15% to 20% of North

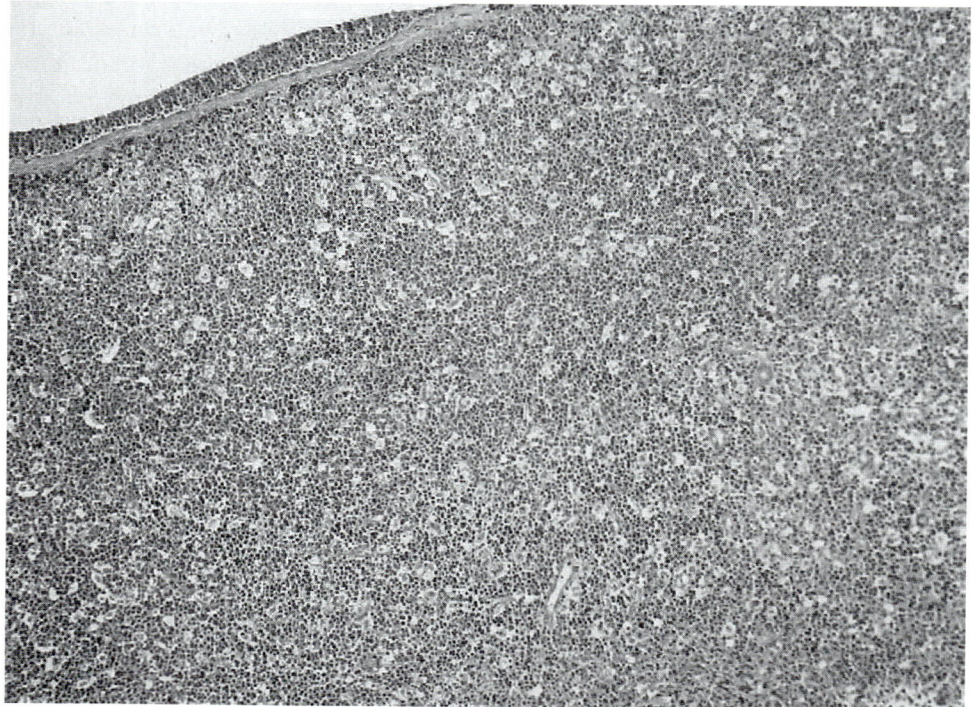

Figure 38-3 Lymph node biopsy of a Burkitt Lymphoma. Overall "starry sky" appearance can be appreciated with this specimen.

TABLE 38-1

Characteristics of Burkitt Lymphoma

	Endemic (equatorial Africa)	Sporadic (western)
Incidence	10/100,000 (50% of pediatric malignancies)	0.2/100,000
EBV	90 + % associated with EBV	20% associated with EBV
Genetics	Chromosome 8 break upstream of c-myc	Chromosome 8 break within c-myc
Presentation	Jaw-abdomen-orbit-paraspinal	Abdomen-bone marrow-nasopharynx-lymph node
Geography	Malaria belt association	No climactic association

EBV, Epstein-Barr virus.

American Burkitt. The mechanism of viral activation is a latent EBV membrane protein which increases expression of bcl-2, a gene responsible for preventing apoptosis. The increased association of EBV with Burkitt lymphoma in Africa over North America is felt to be secondary to multiple reasons. First of all, EBV infection is ubiquitous by 3 years of age in Africa, whereas this does not happen until the late teens in North America. Furthermore, malaria, thought to be a B-cell mitogen and T-cell suppressor, results in more EBV-infected cells in the bloodstream in African children.

Burkitt is a tumor with a very rapid turnover rate, resulting in a very high risk of tumor lysis syndrome when treatment is initiated because of the high tumor burden. Other complications of the tumor itself include CNS involvement, individual organ compromise, and hypercalcemia because of an osteoclast-activating factor often seen with the disease.

There are four different staging systems for Burkitt lymphoma. Prognosis is 60% to 80% disease-free survival at 5 years. This is often related to tumor burden at diagnosis. Treatment involves combination chemotherapy, usually with an alkylating agent. CNS treatment is often recommended, as is timing of the cycles of chemotherapy as close together as possible. Surgical removal is recommended if possible, though debulking alone is not helpful. Radiation is not often performed except for emergent or symptomatic management as with CNS or testicular involvement or venous or urinary obstruction.

Selected References

Abbasoglu L, Gun F, Salman FT, et al. The role of surgery in intraabdominal Burkitt's lymphoma in children. *Eur J Pediatr Surg*. 2003 Aug;13(4):236–239.

Gasparini M, Rottoli L, Massimino M, et al. Curability of advanced Burkitt's lymphoma in children by intensive short-term chemotherapy. *Eur J Cancer*. 1993;29A(5):692–698.

Miller D, Robert B. *Blood Diseases of Infancy and Childhood*. 7th ed. St. Louis, MO: Mobsy; 1995:752z–760.

Pizzo P, Poplack D. *Principles and Practice of Pediatric Oncology*. Philadelphia, PA: Lippincott Williams & Wilkins; 2003:532–556.

29-Year-Old Female with Dyspnea, Chest Pain, and Palpitations

CASE PRESENTATION

A 29-year-old Caucasian female and mother of seven children presented with nonradiating, recurrent, left-sided chest pain, and palpitations. The patient had sudden onset of stabbing chest pain under her left breast of 1 hour's duration while she was attending a physician's appointment at a large community hospital. The patient reports shortness of breath associated with the pain, as well as nausea without vomiting. Deep breaths exacerbated her pain. The patient suffers from these attacks about three times per week, with the symptoms lasting for 3 to 5 minutes and resolving with rest. The patient reports dyspnea on exertion, presyncope, orthostasis, and orthopnea for the past 3 months since giving birth to a term infant male. The patient was diagnosed with thrombophlebitis 2 months prior to admission and was started on Coumadin for Leep vein thrombosis (DVT) prophylaxis by her primary MD. The patient had a computed tomography (CT) scan done at that time for complaints of dyspnea and chest pain that was negative for pulmonary embolus. The patient reports no recent long car rides or recent airplane flights. Other pertinent past history includes mitral valve prolapse diagnosed 3 months ago, migraines, and fibrocystic breast disease. The diagnosis of mitral valve prolapse was made without echocardiography by the patient's primary MD. There was no family history of lupus, pulmonary embolism (PE), DVT, or cardiovascular disease. The patient denies a history of ethyl alcohol use or abuse.

Physical Examination

Patient was slightly anxious appearing, but comfortable and in no acute distress, appearing her stated age. Vital signs: temperature 36°C, pulse 68 beats/min, respiratory rate 16 breaths/min, blood pressure 118/68 mm Hg with room air oxygen saturation of 100%. Head, eyes, ears, nose, and throat: normocephalic, atraumatic; pupils equal, round, reactive to light and accommodation, extraocular movement intact, poor dentition; neck: supple, no lymphadenopathy, no bruit, no jugular venous distension. Cardiovascular: regular rate and rhythm with normal S_1 and S_2, an intermittent gallop and no S_4. No pain on palpation of chest. PMI was nondisplaced but precordium was slightly hyperdynamic, lungs: bibasilar crackles one-third up the chest cavity, abdomen: soft, nontender, normal bowel sounds; no hepatosplenomegaly, extremities: no edema or tenderness, the remainder of the examination was unremarkable.

Laboratory Studies

White blood cell 7.2, hemoglobin and hematocrit 12.4 and 37, respectively, mean corpuscular volume 75, platelets 198, prothrombin time 15.1, international normalized ratio (INR) 1.55, partial prothrombin time 28, cardiac enzymes: creatine kinase 93, CK-MB 2.1, troponin I, 0.08. CT angiogram of chest: negative for PE. D-dimer: negative, lower extremity Doppler: negative for DVT, chest radiograph and electrocardiogram (ECG) are shown in Figs. 39-1 and 39-2.

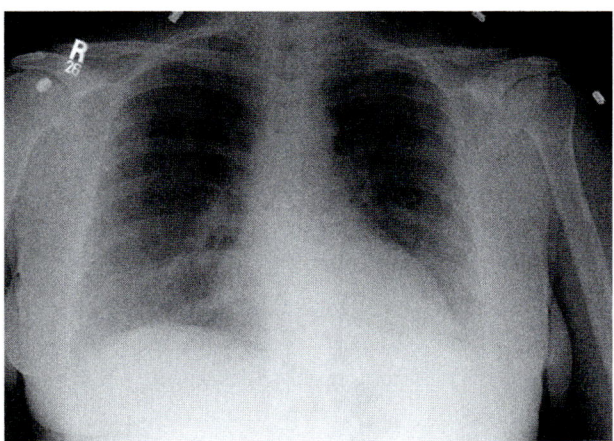

Figure 39-1 Chest radiograph of patient reveals mildly enlarged cardiac silhouette and pulmonary vascular congestion.

Case Resolution

The patient was started on intravenous heparin in the emergency department. This was subsequently discontinued when the patient's CT angiogram, LE Doppler, and D-dimer were all obtained in the emergency department (ED) and found to be negative. The patient's chest pain resolved in the ED and did not return during the hospitalization. The patient had a diagnostic two-dimensional echocardiogram upon leaving the ED that showed a markedly dilated left ventricle with global dysfunction and an ejection fraction (EF) of approximately 20%. There was no left ventricular outflow obstruction. There was a dilated left atrium and mild mitral regurgitation. There was no pulmonary arterial hypertension or evidence of right heart strain. The patient was seen by a cardiologist, started on a digoxin and an angiotensin converting enzyme (ACE) inhibitor, and discharged the next day

with anticoagulation and follow-up with a cardiologist. Thyroid-stimulating hormone (TSH), human immunodeficiency virus (HIV), and iron levels were either normal or negative. Coxsackie viral titers were obtained and reflected no evidence of infection.

Question

What is the most likely explanation of the patient's clinically significant and symptomatic heart failure?

Answer

Although the differential diagnosis of unexplained heart failure is quite broad, given the patient's history, sex, and age, it is most likely peripartum cardiomyopathy (PPCM). Of special note, the patient had no prior history of heart failure or cardiomyopathy of any kind. No other explanation of her cardiomyopathy could be found. Moreover, her illness began to become symptomatic with the parturition of her last child.

Discussion

Congestive heart failure (CHF) is a disease that is frequently encountered by practitioners in all areas of medicine. Myriad etiologies exist for the development of heart failure, including congenital cardiac disease and acquired cardiac valvular abnormalities, obstructive disease such as primary pulmonary hypertension, cor pulmonale from other causes such as untreated obstructive sleep apnea, and most commonly ischemic cardiomyopathy.

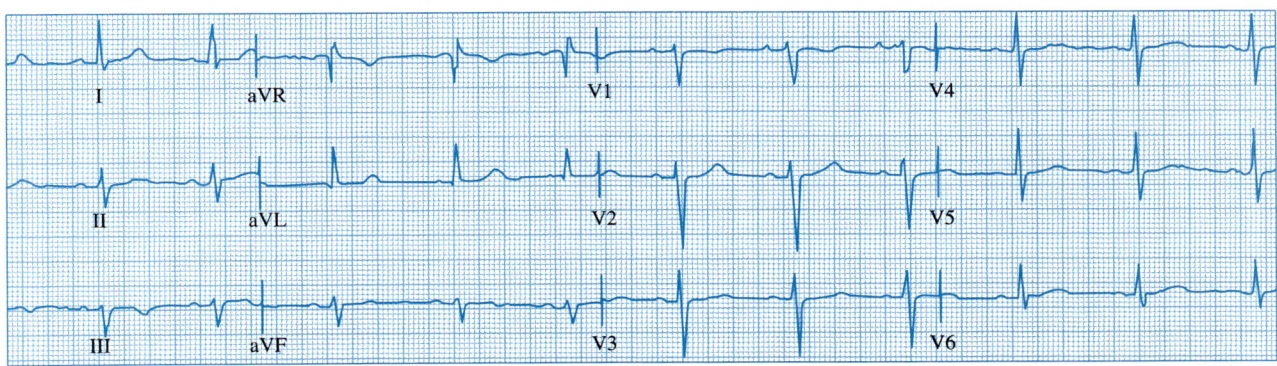

Figure 39-2 12-lead electrocardiogram of patient on presentation shows a largely normal study.

Cardiomyopathy of nonischemic origin is a significant contributor to heart failure worldwide and in the United States. Causes include idiopathic, postinfectious, familial, and toxin-induced cardiomyopathy. For a more complete listing of potential causes and/or types of cardiomyopathy from a large study in year 2000, please see Table 39-1. These types of cardiomyopathy do not necessarily restrict themselves to those in their fifties and sixties as the above case illustrates. Moreover, with advances in neonatal care, the increasing survival of patient receiving successful repair of complex congenital hear diseases, primary care providers such as pediatricians, internists, obstetricians, and family practitioners must understand the etiology, management, and prognosis of heart failure from a multitude of etiologies.

PPCM, formerly known as pregnancy-associated cardiomyopathy, was first recognized in the nineteenth century but was later described in detail as a distinct clinical entity in 1971. Despite significant studies on the potential etiologies, clinical course, and prognosis of the disorder, the disease is incompletely characterized. It is of significant prevalence in women of childbearing age and can bear worrisome rate of morbidity and mortality, especially in subsequent pregnancies.

PPCM is thought to be a distinct clinical and pathophysiologic entity rather than the simple phenomenon of unmasking or accelerating existing cardiomyopathy. Hypotheses as to the etiology/etiologies of the resultant cardiomyopathy are varied and include myocarditis, an abnormal immune response to fetal antigens on chimeric cells in the maternal myocardium, and exaggerated remodeling of the myocardium in response to the hemodynamic changes in pregnancy. Other theories and factors also have been suggested and include the contribution of prolonged tocolysis with terbutaline, myocardial damage from stress-activated TNF-α and IL-1 release as implicated in idiopathic dilated cardiomyopathy, selenium deficiency, and abnormalities in the ovarian hormone relaxin. It is likely that there could be multiple mechanisms of disease in susceptible persons and that there may be common pathologic mechanisms shared by other cardiomyopathies.

Despite a lack of a clear-cut etiology, the currently accepted incidence of PPCM is between 1 in 3000 live births and 1 in 4000 live births in the United States, which translates into about 1000 to 1300 new cases every year. It is interesting that some parts of Africa may have an incidence as high as 1 in 100 live births.

Risk factors analyses on this disorder have uncovered several important risk factors including multiparity, advanced maternal age, multifetal pregnancy, preeclampsia, and pregnancy-induced hypertension. Maternal race is also a risk factor as women of African American heritage are at increased risk of PPCM. Despite these identified risk factors, there are no recommendations for screening at-risk populations for the disease.

PPCM has distinct diagnostic criteria based on both clinical information and patient's history, as well as distinct and echocardiography data. Table 39-2 shows these criteria. These criteria were developed to exclude the diagnosis of PPCM in women with previously undiagnosed heart failure, as these women would likely become clinically apparent earlier than the 36 weeks' gestation. Important is the second criterion that precludes the diagnosis of PPCM until all other potentially identifiable causes have been evaluated (ie, thyroid disease, HIV, iron overload). Because the normal physiologic changes in pregnancy can result in symptoms identical to early CHF, including edema, dyspnea on exertion, and fatigue, it is likely that mild cases go undiagnosed. Symptoms such as chest pain, paroxysmal nocturnal dyspnea, new murmur, and cough should alert the practitioner to early heart failure.

Treatment of patients with PPCM follows standard heart failure guidelines, with the exception of the still-pregnant or lactating female in order to protect the infant

TABLE 39-1

Diagnoses in 1230 Patient with Cardiomyopathy of Initially Unknown Cause

Final diagnosis	% of cohort
Idiopathic CM	50
Myocarditis	9
Ischemic heart disease	7
Infiltrative CM	5
Peripartum CM	4
Hypertensive CM	4
HIV CM	4
CM due to connective tissue disease	3
Toxic (substance abuse) CM	3
Doxorubicin-induced CM	1
Miscellaneous causes of CM	10

CM, cardiomyopathy.
Adapted from Felker GM, Thompson RE, Hare JM, et al. Underlying causes and long-term survival in patients with initially unexplained cardiomyopathy. N Engl J Med. 2000;342:1077–1084.

TABLE 39-2

Criteria for Peripartum Cardiomyopathy

1. Development of cardiac failure in the last month of pregnancy or within 5 months of delivery
2. Absence of an identifiable cause for the cardiac failure
3. Absence of recognizable heart disease prior to the last month of pregnancy
4. Left ventricular systolic dysfunction demonstrated by classic echocardiography criteria (EF < 45% or decreased M mode shortening fraction)

Adapted from Pearson GD, Veille JC, Hsia J, et al. Peripartum cardiomyopathy, National Heart Lung, and Blood Institute and Office of Rare Diseases (NIH): Workshop recommendations and review. JAMA. 2000;283:1183–1188.

from untoward iatrogenic effects. Specifically, diuretics, salt restriction, vasodilators, and digoxin should be initiated. ACE inhibitors are contraindicated in pregnancy, but can and should be used following delivery. Hydralazine and nitrates can be used as safe alternatives until delivery. Because of the negative inotropic effects of calcium channel blockers, these are not usually recommended as first line, although amlodipine may be useful since it has pleiotropic effects on plasma level of the proinflammatory cytokine IL-6 in patients with nonischemic cardiomyopathy. β-Blockers such as carvedilol may have use as this drug conferred a survival benefit in dilated cardiomyopathy. For those patients with markedly decreased ejection fraction (< 35%), anticoagulation may be indicated to prevent systemic emboli from cardiogenic thrombus formation. During pregnancy this would include either heparin or low-molecular-weight-based heparin; while following delivery, warfarin would be the likely choice. Immunosuppressive therapy has not been studied exclusively in patients with PPCM, but it has been suggested if documented biopsy-proven myocarditis exists and patients do not respond to conventional therapy in 2 weeks. Interestingly, intravenous immunoglobulin (IVIG) had some benefit in retrospective studies. For those who fail maximal medical therapy, cardiac transplantation is a final option where survival is similar to other aged matched controls who received cardiac transplantation for other reasons.

A recent large series of patients with PPCM revealed a cardiac transplantation rate of 4% and a mortality rate of 10% at 2 years of follow-up. These rates are considerably lower than previous data suggested. One explanation for this may be the improved survival with optimal medical therapy. Death in women with PPCM was described as sudden half the time, suggesting that these women may benefit from defibrillator implantation. For women with PPCM that did not require transplantation or die, the mean left ventricular ejection fraction increased from 28% at diagnosis to 46% at 2 years. Recovery to an ejection fraction greater than 50% occurred more than half the time; women that presented with an ejection fraction of greater than 30% appeared to have the greatest degree of recovery.

Studies on women with PPCM and subsequent pregnancy have led experts to suggest that women with residual left ventricular dysfunction avoid additional pregnancy. When this is not possible, those women should be followed in high-risk materno–fetal medicine clinics. One study found that 16 women who bore children with existing PPCM had further reduction on ejection fraction. Moreover, overt failure developed in seven patients, premature delivery occurred in six, therapeutic abortion was performed in four, and three women died. In patients whose left ventricular ejection fraction returned to normal following their diagnosis with PPCM, there was significant reduction in ejection fraction, some patients developed overt failure, but there were no deaths.

In summary, although only one cause of non-ischemic cardiomyopathy, PPCM is a significant cause of morbidity and mortality in young women of childbearing age. New signs and symptoms of heart failure in pregnant women and those postpartum should result in a careful analysis of the patient's cardiac status so that appropriate medical management can be initiated and appropriate referral to cardiologists and high-risk obstetricians can be made.

Selected References

1. Pearson GD, Veille JC, Hsia J, et al. Peripartum cardiomyopathy: National Heart Lung, and Blood Institute and Office of Rare Diseases (NIH): Workshop recommendations and review. *JAMA.* 2000;283:1183–1188.
2. Felker GM, Thompson RE, Hare JM, et al. Underlying causes and long-term survival in patients with initially unexplained cardiomyopathy. *N Engl J Med.* 2000;342:1077–1084.
3. Elkayam U, Akhter MW, Singh H, et al. Pregnancy-associated cardiomyopathy: clinical characteristics and comparison between early and late presentation. *Circulation.* 2005;111:2050–2055.
4. Elkayam U, Padmini PT, Kalpana R, et al. Maternal and fetal outcomes of subsequent pregnancies in women with peripartum cardiomyopathy. *N Engl J Med.* 2001;344:1567–1571.

47-Year-Old Male with Acute Renal Failure

CASE PRESENTATION

A 47-year-old Mexican man is carried into a rural emergency department by his friends after 2 days of progressive shortness of breath, fatigue, decreased urine output, progressively worsening mental status, and hemoptysis. Though oriented to person, his significant lethargy and altered mental status rendered him unable to answer more detailed questioning.

Physical Examination

In general, the patient was an awake and alert, but ill-appearing Hispanic male. He displayed Kussmaul respirations and appeared to be in moderate respiratory distress. Vital signs: temperature 37°C, blood pressure 156/94 mm Hg, heart rate 121 beats/min, respiratory rate 34 breaths/min, SpO_2 97% on 100% facemask. The patient's head, eyes, ears, nose, and throat examination revealed dried blood in oropharynx and dry mucous membranes. His neck was supple and with no meningismus, but he had jugular venous distension to the angle of the jaw. Cardiovascular examination revealed a hyperdynamic precordium; tachycardia; no murmurs, gallops, rubs with bounding 2+ distal pulses. The patient's lung examination was notable for tachypnea with diffusely coarse breath sounds and crackles at both lung bases. Abdominal examination was essentially normal, with normal bowel sounds, no hepatosplenomegaly, no tenderness, and without renal bruits. Genitourinary examination was essentially normal except for scant dark urine in the Foley catheter bag. His extremities showed 2+ bilateral pretibial, pitting edema. Neurologically, the patient was altered, oriented to person only. Cranial nerve II to XII were grossly intact, though unable to follow all commands, unable to walk from generalized weakness; reflexes 2+ and symmetric throughout.

Laboratory Studies

Initial arterial blood gas on 100% facemask was pH 7.09, PCO_2 12, PO_2 135, HCO_3 3.6, acid-base balance -24,

lactate 1.3. Electrolytes on presentation included Na 142, K 5.4, Cl 94, HCO_3 < 5, blood urea nitrogen (BUN) 286, creatinine (Cr) 29, glucose 86, Ca 5.3, Mg 3.4, phosphate 12.1. His calculated anion gap >40, aspartate aminotransferase 73, alanine aminotransferase 210, gamma-glutamyltransferase 53, alkaline phosphatase 127, creatine kinase (CK) 10500, CK-MB fraction 70.7, troponin T, 0.170. A complete blood count showed white blood cells 25.8, hemoglobin 12.5, hematocrit 35.8, platelets 118. Urine analysis showed 3+ protein, 3+ blood, many white blood cells while urine sediment contained many oval fat bodies, many fatty casts, and few red cells with normal morphology.

The patient's ECG demonstrated sinus tachycardia with slightly peaked T waves, otherwise unremarkable. A chest x-ray showed prominent bilateral perihilar alveolar opacities. A renal ultrasound obtained several hours later showed mildly echogenic kidneys without obstructive change.

Case Resolution

The patien't was urgently transferred to the ICU after receiving several ampules containing 50 meq of $NaHCO_3$. He became hypotensive upon admission to the ICU. Continuous veno–venous hemodialysis (CVVHD) was initiated because of the patient's labile hemodynamic status. The patient improved dramatically after initiation of dialysis and was transferred to step down within 3 days. When his mental status improved, further questioning found that the patient had emigrated from Mexico 4 days prior to presentation. He walked across the Mexico-Arizona border without water for approximately 20 miles, and then boarded a bus to North Carolina where he was to work as a farm laborer. Renal biopsy ultimately showed pigmented cast nephropathy, consistent with acute myoglobinuric renal failure (Fig. 40-1A, B, and C). After 45 days of slowly tapering intermittent hemodialysis, the patient was discharged home without dialysis, a Cr of 2.8, and modest hypertension.

Question

In the setting of acute renal failure (ARF), which serum and urine markers help to confirm the diagnosis of rhabdomyolysis?

Answer

An elevated serum CK, myoglobin detected in the urine or inferred from heme-positive urine dipstick with an absence of red blood cells on microscopy, as well as hyperkalemia, hyperphosphatemia, hyperuricemia, early hypocalcemia, and a decreased BUN to Cr ratio, all resulting from increased muscle breakdown.

Discussion

ARF is a syndrome caused by the rapid decline, over hours to days, of a patient's glomerular filtration rate (GFR). Retention of nitrogenous waste, referred to as azotemia, the disruption of acid-base homeostasis, and changes in extracellular fluid (ECF) volume are hallmarks of the syndrome. Oliguria, defined at < 400 mL/day of urine, is often present, but is not requisite.

While clinical history often suggests the mechanism of ARF, frequently a clinician must employ a systematic approach to determine the underlying etiology. Classification of ARF is most easily separated into prerenal, intrinsic, and postrenal mechanisms. Prerenal mechanisms account for approximately 55% of ARF, postrenal approximately 5%, and intrinsic approximately 40%.

Once a patient with renal failure is adequately stabilized and life-threatening abnormalities such as hypoxemia, acidosis, hyperkalemia and so on are addressed, the initial approach to a patient with ARF should turn to identifying

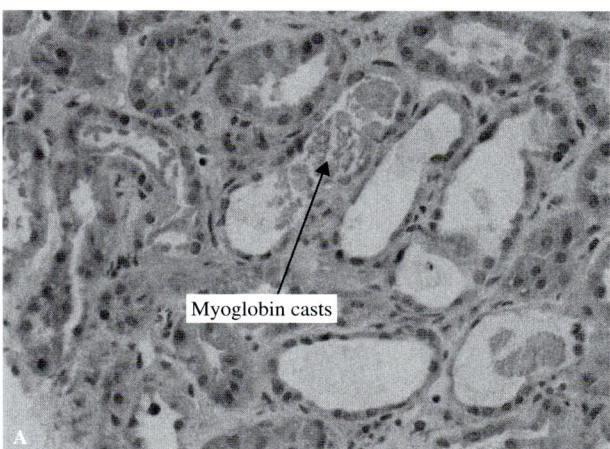

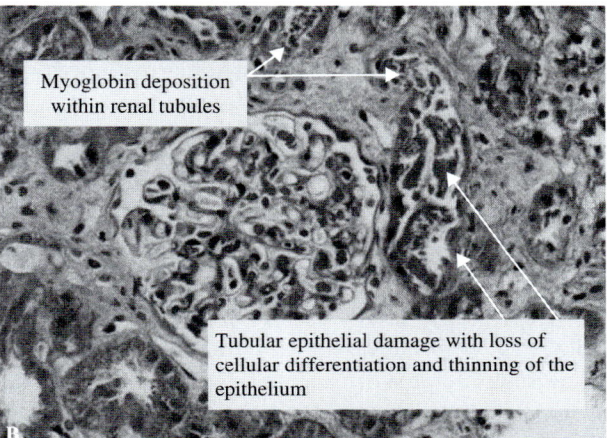

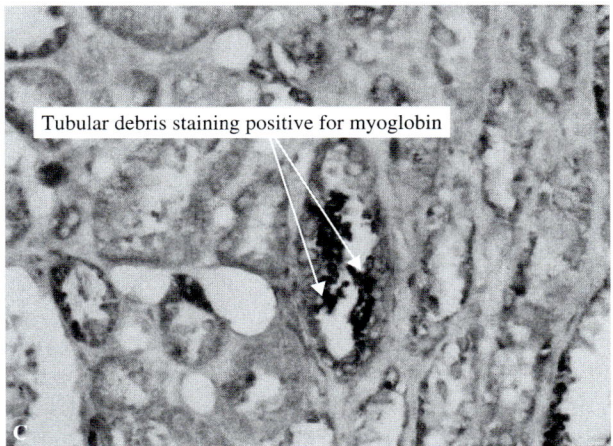

Figure 40-1 Renal biopsy specimens derived from the patient described in the vignette. **(A)** Black arrow identifies myoglobin cast formation within renal collecting tubules. **(B)** Arrows again identifie myoglobin deposition within renal tubules, while tubular epithelial damage with loss of cellular differentiation and thinning of the epithelium is identified by white arrows. **(C)** White arrows identify material and debris dark staining positive for myoglobin indicative of pigmented cast nephropathy. *Photos courtesy of Dr Mathieu Latour, MD, University of North Carolina at Chapel Hill.*

or excluding ARF from either prerenal and postrenal mechanisms. Table 40-1 highlights the pertinent features of these two conditions. Prerenal azotemia is, by definition, rapidly reversible upon restoration of renal blood flow and glomerular ultrafiltration pressure, while postrenal azotemia is oftentimes easily corrected temporarily by bypassing the obstruction unless the obstruction is long standing. Intrinsic ARF, however, often requires more detailed investigation and treatment. Basic elements essential in determining the etiology of ARF include history and physical examination, urinalysis with sediment evaluation, urinary indices including electrolytes and protein concentration, BUN to Cr ratio, and renal ultrasound. Further serum studies, imaging, or even renal biopsy are often necessary, and are obtained as the clinical scenario dictates.

Prerenal ARF occurs with glomerular hypoperfusion from a decrease in effective arterial blood volume. This can be an absolute or relative decline in intravascular volume such as that seen in dehydration, hemorrhage, or arterial occlusion or decreased circulating volume with a normal or elevated ECF such as seen in heart failure, cirrhosis, nephrotic syndrome, or sepsis. In the incipient stages of hypoperfusion, renal compensatory mechanisms are initially able to preserve GFR. However, as circulating intravascular volume continues to decline, the kidney can no longer compensate and GFR falls, leading to ARF. While the spectrum of hypoperfusion can cause both prerenal and intrinsic ARF, with purely prerenal azotemia, there is no parenchymal damage and the renal insult is readily reversed with reperfusion after treatment of the underlying process. Clinical clues pointing to a prerenal etiology include orthostatic symptoms, signs of dehydration including dry mucous membranes, increased thirst, reduced sweating, or stigmata of liver or heart failure. Urine sediment is largely acellular with transparent hyaline casts made mostly of Tamm-Horsfall protein secreted by the loop of Henle. Regardless of the specific insult, urine indices are consistent with salt and water resorption as the kidney attempts to increase circulating blood volume. The calculation of the fractional excretion of sodium (FeNa) can be useful in deducing prerenal azotemia. An FeNa < 1% is usually indicative of prerenal azotemia, although other disease states such as glomerulonephritis can also give an FeNa of < 1%, while diuretic use will skew the FeNa upward making it unreliable. Other urine indices such as osmolality > 500 mOsm, urine Na < 10 mmol/L, urine specific gravity > 1.018, and urine Cr to plasma Cr ratio > 40 are also suggestive of but not specific, for prerenal azotemia. Additionally, a BUN to Cr ratio > 20 may also suggest prerenal azotemia, as antidiuretic hormone acts to resorb both water and urea from the tubular lumen.

Intrinsic ARF is a conglomerate of disease processes that either occur within the kidney or directly cause parenchymal damage. Table 40-2 illustrates the features of common causes of intrinsic ARF. These processes may further be categorized into four major areas: (1) renovascular obstruction including thrombosis, embolism, and aneurysm; (2) glomerular and renal microvasculature disorders including glomerulonephritis (GN), vasculitis, hemolytic-uremic syndrome (HUS), thrombotic thrombocytopenic purpura

TABLE 40-1

Basic Overview of the Clinical Features of ARF from Prerenal and Postrenal Mechanisms

Mechanism of ARF	Physiology	Common causes	Clinical features	Laboratory findings	Urine sediment
Prerenal	Decreased renal blood flow from hypovolemia, systemic vasodilation, or renal vasoconstriction	Dehydration, CHF, sepsis, cirrhosis	Hypotension, dehydration, extravascular fluid accumulation	FENA < 1%, Urine Na < 10 mmol/L, SG > 1.018, BUN:Cr > 20	Hyaline casts
Postrenal	Urinary outflow obstruction	Calculi, compression (cancer, fibrosis), BPH, stricture	Decreased urine output, palpable bladder, prostatic change	Variable	Normal or red blood cells

Adapted from references mentioned at the end of the case.

TABLE 40-2

Basic Classification of Processes Leading to ARF from Intrinsic Renal Mechanisms

Process leading to intrinsic ARF	Mechanism	Common causes	Clinical clues	Urine sediment	Confirmatory testing
Renovascular obstruction	Renal artery/vein obstruction	Atheroembolism	Subcutaneous nodules, digital ischemia, livedo reticularis	Mild proteinuria	Hypocomplementemia, skin biopsy
		Thrombosis	Sudden onset pain, atrial fibrillation, recent myocardial infarction		Renal arteriogram, elevated LDH with normal transaminases
Acute tubular necrosis	Ischemic	Sepsis, recent surgery, hemorrhage	Hypotension	Muddy brown granular casts or tubular epithelial cell casts	None needed
	Exogenous	Contrast dye hemolysis	Recent imaging hemolysis	As above Heme + supernatant	None needed Hyperkalemia, hyperphosphatemia, hypocalcemia
	Toxic	Rhabdomyolysis	Seizure, crush injury, ethanol or cocaine abuse, muscle pain, dark urine	Heme + supernatant	As above, also with elevated creatine kinase and uric acid
	Endogenous	Myeloma	Vertebral fractures, bone pain	Dipstick negative proteinuria (+ sulfacylic acid test)	Circulating or urinary monoclonal spike, light-chain cast nephropathy on renal biopsy
		Tumor lysis	Chemotherapy	Urate crystals	Hyperuricemia, hyperkalemia, hyperphosphatemia
Interstitial nephritis	Allergic medications	β-Lactams, sulfonamides, NSAIDs, diuretics, captopril	Recent medication use, fever, arthralgias, pruritic rash	White cell casts, white cells (often eosinophils)	Systemic eosinophilia, skin biopsy (leukocytoclastic vasculitis), renal biopsy (tubulo-interstitial inflammation)
	Infections	Acute pyelonephritis, leptospirosis, CMV, candidiasis	Fever, flank pain, dysuria, frequency	Leukocytes, WBC clumps, bacteria	Urine and blood cultures
	Infiltrative	Lymphoma, leukemia, sarcoid	Systemic symptoms	Bland	Renal biopsy with special staining, lymph node biopsy, radiologic imaging

(continued)

TABLE 40-2

Basic Classification Of Processes Leading To Arf From Intrinsic Renal Mechanisms (*continued*)

Process leading to intrinsic ARF	Mechanism	Common causes	Clinical clues	Urine sediment	Confirmatory testing
Disorders of glomeruli and renal microvasculature	GN, vasculitis	SLE, Goodpasture, Wegener, postinfectious GN, cryoglobulinemia, membrano-proliferative GN, membranous GN	Oliguria, edema, hypertension, tea-colored urine, skin rash, hepatitis B or C infection, recent infection	Red cell and granular casts, red and white cells	Renal biopsy, C3, C4, ASO, ANA, ANCA, anti-GBM, cryoglobulins, hepatitis serologies
	Miscellaneous	HUS/TTP	Recent gastrointestinal infection, fever, pallor, ecchymoses	Normal or red cells	Renal biopsy, anemia, thrombocytopenia, peripheral smear with schistocytes, elevated LDH, decreased haptoglobin
		Malignant HTN	Severe HTN with headaches, heart failure, retinopathy, papilledema	Proteinuria, red cells, red cell casts	LVH on ECG, retinal examination, resolution of ARF with BP control

ANA, antinuclear antibody test; ANCA, antineutrophil cytoplasmic antibody; GN, glomerulonephritis; HUS, hemolytic-uremic syndrome; TTP, thrombotic thrombocytopenic purpura.

Adapted from references mentioned at the end of the case.

(TTP), disseminated intravascular coagulation, and systemic lupus erythematosus (SLE); (3) acute tubular necrosis from ischemia, toxins, or intratubular obstruction; and (4) interstitial nephritis from allergic reactions, infection, or infiltration with cells of the immune system. Renal allograft rejection is an additional specialized form of intrinsic azotemia. General characteristics of intrinsic ARF include an FeNa > 1%, urine Na > 20 mmol/L, SG < 1.015, BUN to Cr < 20, urine < 500 mOsm, urine to plasma creatinine ratio < 20.

Postrenal ARF is a result of obstruction of the urinary collecting system anywhere along its path. Obstruction results in increased pressure proximal to the lesion, leading to dilation in the proximal ureter, renal pelvis, and calyces. By the time renal failure ensues, dilatory changes are evident on retroperitoneal ultrasound. In order to cause renal failure, ureteral blockages must be bilateral, unless the patient has a solitary functioning kidney, and may be caused by calculi, cancer, or external compression such as surgical ligation or retroperitoneal fibrosis. The bladder neck is the most common site of obstruction as a result of prostatic hypertrophy, neoplasia, infection, as well as neurogenic bladder. Finally, ureteric strictures or valves, or even severe phimosis may lead to postrenal azotemia. A history of nocturia, frequency, and hesitancy may suggest prostatic hypertrophy, and digital rectal examination may demonstrate hypertrophy, tenderness, or neoplasia. Recent anticholinergic medication or autonomic dysfunction along with a palpable bladder may indicate neurogenic bladder. Abdominal or flank pain along with gross or microscopic hematuria may be seen with stones or malignancy. Urine sediment analysis may be useful in determining stone etiology, but is otherwise limited when evaluating postrenal mechanisms. Radiologic studies are useful in locating the obstruction. Plain films or high-resolution CT may demonstrate kidney stones, while intravenous pyelography may be needed to enumerate more subtle processes. Direct imaging via cystourethroscopy may be both diagnostic and therapeutic. Treatment hinges on removing or bypassing the obstructing lesion. Stones are often extracted, ureteral stents are placed when cancer compresses the lumen, and urinary catheters often bypass the prostate or relieve a neurogenic bladder. A postobstruction diuresis of several days duration often accompanies relief of the obstruction with oftentimes return to baseline GFR, depending on the length and severity of the obstruction.

The patient's renal injury described in the vignette above most likely originated from exertional rhabdomyolysis, literally meaning "dissolution of striped muscle." First described as a cause of cast nephropathy in victims of crush injury during the bombing of London in World War II, rhabdomyolysis is a clinical syndrome of acute muscle necrosis, pain, and weakness from a variety of causes (Table 40-3), often presenting with tea-colored urine from pigmented myoglobin. Common causes include severe compartment syndrome, side effect of prescription medicines such as "statins," crush injury, prolonged seizures, prolonged immobility, ethanol or cocaine abuse, metabolic deficiencies, and autoimmune myositis. Besides physical exertion, a variety of infectious insults, toxins, and xenobiotics are associated with rhabdomyolysis.

Renal insufficiency from rhabdomyolysis results from a complex cascade of metabolic derangements as a consequence of muscle breakdown. Myocyte damage releases intracellular contents, resulting in elevated serum myoglobin, CK, aldolase, lactate dehydrogenase, as well as hyperkalemia, hyperphosphatemia, hyperuricemia, and early hypocalcemia. Calcium may be elevated later in the course of the disorder.

Because of often times massive muscle breakdown, the serum BUN to Cr ratio is lower than expected with the acute rise in serum Cr. Urine discoloration from myoglobin often precedes the rise in serum CK. However, because myoglobin is cleared from the serum quickly,

---

TABLE 40-3

Classification of Rhabdomyolysis into Nonexertional and Exertional with Associated and Described Causes and Risk Factors

Type	Cause/risk factors	Examples/remarks
Nonexertional	Drugs	HMG-CoA-reductase inhibitors (statins), colchicine, paralytics, fibric acids, fenfluramine, zidovudine, cyclosporine
	Illicit drugs	ETOH, cocaine, Ecstasy, PCP, LSD
	Toxins	Spider bite, carbon monoxide, methanol
	Metabolic	Hypokalemia, DKA, HONK, RTA, hypophosphatemia, neuroleptic malignant syndrome, serotonin syndrome
	Infectious	Influenza A and B, Coxsackie virus, CMV, adenovirus, HIV, sepsis
	Mechanical	Crush injury, prolonged immobility, prolonged surgery, abuse, lightning strike
	Vascular	Arterial occlusion, venous occlusion, sickle cell disease, emboli, compartment syndrome
	Inflammatory	Burns, fever, hypothermia, pancreatitis hyperthermia, SLE, polymyositis
Exertional	Environmental	High temperature, high humidity, restrictive clothing, high altitude
	Activity type	High-intensity exercise, endurance activity such as marathons etc., maximal weight lifting, basic training in military, law enforcement, or firefighters
	Medical history	Sickle cell trait, family or personal history of exertional rhabdomyolysis, preceding infection prior to event, ETOH or cocaine use, metabolic myopathy
	Condition of participant	Dehydration, poor physical condition, deconditioning, lack of rehydration during event

Adapted from Warren JD, Blumbergs PC, Thompson PD. Rhabdomyolysis: a review. Muscle Nerve. *2002;25:332–347; Line R, Rust G.*
Acute exertional rhabdomyolysis. Am Fam Phy. *1995;52(2):502–506.*

measured elevations in serum and urine myoglobin are often missed because of the presentation of patients suffering from this disorder several days after the initial insult. Renal failure occurs in one-third of all cases. Multiple insults combine to induce myoglobinuric renal failure: (1) direct tubular toxicity from myoglobin, where urate and heme groups lead to free radical formation; (2) direct tubular obstruction with pigmented cast formation; and (3) shock and hypovolemia often from the underlying mechanism of injury or from massive fluid shifts from the vascular space into damaged muscle.

Successful treatment of rhabdomyolysis, regardless of cause, hinges on early recognition and prevention of ARF. This is foremost accomplished by early, extremely aggressive hydration with intravenous volume expansion with agents such as normal saline in an effort to protect renal tubules from the damaging effect of elevated serum myoglobin. Theoretically, alkalinization of the urine by the administration of HCO_3-containing isotonic fluids followed by forced diuresis with mannitol decreases the risk of tubular cast formation, aids with diuresis, and counters the profound metabolic acidosis and hyperkalemia seen frequently with myoglobinuric ARF. There are potential downsides to alkalinization however, especially in the setting of a high-serum phosphate and low calcium, where an alkaline serum can worsen hypocalcemia and promote calcium phosphate precipitation in tissues. It should be noted that the practice of alkalinizing the urine and forcing diuresis with mannitol has not been shown to be any more effective than normal saline at preventing death, progression to hemodialysis, or the development of renal failure in certain studies in trauma patients. It is clear that if urine output cannot be maintained, emergent hemodialysis is often required. Continued administration of copious intravenous fluids in this case could result in further respiratory compromise or compartment syndrome in already damaged muscle beds. As was seen in the case described in the vignette, the majority of rhabdomyolysis patients see a slow return of renal function, though it often does not return to previous baseline.

Selected References

1. Shaver MJ, Shah S. Acute renal failure. In: Dale D, ed. *ACP Medicine.* July 2005. Accessed Dec 2006. www.acpmedicine.com.
2. Slater MS, Mullins RJ. Rhabdomyolysis and myoglobinuric renal failure in trauma and surgical patients: a review. *J Am Coll Surg.* 1998;186:6.
3. Miller M. *Rhabdomyolysis.* UpToDate. Rose B, ed. Accessed Dec 2006. www.uptodate.com
4. Warren JD, Blumbergs PC, Thompson PD. Rhabdomyolysis: a review. *Muscle Nerve.* 2002;25:332–347.
5. Brady HR, Brenner BM. Acute renal failure. In: Kasper D, ed. *Harrison's Principal's of Internal Medicine.* 16th ed. Chap 260. August 2004. Accessed Dec 2006. www.accessmedicine.com.
6. Line R, Rust G. Acute exertional rhabdomyolysis. *Am Fam Phy.* 1995;52(2):502–506.
7. Brown CV, Rhee P, Chan L, et al. Preventing renal failure in patients with rhabdomyolysis: do bicarbonate and mannitol make a difference? *J Trauma.* 2004 Jun;56(6):1191–1196.

42-Year-Old Male with Progressive SOB (Shortness of Breath)

CASE PRESENTATION

A 42-year-old African American man presented to emergency room with dyspnea and pleuritic chest pain. He had been admitted 1 month previously for atypical chest pain and dyspnea. Cardiac evaluation at that point had been unrevealing and he was discharged home. Both his shortness of breath and chest pain had been worsening since discharge. He also reported minimal chills and sweats, mild weight loss, worsening nonproductive cough, three-pillow orthopnea, paroxysmal nocturnal dyspnea, mild edema, presyncope, and epigastric abdominal pain. He denied fevers, nausea, vomiting, or wheezing. His medical history was significant for hypertension, a stab wound to the chest 1 year prior to presentation from which he had residual chest pain less intense than his current chest pain, gonorrhea, and cellulitis treated with cephalexin 1 month ago. His only current medication was aspirin. He denied sick contacts, smoking, or drug abuse. His family history was unremarkable.

Physical Examination

Patient appeared comfortable and was sitting up in bed in no distress. Vital signs: temperature 37°C, pulse 76 to 90 beats/min, respiratory rate 16 breaths/min, blood pressure 90 to 108/40 to 58 mm Hg with room air oxygen saturation of 97%. Head, eyes, ears, nose, and throat: pupils equal, round, reactive to light and accommodation, extraocular movement intact, sclera clear, dentition poor. Neck: supple without lymphadenopathy, jugular venous distension, or bruit. Cardiovascular: regular rhythm and rate, S_1 and S_2 present, without murmurs, heaves, or thrills. Lung: diminished breath sounds at the left base with dullness to percussion, otherwise clear without wheezes, rales, or rhonchi. Respiratory effort was normal without accessory muscle use. Abdomen: diffusely tender without rebound or guarding; bowel sounds normal without organomegaly. Extremities: no cyanosis, clubbing, or edema. Neurologic: alert and oriented × 3 without focal defect. Examination was otherwise unremarkable.

Laboratory Studies

White blood cells 7.7, neutrophils 56%, lymphocytes 25%, hemoglobin/hematocrit 11.7/34, and platelets 289.

Creatine kinase (CK) 211, CK-MB 3.4, and troponin I 0.01; ECG was unchanged from prior studies and chest x-ray (CXR) is shown in Fig 41-1.

Case Resolution

The patient was admitted and underwent human immunodeficiency virus (HIV) testing, purified protein derivative (PPD), and acid-fast bacillus (AFB) smears, which were negative. Sputum culture showed very light *Staphylococcus aureus*. A chest CT revealed bilateral pleural effusions, left greater than right, and small diffuse miliary nodules bilaterally. Thoracentesis was performed, yielding red blood cells 12,375, WBC 1320, 81% lymphocytes, 12% monocytes, glucose 49, protein 4.9, pH 7.61, lactate dehydrogenase (LDH) 309. At that time, serum LDH was 150, protein 7.2, and albumin 3.0. He subsequently underwent bronchoscopy, from which a lymph node biopsy yielded noncaseating granulomas. He was started on prednisone, vitamin D, and calcium.

Question

What is the most likely etiology of the patient's pleural effusion?

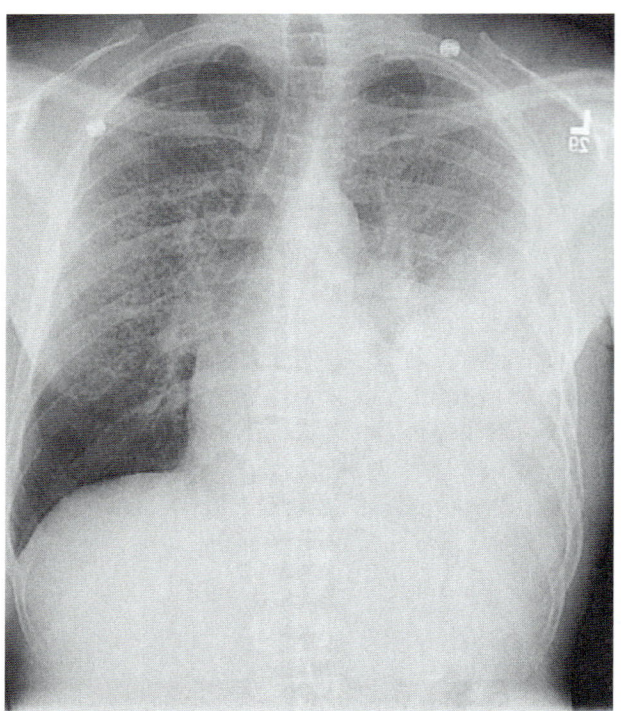 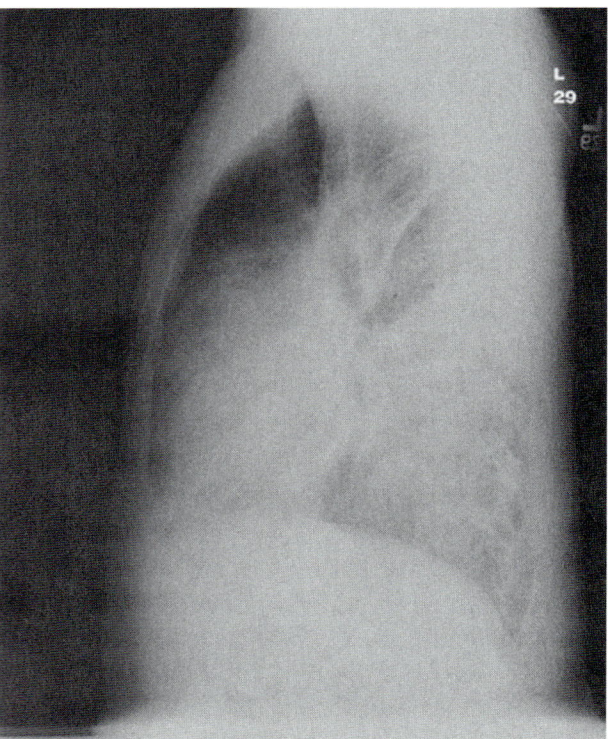

Figure 41-1 Posteroanterior (PA) and lateral chest radiograph on admission notable for significant left pleural effusion and prominent interstitial markings.

Answer

The differential diagnosis of pleural effusions is extremely broad, but the pleural fluid analysis revealed an exudative effusion, which narrows the differential considerably. While the bronchoscopy results lead to a diagnosis of sarcoidosis, this disease itself is a rare cause of pleural effusions. No other cause for an exudative effusions fits with the clinical scenario, and the indolent presentation could easily be one of the varied manifestations of sarcoidosis.

Discussion

Pleural effusions are common findings on patient examination and chest imaging. Often, the practitioner is already aware of a condition which would predispose the patient to pleural effusion, but if a patient has a new pleural effusion larger than 10 mm and not consistent with congestive heart failure or not occurring in the setting of a probable viral pleurisy, further investigation via thoracentesis is warranted.

Before invasive procedures are undertaken, however, a thorough drug and exposure history, focusing on asbestos and tuberculosis, are important. Additionally, HIV risk factors must be assessed, as HIV alters the differential and diagnostic pattern. In HIV, leading causes of effusions are Kaposi sarcoma, pneumonia, and tuberculosis; *Pneumocystis carinii* pneumonia and lymphoma follow. Sputum culture, AFB, PPD, and other studies can be considered. Depending on how the effusion was discovered, posteroanterior, lateral, and decubitus plain films or ultrasonography can be pursued. Further characterization of an effusion with a contrasted CT can also be helpful, and should be performed prior to thoracentesis as it allows better visualization of the pleura for discrimination of benign versus malignant pleural thickening.

Thoracentesis is the next step in the evaluation of pleural effusions, but is contraindicated if mesothelioma is suspected, as seeding of the tract appears to be common. Possible etiologies for pleural effusions are widely varied, but fall into two major categories: transudative and exudative. These categories have been defined based on pleural fluid characteristics, most often using Light criteria (see Table 41-1). Additionally, complex septated, complex non-septated, and homogeneous echogenic patterns on ultrasound are always exudates. A listing of the differential diagnosis of pleural effusions is listed in Table 41-2.

TABLE 41-1

Criteria for Exudative Effusions

Light criteria

Serum/pleural protein > 0.5
Serum/pleural LDH > 0.6
Pleural LDH > 2/3 upper limit of normal for serum

Other characteristics of exudative effusions

Pleural fluid protein > 2.9 g/dL
Cholesterol > 45 mg/dL
LDH > 60% upper limits of normal for serum

The differences in fluid characteristics highlight some of the differences in pathophysiology. Transudative effusions occur when there is an imbalance in the hydrostatic and oncotic pressures of pleural fluid. Autoregulation and precapillary resistance attenuate changes in arterial pressure, so these changes have little influence. However, increased venous pressures, and more importantly increased pulmonary vascular resistance, lead to increasing water concentration of lymph, which eventually overwhelms lymphatic absorptive capacity. This imbalance results in "peribronchial cuffing," fluid accumulation in peribronchial spaces which is not accessible to lymphatics. The fluid then follows pressure gradients to the mediastinum or pleural spaces. A similar process occurs when serum oncotic pressures decrease.

In contrast, exudates arise from pulmonary inflammation which causes protein and fluid leakage from damaged capillaries, and impaired lymphatic drainage. The presence of cytokines, some endocrine conditions, injury from radiation or drugs, lymphatic infiltration, and anatomic abnormalities are all associated with impaired lymphatic contraction. Lymphatics are also subject to external forces altering function; these include decreased respiratory motion, extrinsic compression (eg, pleural fibrosis), blockage of lymphatic stomata, decreased intrapleural pressure, increased systemic venous pressure, and decreased liquid availability.

There are many conditions which can be definitively diagnosed by thoracentesis findings, and specific testing is indicated as it applies in Table 41-2. Some other testing that can be performed on the fluid is listed in Table 41-3. Diagnosis is also aided by the clinical progression of the illness and response to therapy. However, if an effusion remains undiagnosed after these interventions, percutaneous pleural biopsy or thoracoscopy should be performed. Radiation of the biopsy site must be performed in mesothelioma. In general, the yield of bronchoscopy is low in the absence of hemoptysis or signs of bronchial obstruction. Alternatively, idiopathic pleural effusions can be followed for resolution if there is no suspicion for malignancy; the majority resolves spontaneously within a few months, although some will recur over the next few years. A patient with a positive PPD and lymphocytic exudative effusion should be treated for tuberculosis unless pleural fluid adenosine deaminase levels are low (< 43 IU/L). A high pH and the presence of mesothelial cells also argue against a diagnosis of a tuberculous effusion. A high suspicion for pulmonary emboli should always be considered. In general, pleural effusions secondary to pulmonary emboli are less than one-third of a hemithorax and produce dyspnea out of proportion to size, and can be associated with pleuritic chest pain. However, they can have manifold presentations and should always be on the differential diagnosis. In addition to pulmonary embolus, common causes of idiopathic effusions include connective tissue disease, viral pleurisy, and mycoplasmal infection. Thoracostomy or thoracoscopic drainage is thought to be necessary in certain situations. These include presence of pus in aspirated fluid, positive bacterial culture or Gram stain, low pH (<7.2), high LDH (>1000), low glucose (<30), or fluid occupying more than half of the affected hemithorax.

Regarding sarcoid-related pleural effusions, they appear to be rare. The reported incidence ranges from 0.7% to 10%, and right-sided effusions are more common. Those not attributable to other conditions (eg, congestive heart failure or parapneumonic) are more commonly lymphocyte-predominant, paucicellular, and serous. They also seem to be characterized as exudates by protein criteria with mean protein 4.0 IU/dL, but there is often discordance between protein and LDH levels. They are thought to occur secondary to increased capillary permeability rather than inflammation. In one series of 181 patients with sarcoidosis, 1 of 9 patients with an exacerbation developed an effusion as opposed to 1 of 172 who did not have an exacerbation. They are more common in stage 2 disease and regress with progression of disease. Definitive diagnosis is by pleural biopsy. Although they resolve spontaneously, resolution is more rapid with steroid therapy. Other pleural manifestations of sarcoidosis include pneumothorax, pleural thickening, hydropneumothorax, chylothorax, hemothorax, or trapped lung.

Pleural effusions have a variety of etiologies, and should be investigated if the diagnosis is unclear from the

TABLE 41-2

Differential Diagnosis of Pleural Effusions

Type of effusion		Differential (definitive test as applicable)
Transudate		
		Congestive heart failure
		Hepatic hydrothorax
		Nephrotic syndrome
		Hypoalbuminemia
		Peritoneal dialysis
		Urinothorax (pleural fluid/serum creatinine > 1.0)
		Atelectasis
		Superior vena cava syndrome
		Constrictive pericarditis
		Trapped lung
		Hypothyroidism
		Mitral stenosis
		Ovarian hyperstimulation
		Meigs syndrome
Exudate		
	Most common	Infection (empyema – observation, culture, pH; TB – AFB stain, culture; fungal pleurisy – KOH prep, culture)
		Malignancy (positive cytology)
	Less common	Pulmonary infarction
		Rheumatoid arthritis/autoimmune (RA – cytology; SLE – LE cells, ANA > 1.0)
		Benign asbestos effusion
		Post-myocardial infarction syndrome
		Pancreatitis/movement from the abdomen
	Rare	Yellow nail syndrome
		Drugs
	Other	Iatrogenic
		Increased negative pleural pressure
		Lymph disorder/lymphangioleiomyomatosis
		Chylothorax (TG > 110, chylomicrons)
		Trauma (hemothorax – pleural fluid/blood hematocrit > 0.5; esophageal rupture – salivary amylase, low pH)
		Amyloid
		Pseudochylothorax
Either		
		Pulmonary embolus
		Recent significant diuresis
		Sarcoidosis

TABLE 41-3

Testing of Pleural Effusions

Color

Viscosity (high in mesothelioma)

Turbidity (high with inflammation and lipid content)

pH (low in empyema, < 7.2 requires chest tube)

Protein

LDH

Glucose

Albumin

Cell count and differential

Culture

Cytology

Amylase

TB testing

Complement levels

Hematocrit

ANA (a high false-positive rate and generally mirror serum values)

presentation, or if a condition requiring drainage (ie, empyema) may exist. In this case, the patient's presentation with pleural effusion and its investigation lead to a diagnosis of an underlying chronic disease.

Selected References

Light RW. Pleural effusion. *N Engl J Med*. 2002;346: 1971–1977.

Huggins JT, Doelken P, Sahn SA, et al. Pleural effusions in a series of 181 outpatients with sarcoidosis. *Chest*. 2006;129: 1599–1604

Ferrer JS, Munoz. XG, Orriols RM, et al. Evolution of idiopathic pleural effusion: a prospective, long-term follow-up study. *Chest*. 1996;109:1508–1513.

Maskell NA and Butland RJ. British Thoracic Society Guidelines for the investigation of a unilateral pleural effusion in adults. *Thorax*. 2003;58(suppl II):II59–II17.

5-Year-Old Female with 40-hour History of Progressive Lethargy, Nausea, and Yellow Skin

CASE PRESENTATION

A previously healthy 5-year-old Caucasian female presented to the emergency department with a 2-day history of progressive lethargy, nausea, and jaundice. She was well until 2 days prior to presentation, when she first experienced abdominal pain. The next day she began to have emesis and appear "yellow." She was evaluated by her primary care physician 1 day prior to presentation. Given her clinical symptoms, she was thought likely to have hepatitis A and confirmatory laboratory testing was ordered. During the night prior to presentation, the patient's emesis markedly increased. She complained of excessive thirst, but could not tolerate any oral intake. The child was progressively less active. She was noted to have both red urine and stool. The physician was called for advice and she was directed to the emergency room for evaluation. The family reported no fevers, or ill contacts. The child had recovered uneventfully from an upper respiratory tract infection 2 weeks prior. No family members had similar symptoms. There was no history of travel outside of the state or any camping trips. Her emesis was not green or feculent. Her stools were loose but not described as diarrhea. The family denied any history of rashes or swelling.

Physical Examination

In the emergency room, she was noted to be listless but interactive with the examination. Vital signs: she was afebrile with temperature 36.5°C, a pulse of 142 beats/min, respiratory rate of 37 breaths/min, and a blood pressure of 74/39 mm Hg. Her physical examination was significant for jaundice and scleral icterus. Oral examination revealed pale and dry mucous membranes. No cervical, supraclavicular, axillary, or inguinal adenopathy was present. The lung examination was significant for tachypnea but normal auscultation. Her skin was generally pale with pale palmar creases. No other lesions were noted. The heart examination revealed tachycardia with grade 2/6 systolic ejection murmur. Her extremities were cool with a capillary refill time of 4 to 5 seconds. No hepatosplenomegaly was appreciated. She had a nonfocal neurologic examination.

Laboratory Studies

Serum pH 7.16, base deficit 17.3, white blood cells 23.6, hematocrit 8, platelets 274, reticulocyte absolute count 4.5%, blood urea nitrogen (BUN) 36, Cr 0.6, CO_2 13, glucose: 50, total bilirubin: 14.6, lactate dehydrogenase (LDH) 7856, urinalysis hemoglobin: large, red blood cells (RBC) 9.

Case Resolution

In the emergency room, she was fluid resuscitated and transferred to the pediatric intensive care unit for further evaluation and monitoring. Additional laboratory tests of significance included a positive direct Coombs test. She continued to receive aggressive fluid resuscitation, and was given antibiotics after blood and urine cultures were obtained. During the evaluation she became obtunded and emergently received O negative-packed RBC with immediate marked neurologic improvement.

Question

What is the most likely explanation of this patient's profound anemia?

Answer

The patient's decreased energy level and pallor suggest decreased oxygen-carrying capacity of blood. The laboratory results also support this, given the presence of an acidosis which could represent tissue hypoperfusion with resultant lactic acidosis. The presence of jaundice and scleral icterus indicate intravascular breakdown of RBC. The profound anemia is consistent with the historical, clinical, and laboratory features of the case. The positive direct Coombs test in this patient confirms an autoimmune hemolytic anemia (AIHA).

Discussion

The characteristic signs and symptoms of hemolysis are directly related to the degree of anemia. Such signs may include pallor, lethargy, and the laboratory findings of anemia with indirect hyperbilirubinemia and pigmented urine if the hemolysis is brisk. Other laboratory findings that may support hemolysis include an elevated serum LDH, an elevated reticulocyte count, an elevated indirect bilirubin, and a reduced haptoglobin if the hemolysis is intravascular. The clinical presentation of a patient with AIHA can include all the signs and symptoms of hemolysis. An antecedent history of an acute infectious illness can usually be elicited. If the anemia is abrupt and severe, there may be signs of cardiovascular collapse.

AIHA refers to a group of disorders characterized by the presence of antibodies against the patient's RBC [1]. AIHA is relatively rare in children, with an incidence of 1 in 80,000 in the general population [1]. It has a peak incidence at 4 years of age, with a 2 to 1 predilection for females [1]. AIHA is divided into primary and secondary categories.

Primary AIHA refers to the condition of circulating autoantibodies against the RBC without evidence for a systemic condition. Primary AIHA can be further subdivided into warm and cold AIHA (Table 42-1). Warm AIHA is usually caused by IgG antibodies that bind to RBC protein antigens at 37°C and occasionally activate complement. The vast majority of these IgG antibodies are of the IgG 1 subclass, with IgG 3 being the next most common [1]. Cold hemagglutinin disease is caused by IgM autoantibodies binding to polysaccharide antigens on the RBC, and typically may follow an infection with mycoplasma. In that setting, the IgM bind the I/i antigens present on the surface of RBCs [1]. These disorders are generally self-limited.

Secondary AIHA refers to the state where the autoantibodies are a manifestation of a systemic disease, such as lupus, malignancy, immunodeficient states, and drug reactions [1].

In either situation, once the autoantibodies bind to the antigens on the red cells, the Fc portion of the antibody is identified by Fc receptors located throughout the body, including in the spleen and liver. This binding results in incorporation of red cells into the reticuloendothelial system, and ingestion by macrophages. Commonly the ingestion is partial, resulting in the spherocytes which can easily be identified on the peripheral blood smear. Since spherocytes are not as deformable as normal RBCs, they are destroyed in the small vessels of the reticuloendothelial system [1].

The clinical presentation of a patient with AIHA will vary with the rapidity of onset and the degree of anemia. Symptoms usually include the acute onset of fatigue,

TABLE 42-1

Autoimmune Hemolytic Disease and Associated Conditions

Warm hemagglutinin (IgG)
Idiopathic
Post viral
Autoimmune disorders (eg, systemic lupus erythematosus)
Lymphoproliferative diseases (eg, chronic lymphocytic leukemia)
Drugs (eg, penicillin, methyldopa, many others)
allogenic blood transfusions or hematopoietic cell transplantation

Cold hemagglutinin (IgM)
Mycoplasma pneumoniae
Infectious mononucleosis
Lymphoma

pallor, yellow skin, and red urine. The physical examination will reveal the pale mucous membrane, the yellow skin, and can also include hepatosplenomegaly. Laboratory evaluations should be judiciously ordered, given these patients' extreme anemia. Essential laboratory results to be obtained in a patient believed to have AIHA include a type and cross, CBC with differential, peripheral blood smear review, and direct and indirect antiglobulin (Coombs) test.

To complete the direct Coombs test, the patient's RBC are first washed and then mixed with antiserum or monoclonal antibodies, which recognize human immunoglobulins including IgG as well as complement, C3 [2]. The monoclonal antibodies bind to the Fc portion of any IgG bound to the RBC causing agglutination and thus a positive direct Coombs test. If only IgG is present on the RBC, then the hemolysis is because of this antibody alone [2]. If C3 is also found on the RBC, then the IgG was able to fix complement, and the activation of complement may be playing a role in the destruction of the RBC [2]. Another alternative occurs when C3 is identified, but no agglutination occurs with IgG. This usually points to another antibody (IgM or rarely IgA) as the cause of the hemolysis [2] (Table 42-2). The indirect Coombs test is able to detect levels of antibodies in a patient's serum that are not attached to RBC. The patient's serum is mixed with different aliquots of red cells with known antigens on their surface. If antibodies are present in the patient's serum that recognize the antigens on the RBC, an antigen-antibody

complex will form [2]. Antihuman IgG is now added to the sample, and the Fc portion of any bound antibody will be recognized, causing agglutination and a positive indirect Coombs test [2]. Other tests that can be obtained if the patient is stable include a chemistry screen, liver function tests, and a urinalysis.

The peripheral blood smear is very helpful in determining the diagnosis of AIHA. Most commonly, multiple spherocytes can be identified (see Fig. 42-1), as well as polychromatophilic cells. Further evidence supporting the diagnosis of AIHA includes difficulty cross matching blood secondary to antibodies. As a result, identification of the patient's blood type, and the cross-matching of appropriate units can be a long complicated process. Therefore, it is important to discuss the potential diagnosis of AIHA with the blood bank early in the clinical course, and ask the

TABLE 42-2

Patterns of Direct Coombs Testing

Anti-IgG	Anti-C3	Diagnosis
+	−	Warm AIHA, antibody is IgG
+	+	Antibody is IgG which fixes complement
−	+	Cold agglutinins in serum, antibody is IgM

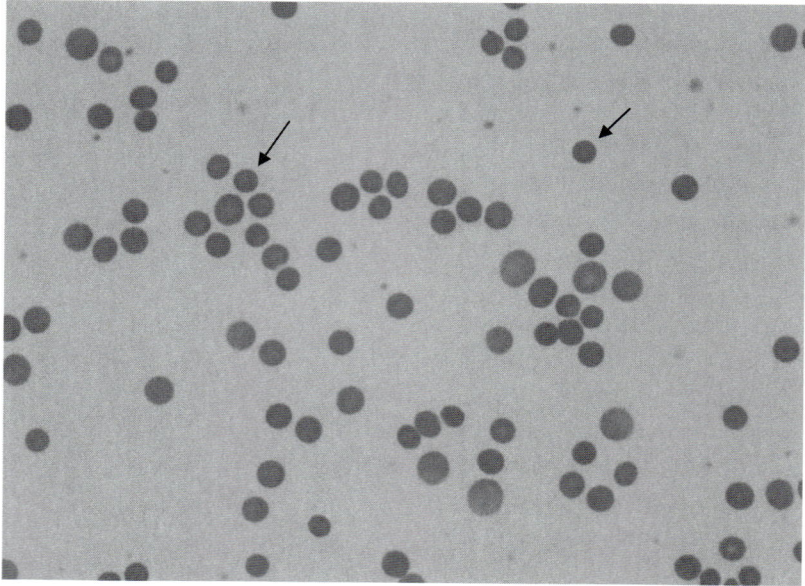

Figure 42-1 Multiple smaller rounded cells (arrows) – spherocytes.

blood bank personnel to identify the closest matched blood they can as soon as possible for the patient. If a cross-matched unit cannot be obtained, giving the best matched unit of blood or an O unit is appropriate. When blood that is not completely cross matched is given to a patient, the blood bank will require a waiver of transfusion card completed by the ordering physician [3].

Treatment involves restoring oxygen-carrying capacity with the closest matched units of blood available, and inhibiting the antibody-mediated destruction of the RBC. One mainstay of therapy is steroids, often at doses as high as 4 to 5 mg/kg/day [4]. Although the exact mechanism of action of steroids in AIHA is not known, it is believed that they may inhibit autoantibody production and downregulate the Fcγ receptor on macrophages, which assists in phagocytosis of coated RBC [5]. Whatever the mechanism of action, the overall affect is to prolong the life span of antibody-coated RBC. If the hemolysis improves after the initiation of IV steroids, then oral steroids can be used at a dose of 1 to 2 mg/kg/day for 2 to 4 weeks, with a slow taper over approximately 3 months. If the process goes on for over a month, the diagnosis of chronic AIHA must be considered. Other potential treatments for AIHA include intravenous immunoglobulin, Rituximab, and splenectomy in nonresponsive or chronic AIHA [6].

Selected References

1. Gehrs BC, Friedberg RC. Autoimmune hemolytic anemia. *Am J Hemat*. 2002;69:258–271.
2. Zarandona JM, Yazer MH. The role of the Coombs test in evaluating hemolysis in adults. *Can Med Assn J*. 2006;174(3):305–307.
3. Reardon JE, Marques MB. Laboratory evaluation and transfusion support of patients with autoimmune hemolytic anemia. *Am J Clin Pathol*. 2006 Jun; 125(suppl):S71–S77.
4. Petz Lawrence D. Treatment of autoimmune hemolytic anemias. *Curr Opin Hematol*. 2001 Nov;8(6):411–416.
5. Rosse WF, Hillmen P, Schreiber AD. Immune-mediated hemolytic anemia. *Hematol Am Soc Hematol Edu Prog*. 2004: 48–62.
6. King NE, Ness PM. Treatment of autoimmune hemolytic anemia. *Semin Hematol*. 2005 Jul;42(3):131–136.

36-Year-Old Male with Lower Extremity Weakness

CASE PRESENTATION

A 36-year-old Caucasian man presented to our hospital complaining of lower extremity weakness for the past month. He reported a long history of having a "sore back," but had specifically noted weakness and leg heaviness in recent weeks. The weakness never went away entirely, but would wax and wane as well as alternate sides. The day of presentation he had fallen down the stairs when his right leg "just stayed behind me" as he walked. On review of systems, he noted occasionally having shooting pains down his legs that were associated with his back pain, a numb feeling over his right anterior chest, weight loss of about 25 lb and night sweats, a "smoker's cough," weekly bitemporal, throbbing headaches, bowel and bladder urgency without frank incontinence, and he thought his memory had worsened over the past month. Though he denied other recent symptoms, he did report a week-long episode 3 years prior of diplopia and having trouble holding water in his mouth when he drank, which had resolved.

His past medical history included an intentional Tylenol overdose 6 years prior, for which he was hospitalized for a few days, a hiatal hernia, and gastroesophageal reflux. He had a family history significant for a brother who had committed suicide, a mother ill with lung cancer, a father who had died of his first myocardial infarction at age 62, and a sister with asthma. The patient himself smoked about a pack a day and had been a heavy drinker for several years, but had cut down to 3 to 4 glasses of beer day in the past several years. He denied any drug use, but had been taking some of his mother's narcotics to treat his back pain. His back pain and weakness had kept him from his construction job for the past several weeks.

Physical Examination

On physical examination, he was afebrile. Vital signs: pulse of 73 beats/min, blood pressure of 123/87 mm Hg, respiratory rate 18 breaths/min with an oxygen saturation of 98% on room air. He was a thin man who appeared worried. His pupils were small bilaterally after having received pain medication and funduscopic examination was limited, but visualized portions of the discs appeared sharp. He had poor dentition, but no other findings on oral examination. He had no lymphadenopathy and his lung examination was normal. Cardiovascular and abdominal examinations were also normal. His neurologic examination was notable for decreased strength in both lower extremities, left greater than right. He had increased, but symmetric reflexes in his lower extremities, upgoing toes bilaterally with three to four beats of clonus on both sides. His gait was unsteady and Romberg was positive; there was no pronator drift. He had decreased sensation over his right, anterior chest without clear dermatomal pattern. The rest of his sensory examination was grossly intact including his perineum.

Laboratory Studies

Initial laboratory data included a complete blood count, chemistries, liver function tests, and a C-reactive protein, which were all within normal limits except for some mild polycythemia. Radiographs of the cervical spine showed mild degenerative disease and a healed right clavicular fracture, but no acute findings from the fall. His noncontrast head CT showed a focal area of decreased attenuation in the subcortical white matter of the mid-left temporal lobe that was concerning for an old contusion, chronic ischemic insult, or possibly a demyelinating disease. He subsequently underwent MRI imaging of both his brain and spine, which met criteria for the diagnosis of multiple sclerosis (MS) (see Fig. 43-1). During the course of his workup, the following tests were all negative or within normal limits: human immunodeficiency virus (HIV) antibody, hepatitis A, B, and C screening serologies, angiotensin-converting enzyme test, antineutrophil cytoplasmic antibody, antinuclear antibody test, Lyme screen, anti-Smith antibodies, anti-myeloperoxidase antibodies, anti-RNA antibodies.

Case Resolution

The patient was treated with high-dose steroids (dexamethasone). He received a total of 12 doses of intravenous dexamethasone that produced a mild improvement in his lower extremity weakness. He was subsequently followed as an outpatient with persistent lower extremity weakness and an uncoordinated gait.

Question

How can this patient be treated to reduce the incidence of relapses?

Answer

Several options exist which have been shown to reduce the incidence of relapses, as well as reduce various imaging based markers of disease. It is unclear if any of these treatments alter the long-term course of the disease. Three formulations of beta-interferon are currently FDA approved for the treatment of relapsing and remitting MS. All three formulations reduce the frequency of exacerbations and improve MRI-based measures of disease activity. Natalizumab is a recombinant humanized monoclonal antibody to certain adhesion molecules expressed on activated lymphocytes and monocytes. This is thought to block their movement across the blood–brain barrier and blunt the inflammatory cascade in MS. Natalizumab has been shown to reduce the frequency of exacerbations both alone and in combination with beta-interferon drugs. Glatiramer acetate, a mixture of synthetic polypeptides is also used to control the frequency of exacerbations. Lastly, studies have suggested that the early treatment of optic neuritis may alter the course of MS. Treatment with high-dose steroids or with intramuscular beta-interferon-1a at the time of first demyelinating event have been shown to reduce the development of clinically definitive MS.

Discussion

MS is a chronic disease that usually begins at a relatively early age. It is characterized by areas of white matter inflammation, demyelination, and glial scarring of the central nervous system (CNS). The key to the diagnosis of MS is objective clinical evidence of multiple CNS lesions occurring in time and space. In other words, the lesions must occur in different areas of the CNS (multiple lesions in space) and must continue to occur (multiple lesions in time). Typically, the disease is relapsing and remitting to begin with and, eventually, permanent neurologic disabilities take hold and do not remit. This typical pattern is relapsing-remitting multiple sclerosis (RRMS) with a secondary progressive course. About 15% of patients have progression from the onset of symptoms and this is called primary progressive multiple sclerosis. The exact causes are unknown, but likely involve an autoimmune process in a genetically and/or environmentally susceptible population.

There are several distinct epidemiologic features of MS. Age of onset is typically between the ages of 20 and 30 years. Women are affected more often than men with a ratio of about 2:1, depending on the case series. The disease occurs more frequently at certain latitudes, specifically those running through northern Europe, northern United States, southern Canada, southern Australia, and New Zealand. It is not certain, however, how race plays into this geographical distribution since white populations are at greatest risk and are also the greatest proportion of people living in those countries. Similarly, it is not certain how environmental factors play into disease risk, but they appear to make a difference. For instance, immigrants moving to higher prevalence areas before the age of 15 years increase their lifetime risk of developing MS after they move. There have also been "epidemics" of MS, which would suggest a specific role for environmental factors.

The signs and symptoms of MS are diverse and reflect the fact that nearly any portion of the CNS can be affected. There are however, certain areas that are more commonly affected, and these include the optic chiasm, brainstem, cerebellum, and posterior and lateral columns of the spinal cord. Optic neuritis is a relatively common early finding and is characterized by early visual impairment, a central or cecocentral scotoma, and orbital or retro-orbital pain precipitated by movement of the affected eye. The diplopia that our patient had experienced was likely because of an internuclear ophthalmoplegia, a result of a lesion affecting the medial longitudinal fasciculus, another ophthalmologic phenomenon that is uncommon in conditions aside from MS, at least among young people. Trigeminal neuralgia is another sign that, when found in young people, should make one consider the diagnosis of MS.

Limb weakness is the most common symptom among those with MS. Interestingly, direct testing of strength frequently does not correlate with the difficulty in walking that the patient may experience, as in our patient's case. This is because of the multiple lesions contributing, which affect not only on muscle strength, but also proprioception and general coordination. Urinary symptoms are relatively common, specifically incontinence. The Lhermitte symptom is a feeling of "electricity" running down the back after the patient flexes his neck and, while classically

associated with MS, it can be associated with other conditions. There is no characteristic pattern as to when or in what order symptoms appear. Similarly, patients may be monosymptomatic or polysymptomatic at onset.

With the variation in clinical presentation and the significance of being diagnosed with MS, health providers must act with caution in making the diagnosis of MS. In fact, there are very specific criteria set out by the International Panel on the Diagnosis of Multiple Sclerosis to guide clinicians in making the diagnosis. There is no specific test for MS, therefore the clinician must rely on the history, neurologic examination, and laboratory tests. If a patient has had two or more "attacks" and has objective clinical evidence of two or more lesions, no further testing necessarily has to be done in order to make the diagnosis (as would be the case with our patient). Magnetic resonance imaging (MRI), however, usually supports the diagnosis and, in those cases which cannot be diagnosed clinically, can make the diagnosis.

Three of four MRI criteria must be met to support the diagnosis of MS: (1) one gadolinium-enhancing lesion or nine T2-hyperintense lesions if there is no gadolinium-enhancing lesion, (2) at least one infratentorial lesion, (3) at least one juxtacortical lesion, and (4) at least three periventricular lesions (Fig 43-1). There are also specific guidelines about the interpretation of spinal lesions and

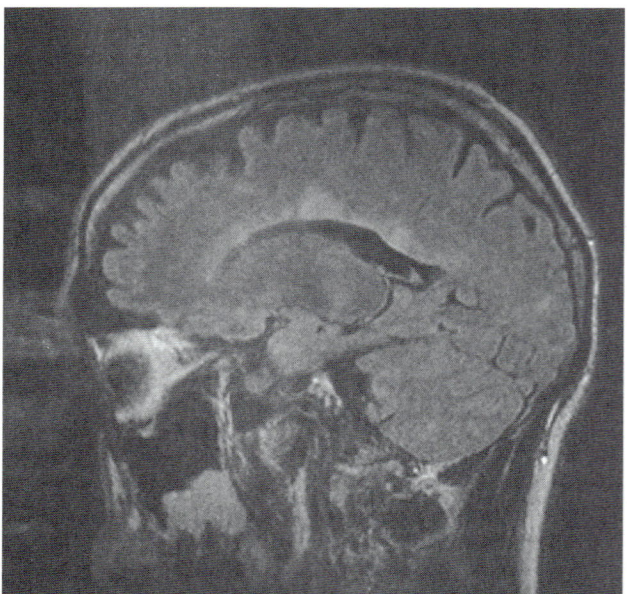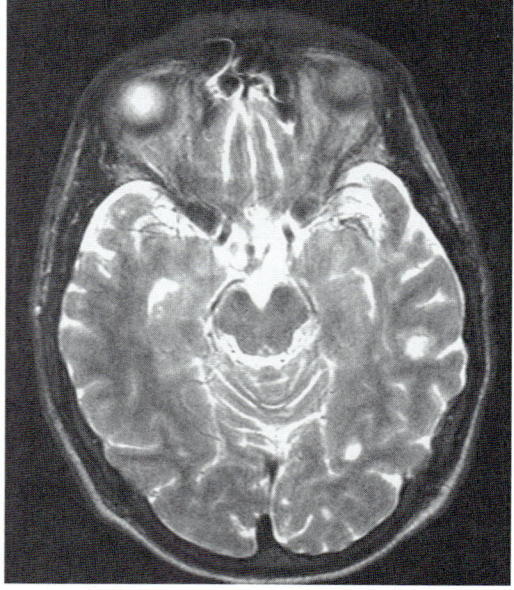

Figure 43-1 On the left is a sagittal *flair* image that shows multiple, deep white matter hyperintensities in a periventricular distribution and involves the lateral aspects of the corpus callosum. On the right is an axial T2 image that shows scattered peripheral white matter hyperintensities involving the juxtacortical white matter.

how they play into these overall criteria. In many cases, the diagnosis may be made on the basis of history, examination, and MRI. Unusual presentations or cases that do not meet the imaging criteria may require cerebrospinal fluid (CSF) analysis and/or visual-evoked potential (VEP) to support the diagnosis. CSF abnormalities relate to the activation of a few antibody-secreting B cells within the CSF in persons with MS, thereby creating oligoclonal IgG bands that differ in the CSF compared to serum and/or an elevated IgG index. When the patient's only clinically-expressed lesion is not visual, abnormal VEP may be used to provide objective data of a second lesion affecting a visual pathway.

In addition to meeting the criteria set out by experts, it is also important to exclude other possible diagnoses. The differential diagnosis is broad and includes acute disseminated encephalomyelitis, Lyme disease, HIV-associated myelopathy, HTLV-I-associated myelopathy, neurosyphilis, progressive multifocal leukoencephalopathy (in immuno-suppressed patients), systemic lupus erythematosus, polyarteritis nodosa, Sjogren syndrome, Behcet disease, sarcoidosis, paraneoplastic syndromes, and other neurologic and miscellaneous conditions. Workup for other conditions can be limited to diagnoses that are at least somewhat likely to affect the patient at hand, but should at least include serologic tests for the infectious etiologies.

The course of MS varies from a benign variant in which patients are nearly asymptomatic to rapid progression and death within a few months. Unfortunately, predicting an individual's course is difficult. The mainstays of treatment are corticosteroids to treat acute attacks and disease-modifying therapy to slow the overall disease process. There are six medications approved for treatment of RRMS; they include three different beta-interferon drugs, glatiramer acetate, mitoxantrone, and natalizumab. Early detection and treatment has been shown to improve prognosis. Treatment of the progressive phase of MS (and for those with primary progressive MS) is more difficult and includes a wide array of immunosuppressive therapies.

Selected References

McDonald WI, Compston A, Edan G, et al. Recommended diagnostic criteria for multiple sclerosis: guidelines from the International Panel on the Diagnosis of Multiple Sclerosis. *Ann Neurol.* 2001;50:121–127 [PMID 11456302].

Polman CH, Reingold SC, Edan G, et al. Diagnostic criteria for multiple sclerosis: 2005 revisions to the "McDonald Criteria." *Ann Neurol.* 2005;58:840–846 [PMID 16283615].

Rowland LP. *Merritt's Neurology.* 11th ed. Books@Ovid; Philadelphia, PA: Lippincott Williams & Wilkins; 2005:941–961.

Frohman, EM, Racke, MK, Raine, CS. Multiple aclerosis—the plague and its pathogenesis. *N Eng J Med.* 2006;354:942–955.

49-Year-Old Female with 24 hours of Right-Sided Numbness and Facial Droop

C
44

CASE PRESENTATION

The patient is a 49-year-old Caucasian female who was in her usual state of excellent health until 48 hours prior to presentation to the emergency department (ED), when she experienced sudden onset of right leg numbness and weakness that lasted about 15 minutes. She had no other symptoms and the "funny" feeling in her leg resolved spontaneously. Twenty-four hours prior to admission and 24 hours following the initial episode, the patient had a recrudescence of these symptoms in her right lower extremity but also had weakness and numbness in her right upper extremity and right side of her face. Because the prior episode resolved spontaneously, the patient went to bed but was alarmed when she awoke the next morning to persistent symptoms or right-sided facial, upper extremity, and lower extremity weakness and numbness. The patient specifically denies headache, slurred speech, vision changes, hearing changes, aura, trauma, palpitations, shortness of breath, chest pain, vertigo, syncope, or presyncope. The patients' past medical history is notable for appendectomy at age 17 and adult rosacea. Her medications include birth control pills, which she has taken for more than 20 years, and minocycline. She does not consume alcohol, does not smoke, and does not use illicit drugs. She works as a paralegal assistant at a local law firm and exercises frequently. Family history is significant for her father having had a myocardial infarct at age 67 and her mother with lupus. There is no history of thrombophilia in her or her family.

Physical Examination

The patient is a middle-aged Caucasian female in no acute distress, who appears her stated age. Vital signs: temperature 36.4°C, pulse 63 beats/min and regular, respiratory rate 18 breaths/min, blood pressure 173/109 mm Hg, and oxygen saturation of 100% on room air. Patient is alert and oriented to person, place, and time and answers questions with appropriate responses. Head, eyes, ears, nose, and throat: normocephalic, atraumatic in nature with pupils equal, round, and reactive to light and accommodation. Extraocular movements are intact. Sclera are clear, neck: supple with no lymphadenopathy or bruits. There is no jugular venous distention and no thyromegaly. Cardiovascular: normal rate and regular rhythm without murmurs, gallops, or rubs; lungs are clear bilaterally. Abdomen: unremarkable with no abdominal bruits. There is no clubbing, cyanosis, or edema of the extremities. Neurologically, the patient has normal function of cranial nerves (CN) II, III, IV, and VI. However, CN V on the right is abnormal with paresthesias and lack of sensation on the right side of the face. CN VII is also abnormal with right facial droop. There is mild tongue deviation to the right but CN VIII, IX, X, and XI appear to be normal. Grossly, the patient has diminished sensation of light touch, and pain on the right side from the knee up. Strength is diminished on the right-upper and right-lower extremities when compared to the left (4/5 vs. 5/5). There is no clonus, and deep tendon reflexes are symmetric and normal. Babinski is downgoing. There is slight pronator drift to the right. Heel to shin and finger to nose are slowed but normal.

Laboratory Studies

Serum chemistries revealed Na 138, K 3.5, Cl 106, HCo$_3$ 26, blood urea nitrogen 9, creatinine 0.8, glucose 110, Ca 8.7, creatine kinase 52, creatine kinase-MB fraction 1.9, troponin 0.01, partial thromboplastin time 24, prothrombin time 10.1, international normalized ratio 1.01. Thyroid-stimulating hormone and complete blood count were normal. A portable anteroposterior (AP) chest x-ray was normal. A 12-lead ECG showed normal sinus rhythm with rate 65, normal axis, and normal intervals. No Q-waves were noted. Isolated t-wave inversion was seen in lead III. No prior ECG available for comparison. Noncontrasted head CT was negative for fracture of bleeding. An MRI/MRA was obtained in the ED and an acute small infarct in the left corona radiata was seen. There were also mild findings of chronic small vessel degenerative white matter disease (Fig. 44-1).

Case Resolution

The patient was admitted for acute stroke, presumably of ischemic origin. She was started on aspirin (ASA) and her birth control pills were stopped. Thrombophilia labs were negative and included a negative Factor V Leiden, normal protein C and protein S, normal homocysteine levels, negative lupus anticoagulant and anticardiolipin antibodies, and negative prothrombin G mutation. The patient's sickle cell screen was also negative. The patient had normal carotid Dopplers, a normal two-dimensional transthoracic echocardiogram (EF 60%) with negative bubble study. Fasting plasma glucose was 101 and antinuclear antibody test was negative. Fasting lipid panel showed total cholesterol of 197, HDL 44, triglycerides 156, low-density lipoprotein (LDL) 122. She was started on pravastatin 40 mg/day and was asked to follow-up with her primary care provider and start an angiotensin-converting enzyme (ACE)-inhibitor, should her blood pressure continue to be elevated. Speech therapist, occupational therapist, and physical therapist as well as neurologist were consulted, who cleared the patient for discharge within 48 hours of admission. She had mild improvement of her paresthesias and weakness, but not her facial droop at discharge.

Question

What therapies are generally recommended for secondary prevention of ischemic stroke so that this patient will have the best chance of living without further cerebrovascular events (CVA)?

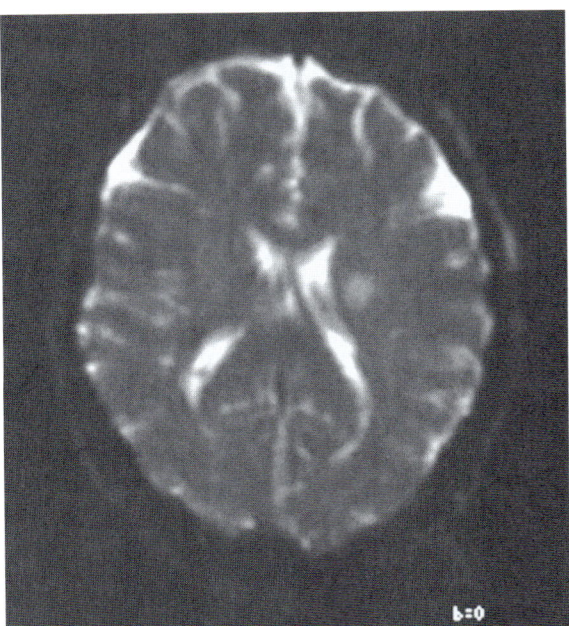
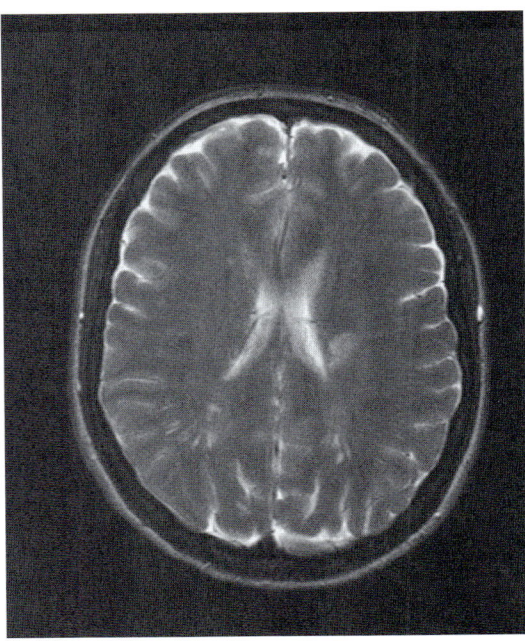

Figure 44-1 Axial diffusion-weighted (A) and T$_2$-weighted (B) MRI images obtained just after admission demonstrating a small 1.1 cm infarct in the corona radiata on the patients left. The initial noncontrasted CT scan of the brain was negative.

Answer

Studies continue to emerge resulting in the production of clinical guidelines with regards to the best medical therapy for secondary prevention of ischemic stroke. Persons with atrial fibrillation and apparent thromboembolic stroke from various thrombophilic conditions are a special circumstance and these therapies do not apply to this patient. Currently, the best evidence exists for the regular use of antiplatelet agents such as extended release dipyridamole combined with ASA twice daily, a daily ASA at between 50 and 325 mg/day, or clopidogrel at 75 mg/day. These agents combined with HMG-CoA reductase inhibitors (statins) and blood pressure control with ACE-inhibitors and/or diuretics are also indicated. Further risk factor modification such as regular exercise, smoking cessation (if she smoked), stopping hormone replacement or birth control pills are also considerations.

Discussion

Stroke is broadly defined by two major processes that lead to neuropathology, namely hemorrhage and ischemia. Hemorrhagic strokes result when blood vessels rupture or leak blood into the intracerebral tissues or subarachnoid space. Ischemic strokes result from a myriad of different processes including thrombosis of large or small vessels, thromboembolism, lipohyalinosis and fibrinoid degeneration of small vessels, or hypo-perfusion of the vessels supplying the brain for other reasons (distributive shock, etc.). A transient ischemic attack (TIA) is classically defined as focal neurologic symptoms or signs that last less than 24 hours. What is implied by this definition is that the lack of blood flow that creates the abnormality resolves in a timely manner, sufficient to avoid injury to tissue from hypoxia. In reality this definition has been questioned as many persons with classic TIA oftentimes have injury of MRI. For this reason, TIA oftentimes is thought of as a harbinger of stroke, but in some cases may represent stroke. Many groups now favor a more restrictive definition to TIA that relies on the lack of evidence for end-organ injury despite resolution of symptoms. Nevertheless, whether a patient is suffering from a TIA or a stroke, many of the same pathologic phenomena responsible for creating the symptoms are at play, including plaque rupture, microembolization of plaque contents, and thrombus formation following platelet activation that leads to symptomatology.

The acute treatment of each of these kinds of strokes is somewhat different and may include diametrically opposed strategies. In the case of hemorrhagic stroke, caregivers may pursue aggressive blood pressure reduction and avoidance of antiplatelet and other anticoagulant medicines. Contrast this to the case of acute ischemic stroke from thrombosis, where treatment may include no blood pressure control in a very hypertensive-stroke patient combined with systemic administration of thrombolytics followed platelet inhibition. An overview of the acute treatment of these conditions is beyond the scope of this discussion, which will focus on primary and secondary prevention of TIA and ischemic stroke.

In the Western world, stroke has been and continues to be a disease of major importance. It is estimated that about 700,000 new strokes occur in the United States each year and that there are more than 4.5 million stroke survivors in the United States at any one time. Moreover, about 160,000 people die per year of stroke, making it the third leading cause of death in the United States. Despite the overall mortality rate of stroke declining, the number of annual deaths from stroke has actually increased of late by 7.7% from 1991 to 2001 because of an increase in prevalence of stroke nationwide. The cost of stroke on society and the individual is enormous; costs are estimated for 2004 to be more than $50 billion in the United States alone and a lifetime more than $140,000 per individual with stroke. Importantly, for those that survive, about 15% to 30% will be permanently disabled and many require institutionalization. Stroke is indeed a life-changing event.

Despite increasingly effective therapies for acute stroke, including thrombolytic drugs, antiplatelet agents, aggressive rehabilitation, and therapy, it is almost universally accepted that primary and secondary prevention of stroke is the best way to lower the stroke burden on individuals and society. Many risk factors that predict stroke are very similar to many which overlap with those for coronary artery disease. Some organizations abdicate the use of the Framingham stroke prediction tool which is very similar to that for coronary artery disease (CAD) and in predicting coronary events. In fact, the collective term cardiovascular disease (CVD) includes coronary artery disease, cerebrovascular disease (stroke/TIA), and peripheral artery disease (PAD). It is not surprising that perusal of most guideline statements will reveal that the processes and pathologies that result in cardiac events, limb ischemia, and stroke are all similar if not identical.

Many risk factors for stroke are modifiable (Table 44-1). In fact most of the decline in CVD mortality seen in the

TABLE 44-1

Major Modifiable Risk Factors for Stroke

Factor	Comments
CVD	
CAD, heart failure, PAD	There is overlap of these with risk factors for stroke
HTN	Biggest modifiable risk factor
Smoking	50% risk reduction within 1 year of stopping
Diabetes	No proven stroke reduction with glycemic controls; however treating HTN and dyslipidemia aggressively markedly decreases risk of stroke
Carotid artery stenosis (asymptomatic)	~50% reduction of risk with appropriate surgery
Atrial fibrillation	Mainly cardioembolic stroke – typically prevented with treatment of dose-adjusted warfarin
Sickle cell disease	Transfusion or exchange treatment of choice
Dyslipidemia	
High total cholesterol	In patients with CAD, HTN, or diabetes markedly reduces risk ~25%. May have further risk reduction if high-dose statin given
Low HDL	
Diet	
High Na	> 2300 mg/day – risk reduction probably relates to blood pressure reduction
Low K	< 4700 mg/day
Obesity	
Physical inactivity	
Hormone therapy	Post menopausal

Adapted with data from Goldstein LB, Adams R, Alberts MJ, et al; American Heart Association/American Stroke Association Stroke Council; Atherosclerotic Peripheral Vascular Disease Interdisciplinary Working Group; Cardiovascular Nursing Council; Clinical Cardiology Council; Nutrition, Physical Activity, and Metabolism Council; Quality of Care and Outcomes Research Interdisciplinary Working Group; American Academy of Neurology. Primary prevention of ischemic stroke: a guideline from the American Heart Association/American Stroke Association Stroke Council: cosponsored by the Atherosclerotic Peripheral Vascular Disease Interdisciplinary Working Group; Cardiovascular Nursing Council; Clinical Cardiology Council; Nutrition, Physical Activity, and Metabolism Council; and the Quality of Care and Outcomes Research Interdisciplinary Working Group: the American Academy of Neurology affirms the value of this guideline. Stroke. 2006 Jun;37(6):1583 and Sacco RL, Adams R, Albers G, et al; American Heart Association; American Stroke Association Council on Stroke; Council on Cardiovascular Radiology and Intervention; American Academy of Neurology. Guidelines for prevention of stroke in patients with ischemic stroke or transient ischemic attack: a statement for healthcare professionals from the American Heart Association/American Stroke Association Council on Stroke: co-sponsored by the Council on Cardiovascular Radiology and Intervention: the American Academy of Neurology affirms the value of this guideline. Stroke. 2006 Feb;37(2):577–617.

recent past 25 to 30 years is attributable to risk factor modification; this is probably mostly attributable to smoking cessation as well as blood pressure reduction via medical therapy and lifestyle modification. Despite these modifiable risk factors, there are factors which are not modifiable (Table 44-2). It behooves generalists and specialists alike to recognize which of their patients are at risk so that adequate and appropriate primary prevention be attempted, as it is estimated that about 70% of all strokes are first strokes.

With any disease with complex contributing factors such as stroke and TIA, primary prevention cannot be expected to remove all risk or the incidence of the disease. Once stroke or TIA has occurred, the individual is at an enormously increased risk for reinfarction. Much of the laboratory and diagnostic workup for a patient that has suffered a first stroke, TIA, or recurrent stroke focuses on identifying modifiable risk factors such as dyslipidemia, diabetes, carotid artery disease, structural heart disease or

TABLE 44-2

Nonmodifiable Risk Factors for Stroke

Factor	Rate/100,000	RR (when known)
Age (rate doubles every 10 years over 50)	Depends on sex and race	N/A
Sex		N/A
Women	122	
Men	174	
Race		N/A
Blacks	233	
Whites	93	
Hispanic	196	
Birth weight	N/A	2.0 for birth weight < 2500 g or > 4000 g
Family history of stroke or TIA	N/A	Paternal 2.2, Maternal 1.4

Adapted from Goldstein LB, Adams R, Alberts MJ, et al; American Heart Association/American Stroke Association Stroke Council; Atherosclerotic Peripheral Vascular Disease Interdisciplinary Working Group; Cardiovascular Nursing Council; Clinical Cardiology Council; Nutrition, Physical Activity, and Metabolism Council; Quality of Care and Outcomes Research Interdisciplinary Working Group; American Academy of Neurology. Primary prevention of ischemic stroke: a guideline from the American Heart Association/American Stroke Association Stroke Council: cosponsored by the Atherosclerotic Peripheral Vascular Disease Interdisciplinary Working Group; Cardiovascular Nursing Council; Clinical Cardiology Council; Nutrition, Physical Activity, and Metabolism Council; and the Quality of Care and Outcomes Research Interdisciplinary Working Group: the American Academy of Neurology affirms the value of this guideline. Stroke. 2006 Jun; 37(6):1583.

clinically silent heart failure, and thrombophilia. Specific therapies have emerged through the use of clinical research and the application of evidence-based review of trials to further reduce the risk of subsequent stroke for those who have suffered a stroke or TIA.

Platelets are central to the many of the mechanisms underlying both acute myocardial infarction (MI) and other acute coronary syndromes (ACS). The vascular pathophysiology that leads to ischemic stroke and TIA of nonthromboembolic origin are thought to at least in part be very similar to MI and ACS. It is no surprise then that in the acute stroke setting just as in MI and ACS antiplatelet agent are useful treatments. By the same token, antiplatelet agents are also one of the mainstays of primary and secondary prevention of stroke just as they are with CAD. Agents used in this regard include ASA, dipyridamole combined with ASA, and in some select patients, clopidogrel. These agents are markedly different from other oral anticoagulants such as warfarin, which are generally indicated is the setting of stroke from atrial fibrillation, thrombophilia, or arterial dissection. Warfarin is generally not recommended for secondary prevention of

stroke in the patient with a history of noncardioembolic stroke or TIA, and will not be discussed further here.

ASA, a drug that has been around in some form for more than two centuries inhibits the enzyme cyclooxygenase in platelets, reducing production of thromboxane A2, a stimulator of platelet aggregation. This interferes with thrombosis by antagonizing platelet function, theoretically reducing the risk of stroke. ASA is already generally recommended for primary (in patients with a 10-year risk of MI of 6% to 10% or greater) and secondary prevention for MI. In an extremely large meta-analysis by the Antithrombotic Trialists' Collaboration (ATC), it was shown conclusively that ASA when given to patients at high risk for CVD events such as MI, stroke, and vascular death, there is a significant reduction of these events. Moreover, in patients who already had a history of stroke or TIA, taking ASA reduced the risk of a second CVD event significantly, including stroke. Currently, recommendation for primary prevention of stroke would support the use of ASA in men who had a sufficiently high 10-year CVD event risk between 6% and 10% or greater, but not specifically to prevent stroke. In meta-analysis, ASA has been shown to be effective in men only to prevent first MI. In women, however, the recommendations are similar, but ASA may technically be used for primary prevention of stoke if the benefits outweigh the risks, as meta-analysis has shown daily ASA to be effective for primary prevention of stroke in women at risk. The use of ASA in the secondary prevention of stroke is well established and studies exist that have found benefit from doses ranging from 30 to 1300 mg/day with no significant benefit from higher doses. Not surprisingly, the risk of gastrointestinal bleeding increased with the use of higher doses of ASA. Currently guidelines would support the use of ASA 50 to 325 mg/day for the secondary prevention of stroke.

ASA combined with extended release dipyridamole (ERDP + ASA) is a second antiplatelet choice which is currently an acceptable alternative to ASA alone. Dipyridamole impairs platelet function by inhibiting the activity of the enzymes adenosine deaminase and phosphodiesterase. Locally within the platelet this causes an accumulation of adenosine, adenine nucleotides, and cyclic AMP, which antagonizes platelet function and inhibits thrombus formation. Dipyridamole may also cause vasodilatation, which could have further anti-ischemic properties. Theoretically, this combination of medicine should provide greater protection from stroke than ASA alone. Two large trials have gone on to bear this out in secondary stroke prevention. The large multicenter ASA plus dipyridamole versus ASA alone after cerebral ischemia of arterial origin (ESPRIT) trial and the European Stroke Prevention Study-2 (ESPS-2) both studied dipyridamole in combination with ASA in the secondary prevention of stroke. The ESPRIT trial also included a meta-analysis that combined the results of disparate trials studying ERDP + ASA. Both studies conclusively showed that the combination of ERDP + ASA has superior secondary protection in patients with history of ischemic stroke or TIA when compared to ASA alone.

A third commonly considered antiplatelet agent is clopidogrel, which inhibits platelets via inhibiting the ADP-dependent platelet activation and aggregation. Clopidogrel is regularly used in patients with coronary artery disease, those suffering from acute coronary syndromes, or those that have received bare-metal or drug-eluting coronary artery stents. In these clinical situations, it is commonly coadministered with a daily ASA. Although it is expensive, it is a recommend alternative for secondary stroke prevention in those persons unable to tolerate ASA. In the large

study called Clopidogrel versus ASA in Patients at Risk of Ischemic Events (CAPRIE), more than 19,000 patients with some type of CVD including history of stroke, CAD, or PAD were randomized to receive ASA at 325 mg/day or 75 mg/day of clopidogrel. Patients were followed for 1 to 3 years and the primary outcome point was a composite of stroke, MI, or vascular death. Not surprisingly, the group that received clopidogrel fared better in this composite endpoint. Despite this, subgroup analysis showed a smaller and statistically insignificant benefit in persons with history of stroke when taking clopidogrel in preventing additional stroke. For a summary of other studies examining the effects of clopidogrel with and without ASA, please see (Table 44-3). Currently, clopidogrel is recommended as a safe alternative to ASA and should be given instead of ASA, but not with ASA for the secondary prevention of stroke.

Besides the use of antiplatelet medicines, another class of medications that has received marked attention for the prevention and secondary prevention of stroke are the HMG-CoA reductase inhibitors or statins. Dyslipidemia is certainly a risk factor for atherosclerosis, MI, PVD, and stroke. With regard to stroke, the association of dyslipidemia with cerebrovascular accidents is probably not as well studied as it is in CAD. Statins have well known cholesterol-lowering properties and are widely used and studied in the setting of CAD for the primary and secondary prevention of MI. What has become clear from multiple studies in patients with CAD is that administration of statins also protects against future stroke in those patients with no history of stroke. This protective effect is oftentimes not explained purely by the lipid-lowering properties of these medications as they may influence plaque stability and inflammation in cerebral vessels, as well as extracranial vessels that supply the brain. A myriad of studies and meta-analysis exist to support the use of statins in the prevention of stroke in those patients without established cerebrovascular disease who also suffer from CAD. What has been less clear, however, is whether patients with no history of CAD would benefit from statins after their first stroke. The recently reported Stroke Prevention by Aggressive Reduction in Cholesterol Levels (SPARCL) trial of more than 4,700 randomly assigned patients with a history of stroke or TIA assigned to take 80 mg of atorvastatin or placebo showed that those persons taking statin therapy had an absolute risk reduction of 2.2% compared to placebo more than 4.9 years median follow-up. Interestingly, there was no mortality benefit from all-cause mortality and there

TABLE 44-3

Studies Examining Clopidogrel with and without ASA vs. ASA for Prevention of Stroke and CVD Events

Study name and year reported	Drugs studied	Groups studied and size of study	Conclusions
Clopidogrel versus Aspirin in Patients at Risk of Ischemic Events (CAPRIE) –1996	Clopidogrel 75 mg/day vs. ASA 325 mg/day	Patients included those with recent stroke, MI, or PAD randomized. Size is over 19,000 patient with ~2-year follow-up	Clopidogrel is more effective and just as safe in reducing the *combined* risk for ischemic stroke, MI, and death from vascular causes. Subgroup of patients enrolled with stroke alone – clopidogrel was no more effective than ASA at reducing stroke risk
Management of Atherothrombosis With Clopidogrel in High Risk Patients With TIA or Stroke (MATCH) –2004	Clopidogrel 75 mg/day vs. clopidogrel 75 mg/day + ASA 75 mg/day	Patients already receiving clopidogrel with previous stroke, TIA or other major risk factors randomized with 18-month follow-up. Size is about 7,600 patients	Clopidogrel + ASA is no more effective at preventing ischemic stroke, MI, vascular death, or hospitalization for acute ischemia (composite endpoint). Major bleeding risk was increased in combination group
Clopidogrel for High Atherothrombotic Risk and Ischemic Stabilization, Management, and Avoidance (CHARISMA) –2006	ASA alone at 75–162 mg/day vs. clopidogrel 75 mg/day + ASA 75– 162 mg/day	Patient with either clinically evident cardiovascular disease or multiple risk factors randomized. Median follow-up is 28 months for some 15,600 patients	Clopidogrel + ASA was not more effective than aspirin alone in reducing the rate of MI, stroke, or death from cardiovascular causes (composite endpoint). Nonsignificant benefit for those with symptomatic atherosclerosis and possible harm to those with multiple risk factors

Adapted from specific study data presented in CAPRIE Steering Committee. A randomised, blinded, trial of clopidogrel versus aspirin in patients at risk of ischemic events (CAPRIE). Lancet. 1996 Nov 16;348(9038):1329–1339; Diener HC, Bogousslavsky J, Brass LM, et al. Aspirin and clopidogrel compared with clopidogrel alone after recent ischemic stroke or transient ischemic attack in high-risk patients (MATCH): randomized, double-blind, placebo-controlled trial. Lancet. 2004 Jul 24;364(9431):331–337; Bhatt DL, Fox KA, Hacke W, et al. Clopidogrel and aspirin versus aspirin alone for the prevention of atherothrombotic events. N Engl J Med. 2006 Apr 20;354(16):1706–1717.

was a slightly increased risk of hemorrhagic stroke in persons taking atorvastatin. Current recommendations include the use of statins in all patients for the secondary prevention of stroke or TIA and in primary prevention of stroke in patients with dyslipidemia. Lifestyle modification and statin therapy is recommended in patients with known CAD and high-risk hypertensive patients even with normal LDL cholesterol. Please see National Cholesterol Education Program's publications and revisions of the Expert Panel on Detection, Evaluation, and Treatment of High Cholesterol in Adults (Adult Treatment Panel III or ATP III) for specific cholesterol target and treatment recommendations, but by and large those patients who have

not had a cerebrovascular event with elevated total cholesterol, or with elevated non–HDL cholesterol in the presence of hypertriglyceridemia should receive lifestyle modification and drug therapy with statins.

Hypertension is probably the most important and highly modifiable risk factor for stroke. There are no absolute cut off values with regards to systolic and diastolic blood pressure and stroke risk. In fact, the association of risk for ischemic stroke and blood pressure is continuous. There is irrefutable clinical evidence to support the treatment of hypertension and even prehypertension for the primary and secondary prevention of stroke. Management of hypertension with the myriad of agents available can be quite confusing, but the cost of not treating hypertension is immense. Many other modifiable risk factors listed above are also tied to elevations in blood pressure. Smoking cessation, exercise, and weight loss, sodium restriction, and moderation or cessation of alcohol consumption are all part of blood pressure reduction therapy. For most patients, lifestyle modification will not suffice and specific antihypertensive therapy will be needed. For primary prevention of stroke current recommendations support the treatment of hypertension following the Seventh Report of the Joint National Committee on Prevention, Detection, Evaluation, and Treatment of High Blood Pressure (JNC-7) guidelines in all persons, and advocate universal screening of all adults for hypertension. Diabetic patients have different goals for therapy for blood pressure reduction as their risk for CVD and CV events is much higher than the general population. For secondary prevention of stroke, similar guidelines apply, although there is a general lack of evidence to fully recommend one antihypertensive agent over another for the secondary prevention of stroke. However a meta-analysis by Rashid et al and two trials, the Heart Outcomes Prevention Evaluation (HOPE) trial and the Perindopril Protection Against Recurrent Stroke Study (PROGRESS) have all suggested that either ACE-I alone or the combination of ACE-I and diuretics may be preferred as blood pressure medication for secondary stroke prevention. What is important to remember is that a decrease in even 10/5 mm Hg may be significant in reducing the risk of stroke.

The epidemic of diabetes that faces the United States today will lead to heretofore unseen numbers of patients suffering from macro- and microvascular complication of the disease including blindness, progression to end-stage renal disease, peripheral vascular disease, amputations, CAD, and stroke. For purposes of risk-stratification for coronary events and to determine lipid goals, blood pressure goals, and need for cardioprotection with ASA, persons with diabetes are considered to have CAD and at high risk for MI and PAD. They have different blood pressure goals and lipid goals set by JNC-7 and ATP III that all practitioners should be aware of. Conventional thinking has been that patient with diabetes take years to develop the macrovascular complications of their disease. Disturbingly however, evidence is emerging from a recent study of more than 12,000 newly diagnosed diabetics that the risk of stroke in persons with even recently diagnosed diabetes is twice that of nondiabetic individuals within 5 years of diagnosis. This should further invigorate diabetes screening and prevention efforts in order to give those with and at risk for diabetes, and therefore stroke, the

additional lipid-lowering and blood pressure reduction therapy that they require.

In summary, stroke places a large and complex burden on patients, caregivers, and society. As hypertension is prevalent in about 50,000,000 Americans and as diabetes surges in prevalence through the young and the old, the outlook can seem bleak. Through primary prevention and secondary prevention it is hoped that the burden of stroke and its associated consequences will continue to respond to efforts of prevention. With the use of specific therapies such as antiplatelet agents, ACE-I, diuretics, and statins, combined with ongoing lifestyle modifications, practitioners are meeting this clinical entity head on.

Selected References

1. Goldstein LB, Adams R, Alberts MJ, et al; American Heart Association/American Stroke Association Stroke Council; Atherosclerotic Peripheral Vascular Disease Interdisciplinary Working Group; Cardiovascular Nursing Council; Clinical Cardiology Council; Nutrition, Physical Activity, and Metabolism Council; Quality of Care and Outcomes Research Interdisciplinary Working Group; American Academy of Neurology. Primary prevention of ischemic stroke: a guideline from the American Heart Association/American Stroke Association Stroke Council: cosponsored by the Atherosclerotic Peripheral Vascular Disease Interdisciplinary Working Group; Cardiovascular Nursing Council; Clinical Cardiology Council; Nutrition, Physical Activity, and Metabolism Council; and the Quality of Care and Outcomes Research Interdisciplinary Working Group: the American Academy of Neurology affirms the value of this guideline. *Stroke*. 2006 Jun;37(6):1583.
2. Sacco RL, Adams R, Albers G, et al; American Heart Association; American Stroke Association Council on Stroke; Council on Cardiovascular Radiology and Intervention; American Academy of Neurology. Guidelines for prevention of stroke in patients with ischemic stroke or transient ischemic attack: a statement for healthcare professionals from the American Heart Association/American Stroke Association Council on Stroke: co-sponsored by the Council on Cardiovascular Radiology and Intervention: the American Academy of Neurology affirms the value of this guideline. *Stroke*. 2006 Feb;37(2):577–617.
3. Albers GW, Caplan LR, Easton JD, et al. Transient ischemic attack—proposal for a new definition. *N Engl J Med*. 2002 Nov 21;347(21):1713–1716.
4. Antithrombotic Trialists' Collaboration. Collaborative meta-analysis of randomised trials of antiplatelet therapy for prevention of death, myocardial infarction, and stroke in high risk patients. *BMJ*. 2002 Jan 12;324(7329):71–86.
5. Diener HC, Cunha L, Forbes C, et al. European Stroke Prevention Study-2. Dipyridamole and acetylsalicylic acid in the secondary prevention of stroke. *J Neurol Sci*. 1996 Nov;143(1–2):1–13.
6. Berger JS, Roncaglioni MC, Avanzini F, et al. Aspirin for the primary prevention of cardiovascular events in women and men:

a sex-specific meta-analysis of randomized controlled trials. *JAMA*. 2006 Jan 18;295(3):306–313.

7. ESPRIT Study Group, Halkes PH, van Gijn J, Kappelle LJ, et al. Aspirin plus dipyridamole versus aspirin alone after cerebral ischemia of arterial origin (ESPRIT): randomised controlled trial. *Lancet*. 2006 May 20;367(9523):1665–1673.

8. CAPRIE Steering Committee. A randomised, blinded, trial of clopidogrel versus aspirin in patients at risk of ischemic events (CAPRIE). *Lancet*. 1996 Nov 16;348(9038):1329–1339.

9. Diener HC, Bogousslavsky J, Brass LM, et al. Aspirin and clopidogrel compared with clopidogrel alone after recent ischemic stroke or transient ischemic attack in high-risk patients (MATCH): randomized, double-blind, placebo-controlled trial. *Lancet*. 2004 Jul 24; 364(9431):331–337.

10. Bhatt DL, Fox KA, Hacke W, et al. Clopidogrel and aspirin versus aspirin alone for the prevention of atherothrombotic events. *N Engl J Med*. 2006 Apr 20;354(16):1706–1717.

11. Amarenco P, Bogousslavsky J, Callahan A, et al; Stroke Prevention by Aggressive Reduction in Cholesterol Levels (SPARCL) Investigators. High-dose atorvastatin after stroke or transient ischemic attack. *N Engl J Med*. 2006;355: 549–559.

12. Svensson P, de Faire U, Sleight P, et al. Comparative effects of ramipril on ambulatory and office blood pressures: a HOPE substudy. *Hypertension*. 2001;38:e28–e32.

13. PROGRESS Collaborative Group. Randomized trial of a perindopril-based blood-pressure-lowering regimen among 6105 individuals with previous stroke or transient ischemic attack. *Lancet*. 2001;358:1033–1041.

14. Rashid P, Leonardi-Bee J, Bath P. Blood pressure reduction and secondary prevention of stroke and other vascular events: a systematic review. *Stroke*. 2003;34:2741–2748.

15. Chobanian AV, Bakris GL, Black HR, et al, for the National Heart, Lung, and Blood Institute Joint National Committee on Prevention, Detection, Evaluation, and Treatment of High Blood Pressure; National High Blood Pressure Education Program Coordinating Committee. The Seventh Report of the Joint National Committee on Prevention, Detection, Evaluation, and Treatment of High Blood Pressure: the JNC 7 report. *JAMA*. 2003;289:2560–2571.

16. Expert Panel on Detection, Evaluation, and Treatment of High Blood Cholesterol in Adults (Adult Treatment Panel III). *The Third Report of the National Cholesterol Education Program (NCEP)*. Bethesda, MD: US National Heart, Lung, and Blood Institute, National Institutes of Health; 2004 (updated). Publication No. 01–3670:1–28.

17. Jeerakathil T, Johnson JA, Simpson SH, et al. Short-term risk for stroke is doubled in persons with newly treated type 2 diabetes compared with persons without diabetes. A population-based cohort study. *Stroke*. 2007;38:1739.

89-Year-Old Female with Dyspnea and Diaphoresis 3 Days After Orthopedic Surgery

CASE PRESENTATION

An urgent medicine consultation is requested for an 89-year-old white female with the sudden onset of shortness of breath and tachycardia. The patient suffered a left displaced femoral neck fracture 6 days earlier and had undergone a cemented left hip hemiarthroplasty. Her hospital course was complicated only by an ileus until post-op day 6 when she suddenly developed shortness of breath while lying in bed. She had no other associated symptoms. She denies chest discomfort currently or at any time in the past. She reports no cough, dyspnea on exertion, orthopnea, or paroxysmal nocturnal dyspnea in the past. Prior to her injury, she lived independently and was able to ambulate throughout her home without any symptoms or difficulty. She has no history of congestive heart failure or lung disease. The patient has a history of mild aortic stenosis, non-insulin-dependent diabetes mellitus, hyperlipidemia, and a 15-pack/year history of tobacco abuse. There is no personal or family history of venous thrombosis or cardiac disease. Her medications include atorvastatin, glipizide, calcium, and a multivitamin.

Physical Examination

Patient was an anxious-appearing elderly female in moderate distress, breathing rapidly but without accessory muscle use. Vital signs: temperature 37.1°C, pulse 128 beats/min, respiratory rate 25 breaths/min, blood pressure 157/96 mm Hg, and room air oxygen saturation of 94%. Head, eyes, ears, nose, and throat: mucous membranes moist. Neck: no thyromegaly, carotid bruits, or jugular venous distention. Cardiovascular: tachycardic, a 3/6 holosystolic murmur is heard best over the right upper sternal border. There is no rub, thrill, or heave. Lungs: mild end-expiratory wheezes bilaterally, no rales or rhonchi. Abdomen: soft, protuberant with hypoactive bowel sounds, nontender on palpation, no hepatosplenomegaly. Extremeties: no clubbing, cyanosis, or edema; left hip bandaged; radial, femoral, and dorsalis pedis pulses 2+ bilaterally. Skin: slightly diaphoretic, no rashes or lesions. Neurologic: alert and oriented to person, place, and time. The remainder of the examination was unremarkable.

Laboratory Studies

White blood cells 9.6, hemoglobin/hematocrit 10.2 and 32, respectively, platelet count 276, K 3.4, blood urea nitrogen 25, Cr 0.9, and glucose 96. First set of cardiac enzymes: creatine kinase (CK) 187, creatine kinase-MB 15.3, and troponin I 2.71. Total cholesterol 260, low-density lipoprotein 190, chest x-ray is shown in Fig. 45-1. Spiral protocol CT of the chest revealed no pulmonary embolism. ECG is shown in Fig. 45-2.

Case Resolution

The differential diagnosis for acute dyspnea postoperatively includes myocardial infarction and pulmonary embolus (fat embolus must also be considered in patients who have undergone an orthopedic procedure). Pneumothorax should be considered in patients who have had cardiothoracic surgery. Sepsis may also cause acute dyspnea and tachypnea

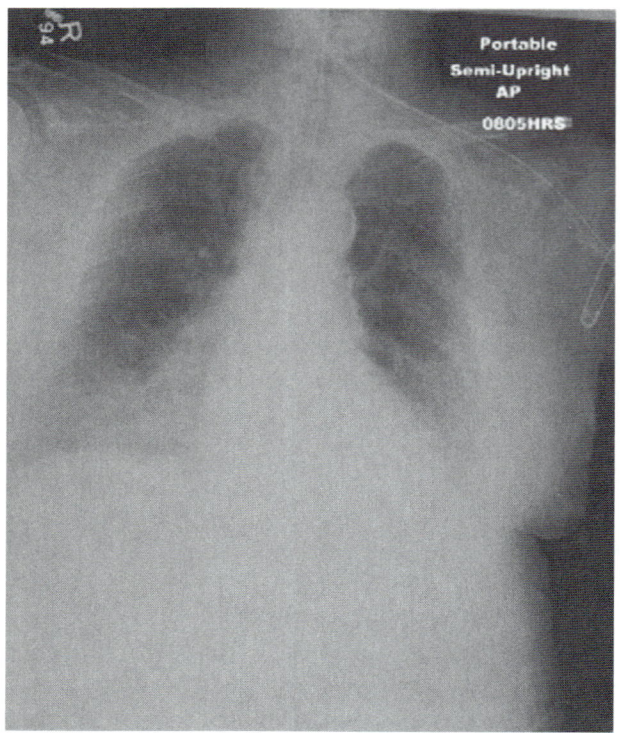

Figure 45-1 Portable chest radiograph taken immediately after the patient complained of shortness of breath shows diffuse interstitial edema.

because of metabolic (lactic) acidosis. Pulmonary edema should be considered in patients with diastolic or systolic left ventricular dysfunction, as many patients receive large volumes of intravenous fluids intraoperatively. Finally, nosocomial pneumonia or aspiration pneumonia can cause the relatively acute onset of dyspnea (Table 45-1).

The patient was immediately started on subcutaneous enoxaparin, aspirin, and metoprolol for an acute non-ST segment elevation myocardial infarction (acute coronary syndrome). The serum CK peaked at 320 and troponin I peaked at 3.71. The possibility of a cardiac catheterization was discussed with the patient, but she refused and wished to be managed medically. A two-dimensional echocardiogram was done 3 days after the infarct, which revealed mild aortic stenosis and a left ventricular ejection fraction of 35% (an echocardiogram done 1 month earlier had shown an ejection fraction of 65%). She was then started on an ACE inhibitor and a low dose of furosemide. A repeat echocardiogram was scheduled to be done as an outpatient 3 months later and the patient was discharged home with no symptoms of heart failure. She planned to attend cardiac rehabilitation as an outpatient.

Question

Should this patient have been on a perioperative β-blocker?

Answer

Yes. Several theories exist to explain the heightened risk of cardiovascular events perioperatively. The pathogenesis related to catecholamine excess supports the plausibility of a benefit from β-blockade. As discussed below, evidence from randomized controlled trials supports the use of perioperative β-blockers particularly in high-risk patients.

Discussion

Knowledge of the management of the perioperative patient undergoing noncardiac surgery is imperative because the proper management can significantly reduce the risk of cardiovascular complications in high-risk patients. As a consequence of the aging population, there are increasing numbers of patients with cardiac disease being brought to the operating room.

Among patients at risk for cardiac complications, 20% to 40% will develop perioperative myocardial ischemia. Numerous studies have concluded that β-blockers reduce the risk of myocardial infarction and death in high-risk patients undergoing noncardiac surgery, as well as coronary artery bypass graft surgery. The utility of β-blockers in the setting of noncardiac surgery will be discussed in this chapter.

In one randomized, double-blind, placebo-controlled trial which included patients with coronary artery disease or who were at risk for atherosclerosis (i.e., patients with two or more risk factors), those who received atenolol perioperatively had a lower overall mortality rate, even 2 years after surgery, and a higher rate of event-free survival. Another randomized trial included patients who were high-risk and had coronary disease (i.e., patients with at least one risk factor and a positive dobutamine stress echocardiogram). Those patients who received bisoprolol pre- and postoperatively had a significantly lower incidence of cardiac mortality or myocardial infarction up to 2 years postoperatively as compared to those patients who did not receive bisoprolol.

The reason β-blockers decrease cardiac mortality perioperatively is likely multifactorial. First, they increase diastolic filling time by lowering the heart rate. It has been well

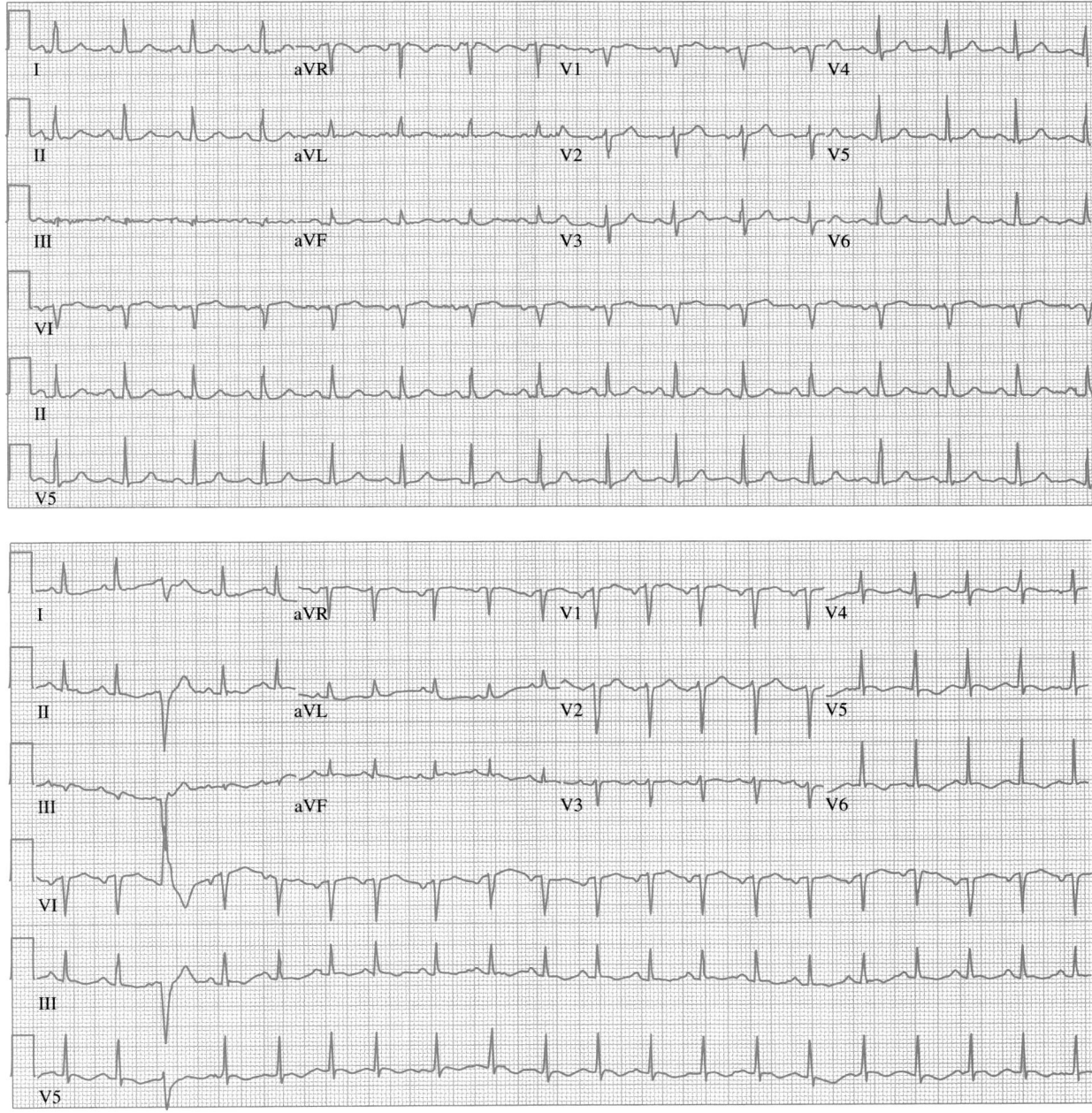

Figure 45-2 A. Preoperative electrocardiogram shows normal sinus rhythm with no evidence of prior infarct. B. Postoperative electrocardiogram obtained during the patient's episode of dyspnea reveals sinus tachycardia, new T-wave inversions in leads V4–V6, and one premature ventricular complex (PVC).

documented that there is an association between an elevated heart rate and postoperative ischemia. Furthermore, studies have suggested that blocking the heart rate response may reduce the risk of myocardial ischemia and/or infarction. Secondly, β-blockers decrease sympathetic tone. Postoperative stress and elevated catecholamine levels correlate with adverse cardiac events because of the imbalance between myocardial oxygen supply and demand. In addition,

secondary plaque rupture can occur in patients with preexisting coronary plaques in the setting of increased myocardial demand. Thus, β-blocker therapy may reduce cardiac events by decreasing myocardial demand. Lastly, β-blockers likely prevent some intra- and postoperative ventricular arrhythmias.

Patients at high risk for perioperative cardiac complications should be started on a perioperative β-blocker

TABLE 45-1

Differential Diagnosis of Acute Postoperative Dyspnea

Atelectasis
Bronchospasm
Pulmonary edema
Pulmonary embolism
Pleural effusion
Pneumothorax
Nosocomial pneumonia
Myocardial infarction
Chemical pneumonitis
Upper airway obstruction
Metabolic acidosis
Abdominal compartment syndrome

unless it is contraindicated (eg, severe chronic obstructive pulmonary disease). Perioperative risk can be determined using the Revised Cardiac Risk Index (RCRI) criteria (see Fig. 45-3). Studies have shown that patients at high risk (i.e., those with an RCRI score of 2 or greater) have a mortality benefit when given perioperative β-blockers. In contrast, patients with an RCRI score of 0 or 1 do not benefit from perioperative β-blockers and, in fact, initiating a perioperative β-blocker in these patients may be detrimental.

According to the RCRI criteria alone, the patient presented above was not at high risk. She did have multiple risk factors for coronary artery disease (age > 65, tobacco abuse, hyperlipidemia, and diabetes mellitus), however, she did not have a history of ischemic heart disease, nor did she demonstrate any symptoms of such prior to her surgery. She also did not report any heart failure symptoms prior to her surgery. She had no history of cerebrovascular disease

or renal insufficiency and, although she was diabetic, her diabetes was controlled with oral medications only. Lastly, her surgery was not considered high risk. Given her RCRI score of 0, she was not at high risk for perioperative cardiac complications. However, the RCRI criteria are only a guideline and should be used as such. According to the RCRI criteria, even a patient with a known history of ischemic heart disease is not considered high risk unless he/she also meets one of the other five criteria. In contrast, the study referenced earlier in the chapter involving administration of atenolol to patients with coronary disease or who were *at risk* for coronary disease showed a mortality benefit of perioperative atenolol in patients who had two or more risk factors for coronary artery disease (see Fig. 45-4). By these criteria, the patient in this case *was* at high risk because she had 4 out of the 5 major risk factors for coronary artery disease. Thus, using the data from this study, a perioperative β-blocker might have prevented her postoperative myocardial infarction.

A meta-analysis published in 2005 looked at twenty-two randomized controlled trials (RCTs), including those discussed above, and concluded that the pooled data from all of these trials was inadequate to definitively lead to a recommendation that patients undergoing noncardiac surgery should be on a β-blocker. This conclusion was largely based on the fact that most of the RCTs were underpowered and there were only a moderate number of major perioperative cardiovascular events among the studies. The authors of this meta-analysis suggest β-blockers may decrease the risk of major cardiovascular event in the perioperative period, in particular with high-risk patients. The authors also highlight that β-blockers lead to higher rates of bradycardia and hypotension requiring treatment. Larger RCTs are needed to further elucidate the role of β-blockers in preventing perioperative

a. History of ischemic heart disease--→ 1 point
b. History of heart failure--→ 1 point
c. History of cerebrovascular disease---------------------------------------→ 1 point
d. Preoperative serum creatinine > 2 mg/dL---------------------------→ 1 point
e. Diabetes mellitus requiring treatment with insulin------------------→ 1 point
f. High risk type of surgery (e.g. intrathoracic or intraperitoneal)---→ 1 point
----
Sum of points = score

Figure 45-3 Revised Cardiac Risk Index (RCRI) criteria. One point is assigned for each risk factor. A patient with a score of 2 or greater is considered at high risk for perioperative cardiac complications.

Adapted from Lindenauer PK, Pekow P, Wang, K et al. Perioperative beta-blocker therapy and mortality after major noncardiac surgery. New Engl J Med. 2005;353:349–361.

1. Age greater than or equal to 65

2. Current smoking

3. Hyperlipidemia (total cholesterol ≥ 240 mg/dL)

4. Diabetes mellitus

5. Hypertension

Figure 45-4 Coronary artery disease risk factors as described by Mangano et al. in their study, "Effect of Atenolol on Mortality and Cardiovascular Morbidity after Noncardiac Surgery." Patients with two or more of these risk factors conferred a mortality benefit from perioperative treatment with atenolol.

Adapted from Mangano DT, Layug EL. Effect of atenolol on mortality and cardiovascular morbidity after noncardiac surgery. New Engl J Med. 1996;335(23):1713–1721.

cardiovascular events in patients of varying levels of risk undergoing noncardiac surgery. The point is that clinicians must consider the data but, more importantly, should do a thorough history and physical examination to determine who might be a high-risk patient.

The optimal length of the course of perioperative β-blocker therapy has not yet been clarified with clear data. Most sources recommend at least 1month of therapy before considering discontinuation. In this patient who had a myocardial infarction, β-blocker therapy will be indefinite. It is important to continue treatment with a β-blocker perioperatively if the patient was already on one for another indication. A β-blocker should never be discontinued acutely before surgery as abrupt discontinuation of β-blockers is associated with adverse cardiac events, including possible myocardial infarction, even in patients who are not undergoing surgery.

Selected References

1. Fleisher LA, Eagle KA. Screening for cardiac disease in patients having noncardiac surgery. *Ann Intern Med.* 1996;124:767–772.
2. Mangano DT, Layug EL. Effect of atenolol on mortality and cardiovascular morbidity after noncardiac surgery. *New Engl J Med.* 1996;335(23):1713–1721.
3. Grayburn PA, Hillis LD. Cardiac events in patients undergoing noncardiac surgery: shifting of the paradigm from noninvasive risk stratification to therapy. *Ann Intern Med.* 2003;138: 506–511.
4. Fleisher LA, Eagle KA. Lowering cardiac risk in noncardiac surgery. *New Engl J Med.* 2001;345(23):1677–1682.
5. Thomas LH, Marcantonio ER. Derivation and prospective validation of a simple index for prediction of cardiac risk of major noncardiac surgery. *Circulation.* 1999;100:1043–1049.
6. Lindenauer PK, Pekow P, Wan K, et al. Perioperative beta-blocker therapy and mortality after major noncardiac surgery. *New Engl J Med.* 2005;353:349–361.
7. Poldermans D, Boersma E, Bax JJ, et al. The effect of bisoprolol on perioperative mortality and myocardial infarction in high-risk patients undergoing vascular surgery. *New Eng J Med.* 1999;341:1789–1794.
8. Devereaux PJ, Beattie WS, Choi PT, et al. How strong is the evidence for the use of perioperative beta blockers in noncardiac surgery? Systematic review and meta-analysis of randomized controlled trials. *BMJ.* 4 July 2005;331:313–321.

46-Year-Old Male with Failure to Thrive

CASE PRESENTATION

A 46-year-old gentleman with a history of chronic substance abuse is brought into the emergency department by his wife for suicidal ideation and 50 lb weight loss over the past 8 months. The patient's wife states that the patient has a history of both methamphetamine as well as amyl nitrate abuse and his use of both substances had been increasing lately. He also has been "acting bizarre," walking unsteadily with some tremors and has also had worsening memory loss over the past year. These symptoms had been getting steadily worse. When asked the last time the patient's wife remembers him being "completely normal" she states it was about 4 years ago. The patient is currently being followed by a physician and had an MRI about 1 month ago that showed a "cyst" on his parotid. He has never had any substance abuse counseling and recently had an HIV test — this was drawn immediately prior to admission and his trip to the hospital.

Physical Examination

The patient is a thin appearing, cachectic male in no acute distress. Vital signs: temperature 37°C, pulse 92 beats/min, respiratory rate 16 breaths/min, blood pressure 127/71 mm Hg, and oxygen saturation on room air was 97%. Head, eyes, ears, nose, and throat examination revealed a neck that was supple without lymphadenopathy, grade 2/6 holosystolic murmur appreciated at the left lower sternal border and apex. There was a normal point of maximal impulse. Lungs were clear to auscultation bilaterally. Abdomen was soft and nontender with normal active bowel sounds and no hepatosplenomegaly. The patient had normal genitalia, rectal tone, and was heme negative. Extremities showed right ankle swelling and right metatarsal swelling with a foot ulcer on his left heel. Multiple 1 to 2 cm skin lesions—dark macular lesions with plaque formation were observed on his lower extremity. Cranial nerve (CN) II to XII grossly intact, strength is 5/5 in all extremities. The patient had normal sensation, although his cerebellar function was normal he had a positive Romberg, poor finger to nose test, no pronator drift. Babinski was downgoing bilaterally. He had 2+ deep tendon reflexes throughout. The patient had a constant level of consciousness that did not wax and wane. Frontal release signs were present—the patient had a present glabellar reflex. Mini mental status examination revealed score of 20/30.

Laboratory Studies

A complete blood count showed white blood cells 2.6, 77% neutrophils, 8% lymphocytes, hemoglobin 7.6 g/dL, and hematocrit 22%, platelets 174, mean corpuscular volume was 90. Chemistry panel was within normal limits. NH_4 normal, urine drug screen was positive for amphetamine and tricyclics. Urinalysis showed pH 6.0, specific gravity 1.023, positive for albumin, hyaline casts, otherwise negative. Liver transaminases, thyroid stimulating hormone B_{12}, and folate were normal. Rapid plasma reagin (RPR) was negative.

Case Resolution

The patient was admitted to the hospital, had a purified protein derivative (PPD) placed, and was started on clindamycin for his foot ulcer. Plain films and bone scan revealed no evidence of osteomyelitis. Lumbar puncture was done that was normal, no evidence of fungal, bacterial, viral, or acid-fast bacillus growth on culture. Heavy metal screen was negative. Esophagogastroduodenoscopy was done and no bleeding source was identified to explain the anemia. White material was seen on his distal esophagus, and biopsy revealed this to be *Candida albicans*. PPD was negative and HIV was positive. Magnetic resonance imaging (MRI) of the brain showed generalized atrophic changes but no masses, lesions, or evidence of prior ischemia. It did show periventricular subcortical T_2 hyperintensity (Fig 46-1). CD4 count was done and found to be 30. The patient was started on highly active antiretroviral therapy (HAART) and antifungal treatment for his *Candida* infection. Additional cerebrospinal fluid (CSF) tests including JC virus polymerase chain reaction were all negative. His mental status did improve during his hospitalization and he was discharged to follow up in the infectious disease clinic for further treatment of his HIV.

Question

What is the most likely cause of this patient's CNS dysfunction and pancytopenia?

Answer

Considering the patient has significant central nervous system dysfunction without change in level of consciousness or lesions seen on brain imaging, this is consistent with a dementia. The most common cause of dementia in young patients is HIV-associated dementia. Other possible causes have been ruled out with imaging, cultures, and further diagnostic procedures. In the setting of HIV infection, this patient's symptoms can be attributed to his severe immune deficiency, bone marrow suppression from HIV, and HIV-associated encephalopathy.

Discussion

Many opportunistic diseases can cause neurologic impairment in HIV-infected patients. However HIV infection itself in the CNS can lead to significant neuropathology. HIV infects T cells, macrophages, dendritic cells, and astrocytes leading to impaired nerve cell function and neuronal death by a variety of mechanisms. The neurologic manifestations of HIV can be grouped into two major categories:

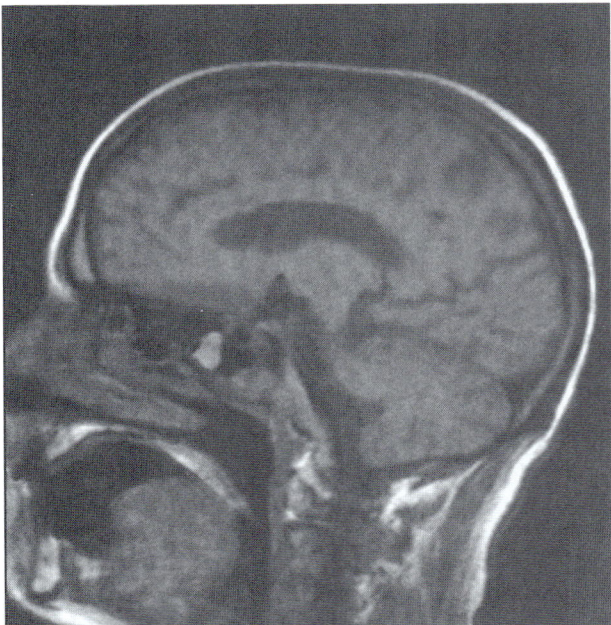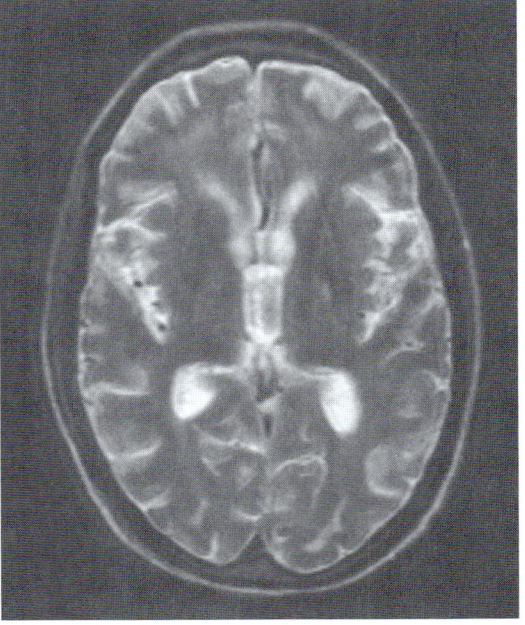

Figure 46-1 Sagital T_1 (A) and axial T_2 (B) weighted MRI images of patient described above showing generalized atrophic changes and periventricular subcortical T_2 hyperintensity.

minor cognitive motor disorder and HIV-associated dementia. HIV-associated dementia is also known as HAD, AIDS dementia complex (ADC), and HIV-1 associated encephalitis (HIVE).

Bizarre behavior and weight loss in a patient with history of drug abuse should prompt the investigation for HIV-related pathologies, including HIV encephalopathy as well as opportunistic infections. HIV encephalopathy is a diagnosis of exclusion after other etiologies have been ruled out.

Neurologic impairment affects approximately 60% of HIV-infected patients. HIV-1 enters the CNS in the early phase of infection and persists in the system for decades. Prior to the introduction of HAART, nearly 30% of the infected population developed HAD in the late stages of HIV/AIDS. With the use of HAART this has reduced to 10%, however, a more subtle form of CNS dysfunction has become more common—termed minor cognitive motor disorder (MCMD). Recently it has been estimated that nearly 30% of patients infected with HIV have MCMD.

The pathophysiology of HIV encephalopathy is complicated and is likely the final common manifestation for a large number of cellular and biochemical derangements in the CNS as a consequence of HIV infection. It is characterized by HIV virions crossing the blood–brain barrier and infecting susceptible constituent cells of the CNS, likely via CD4 and HIV co-receptors (chemokine receptors) found on resident microglial cells and perivascular macrophages. The breach of the blood–brain barrier is likely via infected CD4+ T cells that normally traverse the

CNS, but the exact mechanism is still unclear. Apparently, resident macrophages and microglial cells can produce active infections locally. Importantly, astrocytes appear susceptible to infection as well, despite their lack of CD4 on the cell surface, while oligodendrocytes and brain microvascular endothelial cells show susceptibility to HIV infection *in vitro* (Table 46-1). At the molecular and cellular level, the pathologic consequences of HIV infection in CNS cells results from neuronal death and dysfunction because of the direct effects of viral products on these cells and by an altered inflammatory/excitotoxic microenvironment. Histopathologically, HIV encephalitis is identified on microscopic examination by vascular damage, microglial nodules, lymphocytic infiltrates, diffuse myelin damage (spongy myelinopathy, gliosis), and multinucleated giant cells. It is believed that HIV envelope glycoproteins cause the membranes of HIV-infected macrophages to fuse to form these giant cells. Preliminary clinical data suggests that chronic cocaine or methamphetamine use may increase the permeability of the blood–brain barrier and accelerate HIV-associated encephalopathy, but this is still under investigation.

Minor cognitive motor disorder (MCMD) is the term used for mild cognitive, motor, or behavioral problems associated with HIV, but without serious impairment in daily functioning. Symptoms are impaired attention or coordination, mental slowing, impaired memory, slowed movements, incoordination. Importantly, a clear consciousness is associated with this condition. The findings are subtle and frequently overlooked, and the diagnosis

TABLE 46-1

Susceptibility of Cells of the CNS to Infection from HIV

Cell type	CD4 on surface	Chemokine (HIV coreceptor on surface?)	HIV susceptibility	Productive infection
Perivascular macrophages	Yes	Yes	Yes	Yes
Microglia	Yes	Yes	Yes	Yes
Astrocytes	No	Yes	Yes	No
Oligodendrocytes	No	Yes	In vitro	No
Neurons	No	Yes	No	No
Brain microvascular endothelial cells	No	Yes	In vitro	No

Adapted from Gonzalez-Scarano F, Martin-Garcia J. The neuropathogenesis of AIDS. Nature Rev Immunol. January 2005;69–81.

TABLE 46-2

MCMD Criteria

MCMD criteria

At least two of the following:
  Impaired attention or coordination
  Mental slowing
  Impaired memory
  Slowed movements
  Incoordination
Patients with MCMD have clear consciousness

TABLE 46-3

Stages and Characteristics of HIV-Associated Dementia

Stage	Characteristics
Stage 0 (normal)	Normal mental and motor function
Stage 0.5 (subclinical)	Equivocal symptoms of cognitive or motor dysfunction; no impairment of work or activities of daily living (ADL)
Stage 1 (mild)	Evidence of intellectual or motor impairment, but able to perform most ADL
Stage 2 (moderate)	Unable to work, but can manage self-care
Stage 3 (severe)	Major intellectual incapacity or motor disability
Stage 4 (end-stage)	Nearly vegetative

Adapted from Bartlett JG, Gallant JE. 2005–2006 Medical Management of HIV Infection. Baltimore, MD: Johns Hopkins University Division of Infectious Diseases; 2005.

often requires intensive neuropsychiatric testing, considering the primary disabilities in patients with MCMD are with executive reasoning. The criteria for this diagnosis can be found in Table 46-2. Currently there are no published large randomized controlled trials for the treatment of this condition.

HIV-associated dementia (HAD) is the classic neurologic pathology associated with longstanding HIV infection in the absence of HAART treatment. It is a subcortical dementia associated with memory and psychomotor speed impairment, overall depressive symptoms, as well as movement disorders. This is distinct from higher, cortical dementias such as Alzheimer disease, which are classically associated with aphasia, agnosia, and apraxia.

The classic presentation of HAD is a frontal subcortical demential process. Similar to other frontal insults, this process can be associated with disinhibition—patients may display personality changes as well as physical findings of frontal release including the emergence of the grasp, root, snout, and glabellar reflexes. Mania or psychosis can present in the setting of HIV encephalopathy. The initial findings are often subtle and progressive over time. There is a six-level staging system to quantify the degree of neurologic impairment (Table 46-3). The symptoms can range from mild impairment to a nearly vegetative state.

The treatment for HIV encephalopathy is HAART therapy, aimed at preventing further progression. Long-term prognosis for regaining previous function is not optimistic.

Some drugs may have increased efficacy at preventing HAD because of a higher concentration in the CSF. These drugs include AZT, stavudine, lamivudine, abacavir, nevirapine, and indinavir. Large-scale randomized controlled trials have not yet been conducted to further evaluate these

possibilities. Research has shown a differential in drug concentration from the serum to CSF, which theoretically could promote resistant virus in the CSF despite sensitive virus present in the serum.

Since the advent of HAART therapy, the presentation of HAD is changing. There is research to suggest that the proportion of new HAD cases occurring in patients with higher CD4 counts is increasing. In addition, the type of neuropsychologic impairment is changing. With HAART there is improvement in attention, verbal fluency, visuoconstruction defects, but deterioration in learning efficiency and complex attention.

These findings, along with the studies investigating CSF concentrations of antiretrovirals suggest that HAART may not completely prevent HIV-encephalopathy, but may change the presentation.

Because the signs of HIV encephalopathy can be subtle and are often overlooked, the most definitive way to diagnose is with an HIV test, a thorough evaluation to rule out opportunistic infections, and comprehensive neuropsychologic testing to determine the extent of cognitive impairment and identify contributing factors. The evaluation for other causes of neurologic impairment should include thyroid

TABLE 46-4

International Screening Tool for HIV Dementia

International HIV Dementia Scale (IHDS)

Memory-Registration: Give four words to recall (dog, hat, bean, red) —1 second to say each. Then ask the patient all four words after you have said them. Repeat words if the patient does not recall them all immediately. Tell the patient you will ask for recall of the words again a bit later.

1. Motor speed: Have the patient tap the first two fingers of the nondominant hand as widely and as quickly as possible.
   4 = 15 in 5 seconds
   3 = 11–14 in 5 seconds
   2 = 7–10 in 5 seconds
   1 = 3–6 in 5 seconds
   0 = 0–2 in 5 seconds

2. Psychomotor speed: Have the patient perform the following movements with the nondominant hand as quickly as possible:
(1) Clench hand in fist on flat surface, (2) Put hand flat on surface with palm down, (3) Put hand perpendicular to flat surface on the side of the fifth digit. Demonstrate and have patient perform twice for practice.
   4 = 4 sequences in 10 seconds
   3 = 3 sequences in 10 seconds
   2 = 2 sequences in 10 seconds
   1 = 1 sequence in 10 seconds
   0 = unable to perform

3. Memory recall: Ask the patient to recall the four words. For words not recalled, prompt with a semantic clue as follows: animal (dog); piece of clothing (hat); vegetable (bean); color (red).
   Give 1 point for each word spontaneously recalled
   Give 0.5 points for each correct answer after prompting
   Maximum —4 points

Total International HIV Dementia Scale Score: This is the sum of the scores on items 1–3. The maximum possible score is 12 points. A patient with a score of = 10 should be evaluated further for possible dementia.

Adapted from Berger JR, Brew B. An international screening tool for HIV dementia. AIDS. 2005;19:2165.

testing, CBC, RPR, electrolytes with LFTs, lumbar puncture, brain imaging, review of medications, evaluation for drug or alcohol abuse, and assessment for depression.

The neuropsychologic testing used classically to diagnose is expensive, inefficient, and cumbersome for the typical HIV care provider and bedside screening tests are currently under investigation (Table 46-4).

In summary, a young person who presents with progressive neurologic impairment over time with HIV risk factors should be assessed for HIV encephalopathy. The treatment is aggressive antiretroviral treatment to slow progression of disability.

Selected References

1. Gonzalez-Scarano F, Martin-Garcia J. The neuropathogenesis of AIDS. *Nature Rev Immunol.* January 2005(1);69–81.
2. Ghafouri M, Amini S, Khalili K, et al. HIV-1 associated dementia: symptoms and causes. *Retrovirology.* 2006;3:28.
3. Berger JR, Brew B. An international screening tool for HIV dementia. *AIDS.* 2005;19:2165.
4. Price RW. Neurological complications of HIV infection. *Lancet.* 1996(38);348–445.
5. Bartlett JG, Gallant JE. *2005-2006 Medical Management of HIV Infection.* Baltimore, MD: Johns Hopkins University Division of Infectious Diseases; 2005.

41-Year-Old Male with Palpitations

CASE PRESENTATION

A previously healthy 41-year-old African American male was admitted to the hospital for evaluation of tachycardia. He had woken up at approximately 4 AM feeling his heart racing. This feeling was associated with 7 out of 10 chest tightness and shortness of breath. The discomfort lasted until he came to the emergency room about 12 hours later, at which time it decreased to about 2 out of 10 discomfort. There were no inciting or relieving factors. He had no fevers, weight loss, cough, edema, headache, or dizziness. He had no nausea, vomiting, changes in stool pattern, change in vision, or diaphoresis. He stated that the only time he had ever felt this way before was when he was over-exerting himself with exercise. Past medical history was significant only for vasectomy and right knee replacement several years previously. Family history was significant for a younger brother who had an event very similar to this several years earlier, father with coronary artery disease in his sixties, and a mother who died of a stroke in her seventies. The patient was recently retired and new to the area. He has a 20-pack/year current smoking history and drank alcohol only occasionally.

C

47

Physical Examination

The patient was an overweight male in no distress. Vital signs: temperature 36.8°C, heart rate 128 beats/min, blood pressure 132/80 mm Hg, and respiratory rate 16 breaths/min with oxygen saturation of 98% on room air. Mucous membranes were moist. Pupils were equal and reactive to light. There was no proptosis. Neck was supple with no jugular venous distention, bruits, lymphadenopathy, thyromegaly, or masses. Heart rate was fast and irregularly irregular. There were no murmurs, gallops, or rubs. Chest was clear to auscultation. Abdomen was soft and nontender. No masses were felt. Extremities had no edema or rashes. Neurologic examination was normal.

Laboratory Studies

White blood cells count was 8.2 with a normal differential. Hematocrit was 49 and platelets were 238. Chemistries were normal with a creatinine of 0.9, blood urea nitrogen 17, HCO_3 23, Na 136, K 4.2, Cl 106, and Ca 9. Cardiac enzymes were normal. Thyroid-stimulating hormone (TSH) was normal at 1.02. Total fasting cholesterol was 178, high-density lipoprotein 34, low-density lipoprotein 99, triglycerides 227. Electrocardiogram showed atrial fibrillation with a rate of 97, normal axis, borderline left ventricular hypertrophy.

Case Resolution

This 41-year-old man presented with chest pressure and palpitations secondary to new-onset atrial fibrillation. This led us to question the cause of his fibrillation and whether or not he had experienced paroxysmal atrial fibrillation in the past. Both of these factors would influence his subsequent testing and treatment.

Question

What are some common causes of atrial fibrillation?

Answer

There are many causes of atrial fibrillation. The causes include thyroid disease, ethanol consumption, pericarditis, pulmonary embolism, systemic infection, drugs such as stimulants and cocaine, coronary artery disease, and valvular disease, in particular mitral valve stenosis.

Discussion

Atrial fibrillation is the most common arrhythmia of adulthood, accounting for one-third of hospitalizations for arrhythmia. A predisposing condition exists in up to 90% of cases. Common cardiac associations include rheumatic heart disease, dilated atria, coronary artery disease, hypertension, and congestive heart failure. Given these associations, a patient with new-onset atrial fibrillation should undergo investigation to uncover other associated causes or risk factors, which may warrant additional intervention. After a careful history, this may include a toxicology screen, TSH, and echocardiography with or without stress testing to uncover ischemic disease.

According to Framingham and other data, the risk of stroke in patients with atrial fibrillation is 1% to 5% per year, depending on the presence of other risk factors. Because of its associated morbidity, careful attention has been directed toward management of atrial fibrillation to decrease the incidence of stroke and death.

Given the risk of embolic stroke with atrial fibrillation, the American College of Physicians (ACP)/American Academy of Family Physicians (AAFP) recommend anticoagulation with warfarin for patients to a goal INR of 2 to 3 unless patients have a low risk of stroke or contraindications to anticoagulation. The CHADS2 scoring system has been recommended as a means of stratifying patients' risk for stroke (Table 47-1). The score is calculated by adding one point each for heart failure within the last 100 days, hypertension, age > 75 years, or diabetes. Two points are given for history of stroke or transient ischemic attack. For patients with a lower risk of stroke, meta-analysis by McNamara et al concluded that aspirin alone may be useful, as it does not have the significant risk of bleeding associated with warfarin anticoagulation.

In patients with new onset or symptomatic atrial fibrillation, much research has been conducted on cardioversion to sinus rhythm. According to ACP/AAFP recommendations, there is good evidence to support the use of either

---

TABLE 47-1

CHADS2 Stroke Risk Stratification

Score	Average adjusted stroke rate	Risk level
0	1.9	Low
1	2.9	Low
2	4.0	Moderate
3	5.9	Moderate
4	8.5	High
5	12.5	High
6	18.2	High

---

direct-current or pharmacologic cardioversion. Direct-current cardioversion, for example, appears to be safe and over 90% effective. However, both types of cardioversion show high rates of reversion back to atrial fibrillation. Likewise, both types of cardioversion have the same risk of cardioembolization. Side effects must be considered, including burns or discomfort with direct-current and arrhythmias such as Torsades de point with the use of pharmacologic agents. Pharmacologic maintenance following either type of cardioversion is not recommended, except in cases wherein the rhythm significantly disrupts the patient's life. If direct-current cardioversion in the acute setting is chosen, the ACUTE trial demonstrated that two options exist. Patients may undergo short-term anticoagulation with heparin followed by TEE-guided cardioversion, if no thrombus is seen, and 4 weeks of subsequent anticoagulation. The other option is to anticoagulate 3 weeks before and then again 4 weeks following cardioversion. Rates of bleeding are somewhat higher and the initial cardioversion rate somewhat lower in the second group receiving conventional treatment. However, maintenance of sinus rhythm at 8 weeks, rate of stroke, and rate of embolism did not differ significantly between the groups.

In patients with chronic atrial fibrillation, the physician must decide whether to manage primarily the patient's rhythm or the heart rate. The largest of the studies evaluating rhythm versus rate control was the AFFIRM (Atrial Fibrillation Follow-up Investigation of Rhythm Management) trial, which included more than 4000 patients from 200 clinical sites. Other smaller studies have supported the conclusions of this study. Inclusion criteria for the AFFIRM trial included atrial fibrillation for more than 6 hours plus one additional risk factor for stroke. Patients were randomized to rhythm-control versus rate-control. Both groups were initially started on anticoagulation. Discontinuation of anticoagulation was allowed 1 month following conversion in the rhythm-control group, but it was continued indefinitely in the rate-control group. Although slightly more deaths and cerebrovascular events occurred in the rhythm-control group, the numbers were not statistically significant. Furthermore, approximately 70% of strokes occurred in patients who were no longer therapeutically anticoagulated. Therefore, the ACP and AAFP recommend rate control with anticoagulation for the majority of patients with atrial fibrillation. However, they recognize that rhythm control may be preferable for some patients when taking into consideration other factors such as patient symptoms, exercise tolerance, or comorbidities. In choosing an agent for rate control, β-blockers as calcium channel blockers are usually the preferred medications. Because digoxin will primarily reduce resting heart rate rather than overall heart rate, the ACP/AAFP recommend it only as an adjunct to these medications for rate control.

Selected References

McNamara RL, Tamariz LJ, Segal JB, et al. Management of atrial fibrillation: review of the evidence for the role of pharmacologic therapy, electrical cardioversion, and echocardiography. *Ann Intern Med.* 2003 Dec 16;139(12):1018–1033.

Snow V, Weiss KB, LeFevre M, et al. Management of newly detected atrial fibrillation: a clinical practice guideline from the American Academy of Family Physicians and the American College of Physicians. *Ann Intern Med.* 2003 Dec 16;139(12): 1018–1033.

Brand FN, Abbott RD, Kannel WB, et al. Characteristics and prognosis of lone atrial fibrillation. 30-year follow-up in the Framingham Study. *JAMA.* 1985;254:3449–3453.

Wyse DG, Waldo AL, DiMarco JP, et al. Atrial Fibrillation Follow-up Investigation of Rhythm Management (AFFIRM) Investigators. A comparison of rate control and rhythm control in patients with atrial fibrillation. *N Engl J Med.* 2002 Dec 5;347(23):1825–1833.

Gage BF, Waterman AD, Shannon W, et al. Validation of clinical classification schemes for predicting stroke: results from the National Registry of Atrial Fibrillation. *JAMA.* 2001 Jun 13;285(22):2864–2870.

Klein AL, Grimm RA, Murray RD, et al. Assessment of cardioversion using transesophageal echocardiography investigators. Use of transesophageal echocardiography to guide cardioversion in patients with atrial fibrillation. *N Engl J Med.* 2001 May 10;344(19):1411–1420.

40-Year-Old Female with Dyspnea and Weight Loss

CASE PRESENTATION

A 40-year-old white female presented with 3 months of progressive fatigue, cough, and shortness of breath. Dyspnea initially occurred only with heavy exertion, but in the week prior to admission had limited her ability to work as a forklift operator. There was no history of hemoptysis; the cough was occasionally productive of clear sputum, but was mostly dry. Pleuritic chest pain was present with coughing, but the patient denied angina or heart failure symptoms. The patient denied chills or night sweats, but admitted to fevers for 2 months. The only past medical history was anemia; the patient was divorced and was in a monogamous sexual relationship with her boyfriend of 2 years. Her previous husband had been an intravenous drug user. She reported no history of sexually transmitted disease. She had smoked 1 pack of cigarettes a day for 22 years and did not use alcohol or recreational drugs. She had never traveled outside the southeastern United States. Her father had heart disease; there was no family history of pulmonary or autoimmune disease. Upon further review of systems, she admitted to noticing white plaques in her mouth and on her tongue for several months. She also noted 15 lb weight loss over 6 months, odynophagia, decreased appetite, and heavy menstrual periods.

Physical Examination

Vital signs: temperature 38.4°C, pulse 133 beats/min, blood pressure 93/53 mm Hg, respiratory rate 22 breaths/min, and oxygen saturation of 89% on room air. The patient was thin and in mild respiratory distress, but fully alert and oriented. There was thrush in the oropharynx. Neck was supple without adenopathy. The pulmonary examination was abnormal with diffuse ronchi, inspiratory wheezing, and dry crackles. There was no egophony or dullness to percussion. The heart rate was tachycardic with regular rhythm. The abdomen was soft and nontender, and there was no palpable organomegaly. There was no enlargement of axillary or inguinal lymph nodes; distal pulses were brisk. There was no peripheral edema, no digital clubbing, and no central or peripheral cyanosis.

Laboratory Studies

Arterial blood gas obtained with the patient breathing room air: 7.49/22/53/88.3%, chest x-ray (CXR): diffuse interstitial opacities in both lungs, no hilar adenopathy, no cavitation, no pleural effusion (Fig. 48-1). Chest CT scan: diffuse bilateral ground glass opacities (Fig. 48-2), 12-lead electrocardiogram: sinus tachycardia, rate 141, diffuse low-voltage QRS complexes

Laboratory Values

White blood cell count was 3.9 with neutrophils 3.5, lymphocytes 0.3, monocytes 0.1, basophils 0.0, eosinophils 0.0; hemoglobin 8.6 g/dL; hematocrit 26.7%, mean corpuscular

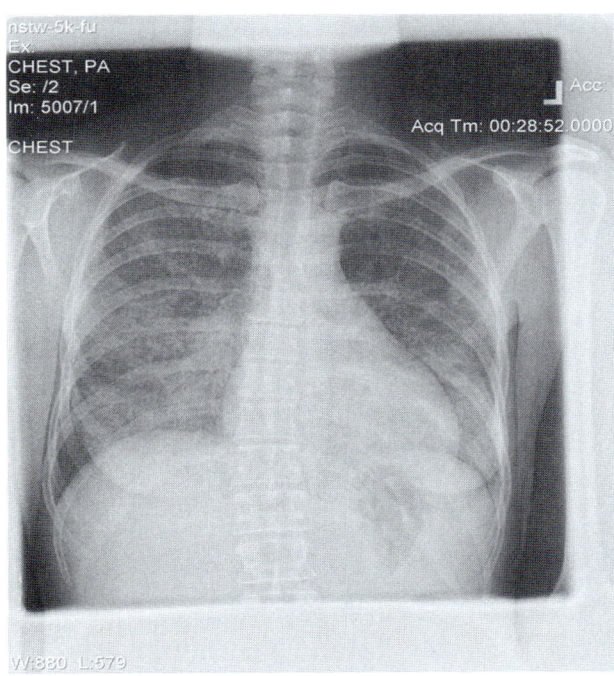

Figure 48-1 PA chest x-ray.

volume 85 FL, reticulocytes 2.3%; platelets 134; Na 139; K 4.4; Cl 117; HCo₃ 22; blood urea nitrogen 18; Cr 0.9; Glucose 113; Mg 1.5; Ca 7.4; P 4.1; LDH 2088 U/L.

Case Resolution

Despite lack of prior diagnosis of human immunodeficiency virus (HIV) infection, several features of the history and physical examination indicated that this patient likely had acquired immunodeficiency syndrome (AIDS) (see Table 48-1).

Opportunistic infection with *Pneumocystis jiroveci* (PCP) (previously pneumocystis carinii) was suspected based on the physical examination findings, CXR findings, hypoxemia, and elevated serum lactate dehydrogenase level. Other diagnoses could not be initially ruled out, however, as 13% to 18% of HIV-infected patients with PCP have another underlying pulmonary process such as tuberculosis, community-acquired pneumonia, or Kaposi sarcoma (1,2). An elevated lactate dehydrogenase level is often seen in cases of PCP, but is not a specific finding (3). The patient's radiographic finding—diffuse bilateral interstitial infiltrates—is the most common pattern seen in patients with PCP; however, PCP can have various other appearances on CXR (2,4,5) (see Table 48-2).

Infectious disease consultation was obtained, and upon their recommendation the patient was placed in respiratory isolation, a purified protein derivative (PPD) was placed, and bronchoscopy was performed to make a definitive diagnosis of PCP. Bronchial alveolar lavage (BAL) specimens stained negative for acid fast bacilli, and polymerase chain reaction was negative for cytomegalovirus and herpes simplex virus. PCP direct immunofluorescent antibody (DFA) tests of sputum and BAL specimen were both positive. Given this weight of evidence, the patient was treated with trimethoprim-sulfamethoxazole (TMP-SMX) and prednisone for PCP. Ceftriaxone and azithromycin were empirically added for community-acquired pneumonia coverage.

BAL culture eventually returned negative for fungi, bacteria including Legionella and Nocardia, viruses, and mycobacteria. HIV enzyme-linked immunosorbent assay (ELISA) and Western blot tests returned positive, and HIV viral load was found to be greater than 750,000 copies per milliliter by PCR. CD4 count was less than 10 cells/UL. Thus, the suspected initial diagnoses—AIDS and PCP—were confirmed.

Despite early and aggressive treatment with intravenous antibiotic therapy, prednisone, bronchodilators, and oxygen, the patient suffered relentless worsening of respiratory status with progressive hypoxemia. She was transferred to the intensive care unit (ICU) 5 days into her stay, and required endotracheal intubation and mechanical ventilation on hospital day 7. She developed acute respiratory distress syndrome and died after a month in the hospital. Tests for several other viral coinfections and opportunistic infections returned negative, including hepatitis B, hepatitis C, rapid plasma reagin, and serum cryptococcal antigen. Multiple blood and sputum cultures taken throughout the hospitalization were negative. The PPD test was nonreactive.

Questions

What is the evidence-based approach to diagnosis and treatment of PCP?

Discussion

The definitive diagnosis of PCP is made primarily by identifying the organism in respiratory secretions—either

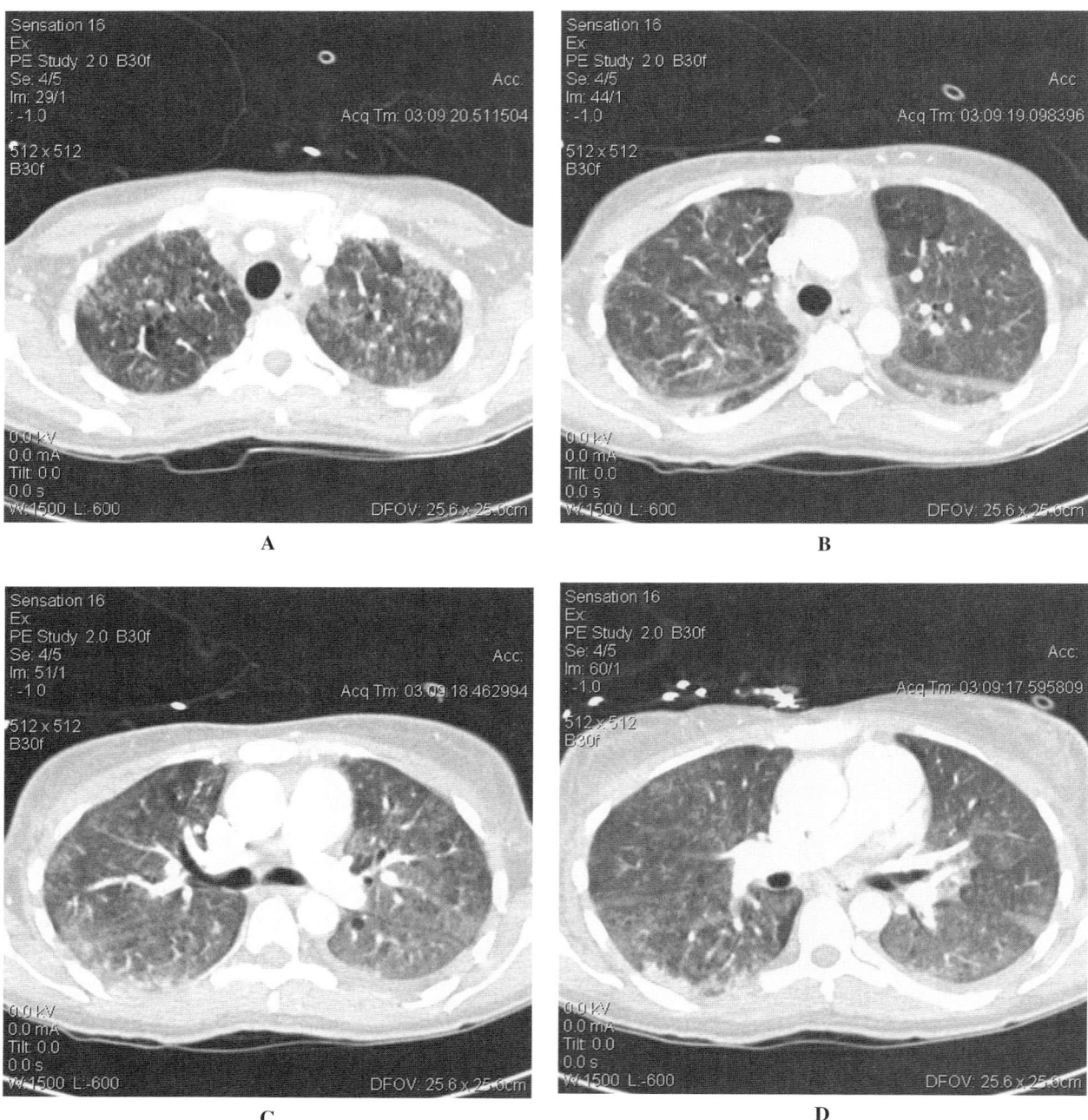

Figure 48-2 Chest CT scan.

sputum, BAL washing, or endotracheal aspirate (2,6). The most common laboratory technique for identifying pneumocystis is DFA staining, in which the antigen is pneumocystis cell wall glycoprotein (7). Expectorated sputum is of lower diagnostic yield than sputum induced by hypertonic saline. A 1993 study from the United Kingdom reported a sensitivity of 95% and specificity of 100% for the diagnosis of PCP, when DFA testing was applied to hypertonic saline-induced sputum (8). This study has limitations, primarily the lack of gold-standard testing, but when combined with data from other similar studies is indicative of the usefulness of induced sputum testing. Given an adequate sample and an experienced laboratory and pathologist, the sensitivity of induced sputum in

TABLE 48-1

Signs and Symptoms of Aids Present in this Case

Findings strongly associated with AIDS

High-risk sexual behavior
Oral thrush/esophagitis
Lymphopenia
Likely opportunistic infection
Findings associated with AIDS

Fatigue
Anemia
Weight loss

diagnosing PCP can be assumed to be as high as 90%; practically, it is somewhat lower, on the order of 55% to 90% (2,6,8).

Bronchoscopy with BAL has high sensitivity and specificity for diagnosis of PCP. The diagnostic yield can be increased even further with addition of transbronchial biopsy and with utilization of site-directed lavage in patients with focal infiltrates (9). In patients not receiving aerosolized pentamidine as PCP prophylaxis, which has been shown to significantly decrease the yield of BAL washings, the sensitivity of bronchoscopy with BAL for

TABLE 48-2

CXR Findings in Patients with PCP

Common CXR findings in PCP

Diffuse interstitial infiltrates
Bilateral infiltrates emanating from the hila
Symmetric infiltrates
Less common CXR findings in PCP

Diffuse alveolar infiltrates
Pneumothorax
Asymmetric disease
Blebs and cysts
Nodules
Upper lobe localization
Normal CXR

diagnosing PCP is close to 100% (10). For patients undergoing mechanical ventilation, endotracheal aspirates have been shown to be 92% sensitive when compared with BAL washing (11). Transbronchial biopsy is considered to be 100% sensitive and specific for the diagnosis of PCP.

In patients such as ours, in whom a diagnosis of AIDS is initially suspected but not definitively known, empirically treating for PCP without making a definitive diagnosis is not recommended (2). Empiric administration of corticosteroids, for example, in a patient suspected to have pneumocystis infection, but actually having mycobacterial infection, could adversely affect the outcome. Obtaining an adequate sample of respiratory secretion—via either induced sputum or bronchoscopy with BAL—that will allow a definitive diagnosis of PCP to be made is recommended prior to commencing therapy (12). If clinical suspicion for PCP is high enough, therapy may be initiated prior to the return of the PCP diagnostic test result (2).

Once a definitive diagnosis of PCP is established in a patient with AIDS, treatment decisions include whether to treat as an inpatient or outpatient, which antipneumocystis regimen to use, whether to use oral or intravenous therapy, whether or not to add corticosteroids, whether or not to treat in the ICU, and the timing of antiretroviral initiation.

In 2004, the Centers for Disease Control and Prevention (CDC) published recommendations on treatment of PCP in HIV-infected patients (2). It is expected that the majority of patients treated for PCP will transiently decline for 2 to 3 days at the onset of therapy. For this reason, all but the most well-appearing HIV-infected patients with PCP are initially treated as inpatients. There is evidence from randomized clinical trials supporting the use of trimethoprim-sulfamethoxazole as the initial treatment of choice for PCP; this drug is given the CDC's highest recommendation in the 2004 report (2). TMP-SMX therapy is highly efficacious both orally and intravenously, as oral absorption is generally very good. Intravenous therapy should be administered if the patient's ability to absorb oral medicine is compromised by infection—such as herpes or candida—or other gastrointestinal malabsorptive process, or if respiratory or metal status is so compromised that the ability to swallow is impaired. Switching from intravenous to oral therapy is recommended once clinical improvement allows it. The recommended dosing regimens for TMP-SMX as well as those for other acceptable, but less preferred treatment regimens are listed in Tables 48-3 and 48-4. Recommended duration of treatment is 21 days (2).

TABLE 48-3

IV Regimens for PCP Treatment

Medication	Dose	Frequency
TMP	15 mg/kg	Q6 or Q8 hours
+	+	
SMX	5:1 ratio with TMP	
Pentamidine	4 mg/kg	Daily
Clindamycin	600 mg	Q8 hours
+	+	+ Daily
Oral primaquine	30 mg	

TABLE 48-5

Risk Ratio Associated with Use of Adjunctive Corticosteroid vs. Placebo in Moderate-Severe PCP

	Mortality at 1 month	Mortality at 3–4 months	Mechanical ventilation
Risk Ratio	0.56; 95% CI, 0.32–0.98	0.68; 95% CI, 0.50–0.94	0.38; 95% CI, 0.20–0.73

For moderate-severe disease, defined as a room air PaO_2 < 70 mm Hg or an alveolar-arterial oxygen gradient > 35 mm Hg, there is evidence that the addition of adjunctive corticosteroids for HIV-infected patients with PCP is beneficial. In 2006, the Cochrane Collaboration reviewed this evidence; six studies were included in the meta-analysis (13). The Cochrane review quantitated the beneficial effects on mortality and prevention of mechanical ventilation associated with using adjunctive corticosteroids in moderate-severe PCP, as summarized in Table 48-5. The recommended dosing regimen for adjunctive corticosteroids is presented in Table 48-6. Intravenous methylprednisolone (at 75% of the prednisone dose) may be substituted for oral prednisone in patients unable to take oral medicines.

The patient presented in this case was treated for respiratory failure in the medical ICU on hospital day number 5, and began mechanical ventilation 7 days into her hospitalization. There is a robust association between respiratory failure requiring ICU care and mortality in HIV-infected patients with PCP. Prior to adjunctive corticosteroid use, mortality in such patients approached 100% (2,14–16). Throughout the 1990s, mortality rates for PCP-associated respiratory failure decreased slightly, and then settled at 60% to 80% (16–19).

In 2003, an intriguing study from San Francisco by Morris et al indicated that initiation of highly active antiretroviral therapy (HAART) either prior to or during hospitalization for PCP conferred a significant decrease in mortality. In this study, the mortality rate for HIV-infected patients with PCP admitted to the ICU for respiratory failure, who received HAART either prior to or during hospitalization, was 25%, while the mortality rate for those not receiving HAART was 63% (OR = 0.14; 95% CI, 0.02 to 0.84). The authors proposed that HAART represented the first therapy since corticosteroids to significantly improve chance of survival in the sickest HIV-infected patients with PCP (18). This paper has several limitations.

TABLE 48-4

Oral Regimens for PCP Treatment

Medication	Dose	Frequency
TMP-SMX	Two double strength tablets	Every 8 hours
TMP	5 mg/kg	tid
+	+	+
Dapsone	100 mg	Daily
Clindamycin	300–450 mg	Q 6 hours
+	+	+
Primaquine	15 mg	Daily
Atovaquone suspension	750 mg	bid

TABLE 48-6

Adjunctive Corticosteroid Regimen for Moderate-Severe PCP

Prednisone 40 mg twice daily for 5 days
then
Prednisone 40 mg daily for 5 days
then
Prednisone 20 mg daily for 11 days

The primary weakness is that it is a retrospective analysis, and while many potential confounders were adjusted with multiple logistic regression analysis, there likely remain important unknown baseline differences between the two groups. Also, only six patients in this study were started on HAART during hospitalization; while only two of these patients died, there could have been substantial bias toward prescribing HAART only for the less ill patients, in whom further care did not seem futile. Finally, there were only 58 patients in this study, and the 95% confidence intervals are thus very wide.

In 2006, a retrospective analysis of 59 patients showed a somewhat improved mortality rate of 53% for HIV-infected patients with PCP admitted to an ICU in London. No patient in this study received HAART prior to or during hospitalization. The authors concluded that improved ICU survival for HIV-infected patients with PCP is independent of HAART therapy, and rather is indicative of the improvements in the overall management of patients with acute lung injury or acute respiratory distress syndrome that have occurred over the past decade, in particular with the advent of ventilation strategies utilizing lower tidal volumes and lower plateau pressures (19).

The 2004 CDC statement recommended that certain patients with AIDS and PCP be offered ICU admission or mechanical ventilation "when appropriate"(2). More recent data indicating improved survival rates for all patients with ARDS (if ventilated properly) suggests that the options of ICU admission and mechanical ventilation are reasonable for most AIDS patients with severe PCP. The timing of HAART initiation remains controversial. There are ongoing prospective, randomized, trials addressing this issue (2).

Selected References

1. Baughman RP, Dohn MN, Frame PT. The continuing utility of bronchoalveolar lavage to diagnose opportunistic infection in AIDS patients. *Am J Med*. 1994;97:515–522.
2. Benson CA, Kaplan JA, Masur H, et al; CDC; National Institutes of Health; Infectious Disease Society of America. Treating opportunistic infections among HIV-infected adults and adolescents: recommendations from CDC, the National Institutes of Health, and the Infectious Diseases Society of America. *MMWR Recomm Rep*. 2004;53(RR-15):1–112.
3. Zaman MK, White DA. Serum lactate dehydrogenase levels and *Pneumocystis carinii* pneumonia: diagnostic and prognostic significance. *Am Rev Respir Dis*. 1988;137:796–800.
4. Opravil M, Marincek B, Fuchs WA, et al. Shortcomings of chest radiography in detecting *Pneumocystis carinii* pneumonia. *J Acquir Immune Defic Syndr*. 1994;7:39–45.
5. DeLorenzo LJ, Huang CT, Maguire GP, et al. Roentgenographic patterns of *Pneumocystis carinii* pneumonia in 104 patients with AIDS. *Chest* 1987;91:323–327.
6. Cruciani M, Marcati P, Malena M, et al. Meta-analysis of diagnostic procedures for *Pneumocystis carinii* pneumonia in HIV-1 infected patients. *Eur Respir J*. 2002;20:982–989.
7. Kovacs JA, Ng VL, Masur H, et al. Diagnosis of *Pneumocystis carinii* pneumonia: improved detection in sputum with use of monoclonal antibodies. *N Engl J Med*. 1988;318:589–593.
8. Willocks L, Burns S, Cossar R, et al. Diagnosis of *Pneumocystis carinii* pneumonia in a population of HIV-positive drug users, with particular reference to sputum induction and fluorescent antibody techniques. *J Infect*. 1993;26:257–264.
9. Levine SJ, Kennedy D, Shelhamer JH, et al. Diagnosis of *Pneumocystis carinii* pneumonia by multiple site-directed bronchoalveolar lavage with immunofluorescent monoclonal antibody staining in human immunodeficiency virus-infected patients receiving aerosolized pentamidine chemoprophylaxis. *Am Rev Respir Dis*. 1992;146:838–843.
10. Jules-Elysee K, Stover DE, Zaman MB, et al. Aerosolized pentamidine: effects on diagnosis and presentation of *Pneumocystis carinii* pneumonia. *Ann Int Med*. 1990;112:750–757.
11. Alvarez F, Bandi V, Stager C, et al. Detection of *Pneumocystis carinii* in tracheal aspirates of intubated patients using calcofluor-white (Fungi-Fluor) and immunofluorescence antibody (Genetic Systems) stains. *Crit Care Med*. 1997;25:948–952.
12. Roger PM, Vandenbos F, Pugliese P, et al. Persistence of *Pneumocystis carinii* after effective treatment of *P. carinii* pneumonia is not related to relapse or survival among patients infected with human immunodeficiency virus. *Clin Infect Dis*. 1998;26:509–510.
13. Briel M, Bucher HC, Boscacci R, et al. Adjunctive corticosteroids for *Pneumocystis jiroveci* pneumonia in patients with HIV-infection (review). *The Cochrane Library*. 2006;4:1–14.
14. Wachter RM, Luce JM, Turner J, et al. Intensive care of patients with the acquired immunodeficiency syndrome. Outcome and changing patterns of utilization. *Am Rev Respir Dis*. 1986;134:891–896.
15. Wachter RM, Russi MB, Bloch DA, et al. *Pneumocystis carinii* pneumonia and refractory respiratory failure in AIDS. *Am Rev Respir Dis*. 1991;143:251–256.
16. Bedos JP, Dumoulin JL, Gachot B, et al. *Pneumocystis carinii* pneumonia requiring intensive care management: survival and prognostic study in 110 patients with human immunodeficiency virus. *Crit Care Med*. 1999;27:1109–1115.
17. Curtis JR, Yarnold PR, Schwartz DN, et al. Improvement in outcomes of acute respiratory failure for patients with human immunodeficiency virus-related *Pneumocystis carinii* pneumonia. *Am J Respir Crit Care Med*. 2000;162:393–398.
18. Morris A, Wachter RM, Luce J, et al. Improved survival with highly active antiretroviral therapy in HIV-infected patients with severe *Pneumocystis carinii* pneumonia. *AIDS*. 2003;17:73–80.
19. Miller RF, Allen E, Copas A, et al. Improved survival for HIV infected patients with severe *Pneumocystis jiroveci* pneumonia is independent of highly active antiretroviral therapy. *Thorax*. 2006;61:716–721.

74-Year-Old Female with "Fullness in the Neck" with Exertion

CASE PRESENTATION

A 74-year-old white female with a past medical history of diabetes mellitus Type II and hypertension came to our emergency room with recurrent episodes of diaphoresis, "fullness" and "pressure" in the throat, and lightheadedness. These unpleasant symptoms first started 1 year prior to admission, and occurred predictably with moderate exertion, such as climbing two flights of stairs. Rest and nitroglycerin usually provided relief; however, on the day of admission symptoms were refractory to these measures. Additionally, symptoms on the day of admission were occurring with minimal exertion, such as walking across the kitchen. The patient denied chest pain, dyspnea, and syncope. The sensation of fullness in the throat was not associated with dysphagia, cough, acid reflux, or stridor. Two of the patient's siblings died of myocardial infarctions (MI) in the sixth decade of life. The patient was a lifelong nonsmoker and denied alcohol use. A recent lipid profile revealed total cholesterol of 166 mg/dL and high-density lipoprotein (HDL) of 33 mg/dL. The patient took metformin and glyburide for diabetes, and recent hemoglobin A1C measured 7.3%. Other medications included aspirin (ASA), lisinopril, hydrochlorothiazide, metoprolol, atorvastatin, and as needed sublingual nitroglycerin.

Physical Examination

The patient was a comfortable white female in no acute distress. Vital signs: temperature 36.1°C, pulse 101 beats/min; blood pressure 120/72 mm Hg, respiratory rate 12 breaths/min; oxygen saturation of 98% while breathing room air. Mucous membranes were moist. Neck was supple with no elevation of jugular venous pressure while at 45° recumbency. Carotid upstrokes were normal and without bruit. Cardiac examination was positive for tachycardia, regular rhythm, normal S_1 and S_2, without S_3 or S_4. Point of maximal impulse was in normal location. Lungs sounded clear with good air exchange. Abdomen was soft and nontender without bruits or hepatomegaly. Extremities were warm with normal capillary refill, no edema, and 2+ pulses at the radial and dorsalis pedal arteries. There was no nystagmus and ocular movements were intact. Further cranial nerve testing was unremarkable. Cerebellar examination and reflexes were normal.

Laboratory Studies

Initial 12-lead electrocardiogram (ECG), recorded by emergency medical services prior to admission: normal sinus rhythm, rate 97, 1-mm ST-depression in leads V4-V6 without evidence of left ventricular hypertrophy. Twelve-lead ECG upon arrival to the emergency department: normal sinus rhythm, rate 95. No evidence of ST depression or elevation, no evidence of LVH. Chest x-ray (CXR): mild cardiomegaly without evidence of vascular congestion.

White blood cells 11.5, hemoglobin 12.2, hematocrit 35.2, platelets 326, Na 136, K 3.5, Cl 97, HCO_3 27, blood urea nitrogen 12, Cr 0.7, glucose 220, Mg 1.6, creatine kinase (CK) 31, creatine kinase MB (CK-MB) 1.6, and troponin T less than 0.029.

Case Resolution

The patient was admitted to the coronary care unit with the diagnosis of unstable angina (UA). She was treated with oxygen, intravenous unfractionated heparin, intravenous metoprolol, subcutaneous insulin, ASA, clopidogrel, lisinopril, atorvastatin, and nitro-paste. She continued to complain of throat fullness and lightheadedness with minimal exertion and occasionally at rest. ECGs were performed every 6 hours, and revealed intermittent ST-segment depression in the anterior and lateral precordial leads. Cardiac biomarkers were drawn every 6 hours and remained within normal limits. Continuous cardiac monitoring was positive for intermittent sinus tachycardia, but

was otherwise unremarkable. On hospital day 1 cardiac catheterization was performed. Angiography revealed severe multi-vessel coronary disease with 60% proximal left anterior descending (LAD) artery stenosis, occluded mid-LAD artery, 90% stenosis of second obtuse marginal artery, and occluded posterior descending artery (see Figs. 49-1 and 49-2). Cardiac surgery consultants felt the patient was a poor candidate for revascularization surgery, given lack of potential distal bypass graft targets. Symptoms improved with addition of long-acting oral nitrates and increased β-blockade, and the patient was discharged in improved condition.

Question

What are the etiologies of UA, how is it characterized, and what is the appropriate evidence-based management strategy?

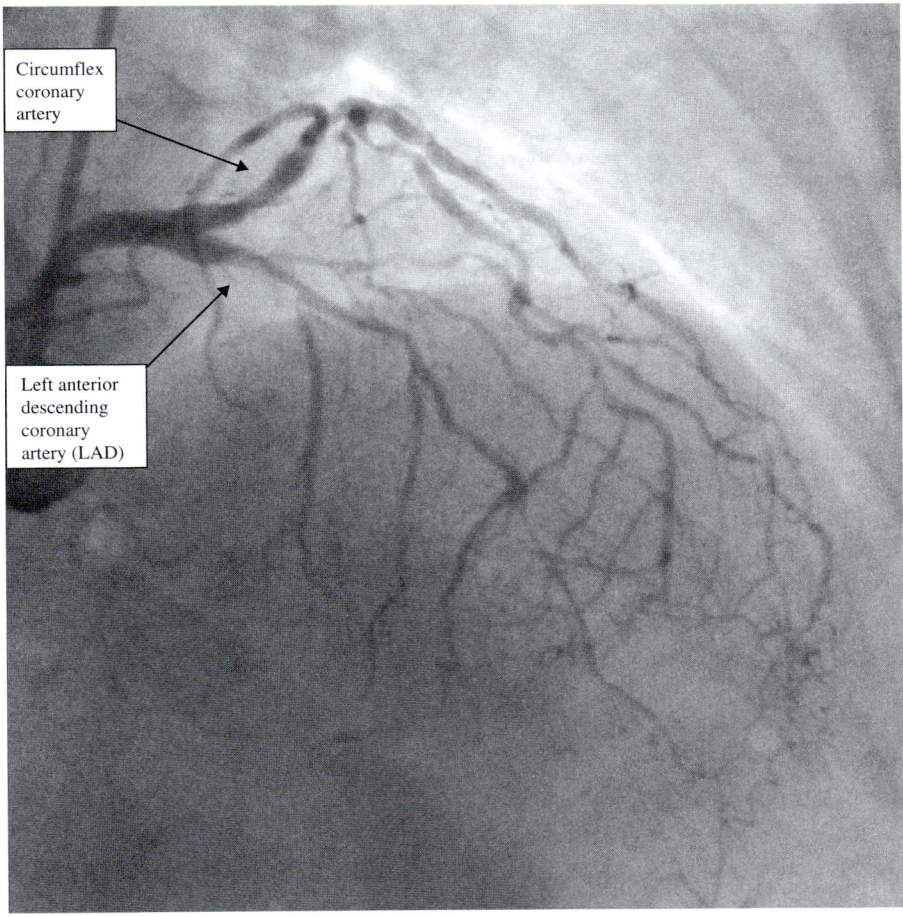

Figure 49-1 AP cranial coronary angiogram revealing diffusely diseased coronary vessels.

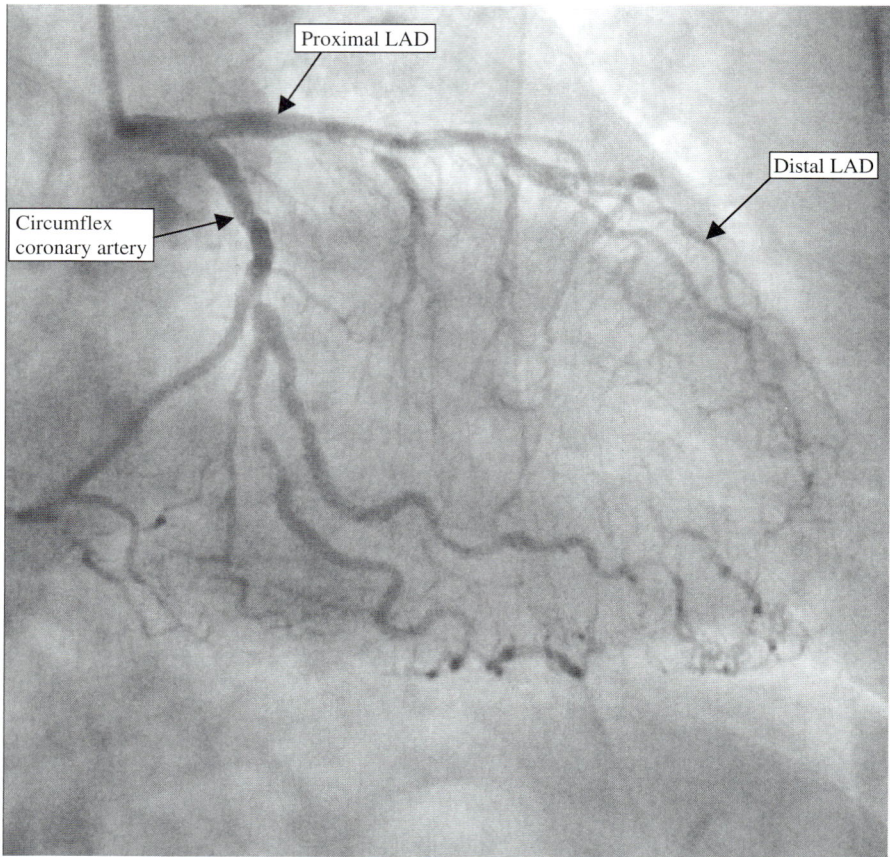

Figure 49-2 RAO caudal coronary angiogram revealing diffusely diseased coronary vessels.

Discussion

Etiologies of Unstable Angina

Angina is a symptom encountered when myocardial oxygen demand exceeds supply for a period of time long enough to induce anaerobic cellular metabolism. Typical angina is substernal in location, brought on by exertion, and relieved with rest. This description is most useful when considering fixed coronary lesions (1). With such "flow-limiting" coronary lesions, myocardial oxygen supply is sufficient at rest, but insufficient with exertion or emotional stress. This is the hallmark pathophysiology of chronic stable angina, which is usually predictable and may be a nuisance, but is rarely acutely life threatening.

Chronic stable angina may thus be thought of as a "demand" problem; as long as the patient is at rest, he is symptom free. UA, in contrast, is most often precipitated by a sudden decrease in myocardial oxygen supply, and thus symptoms may occur at rest. There are five common etiologies of UA (see Table 49-1) (2). Each of the first four

etiologies pertains directly to decreased oxygen supply. Secondary UA refers to conditions that decrease myocardial oxygen supply, such as hypotension and anemia; as well as to conditions that increase myocardial oxygen demand, such as fever, tachycardia, or thyrotoxicosis. Patients with secondary UA usually have underlying coronary artery disease, often significant enough to cause chronic stable

TABLE 49-1

Causes of Unstable Angina

1. Nonocclusive thrombus on preexisting plaque
2. Dynamic obstruction (coronary spasm or vasoconstriction)
3. Progressive mechanical obstruction
4. Inflammation and/or infection
5. Secondary unstable angina

Adapted from Braunwald E. Unstable angina: an etiologic approach to management. Circulation. *1999;98:2219–2222.*

angina. None of the five etiologies presented here are mutually exclusive (2).

In the above case, the patient clearly had progressive mechanical obstruction from severe multi-vessel coronary artery disease. It is also possible that one or more of the diseased vessels was affected by thrombus on preexisting plaque, and relative tachycardia may have been a secondary factor.

Characterization of Unstable Angina

The C7-T4 dermatomes receive afferent innervation from the same segments of the spinal cord as the heart. As such, the discomfort associated with myocardial ischemia may be referred anywhere from the lower jaw to the hands—including the throat, neck, shoulders, arms, back, chest, and upper abdomen (3). Wherever angina is perceived, it is typically not a discrete, stabbing, sharp, or fleeting pain (however, the presence of one or more of these characteristics does not exclude the possibility of angina). Rather, it is usually a sustained visceral discomfort of gradual onset, often described as a feeling of "tightness," "fullness," "squeezing," or "pressure" (4). In the above case, the patient had prominent throat and neck symptoms, but no chest discomfort. Any angina that does not present as substernal chest pressure may be referred to as "atypical angina." Likewise, symptoms other than angina, such as diaphoresis, dyspnea, nausea, and fatigue, may in the appropriate circumstance be considered "anginal equivalents" (5). It is a common observation that the elderly, women, and diabetics often experience "atypical angina" or "anginal equivalents," as occurred in the above case.

The Canadian Cardiovascular Society (CCS) classification was first introduced more than 30 years ago, and remains a useful mechanism for grading angina or anginal equivalents (see Table 49-2) (6).

Angina is generally considered unstable when one of the following conditions is met (see Table 49-3) (7):

UA is one of the acute coronary syndromes (ACS), along with ST-segment elevation myocardial infarction (STEMI) and non-ST-segment elevation myocardial infarction (NSTEMI). The recommended triage protocol is the same for all forms of ACS, and includes a targeted history and physical examination, ECG within 10 minutes of presentation to health care, and measurement of cardiac biomarkers.* The diagnosis of STEMI is made by ECG criteria, while NSTEMI is diagnosed by positive

(*=creatinine kinase [CK], creatinine kinase-myocardial band [CK-MB], troponin I or T).

TABLE 49-2

CCS Staging of Angina

Class I	Ordinary physical activity does not cause angina. Angina occurs with strenuous, rapid, or prolonged exertion.
Class II	Slight limitation of ordinary activity. Angina occurs on walking or climbing stairs rapidly; walking uphill; walking after meals. Angina occurs on walking > 2 blocks on the level and climbing > 1 flight of stairs
Class III	Marked limitations of ordinary physical activity. Angina occurs on walking 1 to 2 blocks on the level and climbing 1 flight of stairs
Class IV	Inability to carry on any physical activity without discomfort — anginal symptoms may be present at rest

Adapted from Campeau L. Letter: grading of angina pectoris. Circulation. 1976;54:522–523.

biomarkers without ST-segment elevation on ECG. UA is a clinical diagnosis, but may feature dynamic ECG changes such as T-wave inversions, ST-segment depressions, or arrhythmia. Together, UA and NSTEMI are referred to as non-ST-segment elevation acute coronary syndrome (NSTE-ACS) (8).

The physical examination of patients with UA may include signs of heart failure, such as tachycardia, abnormal

TABLE 49-3

Principal Presentations of Unstable Angina

Rest angina	Angina occurring at rest and prolonged, usually > 20 minutes
New-onset angina	New-onset angina of at least CCS class III severity
Increasing angina	Previously diagnosed angina that has become distinctly more frequent, longer in duration, or lower in threshold (ie, increased by 1 or more CCS class to at least class III severity)

Adapted from Braunwald E. Unstable angina. A classification. Circulation. 1989;80:410–414.

heart sounds (particularly S3 gallop), rales, elevation of JVP, and lower extremity edema. The presence of examination findings indicative of left ventricular dysfunction confers a higher clinical risk. Other examination findings may indicate that angina is being precipitated by an extra-cardiac condition, such as goiter, tachycardia, and tremor with thyrotoxicosis; heme-occult positive stool and pallor with anemia of gastrointestinal blood loss; and hypoxia, wheezing, and pursed lip breathing with chronic obstructive pulmonary disease. The clinician must seek out physical examination findings that may indicate potentially life-threatening mimics of angina, such as unequal pulses and aortic regurgitation murmur with aortic dissection, pulsus paradoxus with cardiac tamponade, and unequal breath sounds with pneumothorax. In patients presenting with UA, the physical examination is often normal (9).

Risk Stratification and Management of Unstable Angina

Providing the highest quality evidence-based care for patients with UA depends largely on a process of continuous risk stratification. Initially, early risk stratification determines the appropriate level of care. Thereafter, whether to use certain medicines such as glycoprotein IIb/IIIa (GP IIb/IIIa) inhibitors, low-molecular-weight heparin (LMWH), and clopidogrel depends largely on risk stratification. Furthermore, ongoing risk stratification will guide the decision of whether to perform coronary angiography without first obtaining a stress test (the so-called "early invasive" strategy) (10).

Early Risk Stratification, Highest Risk Features (adapted from American College of Cardiology/ American Heart Association [ACC/AHA]* guidelines)

History
1. Prior CAD or MI
2. Prolonged angina at rest
3. Accelerating tempo of angina (more severe pain at a lower threshold)

Physical Examination
1. Hypotension
2. Elevated JVP
3. Pulmonary edema
4. Arrhythmia
5. New or worsened mitral regurgitation murmur

ECG Findings
1. Transient ST-segment elevations
2. ST-segment depressions greater than 0.5 mm while symptomatic
3. Symmetrical precordial T-wave inversions greater than or equal to 2 mm (Wellens sign)

Biomarkers
1. Troponin I elevation
2. Troponin T elevation
3. CK-MB elevation

Early risk stratification is a multifactorial process; the highest risk features from the history, and physical examination are described above. In the absence of ST segment elevations, the two highest risk ECG findings are the presence of ST-segment depressions greater than 0.5 mm while symptomatic, and symmetrical precordial T-wave inversions greater than or equal to 2 mm (11,12). The latter is known as Wellen's sign, and strongly suggests critical stenosis of the left anterior descending artery (13). Other T-wave inversions confer intermediate risk. The presence of elevated cardiac biomarkers in the absence of ST-segment elevations defines NSTEMI. Troponin I and troponin T are more sensitive indicators of myocyte necrosis than CK-MB (14-15). It is estimated that 30% of patients who would otherwise be diagnosed with UA based on negative CK-MB markers actually have NSTEMI, as diagnosed by elevated troponin markers (10). There is great prognostic value in these biomarkers. The GUSTO-IIA investigators showed elevated troponin T level to be the single variable most strongly related to 30-day mortality in patients presenting with acute myocardial ischemia (14). The CK-MB marker remains useful for patients with renal disease, in whom cardiac troponins lose specificity, and for earlier detection of MI. The ACC/AHA recommends repeat CK-MB and troponin biomarker evaluation 6 to 12 hours after the onset of symptoms (10).

The Thrombolysis in Myocardial Infarction (TIMI) score was derived by multivariate logistic regression from two large trials of patients with UA/NSTEMI (ESSENCE and TIMI 11B), and combines features of the history, physical examination, ECG findings, and cardiac biomarker results. It has subsequently been validated in three large trials as a mechanism for risk stratifying patients upon

---

*All ACC/AHA recommendations are class I unless otherwise indicated.

presentation with UA (16). The TIMI risk score is also increasingly useful in determining which patients benefit most from newer therapies such as LMWH, GP IIb/IIIa inhibitors, and early invasive management strategies (described in detail below).

Using the TIMI risk score to define low, intermediate, or high risk is a simple and validated model, however—as the ACC/AHA guidelines emphasize—estimation of risk is a complex and not easily quantifiable problem (10). As such, the TIMI risk score has its potential flaws. For example, a patient with elevated troponin level and ST-depressions, but none of the other findings in Table 49-4, would be considered low risk by the TIMI score. Such a patient would clearly be at increased risk for adverse cardiac events, and for practical purposes should be considered a high-risk patient. Likewise, a patient with either elevated biomarkers or ST-segment depressions, but no other finding from Table 49-4, should be considered at least intermediate risk.

Anti-anginal Therapy

The initial management of UA has two primary goals: relief of anginal symptoms and prevention of infarction or death. Anti-anginal therapy is directed toward improving the oxygen supply to demand ratio. Measures which increase supply include supplemental oxygen and blood transfusion (if angina is secondary to anemia). Measures which decrease demand include β-blocking and calcium channel–blocking drugs. Short-acting dihydropyridines should not be used in the absence of adequate β-blockade, as they have been associated with increased adverse outcomes

(17). Nitroglycerin, morphine, and aortic counterpulsation are therapies that both increase oxygen supply and decrease oxygen demand.

Antiplatelet Therapy

ASA's antiplatelet activity comes from the irreversible inactivation of platelet cyclooxygenase-1, and thus reduction of the prothrombotic cytokine thromboxane A2. Clopidogrel is an antiplatelet agent with a different mechanism of action: irreversible ADP-receptor antagonism. The combination of ASA and clopidogrel is thus referred to as "dual inhibition" of platelet activity (18).

The benefit of ASA for suspected MI was first definitively shown in the ISIS-2 trial (in which the ASA dose was 160 mg) (19). Composite data from multiple trials shows that ASA confers a composite 6.1% absolute risk reduction (ARR) in death or MI over placebo in the setting of NSTE-ACS (see Table 49-5) (10). The ACC/AHA recommends administering 160 to 325 mg of ASA as soon as possible after presentation with suspected UA. Unless contraindicated, ASA should be continued indefinitely (10).

There is evidence from the CURE trial that addition of clopidogrel to ASA reduces the rate of death, stroke, or nonfatal MI in the setting of NSTE-ACS (see Table 49-6). In this trial, clopidogrel was given as a 300-mg loading dose on admission, followed by 75 mg daily thereafter for mean of 9 months. Enrollment criteria included onset of angina within 24 hours, plus either ischemic ECG changes (ST-segment depressions or T-wave inversions) or elevated biomarkers. Importantly, the only component of this

TABLE 49-4

TIMI Risk Factor Score

Risk factors	No of risk factors	% Risk of adverse cardiac event*
1. Age > 65	0–1	4.7
2. = 3 CAD risk factors	2	8.3
3. Prior coronary stenosis = 50%	3	13.2
4. = 2 anginal events in past 24 hrs	4	19.9
5. Aspirin use in past 7 days	5	26.2
6. ST-segment changes	6–7	41
7. Positive cardiac biomarkers		

*Through 14 days after randomization = myocardial infarction, death, severe recurrent ischemia requiring revascularization; CAD risk factors = diabetes, current smoker, hypertension, high cholesterol, family history of CAD; low risk = score 0–2, intermediate risk = score 3–4, high risk = score 5–7.

TABLE 49-5

ASA In Unstable Angina

	Death or MI at variable endpoints*		
ASA	6.4%	ARR	6.1%
Placebo	12.5%	RRR	49%
p value	0.0005	NNT	16.4

RRR, relative risk reduction; NNT, number needed to treat.
*Endpoints range from 5 days to 2 years.

composite endpoint which reached statistical significance was reduction of nonfatal MI. It should also be noted that only 44% of patients in the CURE trial underwent coronary angiography (20). As such, the ACC/AHA recommends initial treatment with clopidogrel in addition to ASA for patients with UA in whom routine angiography is not planned, and to continue clopidogrel for up to 9 months (10). As the inclusion criteria for CURE included either ischemic ST-segment changes or elevated biomarkers, some institutions reserve clopidogrel for patients with at least one of these two findings or an intermediate TIMI risk score.

Of the patients in CURE who underwent angiography, almost half went on to have percutaneous coronary intervention (PCI). This subset of patients was studied in the PCI-CURE trial, in which patients received ASA and clopidogrel versus ASA alone for a median of 10 days prior to PCI (21). All patients then received open-label clopidogrel for 4 weeks after PCI, after which only the study group remained on clopidogrel for a mean of 8 months. The group receiving clopidogrel pretreatment prior to PCI had

TABLE 49-6

Clopidogrel in Unstable Angina

	Cardiovascular death, stroke, or nonfatal MI within 9 months		
Clopidogrel + ASA	9.3%	ARR	2.1%
ASA	11.4%	RRR	20%
p value	<0.001	NNT	47.6

TABLE 49-7

Clopidogrel In Patients with UA Undergoing PCI

	Death or MI at 30 days		
Clopidogrel + ASA	2.9%	ARR	1.5%
ASA	4.4%	RRR	34%
p value	0.04	NNT	66.6

a lower rate of death or MI at 30 days (see Table 49-7). The ACC/AHA recommends treating with clopidogrel in addition to ASA for patients with UA in whom PCI is planned, and to continue treatment for up to 9 months.

In the CURE trial, there was also an increase in major and minor bleeding in the clopidogrel group (see Table 49-8). About 17% of all CURE patients underwent coronary artery bypass graft surgery (CABG); within this group, the risk of major bleeding was greatly increased in the subset of patients who did not stop clopidogrel for at least 5 days prior to CABG. Routine early use of clopidogrel for NSTE-ACS is thus limited primarily by increased major bleeding events in patients undergoing cardiac surgery within 5 days of receiving clopidogrel (20). As such, the

TABLE 49-8

Major Bleeding with Clopidogrel

	Major bleeding in all patients		
Clopidogrel + ASA	3.7%	ARI	1.0%
ASA	2.7%	NNH	100
p value	0.001		
	Major bleeding in surgical patients who stopped taking clopidogrel within 5 days of CABG		
Clopidogrel + ASA	9.6%	ARI	3.3%
ASA	6.3%	NNH	30.3
p value	0.06		

NNH, number needed to harm.

ACC/AHA recommends withholding clopidogrel for at least 5 to 7 days for patients in whom CABG is planned (10). Thus, the practical problem with using clopidogrel routinely in patients with UA is that one cannot predict upon presentation which patients will go on to require CABG. Many institutions who practice routine angiography in UA patients withhold clopidogrel until the coronary anatomy has been visualized.

The GP IIb/IIIa inhibitors abciximab, tirofiban, and eptifibatide inhibit the common final pathway of platelet aggregation—the binding of fibrinogen to platelet GP IIb/IIIa receptors. There is a great body evidence supporting clear benefit of GP IIb/IIIa inhibitors for UA patients undergoing PCI (10). Furthermore, GP IIb/IIIa inhibitors have proven benefits in the medical treatment of UA, but at the expense of increased bleeding complications.

The CAPTURE trial assessed the use of abciximab in UA patients who had received angiography and were awaiting angioplasty (see Table 49-9) (22).

The GUSTO-IV ACS trial failed to show benefit of abciximab in NSTE-ACS populations not undergoing PCI (23). Therefore, abciximab should be reserved for those patients with UA in whom PCI is planned within 24 hours (10).

The PRISM-PLUS trial evaluated the GP IIb/IIIa inhibitor tirofiban, heparin, and their combination in patients with UA. All enrolled patients had angina, plus either ischemic ECG changes or elevated biomarkers. All enrolled patients received concomitant ASA. Patients who received tirofiban got it for 48 hours, and no interventions were done during that time. The group receiving tirofiban alone had excess mortality at 7 days, and this arm of the study was discontinued early. The study showed a mortality/MI

TABLE 49-10

Tirofiban in Unstable Angina

	Death or MI at 30 days		
Tirofiban + heparin + ASA	8.7%	ARR	3.2%
Heparin + ASA	11.9%	RRR	30%
p value	0.03	NNT	31.2

benefit for the group receiving tirofiban plus heparin (see Table 49-10), but also showed a slightly increased risk of major bleeding in this group (see Table 49-11).

Percutaneous transluminal coronary angioplasty (PTCA) was not randomly assigned in this study. However, there was a nonsignificant decrease in death or MI at 30 days in the group of patients receiving the GP IIb/IIIa inhibitor who underwent PTCA (5.9% vs. 10.2%, RR 0.58, CI* 0.29 to 1.09). There was also a nonsignificant decrease of death or MI at 30 days in the group of patients receiving the GP IIb/IIIa inhibitor who did not undergo PTCA (7.8% vs. 10.1%, RR 0.77, CI 0.46 to 1.23) (24).

In 2002, the TIMI risk score was applied to the PRISM-PLUS database. The results show a significant reduction of death or MI at 30 days in patients with TIMI risk score of ≥ 4 who received the IIb/IIIa inhibitor (see Tables 49-12 and 49-13) (25).

In the PURSUIT trial, patients with UA were randomized to standard therapy (heparin plus ASA) or standard therapy plus eptifibatide. All patients had angina, plus either ischemic ECG changes or elevated biomarkers. Patients who received eptifibatide got it for 72 hours or until discharge from hospital, whichever came first. The primary endpoint was the composite of death or MI at 30 days, and fewer patients on the GP IIb/IIIa inhibitor reached the endpoint (see Table 49-14).

About 59% of patients in each group underwent angiography within 72 hours; this was at the physicians' discretion (i.e., not randomized). Nearly 24% of patients in each angiography group went on to receive PTCA. Subgroup analysis showed significant reduction in death or MI at 30 days in favor of the GP IIb/IIIa inhibitor group, who underwent PTCA (11.6% vs. 16.7%, p = 0.01). For the

TABLE 49-9

Abciximab in Patients with Unstable Angina Receiving PTCA

	Death or MI at 30 days		
Abciximab + heparin + ASA	4.8%	ARR	4.2%
Heparin + ASA	9.0%	RRR	47%
p value	0.003	NNT	23.8

*All CIs are 95%.

TABLE 49-11

Major Bleeding with Tirofiban

	Major bleeding		
Tirofiban + heparin + ASA	4.0%	ARI	1.0%
Heparin + ASA	3.0%	NNH	100
p value	0.34	p value	NS

TABLE 49-13

Prism-Plus Patients with TIMI Risk Score < 4

	Death or MI at 30 days
Tirofiban + heparin + ASA	6.3%
Heparin + ASA	6.2%
p value	0.97

group not undergoing PTCA, there was a nonsignificant reduction in death or MI at 30 days favoring the GP IIb/IIIa inhibitor group (14.5% vs. 15.6%, p = 0.23). There was an overall significant increase in major bleeding in patients receiving eptifibatide (see Table 49-15) (26).

A meta-analysis of six trials (more than 31,000 patients) involving GP IIb/IIIa inhibitors was undertaken in 2002. As the utility of GP IIb/IIIa inhibitors before and during PCI has been conclusively proven, this analysis focused only on addressing the utility of these drugs as part of the medical (noninvasive) management of UA. This meta-analysis demonstrated that GP IIb/IIIa inhibitors generate a small but significant reduction in death or MI in all patients with UA, but at the expense of increased risk of major bleeding (see Tables 49-16 and 49-17).

Since there is a relatively small overall benefit associated with use of GP IIb/IIIa inhibitors, subgroup analyses may help determine if certain groups of patients derive greater benefit than others in preventing death or MI. The benefit of GP IIb/IIIa inhibitors appears greater in those patients with elevated troponins, but is not statistically significant (9.3% vs. 11.3%; odds ratio [OR] 0.82; confidence interval [CI] 0.65 to 1.03). Editorials have stated that GP IIb/IIIa inhibitors have only been shown to be beneficial

in UA patients with elevated troponins; indeed, in the subgroup of patients with negative troponins, the OR is greater than 1, indicating potential harm (7.6% vs. 6.9%; OR 1.10; CI 0.84 to 1.43) (27). However, once again this is not a statistically significant finding. Any assumption made from this meta-analysis concerning GP IIb/IIIa and troponins is further flawed by the fact that less than half of patients in the analysis (35%) had this lab value measured.

A more consistent—and perhaps more concerning—subgroup finding is that women treated with GP IIb/IIIa inhibitors seem to have more death or MIs at 30 days than women not treated with this therapy (11.5% vs. 10.4%; OR 1.15; CI 1.01 to 1.30). Further studies are needed to clarify the role of GP IIb/IIIa inhibitors in women with UA.

In the meta-analysis, 24% of patients underwent PCI within 30 days of randomization, and 38% of patients had either PCI or CABG. In this subgroup of revascularized patients, the rate of death or MI at 30 days is significantly in favor of the GP IIb/IIIa inhibitor group (14.9% vs. 16.6%; OR 0.89; CI 0.80 to 0.98). In patients not undergoing PCI or CABG, the OR for death or MI at 30 days is still less than 1, but is not statistically significant (28).

In summary, the ACC/AHA recommends giving GP IIb/IIIa inhibitor therapy to UA patients in whom PCI is planned. This may include patients who have already

TABLE 49-12

Prism-Plus Patients with TIMI Risk Score = 4

	Death or MI at 30 days		
Tirofiban + heparin + ASA	10.3%	ARR	5.2%
Heparin + ASA	15.5%	RRR	33.5%
p value	0.016	NNT	19.2

TABLE 49-14

Eptifibatide in Unstable Angina

	Death or MI at 30 days		
Eptifibatide + heparin + ASA	14.2%	ARR	1.5%
Heparin + ASA	15.7%	RRR	9.6%
p value	0.04	NNT	66.6

TABLE 49-15

Major Bleeding with Eptifibatide

	Major bleeding (TIMI scale)		
Eptifibatide + heparin + ASA	10.6%	ARI	1.5%
Heparin + ASA	9.1%	NNH	66.6
p value	0.02	p value	0.02

TABLE 49-17

Bleeding Associated with GP IIB/IIIA Inhibitors

	Major bleeding		
Therapy including GP IIb/IIIa inhibitor	2.4%	ARI	1.0%
Therapy not including GP IIb/IIIa inhibitor	1.4%	NNH	100
p value	<0.0001		

received a diagnostic angiography and are awaiting PCI, or may involve administering the drug just prior to PCI (ie, in the catheterization laboratory). For UA patients not planning on undergoing PCI, and with a TIMI risk score ≥4, elevated troponins, or continuing ischemia, the weight of evidence is in favor of adding tirofiban or eptifibatide to ASA and heparin therapy (ACC/AHA class IIa recommendation). Substantial controversy exists over whether to use eptifibatide or tirofiban in UA patients without evidence of continuing ischemia or other high-risk features (ACC/AHA class IIb recommendation). The use of abciximab in patients not undergoing PCI is not recommended (ACC/AHA class III recommendation) (10).

Anticoagulation Therapy

Heparins bind to the cofactor antithrombin to cause proteolytic inactivation of clotting factors Xa and thrombin. LMWH predominantly catalyzes the inactivation of factor Xa, and has much less interaction with plasma proteins and endothelial cells than unfractionated heparin. Thus, LMWH may be dosed subcutaneously once or twice a day without regular laboratory monitoring of the partial thromboplastin time, potentially a major advantage over unfractionated heparin.

Several early studies evaluating the potential benefit of anticoagulation in UA compared ASA to unfractionated heparin and showed that either agent used alone is effective in reducing adverse outcomes compared to placebo (29-31). A meta-analysis of six studies evaluating ASA and heparin versus ASA alone in patients with UA showed a nearly significant 33% relative risk reduction (p = 0.06) in favor of the heparin group for MI or death at 2 to 12 weeks (32). The ACC/AHA guidelines committee used a standard endpoint of 1 week, and based on similar data found a statistically significant reduction in MI or death in patients treated with ASA and heparin versus ASA alone (see Table 49-18) (10).

LMWH also has proven benefit in patients with UA (see Table 49-19). The Fragmin in Unstable Coronary Artery Disease (FRISC) study evaluated dalteparin in patients with NSTE-ACS (all of whom received ASA and other anti-ischemic medicines), and found a significant reduction in the primary endpoint of death or MI at 6 days in favor of the dalteparin group (33).

Enoxaparin in patients with NSTE-ACS was compared directly with unfractionated heparin in the ESSENCE and

TABLE 49-16

Results of GP IIb/IIIa Inhibitor Meta-Analysis

	Death or MI at 30 days		
Therapy including GP IIb/IIIa inhibitor	10.8%	ARR	1.0%
Therapy not including GP IIb/IIIa inhibitor	11.8%	RRR	8.5%
p value	0.015	NNT	100

TABLE 49-18

Unfractionated Heparin in Unstable Angina

	Death or MI at 1 week		
Heparin + ASA	2.6%	ARR	2.9%
ASA	5.5%	RRR	53%
p value	0.016	NNT	34.5

TABLE 49-19

Low-Molecular-Weight Heparin in Unstable Angina

	Death or MI at 6 days		
Delteparin + ASA	1.8%	ARR	3%
ASA	4.8%	RRR	63%
p value	0.001	NNT	33.3

TIMI 11B studies, and shows a significant reduction in both studies in the composite endpoint of death, MI, or recurrent angina at 8 (TIMI 11B) to 14 (ESSENCE) days. However, neither study reached statistical significance for the endpoint of death, MI, or both (34,35). Two additional studies (FRIC and FRAXIS) showed no benefit, and even noticed a trend toward poorer outcomes, in NSTE-ACS patients treated with LMWH when compared with patients receiving unfractionated heparin (36,37). LMWH is also less easily reversed with protamine than is unfractionated heparin, and does not facilitate monitoring of activated clotting time in the catheterization laboratory. The ACC/AHA feels that the weight of evidence favors the use LMWH over unfractionated heparin in the initial treatment of UA unless CABG is planned within 24 hours (class IIa recommendation) (10).

In the same paper in which the TIMI risk score is described, it is noted that higher TIMI risk scores correlated with greater benefit of enoxaparin over unfractionated heparin in preventing a composite endpoint of mortality, MI, and severe recurrent ischemia (16).

Early Conservative Versus Early Invasive Management Strategies

Traditionally there has been a general consensus that patients presenting with UA should receive initial medical management for up to 48 hours. As described above, this includes—unless contraindicated—anti-ischemic, antiplatelet, anticoagulant, and β-blocking agents. GP IIb/IIIa agents should be used if indicated. This "cooling off" period of medical management should not be confused with the so called "early conservative" management strategy. In the early conservative strategy, coronary angiography is ischemia driven; that is, only patients who manifest continued signs of ischemia during the "cooling off"

period or who have a positive cardiac stress test undergo coronary angiography. In the early invasive approach, stress testing is bypassed and coronary angiography is performed on all patients after the initial medical management period.

During the initial period of medical management, the patient is continuously reevaluated and risk stratified by physical examination, cardiac monitoring, ECGs, cardiac biomarkers, and response to anti-anginal therapy. There are several high-risk scenarios in which an early invasive strategy has been shown to be beneficial.

The ACC/AHA recommends an early invasive approach if any of the following occurs during the period of initial medical management:

1. Recurrent angina/ischemia at low level of activity despite intensive anti-ischemic therapy

2. Troponin elevation

3. New ST-segment depression

4. Recurrent angina/ischemia with CHF symptoms, an S3 gallop, pulmonary edema, worsening rales, or new or worsening mitral regurgitation

5. Depressed left ventricular systolic function, defined as ejection fraction less than 40%

6. Hemodynamic instability

7. Sustained ventricular tachycardia

In the absence of these findings, and without a history of prior CABG or PCI within the past 6 months, the ACC/AHA recommends either the early conservative or the early invasive management strategies (10). Previous studies showing no benefit to the early invasive strategy may have been skewed by the risk of death or MI because of acute thrombosis or vessel stenosis in the setting of PTCA without stents and GP IIb/IIIa inhibitors (38,39). The more modern FRISC II and TACTICS-TIMI 18 trials provide strong evidence that the early invasive approach reduces the rate of death or MI at 30 days in patients with UA. A prespecified sub-analysis in the TACTICS-TIMI 18 trial showed that patients with TIMI risk score of ≥3 (intermediate or high risk) derived significant benefit from the early invasive approach, while those with low TIMI risk derived equal benefit from either approach (40,41). It is important to note that in the TACTICS-TIMI 18 trial, all patients received "upstream" tirofiban therapy prior to coronary angiography (for an average of 22 hours). The optimum time to start GP IIb/IIIa inhibition prior to early invasive approach remains undefined (10).

Selected References

1. Diamond GA, Forrester JS. Analysis of probability as an aid in the clinical diagnosis of coronary-artery disease. *N Engl J Med.* 1979;300:1350–1358.

2. Braunwald E. Unstable angina: an etiologic approach to management. *Circulation.* 1999;98:2219–2222.

3. Foreman RD. Mechanisms of cardiac pain. *Annu Rev Physiol.* 1999;61:143–167.

4. Lee TH, Cook EF, Weisberg M, et al. Acute chest pain in the emergency room. Identification and examination of low-risk patients. *Arch Intern Med.* 1985;145:65–69.

5. Gibbons RJ, Chatterjee K, Daley J, et al. ACC/AHA/ACP-ASIM guidelines for the management of patients with chronic stable angina. *J Am Coll Cardiol.* 1999;33:2092–2197.

6. Campeau L. Letter: grading of angina pectoris. *Circulation.* 1976;54:522–523.

7. Braunwald E. Unstable angina. A classification. *Circulation.* 1989;80:410–414.

8. Braunwald E, Antman EM, Beasley JW, et al. ACC/AHA guidelines for the management of patients with unstable angina and non-ST-segment elevation myocardial infarction. *J Am Coll Cardiol.* 2000;36:970–1062.

9. Runge MS, Ohman EM. The history and physical examination. In: Runge M, ed. *Netter's Cardiology.* 1st Ed. Teterboro, NJ: Saunders; 2005: chap. 1.

10. Braunwald E, Antman EM, Beasley JW, et al. ACC/AHA 2002 Guideline update for the management of patients with unstable angina and non-ST-segment elevation myocardial infarction. *J Am Coll Cardiol* 2007;50:e1–157.

11. Hyde TA, French JK, Wong CK, et al. Four-year survival of patients with acute coronary syndromes without ST-segment elevation and prognostic significance of 0.5-mm ST-segment depression. *Am J Cardiol.* 1999;84:379–385.

12. Cannon CP, McCabe CH, Stone PH, et al. The electrocardiogram predicts one-year outcome of patients with unstable angina and non-Q wave myocardial infarction: results of the TIMI III Registry ECG Ancillary Study. Thrombolysis in myocardial ischemia. *J Am Coll Cardiol.* 1997;30:133–140.

13. de Zwaan C, Bar FW, Janssen JH, et al. Angiographic and clinical characteristics of patients with unstable angina showing an ECG pattern indicating critical narrowing of the proximal LAD coronary artery. *Am Heart J.* 1989;117:657–665.

14. Ohman EM, Armstrong PW, Christenson RH, et al. for the GUSTO IIA Investigators. Cardiac troponin T levels for risk stratification in acute myocardial ischemia. *N Engl J Med.* 1996;335:1333–1341.

15. Antman EM, Tanasijevic MJ, Thompson B, et al. Cardiac-specific troponin I levels to predict the risk of mortality in patients with acute coronary syndromes. *N Engl J Med.* 1996;335:1342–1349.

16. Antman EM, Cohen M, Bernink PJ, et al. The TIMI risk score for unstable angina/non-ST elevation MI: a method for prognostication and therapeutic decision making. *JAMA.* 2000;284:835–842.

17. Furberg CD, Psaty BM, Meyer JV. Nifedipine: dose-related increase in mortality in patients with coronary heart disease. *Circulation.* 1995;1326–1331.

18. Steinhubl SR, Berger PB, Mann JT, III, et al. for the CREDO Investigators. Early and sustained dual oral antiplatelet therapy following percutaneous coronary intervention. *JAMA.* 2002;288:2411–2420.

19. ISIS-2 Collaborative Group. Randomised trial of intravenous streptokinase, oral aspirin, both, or neither among 17,187 cases of suspected acute myocardial infarction: ISIS-2. *Lancet.* 1988;2:349–360.

20. The CURE Trial Investigators. Effects of clopidogrel in addition to aspirin in patients with acute coronary syndrome without ST-segment elevation. *N Engl J Med.* 2001;345:494–502.

21. Mehta SR, Yusuf S, Peters RJ, et al. Effects of pretreatment with clopidogrel and aspirin followed by long-term therapy in patients undergoing percutaneous coronary intervention: the PCI-CURE study. *Lancet.* 2001;358:527–533.

22. The CAPTURE Investigators. Randomised placebo controlled trial of abciximab before and during coronary intervention in refractory unstable angina: the CAPTURE study. *Lancet.* 1997;349:1429–1435.

23. GUSTO IV-ACS Investigators. Effect of glycoprotein IIb/IIIa receptor blocker abciximab on outcome in patients with acute coronary syndromes without early coronary revascularisation: the GUSTO IV-ACS randomised trial. *Lancet.* 2001;357:1915–1924.

24. The PRISM-PLUS Investigators. Inhibition of the platelet glycoprotein IIb/IIIa receptor with tirofiban in unstable angina and non-Q-wave myocardial infarction. *N Engl J Med.* 1998;338:1488–1497.

25. Morrow DA, Antman EA, Snapinn SM, et al. An integrated clinical approach to predicting the benefit of tirofiban in non-ST elevation acute coronary syndromes. *Eur Heart J.* 2002;23:223–229.

26. The PURSUIT Trial Investigators. Inhibition of platelet glycoprotein IIb/IIIa with eptifibatide in patients with acute coronary syndromes. *N Engl J Med.* 1998;339:436–443.

27. Harding SA, Boon NA, Flapan AD. Antiplatelet treatment in unstable angina: aspirin, clopidogrel, glycoprotein IIb/IIIa antagonist, or all three? *Heart.* 2002;88:11–14.

28. Boersma E, Harrington RA, Moliterno DJ, et al. Platelet glycoprotein IIb/IIIa inhibitors in acute coronary syndromes: a meta-analysis of all major randomized clinical trials. *Lancet.* 2002;359:189–198.

29. Theroux P, Ouimet H, McCans J, et al. Aspirin, heparin, or both to treat acute unstable angina. *N Engl J Med.* 1988;319:1105–1111.

30. The RISC Group. Risk of myocardial infarction and death during treatment with low dose aspirin and intravenous heparin in men with unstable coronary artery disease. *Lancet.* 1990;336:827–830.

31. Cohen M, Adams PC, Parry G, et al. Combination antithrombotic therapy in unstable rest angina and non-Q-wave myocardial infarction in nonprior aspirin users. Primary endpoints from the ATACS trial. *Circulation.* 1994;89:81–88.

32. Oler A, Whooley MA, Oler J, et al. Adding heparin to aspirin reduces the incidence of myocardial infarction and death in patients with unstable angina: a meta-analysis. *JAMA.* 1996;276:811–815.

33. FRISC Study Group. Low-molecular-weight heparin during instability in coronary artery disease. *Lancet.* 1996;347:561–568.

34. Cohen M, Demers C, Gurfinkel EP, et al. A comparison of low-molecular-weight heparin with unfractionated heparin for unstable coronary artery disease. *N Engl J Med.* 1997;337: 447–452.

35. Antman EM, McCabe CH, Gurfinkel EP, et al. Enoxaparin prevents death and cardiac ischemic events in unstable angina/non-Q-wave myocardial infarction. Results of the thrombolysis in myocardial infarction IIB trial. *Circulation.* 1999;100:1593–1601.

36. Klein W, Buchwald A, Hillis SE, et al. Comparison of low-molecular-weight heparin with unfractionated heparin acutely and with placebo for 6 weeks in the management of unstable coronary artery disease. Fragmin in unstable coronary artery disease (FRISC) study. *Circulation.* 1997;96:61–68.

37. The FRAX.I.S. Study Group. Comparison of two treatment durations (6 days and 14 days) of a low molecular weight heparin with a 6-day treatment of unfractionated heparin in the initial management of unstable angina or non-Q wave myocardial infarction: FRAX.I.S. (FRAxiparine in Ischaemic Syndrome). *Eur Heart J.* 1999;20:1553–1562.

38. Boden WE, O'Rourke RA, Crawford MH, et al for the VANQWISH Trial Investigators. Outcomes in patients with acute non-Q-wave myocardial infarction randomly assigned to an invasive as compared with a conservative management strategy. *N Engl J Med.* 1998;338:1785–1792.

39. McCullough PA, O'Neill WW, Graham M, et al. A prospective randomized trial of triage angiography in acute coronary syndromes ineligible for thrombolytic therapy. Results of the MATE trial. *J Am Coll Cardiol.* 1998;32:596–605.

40. FRISC II Investigators. Long-term low-molecular-mass heparin in unstable coronary-artery disease: FRISC II prospective randomised multicentre study. *Lancet.* 1999;354: 701–707.

41. Cannon C, Weintraub WS, Demopoulos LA, et al for the TACTICS-TIMI 18 Investigators. Comparison of early invasive and conservative strategies in patients with unstable coronary syndromes treated with the glycoprotein IIb/IIIa inhibitor tirofiban. *N Engl J Med.* 2001;344:1879–1887.

54-Year-Old Female with Shortness of Breath and Fatigue

CASE PRESENTATION

A 54-year-old female with a history of diabetes mellitus, hypothyroidism, hypertension, and longstanding medical noncompliance presented to her primary care physician with a 3-day history of shortness of breath, altered mental status, and fatigue. She and her family denied any history of chest discomfort, long distance travel, changes in medication, sick contacts, headache, fevers, or chills. Initial vital signs were reportedly unremarkable, but routine chemistries revealed acute on chronic renal failure and anion gap acidosis. She was sent to the emergency department for further evaluation and treatment.

Physical Examination

Patient was an obese female in bed, lethargic and incoherent. Vital signs: temperature 32.7°C, pulse 110 beats/min, respiratory rate 20 breaths/min, blood pressure 108/72 mm Hg, oxygen saturation 92% on 4 L nasal canula. Head, eyes, ears, nose, and throat examination revealed a large tongue; no lymphadenopathy or thyroid masses were noted. Heart examination revealed tachycardia, and lung examination revealed faint crackles in bilateral bases. No organomegaly or peritoneal signs. Nonpitting edema was noted over the patient's lower extremities and abdomen. Reflexes could not be elicited, and Babinski was absent bilaterally. Otherwise, examination was unremarkable.

Laboratory Studies

Arterial blood gas on 4 L oxygen/minute via nasal cannula showed a pH of 7.01, PCO_2 of 14, PO_2 of 87, and base balance of −25.7. White blood cells count was 9.6 with absolute neutrophil count of 7.7, hematocrit 27.0, platelets 239. Chemistries: Na 140, K 4.8, Cl 109, CO_2 of 10, blood urea nitrogen 96, creatinine 10.6, Ca 7.1, P 9.8, thyroid-stimulating hormone (TSH) 81.60, Pro-brain natriuretic peptide greater than 70,000, creatine kinase (CK) 451, creatine kinase MB (CK-MB) 8.0, troponin T 0.201. Chest x-ray revealed mild cardiomegaly without evidence of significant infiltrate or pulmonary vascular congestion.

Case Resolution

Nephrology was consulted to initiate urgent hemodialysis and she was started on broad antibiotic coverage for presumed sepsis. She received IV fluids containing sodium bicarbonate ($NaHCO_3$), and IV methylprednisolone and levothyroxine were given. Within hours of her presentation, she became progressively hypotensive and hypoxic despite adequate resuscitative measures. She was intubated, had central venous access established and arterial cannulation was performed for invasive blood pressure monitoring. The patient subsequently received vasopressors, including dobutamine, levophed, vasopressin, and epinephrine. Despite aggressive measures, she expired within 24 hours of presentation from presumed myxedema coma.

Question

What is the classic triad associated with myxedema coma?

Answer

Myxedema coma is hypothyroidism with associated (1) altered mental status, (2) defective thermoregulation, and (3) precipitating event or illness. Altered mental status can be mild to severe. Defective thermoregulation may present as hypothermia or inappropriate normal body temperature.

Precipitating event can be anything from infection to drugs to trauma, but infections, particularly pneumonia, is the most common event.

Discussion

Thyroid disorders are common chronic medical problems encountered in many general medicine outpatient clinics. Hypothyroidism in particular occurs in approximately 1.5% of women and 0.2% of men (1). This incidence increases with age; women and men older than age 60 have a prevalence hypothyroidism (by measurement of TSH greater than twice the upper limit of normal) of 6% and 2.5%, respectively (3). Levothyroxine is currently the third most commonly prescribed drug in the United States (2). Given the ubiquity of hypothyroidism, the primary care physician must know how to appropriately recognize and treat thyroid-associated emergencies.

Myxedema coma is understood to be the result of decompensated hypothyroidism. Typical patients are untreated or inadequately treated elderly females. It is more likely to present in the winter months (4). Etiologies vary, but post-ablative hypothyroidism is a less common cause. Occasionally, therapeutic patients may convert to hypothyroid (and subsequent myxedema coma) after the addition of amiodarone or lithium to a patient's medical regimen (5–7).

Since clinical presentations vary, myxedema coma can be recognized by the triad of mental status changes, and hypothermia with a precipitating event. Mental status changes may range from apathy or neglect to psychosis. Only rarely does the patient present with coma. Family may relate a gradual decline in mental status over weeks to months.

Hypothermia can be mild to severe, though usually measured temperature on presentation is less than 35.5°C (95.9°F). This is related to impaired thermoregulation, and in part explains why the incidence of myxedema coma is higher in winter months. Presenting temperature may be normal, however, especially in the setting of an infectious cause as the precipitating event.

Precipitating events vary (see Table 50-1); in addition to infection (pneumonia is most common), other causes include cold exposure, myocardial infarctions (MI), congestive heart failure, cerebrovascular accident, blood loss, or respiratory depression from drugs such as anesthetics or sedatives, especially opiates.

Physical examination will likely reveal sequelae of long-standing hypothyroidism, including dry skin, nonpitting

TABLE 50-1

Precipitating Events in Myxedema Coma

Infectious — bacterial pneumonia, sepsis, urinary tract infection (UTI), influenza

Cardiovascular — MI, CHF exacerbation, CVA

Physical — trauma, surgical procedure

Hypothermia

Hypoglycemia

Medicines — amiodarone, anesthesia, barbiturates, β-blockers, diuretics, lithium, narcotics, phenothiazines, phenytoin, rifampin, tranquilizers

Adapted from Myxedema coma: diagnosis and treatment. Am Fam Physician. *2000 Dec 1;62(11):2485–2490.*

body edema, periorbital edema, delayed relaxation of motor reflexes, loss of eyebrows, pleural/pericardial effusions, and ascites. Routine laboratory examinations may reveal signs of hypoventilation, which is thought to be secondary to decreased respiratory drive to hypercapnia and hypoxia. Hyponatremia, a common finding, is secondary to elevated vasopressin levels.

Most patients with myxedema coma require intensive care unit (ICU) care. Intensive supportive measures, including mechanical ventilation, invasive blood pressure monitoring, vasopressor support, and emergent hemodialysis for refractory acidosis is often warranted. The mainstay of therapy, however, must include intravenous thyroid hormone replacement. Most sources recommend IV T4, given as a 400 mcg IV load, followed by 100 mcg daily. Stress dose glucocorticoids are also indicated until adrenal insufficiency has been ruled out. The patient should be warmed gradually. Warming blankets should be avoided, as resulting vasodilation can worsen the likely hypovolemic state.

With adequate therapy, mortality from myxedema coma has decreased from 80% to 20%–30% (8). Severe vital sign abnormalities, advanced age, bradycardia, persistent hypothermia is all associated with a worse prognosis.

Selected References

1. Tunbridge WM, Evered DC, Hall R, et al. The spectrum of thyroid disease in a community: the Whickham survey. *Clin Endocrinol (Oxf).* 1977;7:481–493.
2. Wysowski DK, Governale LA, Swann J. Trends in outpatient prescription drug use and related costs in the US: 1998–2003. *Pharmacoeconomics.* 2006;24(3):233–236.

3. Sawin CT, Castelli WP, Hershman JM, et al. The aging thyroid. Thyroid deficiency in the Framingham Study. *Arch Intern Med.* 1985;145:1386–1388.

4. Davis PJ, Davis FB. Hypothyroidism in the elderly. *Compr Ther.* 1984;10:17–23.

5. Santiago R, Rashkin MC. Lithium toxicity and myxedema coma in an elderly woman. *J Emerg Med.* 1990;8:63.

6. Waldman SA, Park D. Myxedema coma associated with lithium therapy. *Am J Med.* 1989;87:355.

7. Mazonson PD, Williams ML, Cantley LK, et al. Myxedema coma during long-term amiodarone therapy. *Am J Med.* 1984;77:751.

8. Jordan RM. Myxedema coma. Pathophysiology, therapy, and factors affecting prognosis. *Med Clin N Am.* 1995;79:185–194.

60-Year-Old Female with Palpitations, Fatigue, and Night Sweats

CASE PRESENTATION

A 60-year-old woman with a history of coronary artery disease, hyperlipidemia, and atrial fibrillation presents to a local emergency department with three episodes of heart palpitations. The patient recognizes these episodes as atrial fibrillation, and she has not experienced any other symptoms, including presyncope, shortness of breath, or chest pain. The episodes lasted between 1 and 6 hours each and they resolved spontaneously. She was diagnosed with atrial fibrillation about 18 months ago and was started on amiodarone therapy, and since converting to normal sinus rhythm she has been asymptomatic until these most recent episodes. She normally works during the day and then leads an active life at home. For example, she regularly mows the lawn and cares for her granddaughter. In contrast, she feels increasingly "run down" over the past 2 weeks, stating, "I've gone to bed at 7:30 for the past few nights." She has not gone to work for the past week because of the fatigue. She denies any acute shortness of breath, but says that she does become dyspneic with exertion more than usual during the present illness. She denies wheezing, cough, and edema. The patient has not experienced flushing, tachycardia, except during the episodes of atrial fibrillation, fevers, tremor, or vision changes. She has some sweating at night and has lost 3 or 4 lb in the last 2 weeks. The patient does not have a prior history of thyroid dysfunction, and the only significant family history includes early-onset coronary artery disease in the patient's father. She has a 20-pack/year smoking history, but quit 10 years ago after she received a bare-metal coronary artery stent. The patient does not use alcohol or illicit drugs. The patient takes warfarin for her history of atrial fibrillation.

Physical Examination

The patient is well-appearing and in no acute distress. Vital signs: temperature 36.4°C, blood pressure 110/65 mm Hg, pulse 78 beats/min (regular), respiratory rate 16 breaths/min, oxygen saturation while breathing room air 95%. Head, eyes, ears, nose, and throat examination is normocephalic, atraumatic, pupils equal, round, and reactive to light, mucous membranes moist, oropharynx is without erythema or exudate, partial denture is intact, sclerae are non-icteric. Neck is supple, carotid pulses 2+ bilaterally, no bruits. Thyroid is mildly enlarged, nontender, no palpable nodules. There was no lymphadenopathy in the submandibular, anterior cervical, posterior cervical, axillary, or inguinal areas. Cardiovascular examination demonstrates regular rate and rhythm, no murmurs, rubs or gallops, normal S_1 and S_2, pulses 2+ bilaterally in radials and dorsalis pedis. Lungs are clear to auscultation bilaterally with normal work of breathing. Abdomen is soft, nontender, and nondistended, normal active bowel sound auscultated, no organomegaly. Extremities show no edema. Neurologically the patient's cranial nerve II to XII intact grossly, strength 5/5 bilaterally in upper and lower extremities, sensation intact throughout, however deep tendon reflexes in bilateral patellar, biceps, and Achilles tendons are 3+.

Laboratory Studies

Serum chemistries show Na 143, K 3.7, Cl 110, HCo_3 27, blood urea nitrogen 19, creatinine (Cr) 0.8, glucose 105, calcium 9.2, magnesium (Mg) 1.9, phosphorous 3.9, total protein 6.1, albumin 2.9, prothrombin time 40.5, international normalized ratio 3.9, partial thromboplastin time 47.5, thyroid-stimulating hormone (TSH) less than 0.01, total thyroxine (T4) 22.5 mcg/dL (elevated), free T4 11.7 (elevated), antithyroid microsomal antibody negative, thyroid-stimulating antibody negative, IL-6 normal. Chest x-ray is normal. Thyroid ultrasound shows an enlarged gland with no abnormal blood flow and no nodules.

Case Resolution

The patient was started on methimazole and prednisone and monitored for hyperthyroid crisis (thyroid storm). She did not develop tachycardia, further episodes of atrial fibrillation, vomiting, diarrhea, fever, or mental status changes. The patient's T4 and T3 levels did not decline despite the therapeutic interventions, so a thyroidectomy was performed. She is now taking levothyroxine and is without significant symptoms, including atrial fibrillation.

Question

What caused this patient's thyrotoxicosis?

Answer

The differential diagnosis for thyrotoxicosis includes amiodarone-induced thyrotoxicosis (AIT), autoimmune thyroid disease (Graves disease), autonomous thyroid tissue (toxic adenoma, toxic multinodular goiter), TSH-producing pituitary adenoma, subacute granulomatous or lymphocytic thyroiditis, exogenous thyroid hormone administration, and metastatic follicular thyroid cancer. In this patient's case, the cause is most likely to be amiodarone, but she may also have other underlying thyroid disease.

Discussion

The differential diagnosis of thyrotoxicosis, defined as a state of thyroid hormone excess, is broad (Table 51-1). In many cases however, a good history and physical examination can help narrow the possibilities. Thyrotoxicosis is not necessarily synonymous with hyperthyroidism, although hyperthyroidism can cause thyrotoxicosis. Thyrotoxicosis is diagnosed by measuring a low serum value for TSH combined with an elevation of free T4, free T3, or free thyroxine index. Once the diagnosis of thyrotoxicosis is made, a radioactive iodine uptake scan can be performed which may be helpful in delineating a cause (Table 51-1).

In this case, the patient is taking a medicine known to cause multiple toxicities including thyroid disease. Amiodarone, which contains iodine, causes thyroid disease (both hypo- and hyperthyroidism) both by intrinsic effects of the drug and by serving as a source of iodine; the resulting thyroid disorder depends partly on the presence of any underlying thyroid disease. In early studies of higher dose amiodarone therapy, the incidence of AIT is as high as 15% to 20%, but studies of lower doses like those used in this patient show an incidence of 3.7% with at least 1 year of therapy.

The intrinsic effects of amiodarone on thyroid function include inhibition of T4 conversion to T3, blocking of nuclear T3 receptors, and a direct thyrotoxic effect that leads to a destructive thyroiditis. The first two actions contribute directly to clinical hypothyroidism; the third action leads first to hyperthyroidism, usually followed by a hypothyroid period and eventual recovery to a euthyroid state. The hyperthyroid period caused by an amiodarone-induced destructive thyroiditis is categorized as a Type II AIT (Table 51-2).

In addition to its intrinsic effects, amiodarone also affects thyroid function by supplying iodine. The average daily dietary intake of iodine is 0.3 mg; taking 200 mg of amiodarone per day increases the daily intake to approximately 6 mg. This iodine affects the thyroid in different ways, depending on individual genetic susceptibility as well as the presence of underlying disease. In some individuals, increased iodine intake can lead to Hashimotos thyroiditis; in those who already have Hashimotos disease, increased iodine can worsen their hypothyroidism by exacerbating the autoimmune response against the thyroid. In those with Graves disease, increased iodine can also cause an autoimmune response against the thyroid, which can lead to relief of the hyperthyroidism. In those with autonomous thyroid tissue, such as in nodular goiter, increased iodine intake leads to unregulated increases in production of both T3 and T4. This iodine-induced hyperthyroidism is categorized as Type I AIT.

TABLE 51-1

Causes of Thyrotoxicosis

Etiology	Comments
Thyrotoxicosis from hyperthyroidism	
1. Hyperthyroidism	
Common	
Graves disease	Autoimmune – presence of thyroid-stimulating immunoglobulin in serum. Increased and diffuse uptake on radioactive iodine uptake scan. May have ophthalmopathy. About 60% to 80% cases of thyrotoxicosis
Toxic multinodular goiter	Normal to increased radioactive iodine uptake by thyroid with areas of increased and decreased uptake. Thyroperoxidase antibodies absent
Toxic adenoma	Normal to increased radioactive iodine uptake by thyroid with "hot" area on scan. Thyroperoxidase antibodies absent
Rare	
Excess iodine	
Thyroid cancer metastases	
Struma ovarii	Ovarian teratoma that differentiates into thyroid tissue
2. Hyperthyroidism	
Molar pregnancy	Human chorionic gonadotropin (β-HCG) stimulates thyroid gland
Gestational thyrotoxicosis	β-HCG stimulates thyroid gland. Scan contraindicated in pregnancy
TSH-secreting pituitary lesion	Usually an adenoma of the pituitary gland
Thyrotoxicosis without hyperthyroidism	
Excess exogenous thyroid hormone administration	*Thyrotoxicosis facticia* produces low-to-undetectable radioactive iodine uptake by thyroid and low serum thymoglobulin values
Subacute thyroiditis	Low-to-undetectable radioactive iodine uptake by thyroid
Amiodarone-induced thyrotoxicosis	Low-to-undetectable radioactive iodine uptake by thyroid with history of amiodarone ingestion (see Table 51-2)
Postpartum thyroiditis (lymphocytic)	Low-to-undetectable radioactive iodine uptake by thyroid and present thyroperoxidase antibodies
Other drug induced	Lithium, interferon
Other causes of thyroid destruction	Radiation, destruction via infarction. Low-to-undetectable radioactive iodine uptake by thyroid

The typical clinical presentation of AIT includes recurrence of arrhythmias including atrial fibrillation, exacerbation of ischemic heart disease, congestive heart failure (CHF) exacerbations, weight loss, restlessness, and fever. These symptoms can sometimes be masked by amiodarone's β-blocking activity, as well as amiodarone's intrinsic ability to block T3 production and receptor activity, as mentioned above. This fact often makes it difficult to distinguish between Type I and Type II AIT.

Several methods of distinguishing between the two types of AIT have been described (Table 51-2). Radioactive iodine uptake is usually decreased or absent in Type II, so normal uptake suggests Type I AIT. Similarly, decreased thyroid vascularity as measured by color flow Doppler ultrasonography is associated with Type II. Type II is less commonly associated with a large goiter. Serum thyroglobulin is usually increased in Type I, while markedly increased serum IL-6 levels suggest Type II disease. Presence of antithyroid antibodies are associated with Type I disease. Our patient does not have a large goiter on examination. She had a thyroid ultrasound (U/S) that did not show increased vascularity; her serum IL-6 was normal; and her anti-thyroid

TABLE 51-2

Classification of Amiodarone-Induced Thyrotoxicosis

	Type I AIT	Type II AIT
Length of amiodarone therapy	1–2 years	> 2 years
Goiter on examination	Yes with nodules	Normal thyroid that may be tender
Preexisting thyroid disease	Yes — toxic multinodular goiter or Graves disease	Oftentimes no
Thyroid autoantibodies	Usually absent unless Graves disease is present	Usually absent
Doppler	Increased blood flow	Normal or decreased blood flow
Radioactive iodine uptake	Any pattern	Low
Serum IL-6	Slightly increased	Markedly increased
Responds to thionamides or perchlorate	Yes	No
Responds to glucocorticoids	No	Yes
Hypothyroidism after resolution	No	Often

Adapted from Daniels GH. Amiodarone-induced thyrotoxicosis. J Clin Endocrinol Metab. *2001;85(1):3–8; Basaria S, Cooper DS.* Amiodarone and the thyroid. Am J Med. *2005 Jul;118(7):706–714.*

antibody tests were negative. Treatment depends on the type of AIT. In either case, amiodarone therapy should be stopped if it is not absolutely essential. However, the long half-life (~100 days) of amiodarone means that simply stopping the medication will not have any effect on AIT in the short term. Therefore, Type I is treated with an antithyroid medication such as methimazole, and potassium perchlorate can also be added to this regimen. Type II is treated with glucocorticoids. In a small prospective study of 24 patients with AIT, those with Type I were shown to return to normal free T3 levels in 4 weeks with methimazole and potassium perchlorate therapy. Those with Type II recovered more quickly, taking an average of 8 days to return to normal T3 levels. Since it was not immediately clear from which type of AIT the patient described above was suffering, she was treated with both methimazole and prednisone. If she had responded rapidly (ie, free T3 levels decrease within the next few days), she would have been more likely to have Type II AIT. Because she did not respond within 2 to 3 days and continued to have very high levels of circulating thyroid hormone, surgery was consulted for consideration of a thyroidectomy.

Another important consideration in management of this patient is monitoring for thyroid crisis, also known as thyroid storm. This would be manifested as tachycardia, possible atrial fibrillation, nausea/vomiting, diarrhea, hepatic failure, jaundice, fever, and mental status changes. Treatment, which would necessitate close monitoring in an intensive care unit, would include some combination of high-dose methimazole and steroids, a β-blocker, an iodinated radiocontrast agent (to reduce peripheral conversion of T4 to T3), and infusion of iodine solution (to decrease thyroid release of T4 and T3).

In summary, amiodarone is a commonly used antiarrhythmic agent with various serious side effects that include thyroid dysfunction. Recurrence of arrhythmias after being on amiodarone for a prolonged period of time should prompt clinicians to evaluate the thyroid as part of the patient's diagnostic workup. Treatment of AIT, if present, depends on the clinical subtype, so further studies are usually necessary to guide therapy.

Selected References

1. Trip MD, Wiersinga W, Plomp TA. Incidence, predictability, and pathogenesis of amiodarone-induced thyrotoxicosis and hypothyroidism. *Am J Med.* 1991 Nov;91(5):507–511.
2. Daniels GH. Amiodarone-induced thyrotoxicosis. *J Clin Endocrinol Metab.* 2001;85(1):3–8.
3. Pearce EN. Diagnosis and management of thyrotoxicosis. *BMJ.* 2006 Jun 10;332(7554):1369–1373.
4. Bartalena L, Brogioni S, Grasso L, et al. Treatment of amiodarone-induced thyrotoxicosis, a difficult challenge: Results of a prospective study. *J Clin Endocrinol Metab.* 1996 Aug;81(8):2930–2933.
5. Jameson JL, Weetman AP. Disorders of the thyroid gland. In: Kasper DL, Braunwald E, Fauci AS, et al. (eds) *Harrison's Principles of Internal Medicine.* 16th ed. New York: McGraw Hill; 2005: 2104–2127: chap. 320.
6. Basaria S, Cooper DS. Amiodarone and the thyroid. *Am J Med.* 2005 Jul;118(7):706–714.

2-Year-Old Female with Fever and Nystagmus

CASE PRESENTATION

You are called by the emergency department to admit a 2-year-old female with suspected meningitis. According to the mother, a poor historian, the toddler has been healthy until 14 days ago, when the child had poor oral intake and diminished activity. The mother took the child to her primary doctor. The child was diagnosed with streptococcal pharyngitis without throat culture or rapid antigen testing, and given a prescription for penicillin VK. Mother gave the child approximately half of the prescription of the antibiotic, but stopped it when the child appeared to have recovered from the initial illness. She now comes to the emergency room (ER) because the child "felt warm, is crying all the time, and is extra sleepy." Further history elicits that the child has had normal growth and development, immunizations are up-to-date, and no prior serious illnesses or hospitalizations. Family history is noncontributory, and there are four other children in the house who have all been healthy (ages 5 to 15). Review of systems reveals decreased oral intake but good urine output, no viral symptoms except a little rhinorrhea, and difficulty walking for 3 to 4 days. No fevers, diarrhea, or cough have been present.

Physical Examination

The patient is a mildly ill-appearing African American female. She is irritable with a strong cry, and makes good eye contact. Vital signs: temperature 37.3°C, heart rate 146 beats/min, blood pressure 96/68 mm Hg, respiratory rate 26 breaths/min. Head, eyes, ears, nose, and throat examination shows an erythematous oropharynx without tonsillar enlargement or exudates. Multiple small posterior cervical lymph nodes are present. The infant does appear to have meningismus (holds her neck stiff and resists active cervical range of motion testing), but her irritability makes for a difficult examination. Heart, lung, and abdominal examinations are normal. Skin examination shows poorly treated eczema but no other rash, petechiae, or other lesions. Neurologic examination is significant for no focal deficits, brisk reflexes in the lower extremities (2–3+), and the child refuses to walk in the ER.

Laboratory Studies

Complete blood count shows a white blood cell (WBC) count of 15.8, with normal hematocrit and platelets. Electrolytes are also normal. Blood and cerebrospinal fluid (CSF) cultures are obtained. CSF studies show 1 red blood cell and 250 WBC, with no organisms on Gram stain. Differential of the CSF white cells is 43% polymorphonuclear cells, 37% lymphocytes, and 20% monocytes. CSF glucose is 52 and protein was 68.

Case Resolution

The patient was admitted with a presumptive diagnosis of partially treated bacterial meningitis, and started on broad spectrum antibiotics. The next morning the patient developed horizontal nystagmus and bilateral clonus (4–6 beats.) The child is still irritable, but continues to make eye contact and responds to her mother's voice. An MRI of the brain (Fig. 52-1) shows patchy T2 hyperintensities of periventricular and subcortical white matter of bilateral cerebral hemispheres, bilateral basal ganglia, and right cerebellar deep white matter.

Question

What is the correct diagnosis?

Answer

The history and MRI findings are consistent with acute disseminated encephalomyelitis. The child was treated with intravenous immunoglobulin (IVIG) 2 g/kg over 48 hours and showed resolution of the nystagmus and clonus, but still refused to walk. The child was discharged on a slow steroid taper over the next 4 weeks, and made a full recovery over this time period.

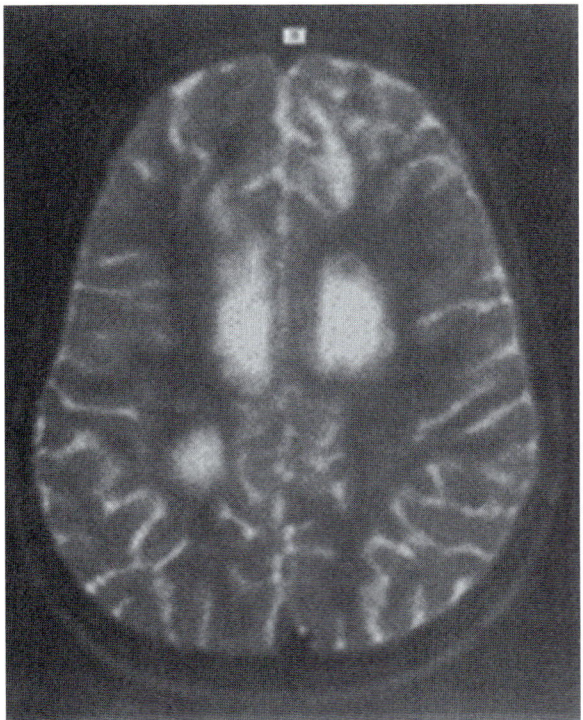

Figure 52-1 MRI showing ADEM. Note the patchy, asymmetric hyperintense lesions scattered throughout the white matter, representing focal areas of inflammation and demyelination.

Discussion

Acute disseminating encephalomyelitis (ADEM), once called postinfectious encephalomyelitis, is an autoimmune disease affecting myelinated fibers within the nervous systems of children. While pathologically indistinguishable from multiple sclerosis (MS), it is markedly different in its epidemiology and prognosis (Table 51-1). ADEM is most common in preadolescent children, affecting males and females equally and usually presents with multiple or generalized neurologic manifestations. Conversely, MS affects adolescent and young adult females most frequently and usually presents as a single neurologic deficit. ADEM always follows an infection, vaccination, or some other assault on the immune system. Prodromal symptoms of infection are present in up to 80% of cases. It is believed that these infectious agents share antigenic structure with myelin proteins (including myelin basic protein, proteolipid protein, and myelin oligodendrocyte protein) and thus, following an infection, the immune system may also inadvertently attack myelinated cells.

Many different infectious agents have been associated with the development of ADEM. Viruses include influenza, measles, mumps, Epstein-Barr virus (EBV), herpes simplex virus (HSV), cytomegalovirus (CMV), human herpesvirus type-6 (HHV-6), varicella, and Coxsackie viruses, while bacteria include *Mycoplasma, Chlamydia, Campylobacter, group A Streptococcus,* and *Salmonella.* Immunization has also been implicated, including the Hepatitis B, DTaP, and MMR vaccines. Not surprisingly, seasonal peaks in incidence have also been reported, further supporting a postinfectious pathogenesis.

TABLE 52-1

Selected Differences Between ADEM and Multiple Sclerosis

ADEM	Multiple sclerosis
Usually preadolescent	Late adolescent and adult
Viral prodrome or recent immunizations	No prodrome
Relapses rare, closely follow illness	Relapses common
Ataxia common	Ataxia rare
Thalamic lesions 40%	Thalamic lesions rare
MRI lesions same age	MRI lesions different ages

Due to a variety of presentations, the diagnosis of ADEM is often made after a lingering illness; that is, several other diagnoses are often worked up prior to making the correct diagnosis. In addition to recent infection, the most common findings are altered mental status and motor deficits, each present in between 60% and 70% of patients. Other nonspecific symptoms such as headache and fever are present in less than 60% of patients, and ADEM may present as seizures in up to 10% to 15% of patients. In our patient presentation, with a questionable diagnosis of partially treated streptococcal pharyngitis, several other diagnoses should be considered for a febrile, irritable child. The most serious of these include partially treated bacterial meningitis, retropharyngeal abscess, and peritonsillar abscess. The development of nystagmus and clonus, of course, warrants further investigation for a variety of intracranial processes.

Laboratory workup is rarely helpful in the diagnosis of ADEM, with the exception of CSF pleocytosis in two-thirds of patients. The patient may also have a lymphocytosis and elevated sedimentation rate and C-reactive protein. Brain MRI is the standard for diagnosis. While head CT may be normal, MRI will show demyelinating lesions more than 90% of the time in the white matter and subcortical gray matter. There may also be lesions of the periventricular white matter, corpus callosum, brainstem, and spinal cord. In addition to the patient's history, imaging can be helpful in differentiating MS from ADEM. While lesions of the basal ganglia and thalamus are common in ADEM (up to 40%), they are rare in MS. Lesions in ADEM are all of the same age, as opposed to lesions of different ages in multiple sclerosis. EEG may also be helpful in diagnosis, often showing a background of slow wave activity consistent with encephalitis.

Treatment of ADEM is somewhat controversial. Each type of treatment advocated for ADEM addresses the autoimmune and inflammatory nature of the disease. No randomized controlled trials currently exist to separate different therapies. One modality involves a high-dose steroid burst (up to 30 mg/kg/day, maximum 1 g) for 5 days, without a taper. Other treatment modalities involve IVIG with or without a prolonged steroid taper, or plasmaphoresis. Recovery usually occurs slowly over the next 4 to 6 weeks. Because bacterial meningitis and herpes encephalitis may also present with a variety of neurologic deficits, it is prudent to cover the patient with broad spectrum antibiotics and acyclovir until the diagnosis is certain. However these disease entities do not often produce the patterns of lesions seen on MRI with ADEM.

Overall mortality rate with ADEM was once 20%, but has now fallen to less than 5%, and more than 80% of children have full recovery. The remainder of those will have mild-to-severe prolonged neurologic deficits, and the risk for residual deficits is higher in children less than 2 years of age. There is still some thought that ADEM and MS may be diseases along the same continuum, as lifetime risk for MS is 6% to 15% after a diagnosis of ADEM, which is greater than the general population risk. This risk is even higher for children who are older than 12 at presentation with ADEM. These children have a 50% lifetime risk of MS. Relapse rate is the other significant difference between the ADEM and MS, with relapses being common for MS and rare with ADEM. When relapses occur shortly after treatment, it is called multiphasic ADEM, and those children have an increased 33% lifetime risk of developing MS.

Selected References

1. Goetz CG. *Textbook of Clinical Neurology*. 2nd ed. Philadelphia, PA: WB Saunders; 2003.
2. Hynson JL, Komberg AJ, Coleman LT, et al. Clinical and neuroradiologic features of acute disseminated encephalomyelitis in children. *Neurology*. 2001 May 22;56(10):1308–1312.
3. Hartung, Hans–Peter. ADEM: distinct disease or part of the MS spectrum? *Neurology*. 2001 May 22;56(10):1257–1260.
4. Stonehouse M, Gupte G, Wassmer E, et al. Acute disseminated encephalomyelitis: recognition in the hands of general pediatricians. *Arch Dis Child*. 2003;88:122.

54-Year-Old Male with Fever, Rash

CASE PRESENTATION

A 52-year-old man with acute myelogenous leukemia status post–autologous bone marrow transplant with relapse was admitted to the hospital for completion of day 8 and 9 of high-dose cytarabine salvage chemotherapy. Upon admission, his absolute neutrophil count was 0.0. On day 13 following initiation of chemotherapy (day 6 of the hospitalization), he developed a fever to 38.4°C, became hypotensive, and was started on cefepime and vancomycin. On day 17, (day 4 of fever) the patient developed a diffuse papular rash on his trunk, back, arms, and legs. He denied oral pain, odynophagia, dyspnea, chest pain, or leg swelling.

Physical Examination (on day 17)

The patient was febrile to 38.9°C, the blood pressure was 89/58 mm Hg, and oxygen saturations were 99% on room air. The patient was uncomfortable appearing in mild distress. His head, eyes, ears, nose, and throat examination revealed no oral lesions, the lung examination was clear with no rhonchi, the abdominal examination was benign, and the spleen tip and liver were not palpable. The extremity examination revealed 1+ edema at the dorsum of the feet bilaterally. Skin examination revealed diffuse, circumscribed papular erythematous lesions that were blanching on the arms, trunk, legs, and face.

Case Resolution

Intravenous voriconazole was initiated on the fourth day of fever. The next day, a blood culture returned positive for Candida species. Biopsy of the skin lesions revealed *Candida tropicalis*. The central venous catheter was removed; the patient remained febrile and developed adult respiratory distress syndrome. He eventually required mechanical ventilation. Later he developed a large cerebral vascular accident in the distribution of the middle cerebral artery resulting from severe sepsis. In recognition of his exceptionally poor prognosis, the family decided to withdraw support. He passed away on day 42 following initiation of chemotherapy.

Question

What organisms should one suspect in febrile neutropenic patients and how should this suspicion guide antibiotic therapy?

Answer

Gram-positive organisms constitute the bulk of infections among patients with neutropenic fever (61%), but gram-negative infections still remain a significant source (25%) with increased morbidity and mortality. Likewise, fungal infections, though a small proportion of sources for neutropenic fever (9%), as demonstrated in this case, can lead to poor outcomes. Antibiotic coverage must begin promptly upon recognition of the fever and initially cover gram-negative organisms. Additional gram-positive coverage and fungal coverage can be added in certain clinical circumstances or if the fever persists.

Discussion

While potent chemotherapeutic agents have led to decreased rates of death among individuals with cancer, they are fraught with the side effect of hampering the body's innate and acquired immunity. While lapses in cell-mediated immunity can lead to poor outcomes due to overwhelming viral infections, bacterial infections remain the biggest cause of chemotherapy-associated deaths.

Neutropenia is defined by the Infectious Disease Society of America as an absolute neutrophil count of less than 500 cells/mm³, or a count of less than 1000 cells/mm³ with a predicted fall to less than 500 cells/mm³. A fever is defined as a single oral temperature of greater than or equal to 38.9°C (101°F) or a temperature greater than or equal to 38.0°C (100.4°F) lasting more than 1 hour.

A review of organisms recovered from chemotherapy-related neutropenic patients with fever found that gram-positive organisms cause the bulk of documented blood stream infections in patients with cancer and neutropenic fever. Coagulase-negative *Staphylococcus aureus* is the most common gram-positive organism. Among gram-negative documented infections, *Escherichia coli* is the most common. Mortality rates for selected organisms are listed in Table 53-1.

Once it has been determined that the patient has neutropenic fever, a risk assessment can be performed to determine if the patient is at low risk for complications and can be considered for outpatient therapy with oral antibiotics or if inpatient therapy with intravenous antibiotics is warranted.

Patients with no known focus for bacterial infection, no symptoms or signs suggesting systemic illness other than fever may be carefully selected for outpatient therapy. If the patient meets the criteria listed in Table 53-2, can reliably fill prescriptions, comply with antibiotic regimen, and has rapid access to medical care 24 hours/day, the patient may be managed as an outpatient with an oral quinolone and amoxicillin/clavulanate.

For patients who do not meet outpatient treatment criteria, inpatient admission is required. Initial selection of antibiotics is recommended as a single agent, broad spectrum antibiotic with anti-pseudomonal coverage, generally an intravenous third-generation cephalosporin such as cefepime or ceftazidime, or a carbapenem such as imipenem or meropenem. Vancomycin should not be added empirically initially unless one of the following conditions exists: (1) clinically suspicion of a serious catheter-related infection, (2) history of colonization with penicillin and cephalosporin-resistant pneumococci or methicillin resistant *S. aureus*, (3) positive results of gram-positive bacteria prior to specific sensitivities returning, (4) hypotension or other evidence of cardiovascular impairment.

As with this case presentation, persistent fever throughout the first 3 to 5 days of therapy should trigger further

TABLE 53-1

Selected Prevalence and Mortality Rates for Patients with Malignancies and Neutropenic Fever by Recovered Organism

Organism	Prevalence %	Mortality
Gram-positive	61.0 (total)	
Coagulase-negative S. aureus	31.6	33.5
S. aureus	12.3	20.7 (MSSA) 28.6 (MRSA)
Enterococcus faecalis	3.1	30.0 (vancomycin susceptible) 66.7 (vancomycin resistant)
Gram-negative	24.9 (total)	
E. coli	7.3	38.1
Klebsiella sp.	5.4	20.0
Pseudomonas aeruginosa	3.6	47.8
Fungal	9.3 (total)	
Candida species	8.6	48.2

MSSA, methicillin-sensitive *Staphylococcus aureus;* MRSA, methicillin-resistant *Staphylococcus aureus.*
Adapted from Wisplinghoff H, Seifert H, Wenzel RP, et al. Current trends in epidemiology of nosocomial bloodstream infections in patients with hematological malignancies and solid neoplasms in hospitals in the United States. Clin Infect Dis. 2003;36(10):1103–1110.

evaluation and potential change in management. Possible reasons for persistent fever include: nonbacterial illness (i.e., viral, fungal), bacterial illness resistant or slow to respond to current antibiotic therapies, a second infection, inadequate tissue penetration of antibiotics or abscess formation, or drug fever. Repeat cultures and meticulous physical examination should be performed during this time period to evaluate for the potential causes for persistent fever. Consideration for adding therapy, either vancomycin if patient meets the criteria above or, specifically, antifungal coverage if the neutropenia is expected to persist.

In this case, the patient was high risk for neutropenic fever as he developed his fever in the hospital and was hypotensive. He was initially started on appropriate antibiotic coverage

TABLE 53-2

Multinational Association for Supportive Care in Cancer (MASCC) Risk Index Scoring System to Identify Low-Risk Febrile Neutropenic Adults

Characteristic	Score
Extent of illness (choose one)	
No symptoms	5
Mild symptoms	5
Moderate symptoms	3
No hypotension	5
No chronic obstructive pulmonary disease	4
Solid tumor or no fungal infection	4
No dehydration	3
Outpatient at onset of fever	3
Age < 60 years	2

The highest theoretical score is 26. A risk index ≥ 21 indicated the patient is at low risk for the development if complications and morbidity.

Adapted from Klastersky J, Paesmans M, Rubenstein EB, et al. The Multinational Association for Supportive Care in Cancer risk index: a multinational scoring system for identifying low-risk febrile neutropenic cancer patients. J Clin Oncol. *2000;18: 3038–3051.*

with the addition of vancomycin due to his hypotension. When a rash developed and he was persistently febrile, fungemia was suspected and broad antifungal coverage was initiated. When his blood culture returned positive for fungemia, his catheter site was changed. Despite this aggressive treatment, the patient died from complications of sepsis resulting from his *C. tropicalis* infection. This case illustrates the high mortality (near 50%) of candidal infections in febrile neutropenic patients with underlying malignancy.

Selected References

Hughes WT, Armstrong A, Bodey GP, et al. 2002 Guidelines for the use of antimicrobial agents in neutropenic patients with cancer. *Clin Infect Dis.* 2002:34:730–751.

Klastersky J, Paesmans M, Rubenstein EB, et al. The Multinational Association for Supportive Care in Cancer risk index: a multinational scoring system for identifying low-risk febrile neutropenic cancer patients. *J Clin Oncol.* 2000;18:3038–3051.

Sipsas NV, Bodey GP, Kontoyiannis DP. Perspectives for the management of febrile neutropenic patients with cancer in the 21st century. *Cancer.* 2005;103(6):1103–1113.

Wisplinghoff H, Seifert H, Wenzel RP, et al. Current trends in epidemiology of nosocomial bloodstream infections in patients with hematological malignancies and solid neoplasms in hospitals in the United States. *Clin Infect Dis.* 2003;36(10):1103–1110.

15-Year-Old Male with Rash and Abnormal Renal Function

CASE PRESENTATION

A 15-year-old male was transferred to the pediatric intensive care unit (PICU) from an outside hospital with limited pediatric services because of fever and renal failure. His illness began 2 weeks prior when he complained of fever and a sore throat. He was taken to a local emergency department where he was diagnosed with streptococcal pharyngitis. He was started on a treatment course of amoxicillin, which he completed. Several days after starting the antibiotic, he developed a diffuse rash over his arms, legs, back, and trunk. His fevers also returned and he became very tired. His mother brought him back to the emergency department where he was found to have an elevated creatinine. He was admitted to the outside hospital where his creatinine did not improve, but worsened with overnight hydration and he was found to have hypotension. At this point he was transferred to a tertiary care hospital for further care. The patient's past medical history was significant for cognitive dysfunction with some aggressive behavioral features. He lived in a group home and was on phenytoin and olanzapine. He had no known drug allergies and did not use any alcohol, tobacco, or illicit drugs.

Physical Examination

Upon arrival to the PICU, he was found to be febrile. Vital signs: temperature 38.8°C, tachycardic with a heart rate of 116 beats/min, blood pressure of 82/50 mm Hg, and respiratory rate 16 breaths/min. He was saturating 98% on room air. He was somnolent, had periorbital swelling, but no conjunctivitis. He had cracked lips, but no intraoral lesions. His cardiac examinations revealed regular tachycardic rhythm, normal S_1 and S_2 without murmurs. His lung examination was unremarkable. His abdominal examination revealed a liver edge palpable 2 cm below the right costal margin, but no palpable spleen. He had hypoactive bowel sounds. The genitourinary examination was unremarkable and without ulcerations. His skin examination revealed a diffuse erythematous papular rash (Fig. 54-1). Discrete areas on the forearms and thighs were peeling with erythematous skin underneath the peeling. There was no peeling in response to application of pressure (negative Nikolsky sign).

Laboratory studies

White blood cell count of 17,000 (11,000 neutrophils, 4,000 lymphocytes, 2,000 eosinophils), hemoglobin 13.6, platelets 296,000, sodium 142, potassium 3.7, chloride 105, bicarbonate 16, blood urea nitrogen 49, creatinine 2.4, alanine transferase 256, aspartate transferase 340.

Case Resolution

Initially, the patient was treated with broad spectrum antibiotics for presumed toxic shock syndrome, his home medications held, and started on corticosteroids for persistent hypotension. He initially improved with these treatments. On the seventh hospital day, he was transferred from the PICU to the pediatric floor and his home medications were resumed and antibiotics discontinued. Within 2 days, he again became hypotensive and febrile and was transferred back to the PICU. Despite aggressive

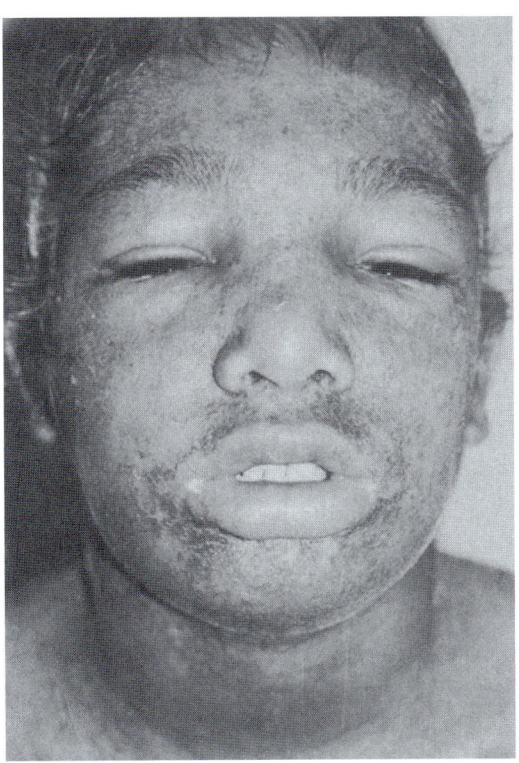

Figure 54-1 Patient with DRESS syndrome. Note maculopapu-lar rash and facial edema.

Adapted from Kaur S, Sarkar R, Thami GP. Anticonvulsant hypersensitivity syndrome. Pediat Dermatol. *2002;19(2):142–145.*

treatment with broad spectrum antibiotics and fluid resuscitation, he went into renal failure, was started on dialysis, continued to be profoundly hypotensive and underwent cardiac arrest, and could not be resuscitated. On the day he passed away, the clinical diagnosis was made of anticonvulsant hypersensitivity syndrome (DRESS syndrome—drug reaction eosinophilia and systemic symptoms) to carbamazepine which, upon obtaining further history, had been started 4 weeks earlier.

Question

What are the different types of drug eruptions and when should they be suspected in patients?

Answer

There are four broad categories of drug-induced skin eruptions: generalized, anaphylactic, DRESS, Stevens-Johnson/

TEN. These syndromes have several distinguishing features. They differ in pattern of eruption, temporal relationship to inciting antigen, and immunologic pathogenesis (see Table 54-1).

Discussion

A brilliant clinician is not typically required to diagnose a classic, dramatic, anaphylactic reaction to a drug that occurs within 1 hour of the second exposure to a medication. These reactions are fairly easily recognized, though the offending agent may not be obvious. Other, more subtle and difficult to recognize forms of medication reactions can also occur and lead to significant morbidity and even mortality as evidenced in the above case. An astute history, a thorough physical examination, and an elevated index of suspicion will lead to earlier diagnosis of more subtle forms of drug reactions.

Generalized maculopapular or erythematous drug eruptions are common, affecting 1% to 3% of users of new medications. These reactions are idiosyncratic and unpredictable, mediated through activated CD4+ T lymphocyte mechanisms. These reactions are frequently seen in the setting of a viral illness. The rashes are similar to typical viral exanthems. When antibiotics are used in the setting of a viral illness, these reactions lead to patients being labeled with an "allergy" to a medication. Less than one in five patients reporting an allergy to penicillin will actually react to a skin test with a penicillin allergen. Thus, it is important to question patients concerning the symptoms of their reaction and the time course in relation to the initiation of the medication to distinguish generalized drug eruptions whereby the drug may be safely administered without anaphylactic reactions. True maculopapular drug eruptions will recur with repeated exposure to the medication but without any other systemic findings.

The onset of anaphylactic reactions is typically within minutes of exposure to the antigen. While 2% to 3% of hospitalized patients will experience a drug reaction, only one in 2700 will experience anaphylaxis. Its hallmarks are laryngeal edema and hypotension. Anaphylaxis is easily reversed by epinephrine within minutes of administration and treatment is then followed by corticosteroids and antihistamines. For this reason, patients with identified anaphylactic reactions to common allergens, such as peanut butter or insect stings, carry epinephrine that may be self-administered in case of exposure. For specific sets of

TABLE 54-1

Overview of Common Types of Drug Reactions

	Clinical features	Time course	Immunologic pathway	Most common offending agents
Generalized eruption	Transient, benign, erythema or diffuse maculopapular rash often starting on the trunk or upper extremities and coalesce	4–14 days with first exposure, 2–3 days with repeat exposure	CD4 activated, T lymphocyte mediated	Allopurinol, penicillins, cephalosporins, antiepileptic agents, antibacterial sulfonamides, viruses (EBV, CMV, HHV6, parvovirus B19)
Anaphylaxis	Urticaria, facial swelling (angioedema), buccal mucosa, tongue, upper airway, respiratory collapse, shock	Begins within 1 hour, Lasts < 24 hours	Type I hypersensitivity reaction, IgE mediated	Immune modulators, monoclonal antibodies, penicillins, general anesthetics, insect stings, radiocontrast media*
DRESS†	Exfoliative dermatitis, fever, eosinophilia, leukocytosis, elevated LFTs, enlarged lymph nodes, interstitial nephritis, arthralgias, pulmonary infiltrates	2–6 weeks	CD4 activated, T lymphocyte mediated, cytokines IL-5 and eotaxin predominate	Aromatic antiepileptic agents (phenobarbital, carbamazepine, phenytoin), minocycline, allopurinol, sulfonamides, gold salts, dapsone
Stevens-Johnson Syndrome/ TEN‡	Fever, mucosal involvement (conjunctival, oral, or penile/vaginal) severe, diffuse rash, positive Nikolsky sign§, with hepatic, renal or GI involvement	1–8 weeks	CD8 activated, T lymphocyte mediated, cytokines Fas-L and TNF-α predominate	Antibacterial sulfonamides, anticonvulsants, NSAIDs, allopurinol, nevirapine

*NSAIDs and ACE inhibitor-associated angioedema is not a Type I IgE-mediated hypersensitivity reaction, but clinical features are similar.

†Drug reaction eosinophilia and systemic symptoms.

‡Toxic epidermal necrolysis, differentiation between the two is determined by the extent of skin involvement (<10% defines Stevens-Johnson, >30% constitutes TEN).

§Sloughing of the skin following superficial application of pressure.

patients with medication allergies without alternative drug agents available (ie, patients with cystic fibrosis and multiple drug-resistant strains of bacterial lung infections) desensitization may be undertaken using initially very small, then incrementally increasing doses of the medication in a monitored ICU setting. Similarly, allergen desensitization can occur for bee and wasp venom in the outpatient setting.

As noted in the above case, significant systemic symptoms can be present from a drug reaction involving every organ system. Hepatitis, renal failure because of interstitial nephritis or other causes, lymphadenopathy, encephalitis, hypersensitivity myocarditis, arthralgias, fever, and thyroiditis can all be manifestations of drug toxicity. This broad range of symptomatology frequently mimics infectious

illnesses. The most common medications to cause these systemic reactions are aromatic antiepileptic medications. Incident estimates are 1 reaction per 3000 exposures. The aromatic anticonvulsants include carbamazepine, phenytoin, phenobarbital, and primidone. Additionally, lamotrigine, which is a nonaromatic anticonvulsant, has also been associated with DRESS syndrome. Keys to the diagnosis include the prominent eosinophilia, multisystem involvement, and the presence of exposure to a high-risk medication. Familial associations have been described and it is felt that a genetic inability to process intermediate metabolites of the aromatic compounds leads to the buildup of toxic metabolites that then bind cellular macromolecules and lead to cell necrosis and secondary immune response.

As with all drug reactions, removal of the offending agent remains the mainstay of treatment. Additionally, case reports have been published using corticosteroids for severe cases; IVIG and plasma exchange have also been reported as useful. Even with these modalities, 10% mortality rate exists for individuals with this syndrome.

Representing the most serious and most rare of drug reactions are Stevens-Johnson syndrome and toxic epidermal necrolysis (TEN) with an estimated prevalence of 0.4 to 0.5 per million people and 1.2 to 6 per million people per year, respectively. These syndromes are characterized by diffuse erythematous or purpuric macules, blistering of skin, and target lesions. Unlike the DRESS or other drug reactions, Stevens-Johnson/TEN also has mucosal lesions present as stomatitis, conjunctivitis, or urethritis. Additionally, systemic symptoms may arise with hepatic, renal, or gastrointestinal involvement. When less than 10% of the body surface area is involved, the diagnosis of Stevens-Johnson syndrome is made. If more than 30% of the body surface area is affected, toxic epidermal necrolysis is diagnosed. Most commonly, these syndromes are in response to antibacterial sulfonamide medications, antiepileptics, or penicillins. Stevens-Johnson/TEN are rapidly progressive and frequently fatal conditions with a mortality rate of 5% for Stevens-Johnson syndrome and 30% for TEN. These conditions continue to progress after withdrawal of the offending medication. For these reasons, rapid diagnosis and transfer to a center with capabilities to handle patients with severe burns is essential.

Drug reactions of various sorts are common in all areas of clinical practice. Learning to distinguish the common, benign, maculopapular drug eruptions from more serious drug reactions and apparent systemic illnesses that may be because of exposure to a medication will allow for earlier removal of offending agents and quicker provision of appropriate care.

Selected References

Arevalo-Lorido JC, Carretero-Gomez J, Bureo-Dacal JC. Antiepileptic hypersensitivity syndrome in patient treated with valproate. *Br J Clin Pharmacol*. 2003;55:413–416.

Gomes ER, Demoly P. Epidemiology of hypersensitivity drug reactions. *Curr Opin Aller Clin Immunol*. 2005;5(4):309–316.

Greenberger PA. Drug Allergy. *J Allergy Clin Immunol*. 2006;117(2): S464–S470.

Karakas MB, Aksungur VL, Homan S. The anticonvulsant hypersensitivity syndrome. *J Eur Acad Derm Vener*. 2003;17:399–401.

Kaur S, Sarkar R, Thami GP. Anticonvulsant hypersensitivity syndrome. *Pediat Dermatol*. 2002;19(2):142–145.

Kay AB. Advances in immunology: allergy and allergic diseases. *NEJM*. 2001;344(2):109–113.

Mahadeva U, Al-Mrayat SK. Fatal phenytoin hypersensitivity syndrome. *Postgrad Med J*. 1999;75(890):734–736.

Mostella J, Pieroni R, Jones R. Anticonvulsant hypersensitivity syndrome: treatment with corticosteroids and intravenous immunoglobulin. *South Med J*. 2004;97(3):319–321.

Roujeau JC. Clinical heterogeneity of drug hypersensitivity. *Toxicology*. 2005;209:123–129.

Scully RE, Mark EJ, McNeely WF. Case reports of the Massachusetts General Hospital. Case 26. *N Engl J Med*. 1996;335(8):577–584.

Shaw NH, Spielberg SP. Anticonvulsant hypersensitivity syndrome. *J Clin Invest*. 1988;82:1826–1832.

Verotta A, Trotta D, Salladini C. Anticonvulsant hypersensitivity syndrome in children. *CNS Drug*. 2002;16(3):197–205.

Yawalker N. Drug-induced exanthems. *Toxicology*. 2005;3:131–134.

52-Year-Old Woman with Chest Pain, Arm Numbness

CASE PRESENTATION

A 51-year-old woman with a history of hypertension presented to the emergency department (ED) of a tertiary care medical center with a 2-month history of intermittent chest pain. The patient described the pain as being located in her sternum and radiating below her left breast, to her left shoulder, down her left arm, and down her left leg. She does report that the pain is associated with left-sided numbness. The pain is relieved with aspirin and diphenhydramine. The pain occurs two to three times per day and lasts about 1 hour. It has been occurring in this pattern for the past 2 to 3 months. There is no association with activity. She does endorse occasional shortness of breath, but no diaphoresis, syncope, or presyncope. The pain was worse the day that prompted the patient to come to the ED for evaluation. In the ED, the pain was initially 10/10, decreased to 7/10 with nitroglycerin, and then it was 3/10 with morphine. Her home medications included atenolol, omeprazole, aspirin, and occasional diphenhydramine. She was temporarily living in the area with her husband, who was retired from the military and performing contract work. He was present during her ED evaluation. She denied tobacco, alcohol, or drug use. Her father had a myocardial infarction in his forties and she had two brothers who also had myocardial infarctions in their forties.

Physical Examination

Vital signs: patient was afebrile, heart rate 65 beats/min, blood pressure 138/79 mm Hg, pulse oxygen saturation 100% on room air. She was in no distress. Ear, nose, throat examination was unremarkable. Neck is supple without lymphadenopathy, no thyromegaly, no jugular venous distention. She had a regular heart rate and rhythm, with no murmurs, rubs, or gallops. Her pulses were 2+ and symmetric at the radial arteries and she had a normal point of maximal impulse. Lung examination was unremarkable. Her musculoskeletal examination revealed tenderness to palpation along the trapezius muscle and tenderness to palpation along the anterior shoulder, which the patient stated reproduced her symptoms. The patient's neurologic examination revealed normal cranial nerves, strength 4+/5 throughout upper and lower extremities, but symmetric and sensation to light touch and vibratory sense symmetric and intact throughout.

Deep tendon reflexes are 2+ symmetric at patellar tendon, triceps tendon. Babinski was negative bilaterally. Romberg test was normal.

Laboratory Studies

Chest x-ray revealed no infiltrates and normal cardiac contour. Electrocardiogram revealed rate of 65, PR interval of 205, normal qrs and axis and no ST-segment changes. Complete blood count showed white blood cell count 6.7, hemoglobin 14.4, hematocrit 41.1, and platelets 277. Routine metabolic panel showed Na 144, K 4.0, Cl 102, HCO_3 30, blood urea nitrogen 12, creatinine 0.6, glucose 130. Creatinine kinase 174, creatine kinase-MB 2.6, and troponin less than 0.029. Calcium 9.5, magnesium 1.6, phosphorus 2.3, partial thromboplastin time 25.9, prothrombin time 10.2, international normalized ratio 0.8. Serial cardiac enzymes over the next 24 hours were normal. Treadmill sestamibi examination was normal. A brain magnetic resonance imaging was also performed, given her unusual neurologic complaints, which was normal. She was discharged from the hospital with a diagnosis of atypical, noncardiac chest pain and scheduled for a follow-up appointment in 2 weeks to discuss apparent symptoms of depression that were noted while she was an inpatient.

Case Resolution

Two weeks later, the patient returned for a follow-up clinic appointment. When she was asked about her sleep, she began to cry. She revealed that her husband had been physically abusive and that several weeks prior to her presentation in the ED, had thrown her down a flight of stairs and while she was lying on the ground, he reportedly placed his foot on her neck and applied pressure. She was referred to the local domestic violence assistance line and lost to follow up for 1 year. When contact was reestablished with the patient, she was physically separated from her husband and had accessed local resources working against domestic violence.

Question

In what clinical circumstances should domestic violence be suspected?

Answer

The prevalence of domestic violence is such that screening in all clinical encounters is warranted. Particular somatic complaints that can be suggestive of abuse include chronic abdominal, chest, or pelvic pain and, as with this patient, musculoskeletal injuries resultant from abuse.

Discussion

Domestic violence is the most common cause of nonfatal injury to women in the United States. One in four women report physical abuse at some point in her lifetime and one in seven report abuse within the preceding year.

Nearly 1 in 10 women will sustain a severe injury as a result of domestic abuse, though less than 1 in 3 women seek care for injuries sustained as a result of domestic violence. Victims of domestic abuse have higher rates of seeking medical care because of both physical injuries sustained from domestic violence, worsening of chronic medical conditions, and the presence of somatic complaints when compared to their nonabused peers. The medical encounter is an appropriate place to screen for and aid victims of abuse as it provides a safe environment away from the home and victims may feel more comfortable discussing sensitive issues with their healthcare provider than other members of their social networks.

Epidemiologically, no specific race or socioeconomic group reliably predicts a predilection toward domestic violence. Prevalence estimates of domestic violence in clinical settings range from one in seven women in primary care offices who have been abused in the past 12 months to one in six pregnant women who are currently being abused to one in four women seen in the ED with any complaint (Table 55-1). Partner factors that have been associated with

TABLE 55-1

Prevalence Estimates of Domestic Violence by Practice Setting

Primary Care

One in four women reports being abused in her lifetime
One in seven women reports being abused in the prior 12 months

Obstetrics & Gynecology

One in six pregnant women is abused during her pregnancy

Emergency Medicine

One in four women presenting to emergency department is undergoing domestic violence
One in three women with traumatic injuries were injured by their partners

Psychiatry

One in four women who attempt suicide is a victim of domestic violence
One in four women seeking psychiatric care for any reason is a victim of domestic violence

Adapted from Eisenstat SA, Bancroft L. Domestic violence. New Engl J Med. 1999;(341):886–892

TABLE 55-2

Clinical Factors Raising Suspicion of Domestic Violence

Physical Findings

Dental trauma

Any traumatic injury, particularly to head and neck, any fatal injury

Centrally distributed injuries or injuries in multiple locations

Defensive injuries of forearms

Bruises in multiple stages of healing

Unexplained stroke in a young woman

Subjective Complaints

Chronic abdominal, pelvic, or chest pain, joint or back pain, headaches, numbness

Somatic disorders

Irritable bowel syndrome

Chronic gynecologic complaints

STDs and exposure to HIV through sexual coercion

Exacerbation of a chronic disease such as asthma, coronary artery disease

Medical noncompliance

Psychologic Complaints

Depression and suicidal ideation

Anxiety symptoms, panic disorder

Eating disorder

Substance abuse

Posttraumatic stress disorder

Incidental Findings

Delay in seeking care for or inconsistent stories for injuries

Repeated visits to clinics or ED for clinically unclear reasons

Evasiveness of patient, emotional lability

Overly attentive or verbally abusive partner

Abuse of a child or elderly adult in household

Adapted from Eisenstat SA, Bancroft L. Domestic violence. New Engl J Med. 1999;(341):886–892.

women who seek care in the ED for injuries resulting from domestic violence include alcohol and drug abuse, intermittent or lack of employment, having less than a high school education, and being a former or estranged partner.

Patients suffering from the ravages of domestic violence can present as any one of many clinical scenarios, including injuries resulting from abuse, exacerbations of chronic illnesses, or somatic complaints (Table 55-2). Screening should take place in private with only the patient and the clinician present. The provider should explain to anyone else initially present in the clinical encounter that each clinician needs a few minutes alone with the patient for the examination and ask the other individuals present to wait in the waiting room. Simple screening questions can be preceded with a broad, general statement such as "We're concerned about the health effects of domestic abuse so we now ask a few questions of all of our patients. . ." The screening questions "Do you ever feel unsafe at home?" and "Has anyone at home hit you or tried to injure you in any way?" when used together, have a 71% sensitivity for detecting domestic abuse and a specificity of almost 85%. In the event of a positive screen, the clinician should obtain details as to the nature of the abuse, the injuries sustained, and the timing of abuses. Additionally, clinicians should follow-up a positive screen with a supportive statement such as "I believe what you are telling me" and be aware of resources against domestic violence that are available in the area for the patient.

Routine screening for domestic violence is recommended by the major professional medical organizations including the American Academy of Pediatrics, the American Academy of Family Physicians, the American College of Emergency Physicians, the American College of Obstetrics and Gynecology, and the American Medical Association. The goal of screening for domestic violence is early recognition and intervention. Most local communities have area resources available. There is a national hotline 1-800-799-SAFE that can make referrals to local domestic violence resources.

Selected References

Eisenstat SA, Bancroft L. Primary care: domestic violence. *New Engl J Med.* 1999;341(12):886–892.

Hathaway J. Use of medical care, police assistance, and restraining orders by women reporting intimate partner violence—Massachusetts 1996–1997. *MMWR.* 2000;284(5):558–560.

Kyriacou DN, Anglin D, Taliaferro E, et al. Risk factors for injury to women from domestic violence. *New Engl J Med.* 1999;341(25):1892–1898.

Rhodes KV, Levinson W. Interventions for intimate partner violence against women: clinical applications. *JAMA.* 2003;289(5):601–605.

62-Year-Old Male with Chronic Cough and Weight Loss

CASE PRESENTATION

A 62-year-old-man with mild mental retardation presented to an outpatient clinic with a chief complaint of "coughing for months." The cough was worse at night and productive of greenish sputum, but the patient denied hemoptysis or blood-tinged sputum. He reported occasional night sweats and exertional dyspnea. He had no fevers, weight loss, fatigue, chest pain, shortness of breath, congestion, heartburn, or recent viral illnesses. He had not been out of the country or imprisoned, and he denied any known contacts with tuberculosis. Medical history was notable for tonsillectomy and pneumonia, requiring chest tube placement, about 20 or 30 years prior. He reported no medications or allergies. He had smoked about one-half pack per day of cigarettes for the last 20 years and drank about 40 ounces of beer each night.

Physical Examination

Patient was a thin-appearing, but not cachectic, male in no acute distress. Vital signs: temperature 36.1°C, pulse of 81 beats/min, blood pressure 103/61 mm Hg, respirations of 20 breaths/min, and an oxygen saturation of 82% on room air, which improved to 100% on 2 L of nasal cannula oxygen. Nasal pharynx was clear and oral pharynx was only notable for poor dentition. Lungs had diffuse rhonchorous breath sounds, which cleared after coughing. Cardiac examination revealed a regular rate and rhythm without murmurs, rubs, or gallops. Abdomen was nontender and without hepatosplenomegaly. Extremities revealed mild clubbing of the fingernails. No cervical or axillary lymphadenopathy was evident.

Laboratory Studies

White blood cells 6.0, hematocrit 43.5, and platelets 239. Na 141, K 4.8, Cl 102, CO_2 34, blood urea nitrogen 14, creatinine (Cr) 1.2, glucose 67, Ca 9.7, Mg 2.3, P 3.7, total bilirubin 0.3, aspartate aminotransferase 34, alanine aminotransferase 32, alkaline phosphatase 83, gamma-glutamyltransferase 32, lactate dehydrogenase 639, total protein 7.4, albumin 4.2. Partial thromboplastin time 28.5, prothrombin time 12, and international normalized ratio 1. Chest radiograph (Fig.56-1) showed right hilar mass and reticular nodular changes at the right apex. Chest CT (Fig. 56-2) showed a 4 cm by 3 cm right hilar mass abutting the right pulmonary artery, mainstem bronchus, and superior vena cava; right paratracheal lymphadenopathy; multiple small (<5 mm) nodular opacities in the periphery of both lungs; and many, tiny, low-density areas in the liver which were too small to characterize by CT. The differential for these radiographic findings was small cell lung cancer, tuberculosis, sarcoidosis, or mycobacterium avium intracellularae. His purified protein derivative (PPD) was positive and patient subsequently had three sputum samples which were negative for acid fast bacilli by smear. Patient then underwent bronchoscopy.

Case Resolution

Endobronchial biopsy from the right upper lobe revealed small cell undifferentiated carcinoma. The patient was diagnosed with limited stage small cell lung cancer and underwent combined modality treatment with chemotherapy and radiation therapy. He did well for about 1 year and then, a new left upper lobe nodule was detected.

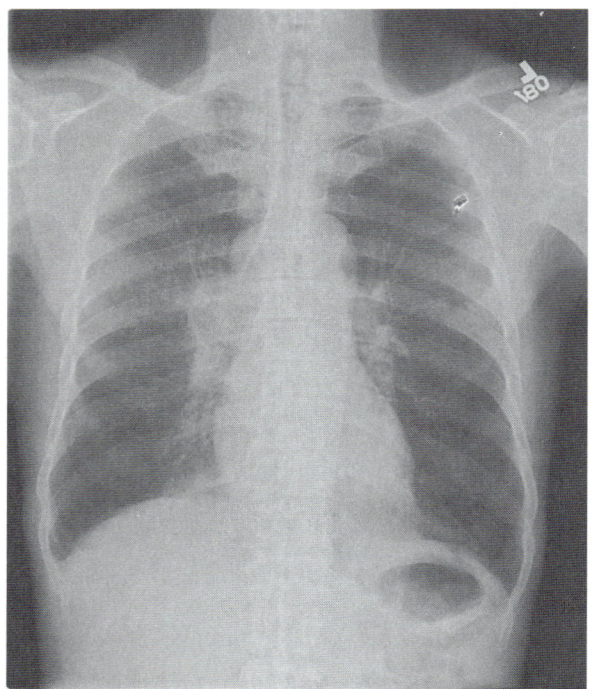

Figure 56-1 Chest radiograph shows a right hilar mass.

He underwent left upper lobe wedge resection which showed poorly differentiated adenocarcinoma (stage I). He continued to well following resection of this second primary lung cancer.

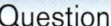

Question

What diseases present as chronic cough?

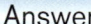

Answer

The most common causes of chronic cough include post-nasal drip syndrome or upper airway cough syndrome, asthma, and gastroesophageal reflux disease (GERD). In smokers diagnosed with lung cancer, cough is present at the time of diagnosis in less than 65% of patients. Lung cancers which arise centrally in the airways, such as squamous cell cancer and small cell undifferentiated lung cancer, are more likely to cause cough than more peripherally located lung cancers. However, when evaluating all patients with chronic cough, lung cancer accounts for less than 2% of patients.

Discussion

Chronic cough is defined as cough lasting at least 8 weeks, while acute cough is defined as lasting less than 3 weeks, subacute cough as lasting 3 to 8 weeks. About 10% to 20% of adults report chronic cough and it is more common in females and obese patients. Cough is often a presenting complaint for visits to both primary care physicians and a

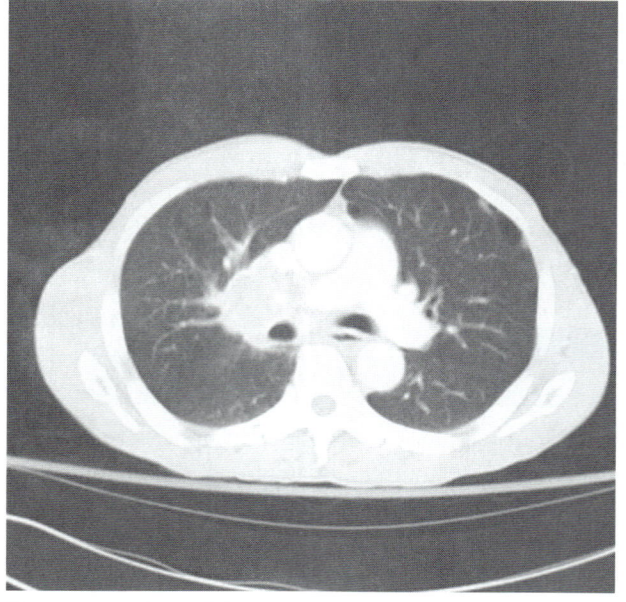

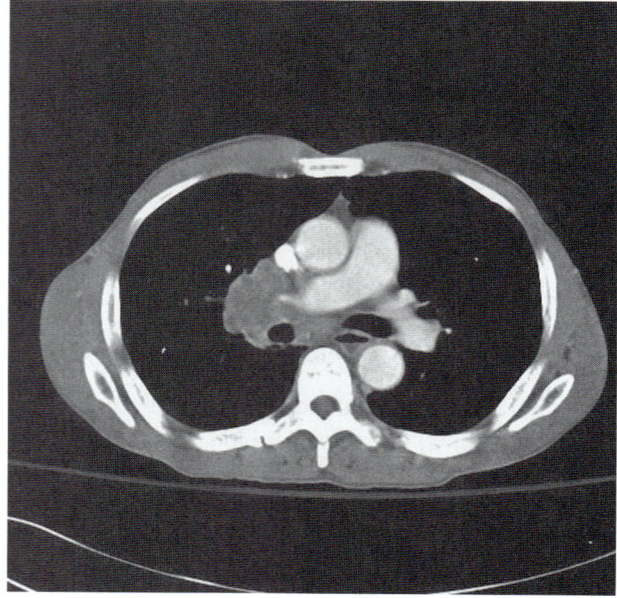

Figure 56-2 Chest CT shows a 3 cm by 4 cm right hilar mass in the right hilum.

leading cause of referral to pulmonologists. With chronic cough, the etiology can be determined in 88% to 100% of patients.

The three most common etiologies of chronic cough include postnasal drip syndrome, asthma, and GERD. However, these entities may present with no other symptoms than cough. In prospective studies, patients who were nonsmokers, were not on an angiotension-converting-enzyme (ACE) inhibitor, and who had normal chest radiographs were found to have postnasal drip syndrome, asthma, GERD, or a combination of those etiologies in 92% to 100% of cases.

Other less common causes of chronic cough include chronic bronchitis, bronchiectasis, and nonasthmatic eosinophilic bronchitis (NAEB). In series outside of the United States, the prevalence of NAEB ranges from 13% to 33%. The rarer etiologies of chronic cough include bronchogenic carcinoma, carcinomatosis, sarcoidosis, left ventricular failure, infection with *Mycobacterium tuberculosis*, or chronic aspiration.

The history and physical examination can be useful in determining the cause of chronic cough. Patients should be asked about smoking or exposure to other irritants, and medications, especially ACE inhibitors. Interestingly, the character and timing of the cough have not been shown to be useful for diagnosis. Patients should be asked about symptoms of postnasal drip syndrome, asthma, and GERD. However, as mentioned previously, many patients with these etiologies present with cough as their only symptom. Patients should also be asked about travel to areas where tuberculosis is endemic and about known contacts with tuberculosis. Additionally, patients should be asked about history of cancer, tuberculosis, or HIV/AIDS. It is important to know if patients have had hemoptysis or systemic symptoms such as fever, weight loss, or night sweats. On physical examination, particular attention should be paid to both the upper and lower respiratory tracts. Based on the PPD status of the patient, placing a PPD test may also be warranted.

A key diagnostic examination in the evaluation of chronic cough is chest radiograph. A normal radiographic examination in an immunocompetent patient points toward a diagnosis of postnasal drip syndrome, asthma, GERD, chronic bronchitis, or NAEB. Patients with hemoptysis, weight loss, night sweats, fevers, or risk factors for immunosuppression warrant a more extensive evaluation and referral to a specialist.

Additional diagnostic evaluation and treatment should be based on the history and physical examination. In patients with chronic cough who are nonsmokers, are not on ACE inhibitors, and have a normal chest radiograph, the clinician should focus the diagnosis and treatment of the most common causes of cough which include postnasal drip syndrome, asthma, GERD, and NAEB. Peak flow monitoring or spirometry may be useful to establish the diagnosis of asthma. For suspected postnasal drip syndrome and GERD, a trial of therapeutics may improve symptoms and help establish the diagnosis. In many cases, patients may have a combination of these etiologies. The diagnosis of NAEB can be made by evaluating eosinophils in induced sputum and it can be treated with inhaled corticosteroids. Table 56-1 provides treatment options for these common causes of chronic cough.

In smokers, cough can also be because of multiple etiologies. Many smokers have chronic cough because of irritation and the cough should improve after about 4 weeks of smoking cessation. Although any types of lung cancer can present as chronic cough, lung cancers which involve the airways are more likely to present as cough owing to the location of cough receptors. The most common types of lung cancer include adenocarcinoma, squamous cell carcinoma, small cell carcinoma, and large cell carcinoma. Even though cough is present at diagnosis in no more than 65% of patients with lung cancer, lung cancer accounts for less than or equal to 2% of all patients who present with chronic cough. Other common complaints related to primary lung cancers include chest discomfort, dyspnea, and hemoptysis. Lung cancer should be suspected in any

TABLE 56-1

Common Causes of Chronic Cough and Treatment Options

Cause	Treatment options
Postnasal drip syndrome	Antihistamine-decongestant combination
	Nasal steroid or anticholinergic agent
Asthma	Bronchodilators
	Inhaled corticosteroids
GERD	Modification of diet and lifestyle
	Acid suppression
	Prokinetic therapy
NAEB	Inhaled corticosteroids

smoker who presents with new-onset cough, a change in the nature of their chronic cough, or with hemoptysis. All smokers with these complaints should be evaluated by chest radiograph. Patients with abnormal chest radiographs often require CT imaging for further evaluation. A normal radiograph reduces but does not eliminate the question of lung cancer, and CT imaging may detect a cancer that was not visible by chest radiograph. In patients with a suspected diagnosis of lung cancer by chest radiograph or CT imaging, expectorated or induced sputum samples should be collected for cytologic examination. Although sputum cytology may provide the diagnosis, patients often require other methods for diagnosis. Table 56-2 presents the sensitivities and specificities of several diagnostic methods. Patients presenting with cough and hemoptysis, in which the cancer is felt to involve the airways, should also undergo bronchoscopy. Additional methods for diagnosis of lung cancer include biopsy of an involved accessible lymph node, thoracentesis of a pleural effusion, transthoracic needle aspiration guided by fluoroscopy or CT, and surgical excision.

In summary, cough is one of the most common presenting symptoms to primary care physicians. Chronic cough is defined as lasting more than 8 weeks. In non-smokers, the most common causes of cough include postnasal drip syndrome, asthma, and GERD. Although lung cancer accounts for a very small percentage of patients presenting with chronic cough, it is often present at the diagnosis of lung cancer. Smokers with chronic cough or a change in the nature of their chronic cough warrant further evaluation with chest radiograph. Importantly, the cause of chronic cough can be identified in most patients.

TABLE 56-2

Diagnostic Methods for Lung Cancer

Method	Sensitivity (%)	Specificity (%)
Sputum cytology (3 specimens)	Central cancers: 71 Peripheral cancers: < 50	99
Thoracocentesis (of pleural effusion)	80	> 90
Bronchoscopy	Central cancers: 88 Peripheral cancers: 60–70	90
Transthoracic needle aspiration	Peripheral: 90	97

Adapted from Collins LG, Haines C, Perkel R, et al. Lung cancer: diagnosis and management. Am Fam Phy. 2007;75;56–63.

Selected References

1. Collins LG, Haines C, Perkel R, et al. Lung cancer: diagnosis and management. *Am Fam Phy*. 2007;75:56–63.
2. Currie GP, Gray RD, McKay J. Chronic cough. *BMJ*. 2003;326:261.
3. Irwin RS, Madison JM. The diagnosis and treatment of cough. *New Engl J Med*. 2000;343:1715–1721.
4. Kvale PA. Chronic cough due to lung tumors. ACCP evidence-based clinical practice guidelines. *Chest*. 2006;129 supplement: 147S–153S.
5. Morice AH, McGarvey L, Pavord I. Recommendations for the management of cough in adults. *Thorax*. 2006;61:1–24.
6. Pratter MR. Overview of common causes of chronic cough. ACCP evidence-based clinical practice guidelines. *Chest*. 2006;129 supplement; 59S–62S.

7-Month-Old Female with Rash and Failure to Thrive

CASE PRESENTATION

A 7-month-old female was referred to a tertiary care children's hospital for zinc deficiency detected on routine laboratory testing, 3 weeks of worsening rash, and poor growth. Past medical history revealed normal birth weight with growth parameters between the 25th and 50th percentiles at 2 months of age, falling to below the 5th percentile by 6 months. Past infections included three cases of otitis media and one episode of thrush. She was admitted to the general pediatric service and a diagnostic workup was initiated for immune dysfunction, metabolic defects, and gastrointestinal disorders.

Physical Examination

At presentation, the infant was irritable but consolable. Vital signs: temperature 37.1°C, pulse 144 beats/min, respiratory rate was 30 breaths/min, and pulse oxygen saturation of 98% on room air. Weight, height, and head circumference were all below the 3rd percentile. Abdomen was soft, nondistended without hepatosplenomegaly or masses palpated. Chest was clear to auscultation without retractions. Diffuse anasarca was noted. She had a diffuse scaly erythematous rash sparing the head, upper back, and skin folds.

Laboratory Values

Albumin 1.5 (3.5–5.0, normal), Na 32, K 6.0, Cl 110, HCO_3 23, glucose 83, aspartate aminotransferase 366, alanine aminotransferase 190, alkaline phosphate 251, gamma-glutamyltransferase: 151; white blood cells 19.7; hemoglobin 11.7, platelets 490, prothrombin time 15.9 sec, partial thromboplastin time 36.3 seconds. Chest radiograph demonstrated slightly increased bilateral perihilar and peribronchial markings.

Case Resolution

Acrodermatitis enteropathica was confirmed by skin biopsy performed by the Pediatric Dermatology service.

The rash became more excoriated and extended to include 70% of her body surface area. Electrolyte abnormalities worsened, albumin fell to less than 1 g/dL and vitamin A and E levels were extremely low at 126 ug/L and 1.2 mg/L respectively. On hospital day 6, the infant became lethargic, hypoglycemic, hypothermic, and hypotensive. She was transferred to the pediatric intensive care unit (PICU) for treatment of septic shock and respiratory failure. Blood cultures grew *Pseudomonas aeruginosa*. Despite cardiovascular support, appropriate antibiotic therapy for presumed pseudomonal sepsis, and oscillatory ventilation, the patient expired on hospital day 8.

Autopsy findings were consistent with pseudomonal sepsis and cystic fibrosis. Necrotic skin areas were overgrown with gram-negative rods and represented the likely source of infection. The pancreas was fibrotic with acinar atrophy, which is a classic finding in cystic fibrosis. Lung specimens grew *Pseudomonas* and *Staphylococcus* species but otherwise had no discernible changes consistent with cystic fibrosis (CF). Frozen spleen sections were sent for CF genotyping revealing the infant was homozygous for the delta F508 mutation.

Question

What are the presenting symptoms of CF in infancy?

Answer

See Table 57-1.

Discussion

Failure to thrive is a common diagnostic dilemma faced by pediatric practitioners. The differential diagnosis is broad (Table 57-2),[1] and must be tailored to the individual patient's history and physical examination. However, the incidence of CF is approximately 1 in 2500 live births,[2] making it the most common inherited disorder in the Caucasian population and therefore an important diagnostic consideration. The classic presentation of CF is recurrent respiratory symptoms and failure to thrive with malabsorptive stools secondary to pancreatic insufficiency. Rarely, as in the case described above in the vignette, is CF diagnosed after severe complications from nutritional deficiencies. This discussion will focus on common presenting features of CF, an introduction to CF newborn screening, and the process of appropriate referral and initial management for patients with a suspected diagnosis.

Newborn screening for CF consists of elevated blood immunoreactive trypsinogen levels and is currently available

TABLE 57-1

Clinical Features in the Infant Suggestive of CF

Clinical feature	Approximate incidence (%)
Meconium ileus	10–20
Malabsorptive stools (pancreatic insufficiency)	85
Failure to thrive	40–50
Respiratory symptoms	40–50
Hypochloremic/hyponatremic alkalosis	5
Nasal polyps/sinus disease	3–5
Hypoproteinemia	1–30
Deficiency of fat-soluble vitamins	40–50
Rectal prolapse	3
Biliary cirrhosis	<1
Anemia	5
Acrodermatitis enteropathica	Rare

TABLE 57-2

Differential Diagnosis for Failure to Thrive in the Infant

Inadequate intake	Poor absorption	Increased metabolism/ defective utilization
Neglect	Cystic fibrosis	Heart failure
Food shortage	Diarrhea	Chronic inflammation
Developmental anomalies	Milk protein allergy	Malignancy
Improper formula preparation	Celiac disease	Chronic infection
Reflux, vomiting	Biliary atresia/ liver disease	Chronic hypoxemia (CLD)
Pain	Growth hormone deficiency	Metabolic disorders
Cleft palate	Hypothyroidism	Renal failure/RTA
Neuromuscular weakness		Hyperthyroidism

in approximately 30 states[3] as a blood spot test. There is still some controversy over absolute benefits of CF diagnosis soon after birth on long-term health and life expectancy. Grosse et al.[4] systematically reviewed mortality rate differences between screened and nonscreened groups of patients with classic CF without meconium ileus up to age 10 years in the United States and other countries. Non-US data demonstrated a significant reduction in CF-related mortality risk through newborn screening, though this effect was not seen with the US data. In the United State, there was an absolute mortality risk difference between states with and without CF newborn screening of 2.0 per 100 children with CF. The lack of significance may be because of the stringent follow-up and protocolized care provided to the Wisconsin group of screened and nonscreened patients. In 2001, Farrell et al.[5] described the Wisconsin Cystic Fibrosis Neonatal Screening Project and strong evidence that growth parameters were significantly better in the NBS group, even with that group's higher proportion of pancreatic insufficient patients. These growth parameters remained significantly better in the screened group throughout the 13-year follow-up period.

If CF is strongly suspected, the patient should be referred to a pediatric pulmonologist at an accredited CF center. In the case described above, sweat chloride (quantitative pilocarpine iontophoresis) testing had been attempted without success at an outside facility. In addition, the degree of skin involvement precluded repeat sweat testing at our facility. To ensure accuracy, it must be performed at a CF center where technicians are accredited and experienced in sweat testing. If sweat chloride testing is not possible secondary to skin lesions, prematurity (<36 weeks postmenstrual age), size (<2 kg), or mechanical ventilation,[6,7] the next step should be a serum CF genotype. At the institution where this patient was admitted, a 32 mutation screen is routinely used unless a specific mutation is suspected based on family history, ethnicity, or unusual presenting signs and symptoms.

In this case, the clinical pearl is involvement of supporting services, who are experts in CF care, as soon as possible. A CF team, such as that found at an accredited CF center, would likely have sent a genotype at presentation, initiated pancreatic enzyme therapy, administered fat-soluble vitamins to replete those found to be deficient and supported nutrition with 120% to 150% of FDA-suggested caloric intake for age, using aggressive nasogastric tube feedings and parenteral nutrition. In addition, recognition of susceptibility to possible infected gram-negative rods in such a malnourished at-risk infant is crucial for initiation of adequate anti-pseudomonal antibiotic coverage.

Evidence supports the critical role of dietary supplementation in patients with CF, not only for micro- and macronutrient repletion, but also for improved pulmonary function and cognitive scores. Pedreira et al.[8] demonstrated a strong association between FEV_1 percent predicted (forced expiratory volume in 1 second percent predicted) and BMI in a group of CF patients aged 7.7 to 16.7 years with pancreatic insufficiency and generally mild lung disease. For each 1.0 Z-score difference in BMI, there was an 11% difference in FEV_1 percent predicted. Koscik et al.[9] compared cognitive performance in control CF subjects with late diagnosis (no newborn screening) to those screened subjects diagnosed via CF newborn screening. Their results demonstrated that children with poor nutritional status (< 10th percentile) at diagnosis, and at 3 and 6 months after diagnosis, had lower cognitive assessments. In addition, the control group (no newborn screening) who had vitamin E deficiency had lower scores in cognitive testing than those control subjects with normal vitamin E levels and those screened subjects with normal or low vitamin E levels at diagnosis.

In conclusion, CF can present with severe nutritional failure and vitamin deficiencies. CF should always be included in the differential diagnosis for failure to thrive, especially when accompanied by malabsorptive stools and/or respiratory symptoms. It is most appropriate to then refer the patient to a pediatric pulmonologist at an accredited CF center for further specific testing. The median survival for CF is now 37 years of age, and we hope to further increase survival through newborn screening, protocolized care, and novel therapies aimed to improve mucociliary clearance, prevent chronic infection, and prevent loss of lung function.

Selected References

1. Chernick V, Boat TF, Kendig EL Jr, eds. *Kendig's Disorders of the Respiratory Tract in Children*. 6th ed. Philadelphia, PA: Elsevier Science; 1998: 849.
2. FitzSimmons SC. The changing epidemiology of cystic fibrosis. *J Pediatr*. 1993;122:1–9.
3. Cystic Fibrosis Foundation. Newborn screening. www.cff.org. Accessed Mar 23, 2008
4. Grosse SD, Rosenfeld M, Devine OJ, et al. Potential impact of newborn screening for cystic fibrosis on child survival: a systematic review and analysis. *J Pediatr*. 2006;149:362–366.
5. Farrell PM, Kosorok MR, Rock MJ, et al, Wisconsin Cystic Fibrosis Neonatal Screening Study Group. Early diagnosis of cystic fibrosis through neonatal screening prevents severe malnutrition and improves long-term growth. *Pediatrics*. 2001; 107:1–13.
6. LeGrys VA. Sweat testing for the diagnosis of cystic fibrosis: practical considerations. *J Pediatr*. 1996;129:892–897.
7. Eng W, LeGrys VA, Schechter MS, et al. Sweat-testing in preterm and full-term infants less than 6 weeks of age. *Pediatr Pulmonol*. 2005;40:64–67.
8. Pedreira CC, Robert RGD, Dalton V, et al. Association of body composition and lung function in children with cystic fibrosis. *Pediatr Pulmonol*. 2005;39:276–280.
9. Koscik RL, Farrell PM, Kosorok MR, et al. Cognitive function of children with cystic fibrosis: deleterious effect of early malnutrition. *Pediatrics*. 2004;113:1549–1558.

5-Year-Old Boy with Fever and Sore Throat

CASE PRESENTATION

A 5-year-old, previously well, Indian boy presented to his primary physician with a fever and sore throat. His mother was reassured that this was most likely a viral illness and he was sent home. Over the course of the next 2 weeks, he returned three times, with similar, nonspecific complaints. At the most recent visit, a complete blood count and chest x-ray were obtained. The cardiomediastinal silhouette was greatly enlarged. He was referred to the local University Children's Hospital for evaluation of a presumed pericardial effusion. The patient denied chest pain, shortness of breath, dizziness, or syncope. He had nausea and a few episodes of emesis. His parents had noticed decreased appetite and overall decreased energy. He had a nonproductive cough, which seemed to be worsening. He had near daily fevers ranging from 37.8°C to 39°C.

The patient had a past medical history of allergies, controlled with montelukast and cetirizine. He had an isolated febrile seizure at age 3. Pertinent family history included a cousin with a "hole" in the heart requiring surgery and his father having tuberculosis as a child. The patient was born in the United States and lives with his mother, father, and 1-year-old brother. Although he has never traveled abroad, his father returns to India several times a year. They have no pets. His vaccines are up-to-date. Other than those noted above, review of systems was negative.

Physical Examination

Vital signs: temperature 37.3°C, pulse 128 beats/min, respiratory rate 24 breaths/min, blood pressure 101/61 mm Hg. Height was 122.5 cm (95th percentile for age) and weight 27.4 kg (95th percentile).

Physical examination was remarkable for a well-appearing young boy in no apparent distress. He had mildly erythematous oropharynx with mobile subcentimeter anterior neck lymphadenopathy. Cardiovascular examination revealed muffled heart sounds, but a regular rate and rhythm with normal S_1 and S_2. A biphasic, "scratchy" rub was heard at the left lower sternal border. There was no jugular venous distension or pulsus paradoxus. Pulses were strong and equal in the upper and lower extremities. His lungs were clear. Abdominal examination was positive for a palpable liver edge and a nontender spleen tip. Physical examination was otherwise normal.

Laboratory Studies

The patient was admitted to the hospital for further workup. Initial echocardiogram showed a large pericardial effusion, with no tamponade physiology. Initial laboratory workup included normal electrolytes, white blood cell count 12,600, absolute neutrophile count 7900, C-reactive protein as 5.4, and erythrocyte sediment rate was 60. Creatine kinase was 39 and troponin T was less than 0.029. His electrocardiogram was normal. He initially underwent a pericardiocentesis, which drained approximately 300 mL of sanguineous fluid. He was started on ibuprofen and broad spectrum antibiotics. Enterovirus polymerase chain reaction (PCR) on the pericardial fluid was positive for Coxsackie B virus. Antibiotics were discontinued. Patient remained hemodynamically stable. At the time of discharge, his echocardiogram showed normal left ventricular function and a small residual pericardial effusion at the apex of the heart. At follow-up 1 year later, he continued to do well, with a normal cardiovascular examination and a normal echocardiogram.

Question

What is pulsus paradoxus and how is it measured?

Answer

Systemic arterial pressure normally falls with inspiration. Intraarterial cannulation reveals a drop of up to 10 mm Hg of arterial pressure during inspiration. Pulsus paradoxus is an exaggerated fall of systolic pressure with inspiration. This is not necessarily paradoxical but rather an exaggeration of a normal phenomenon.

The initial Korotkoff sound is heard only during expiration. With further deflation of the sphygmomanometer cuff, the Korotkoff sounds are heard throughout the respiratory cycle. The difference between systolic pressure at which the first Korotkoff sound heard during expiration and the pressure the Korotkoff sounds are heard throughout the respiratory cycle is the measurement of pulsus paradoxus.

The reason for an exaggerated fall in systolic blood pressure is related to ventricular filling. In the setting of increased pericardial pressure or reduced compliance, the normal increase in right ventricular filling with inspiration will cause a bowing of the interventricular septum. This leads to a reduced left ventricular stroke volume and an exaggerated drop in systolic blood pressure during inspiration. This is measured as a greater difference between the first Korotkoff sound and the pressure at which the sound is heard throughout the respiratory cycle.

Discussion

Diseases of the pericardium can be divided into four broad categories: (1) acute pericarditis, (2) chronic pericarditis, (3) constrictive pericarditis, and (4) pericardial effusions. See Table 58-1 for the different etiologies of pericardial disease. In this discussion, I will focus on acute pericarditis and pericardial effusions.

The pericardium is a fibrous sac that is well innervated but relatively avascular and inelastic. It consists of both a

TABLE 58-1

Etiologies of Pericardial Disease

Congenital anomalies	Metabolic-endocrine
Absence (partial, complete)	Uremia
Cysts	Hypothyroidism
Mulibrey nanism (*muscle, liver, brain, eye*) with congenital pericardial thickening and constriction	Chylopericardium

visceral and a parietal layer, which are separated by a potential space. This space normally contains 15 mL to 35 mL of serous fluid. It is thought that the pericardium serves three main functions: (1) fixing the heart within the mediastinum, (2) limiting cardiac distension during increases in intracardiac volume, and (3) limiting the spread of infection from the adjacent lungs. Despite these important functions, children born with a congenital absence of the pericardium tend to do well.

Pericarditis simply implies inflammation of the pericardium. Although acute inflammation can be caused by a variety of etiologies, the vast majority are idiopathic or viral. Tuberculous and bacterial infections of the pericardium have declined in prevalence. Acute pericarditis is more common in men than women, and in adults compared to children. In general, pericarditis is a self-limited disease and that readily responds to treatment and infrequently necessitates hospital admission.

The clinical presentation of acute pericarditis is typically severe, sharp retrosternal chest pain. The pain is worse with inspiration and when supine, relieved with sitting forward. Because of likely irritation of the phrenic nerves, the pain can refer to the scapular ridge. Other symptoms can include shortness of breath, palpitations, and a fever. Many patients have a history of a viral prodrome. On physical examination, a pericardial friction rub is almost always present. It is high-pitched and scratchy sounding. It can have 1, 2, or 3 components, representing atrial systole, ventricular systole, and rapid ventricular filling during early diastole. It is typically heard best along the lower left sternal border. A pericardial friction rub will be unaffected by respirations, helping to differentiate it from a pleural rub, which is absent during suspended respiration. The etiology of the rub is not clear, as even patients with large pleural effusions lubricating the two layers can have an audible rub.

Further physical examination findings may provide clues to the etiology of the pericarditis, such as obvious trauma, or evidence of systemic autoimmune disease.

The initial workup of pericarditis typically includes a chest radiograph, basic laboratory studies, an electrocardiogram, and an echocardiogram. Potentially, all four can be normal; particularly the radiograph if there is not a large effusion. Laboratory studies typically only show nonspecific signs of inflammation, including an elevated white blood cell count, elevated erythrocyte sedimentation rate, and increased C-reactive protein, as well as potentially concurrent myocarditis with elevation of cardiac biomarkers. Although the ECG can be normal, approximately 90% of patients will have an abnormality. The classic ECG findings are diffuse concave ST elevation with PR depression. These changes are present with the onset of chest pain and remain for a few days. Then, the ST segment normalizes. Later, widespread T-wave inversion develops. Eventually, there is resolution and normalization of the T waves. Echocardiogram will usually demonstrate at least a small pericardial effusion and is useful in evaluating for tamponade.

The treatment of acute pericarditis is to treat any known underlying disease if possible. Most forms of idiopathic and viral pericarditis are self-limited and respond to nonsteroidal anti-inflammatory agents. In adults, aspirin is a preferred agent, often in combination with colchicine. Although steroids are effective, their use may be associated with an increased risk of relapse. One long-term risk of acute pericarditis is constrictive pericarditis, a chronic disease that can respond to pericardiectomy but is still associated with increased mortality.

Many types of injury to the pericardium, including but not limited to, acute pericarditis, can lead to a pericardial effusion. The most common causes which eventually lead to pericardiocentesis include malignancy, postoperative causes, cardiac perforation during a percutaneous procedure, idiopathic etiologies, connective tissue disorders, and infection. Other causes include renal failure, coagulopathy, hypothyroidism, trauma, postradiation, HIV, and myocardial infarction.

Patients with pericardial effusions can vary dramatically in their clinical presentation, based on the amount and the rate of fluid accumulation in the pericardial sac. Rapid accumulation of as little as 80 mL of fluid can elevate intrapericardial pressures. Slow accumulation of up to 2 L of fluid can be asymptomatic. Symptoms of effusions include dyspnea, coughing, orthopnea, and chest pain. Patients may have muffled heart sounds. Signs such as paradoxic pulse, tachypnea, tachycardia, hypotension, and peripheral edema are worrisome for potential tamponade, an emergent condition that necessitates intervention. The classic triad of tamponade includes hypotension, muffled heart sounds, and jugular venous distension. Pulsus paradoxus is an exaggeration of physiologic respiratory variation in systemic blood pressure (SBP) and is defined as a decrease in the SBP of more than 10 mm Hg with inspiration. Pulsus paradoxus is neither sensitive nor specific for cardiac tamponade.

Evaluations of pericardial effusion typically rely on echocardiography. In tamponade, diastolic collapse of the right atrium and ventricle may be evident. Doppler studies demonstrate marked respiratory variation in the flow across the tricuspid and mitral valves. Although not perfect, echocardiography is typically sufficient to evaluate effusions. Computed tomography can detect small effusions, but does not typically help with the workup. Magnetic resonance imaging can be used as it can distinguish between hemorrhagic and nonhemorrhagic effusions.

Small effusions can typically be managed with observation along, as most will resolve without drainage. Indication for pericardiocentesis include a clinical diagnosis of cardiac tamponade, a suspicion of infection, or a large effusion (>20 mm on echocardiography) that has been present for less than 1 month or is associated with diastolic right-sided collapse. Shorter duration and evidence of collapse are both associated with increased risk of progressing to tamponade. The primary indication for the procedure is to treat or avoid tamponade, as it will not lead to a diagnosis in most patients.

In summary, although pericardial disease is not common in children, it is important to remember the clinical presentation of pericarditis and the evaluation of pericardial effusions.

Selected References

Chiles CD, Stouffer GA. Pericardial disease: clinical features and treatment. In: Runge MS, Ohman EM, eds. *Netter's Cardiology*. 1st ed. Teterboro, NJ: WB Saunders; 2004: 334–345.

Little WC, Freeman GL. Pericardial disease. *Circulation*. 2006;113: 1622–1632.

Bernstein D. Diseases of the pericardium. In: Behrman RE, Kliegman RM, Jenson HB, eds. *Nelson Textbook of Pediatrics*. 17th ed. Philadelphia, PA: WB Saunders; 2004: 1579–1581.

9-Month-Old with Cough and Labored Breathing

CASE PRESENTATION

A 9-month-old African American female was in her usual state of health until 10 days prior to presentation. At that time she began to develop cough and coryza. Her parents began to notice that she was becoming less active and taking less oral intake. After 3 days of these symptoms, her parents took her to the primary physician. There she was found to have adequate hydration and to be slightly irritable but consolable. Her clinical scenario was felt to be most consistent with a viral syndrome. Her symptoms persisted over the next 7 days. In addition, her parents noted her to have increasingly labored breathing. Her breathing became so fast that they found it hard to feed her. At this point they sought care at our emergency department.

Her past medical history was unremarkable. She was born at term after an uncomplicated gestation. There were no perinatal complications. Her growth and development had been normal up to the point of her presentation. She was able to sit unsupported, pull to a stand, and interacted well socially. The parents denied any history of hereditary diseases. They lived in a home with no pets and city water. The child was cared for at home by the mother.

Physical Examination

Vital signs: pulse 185 beats/min, respiratory rate 48 breaths/min, temperature 37.2°C, blood pressure 68/42 mm Hg, and pulse oxymetry was 91%. In general, the infant was pale, listless, and in obvious respiratory distress. Mucus membranes were dry. Scleras were nonicteric. No lymphadenopathy could be appreciated in the cervical, supraclavicular, axillary, or femoral chains. Lungs were clear to auscultation, but significant use of accessory muscles and tachypnea was present. Cardiac examination revealed no murmurs but tachycardia. No abdominal tenderness, hepatosplenomegaly, or abdominal distension was present. Skin examination revealed no jaundice, petechiae, or other rash. The remainder of the physical examination was unremarkable.

Laboratory Studies

Laboratory evaluation on presentation: Arterial blood gas (ABG) 6.7/19.4/77.9/2.4/−3.7, white blood cells (WBC) 12.9, hemoglobin (Hgb) 2.2, hematocrit (Hct) 6.8, platelet 561, and mean corpuscular volume (MCV) 90. Peripheral blood smear was normal with no spherocytes or schistocytes. Na 145, K 4.5, Cl 109, HCO_3 less than 5, blood urea nitrogen 35, creatinine 1.2, total bilirubin (Tbili) 0.4, aspartate aminotransferase 385, alanine aminotransferase 280, gamma-glutamyltransferase 46, and alkaline phosphatase 308. After a transfusion of fluids and packed red blood cells (PRBCs), ABG 7.41/31/121/21/−4.6, WBC 15.9, Hgb 11.8, Hct 32.2, platelet 243, absolute neutrophil count 12.9, and reticulocyte count 1.2%.

Other Studies

CTs of abdomen, pelvis, and head to evaluate for possible traumatic causes of blood loss were normal. Stool was guaiac negative. Skeletal survey and ophthalmologic examination to evaluate for nonaccidental trauma were also negative. Blood, urine, and sputum cultures were negative. Parvovirus B19 titers were negative. Magnetic resonance imaging (MRI) revealed bilateral internal carotid artery watershed territory ischemic lesions and acute ischemia within the posterior division of the right middle cerebral artery, thought to be the sequelae of cerebral anoxia secondary to severe anemia.

Case Resolution

In the emergency department intravenous access was obtained and fluid resuscitation was begun. She was intubated for respiratory failure and transferred to the pediatric intensive care unit. Initial laboratory studies revealed profound metabolic acidosis and Hgb of 2.2. She was transfused immediately with 40 mL/kg of packed red blood cells. The patient initially had a profound normocytic anemia which resolved with transfusion, and hemoglobin remained stable throughout her hospitalization. Her acidosis resolved and creatinine and liver function tests (LFTs) returned to normal, thought all to be secondary to initial shock. No other source besides profound anemia, including sepsis, was found for this episode of shock. She was treated with a course of Ceftriaxone for lung infiltrates that developed after her intubation, but never had fever and pneumonia was not thought to be initially present. Her mental status returned to normal after extubation and she was discharged home after a presumptive diagnosis was made.

On follow-up with hematology 1 month later, she was found to have an Hgb of 4.9 and reticulocyte count of 0.3%. Hgb electrophoresis at this time was normal. She was transfused 15 mL/kg at this time and on follow-up 2 months later had an Hgb of 12.6 and a reticulocyte count of 0.9%. The patient initially did well, but she was noted to have some developmental delay. She presented to the hospital 19 months after the first episode with status epilepticus, thought to be secondary to encephalomalacia in the area of her old watershed infarcts. CBC at this time remained normal.

Question

What is the cause of this child's anemia, and how do you establish the diagnosis of this and other anemias in children?

Answer

This patient has transient erythroblastopenia of childhood, or TEC, a self-limited anemia in previously healthy children secondary to temporary cessation of erythrocyte production.

The etiology of TEC is uncertain, but may be because of either viral or immune-mediated suppression of erythropoiesis. Presentation is at 1 to 4 years of age with gradual, often asymptomatic, onset of pallor in an otherwise normal child. Normocytic, normochromic anemia with very low reticulocyte count is found on the peripheral smear. The anemia is self-limited, resolving within a few months with no sequelae. Treatment is not recommended or required. It is important to know that this case illustrates an atypical presentation of this disease, as TEC usually has a benign course.

Because this patient did not have a typical presentation for TEC, her diagnosis was established by ruling out other causes of normocytic anemia. CT scans and stool guaiac revealed no source of blood loss. She had no sign of increased RBC destruction, given her normal bilirubin, lactate dehydrogenase (LDH), and peripheral smear. In addition, her reticulocyte count was low, consistent with decreased production. WBC count and platelets were normal, indicating that only the RBC lines were affected, making bone marrow infiltration or malignancy such as leukemia or lymphoma unlikely. Children with this disorder can usually be followed by their primary pediatrician with no need for bone marrow biopsy to establish the diagnosis. Hospitalization is not generally required. However, this case illustrates the importance of close monitoring of hemoglobin and symptoms, as the anemia occasionally becomes severe enough to require transfusion, without which they can develop severe sequelae.

Discussion

Anemia, defined as hemoglobin level below the age and sex-adjusted normal range, is a common finding in children and adolescents. To diagnose anemia, one must be familiar with these norms, recognizing that Hgb is the highest at birth, up to 17 g/dL. By approximately 6 weeks of age, infants reach their physiologic nadir, dropping as low as 9.5 g/dL. The Hgb then gradually increases throughout infancy and childhood to reach standard adult values. The differential diagnosis of anemia is vast, but a stepwise, systematic approach including components of history, physical examination, and laboratory workup can be helpful in determining the etiology.

History

Anemic infants will commonly present with irritability and poor feeding, whereas an older child may have decreased activity or complain of fatigue or headaches. Pallor may also be noted. Children may be asymptomatic more often than adults, because they have more reserve and greater ability to compensate hemodynamically, particularly if the anemia has been chronic.

Key components of the history include the following:

Jaundice, dark urine, or need for transfusion in neonatal period may indicate hemolytic process.

Prior episodes of anemia.

Family history of anemia, gallstones, or splenectomy may point toward a hereditary hemolytic disorder.

Ethnicity: Asian/Mediterranean ethnicity may increase suspicion for thalassemia, while sickle cell is more common in those of African descent.

Evidence of blood loss, such as melena, bright red blood per rectum (BRBPR), or heavy menses.

Infectious symptoms (i.e., fever, malaise) or recent travel to areas where hepatitis or malaria are endemic increase suspicion for infectious cause.

Other systemic symptoms may indicate underlying inflammatory disease.

Drug or toxin exposure: risk factors for lead exposure such as old home with chipping paint, increased symptoms after taking a sulfa drug.

Diet: strict vegetarian diet or excessive cow's milk intake in a toddler predispose to iron deficiency.

Physical Examination

Pallor, flow murmur, tachycardia.

Minimal symptoms usually indicate a more chronic, well-compensated anemia.

Jaundice, scleral icterus, splenomegaly may be found in hemolytic processes.

Petechiae, purpura indicates concurrent thrombocytopenia. This suggests more global bone marrow suppression. If hepatosplenomegaly is also present, it should raise suspicion for leukemia or lymphoma.

Approach to Laboratory Workup

The history and physical may provide important clues, but definitive diagnosis generally requires a basic laboratory workup. There are essentially two categories of anemia: inadequate production and increased destruction or loss. The easiest way to distinguish these is with the reticulocyte count, a marker of red cell production. It is important

to determine if the reticulocytosis is appropriate for the degree of anemia, which can be done by calculating the reticulocyte production index, or RPI:

$$RPI = \frac{\text{Retic. Ct} \times \text{Hgb (observed)} \times 0.5}{\text{Hgb (normal)}}$$

If the RPI is greater than 3, then production is adequate, indicating that the anemia is secondary to RBC destruction or loss. If the RPI is less than 2, marrow production is inadequate for the degree of anemia. Once this is determined, the mean corpuscular volume, a marker of red cell size, can help to further distinguish causes secondary to inadequate production. For a pictorial approach to anemia and summary of selected types of anemia please see Fig. 59-1 and Table 59-1, respectively.

Anemia with Adequate Reticulocyte Count (RPI > 3)

Initially, blood loss should be ruled out. If there is no sign of this, evaluate for hemolysis with LDH, total bilirubin, and/or haptoglobin. If LDH and bilirubin are elevated with a low haptoglobin, and/or schistocytes are seen on peripheral smear, there is likely RBC destruction and the following studies can elucidate the etiology:

Positive direct Coombs test: immune hemolytic anemia

Abnormal Hgb electrophoresis: sickle cell disease or sickle beta-thalassemia (see below)

Abnormal RBC glucose-6-phosphate dehydrogenase (G6PD) or pyruvate kinase enzyme assay: G6PD or pyruvate kinase deficiency (see below)

Positive osmotic fragility test: hereditary spherocytosis

Disseminated intravascular coagulation (DIC) panel: sepsis, thrombotic thrombocytopenic purpura (TTP), hemolytic uremic syndrome (HUS), often low platelets are seen as well

Sickle cell disease

Sickle cell disease is caused by abnormalities in the β-chain of hemoglobin, causing chronic anemia, painful vaso-occlusive symptoms from sickling, and susceptibility to infection secondary to auto-infarction of the spleen. It is usually detected on state newborn screen, but if not, will usually present in the second half of the first year of life, when the change from fetal Hgb to β-chain production is nearly complete.

G6PD deficiency

Glucose-6-phosphate dehydrogenase deficiency predisposes to red cell destruction by preventing maintenance of reduced

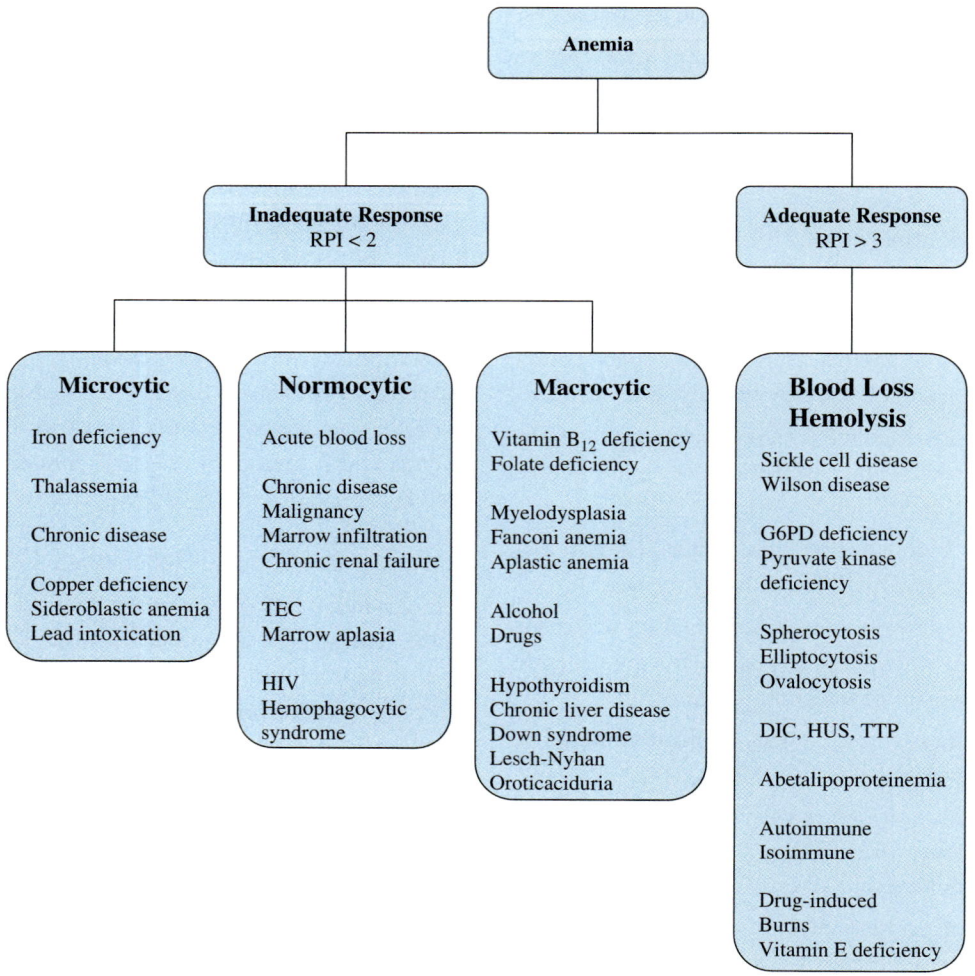

Figure 59-1 Approach to anemia.

RBC glutathione. Thus, in situations of oxidant stress, such as illness (especially hepatitis, diabetic acidosis, other infections) or antioxidant drugs/toxins (such as sulfa, antimalarial drugs, or fava beans), a hemolytic anemia results. This can lead to jaundice, fatigue, and even cardiovascular collapse. It most commonly presents as neonatal jaundice or later in life when an exposure to any of the above occurs. It is most commonly found in African American males and those of Mediterranean descent. Diagnosis is established with an abnormal G6PD enzyme assay. However, this test may be falsely normal during a hemolytic episode because more of the affected cells have been hemolyzed; thus, the test should be repeated once the Hgb has returned to normal.

Anemia with Low Reticulocyte Count (RPI < 2)

Microcytic (low MCV), hypochromic

The most common cause of microcytic anemia in any age is iron deficiency. Iron studies revealing a low iron level and low ferritin with a normal to high total iron binding capacity (TIBC) confirm this diagnosis. History is the key to establishing the etiology of the deficiency. Positive stool guaiac indicates occult gastrointestinal (GI) bleeding as a possible cause. Heavy menses in an adolescent female may also be the cause. Pure dietary deficiency is a rare cause in children. However, toddlers commonly develop iron deficiency anemia from excessive cow milk intake.

Iron deficiency from excessive cow milk intake

This typically presents with gradual onset of pallor in a child aged 1 to 3 years, as a result of cow milk being a major component of the child's diet. Cow milk is low in iron, and excessive intake, usually greater than 16 oz a day, can induce satiety and prevent children from ingesting other iron-rich foods. Very excessive intake can lead to mild occult GI blood loss from allergy-induced GI mucosal damage, adding to the iron deficiency anemia.

If iron studies are normal, one should consider thalassemia, particularly in a patient of African American,

TABLE 59-1

Selected Anemias

Disease	Presentation	Diagnosis	Management
Sickle cell	- Episodes of jaundice - Pain crises - Splenomegaly early, followed by autoinfarction by age 5 - Acute chest - Priapism	- Normocytic anemia with evidence of hemolysis and increased reticulocyte count during crises - Abnormal Hgb electrophoresis	- Folate supplementation and penicillin prophylaxis - Analgesia, hydration, oxygen during crises - Transfusion if necessary - Hydroxyurea to increase fetal Hgb in severe cases
G6PD deficiency	- Neonatal jaundice - Pallor, jaundice during oxidant stress; otherwise, asymptomatic or with chronic anemia	- Increased reticulocyte count and hemolytic anemia during oxidant stress - Abnormal G6PD assay after acute hemolytic episode has resolved	- Avoid precipitating agent - Supportive care, including transfusion if necessary
Iron deficiency	- Pallor, fatigue, irritability, poor feeding - Excessive intake of cow milk or occult bleeding	- Microcytic anemia - Low percent of serum iron, ferritin saturation - Increased TIBC	- Correct diet - Identify and eliminate source of bleeding - Iron supplementation
Thalassemia trait	- Pallor or asymptomatic	- Microcytic anemia - Beta-thalassemia trait: increased A_2 Hgb on electrophoresis and basophilic stippling beta-thalassemia trait	- Avoid iron therapy - Genetic counseling
Transient erythroblastopenia of childhood (TEC)	- Pallor - Asymptomatic or fatigue, irritability	- Profound normocytic anemia - Low reticulocyte count	- Close monitoring of Hgb - Transfusion if necessary
Aplastic crisis	- Pallor and fatigue in a patient with underlying sickle cell or other hemolytic disorder	- Normocytic anemia with low reticulocyte count - May have positive parvovirus B19 titers	- Close monitoring of Hgb - Transfusion if necessary
Vitamin B_{12}/folate deficiency	- May have history of drug exposure, ileal resection, malabsorption - May have neurologic sx if long hx of B_{12} deficiency	- Macrocytic anemia - Other cell lines normal	- Remove offending drug - Others need lifelong folate or vitamin B_{12} supplementation - If vitamin B_{12} deficiency, do Schilling test to evaluate for pernicious anemia: will need vitamin B_{12} injections if present

South Asian, or Mediterranean descent. Hemoglobin electrophoresis revealing elevated Hgb A_2 or F indicates beta-thalassemia trait. There is no convenient test for alpha-thalassemia, however.

If the above studies are normal, consider more rare conditions such as sideroblastic anemia, lead poisoning, and copper deficiency.

Normocytic (normal MCV), normochromic

First, evaluate for signs of infection or systemic illness. If a patient has an elevated WBC count and infectious symptoms such as fever and malaise, viral suppression may be the cause. In particular, one should consider aplastic crisis in a patient with underlying hemolytic disease.

Aplastic crisis: Parvovirus B19 is responsible for fifth disease in children, and may produce transient erythroid aplasia. In healthy children with a normal RBC lifespan, this does not cause anemia. However, in those with underlying hemolytic disease, such as G6PD deficiency or sickle cell disease, it can cause an aplastic crisis with low reticulocyte count, often requiring transfusion until the marrow recovers. Parvovirus B19 titers can be sent to confirm the diagnosis.

If the patient has systemic illness such as HIV, inflammatory bowel disease (IBD) collagen-vascular disease, or others, consider anemia of chronic disease. Iron studies will reveal decreased TIBC with normal-to-high iron and ferritin. If the anemia is accompanied by low platelets and WBC, consider a more extensive bone marrow process such as marrow infiltration, aplastic anemia, or hematologic malignancy such as leukemia or lymphoma.

If none of the above findings are present, and the patient is a young, otherwise healthy child, the most likely diagnosis is *TEC*. However, other rare congenital marrow failure syndromes, such as Diamond-Blackfan anemia, should be considered if the anemia does not resolve within a few months.

Macrocytic (elevated MCV)

Low folate or vitamin B_{12}

Folate or vitamin B_{12} deficiency from inadequate dietary intake is very rare. It is more commonly secondary to malabsorption or impaired metabolism. Vitamin B_{12} deficiency can be found in patients with pernicious anemia and ileal resection, as well as cobalamin transport deficiencies. Folate deficiency often results from drugs that interfere with folate such as methotrexate, phenytoin, sulfa, or alcohol.

If folate/vitamin B_{12} levels are normal, think of other systemic diseases, such as hypothyroidism, inborn errors of metabolism, liver disease, or Down syndrome. Consider other marrow failure syndromes like Fanconi anemia, myelodysplasia, Diamond-Blackfan, recognizing that these may affect WBC and platelets as well.

Selected References

Behrman RE, Kliegman RM. *Nelson's Essential's of Pediatrics*. 3rd ed. Philadelphia, PA: WB Saunders Company; 1998.

Segel GB, Hirsh MG, Feig SA. Managing anemia in pediatric office practice: part 1. *Pediat Rev.* 2002 March;23(3):75–84.

Segel GB, Hirsh MG, Feig SA. Managing anemia in pediatric office practice: part 2. *Pediat Rev.* 2002 April;23(4):111–121.

33-Year-Old Male with 1-day History of Lower Extremity Weakness and Inability to Walk

CASE PRESENTATION

A 33-year-old Hispanic male presented to the emergency department after awakening one morning with weakness in his arms and legs. His legs are much weaker than his arms. It has progressed throughout the morning to the point where the patient is unable to move his legs or ambulate. The patient had awakened hours previously with leg cramps, which were relieved with walking. He denies any similar episodes in the past. No recent illnesses, no fevers, chills, vomiting, or diarrhea. He does report finding a tick 2 weeks ago, which was subsequently removed. He denies any recent travels or any visual disturbances or back pain. No bowel or bladder incontinence. Patient is otherwise healthy. He takes no medication, including herbals or other supplements. He denies tobacco use or other drug use, but does drink occasionally. He is originally from Guatemala but has lived in the United States for the past 5 years. Family history is negative for neurologic processes or paralysis. Review of symptoms is positive only for mild shortness of breath and heat intolerance.

Physical Examination

Patient was alert and oriented, and did not appear ill. Vital signs: temperature 98.3°C, pulse 77 beats/min, respiratory rate 18 breaths/min, blood pressure 127/95 mm Hg, and oxygen saturations of 100% on room air. Head, eyes, ears, nose, and throat: normocephalic, atraumatic, pupils equal, round, reactive to light and accommodation, extraocular movement intact, sclera nonicteric. Neck: supple without lymphadenopathy, no bruit, no jugular venous distension, no thyroid nodules or bruits. Cardiovascular: regular rate and rhythm (RRR) with no murmur, gallops, or rubs. The first and second heart sounds were normal. Lungs: clear to auscultation bilaterally with a normal work of breathing. Abdomen: soft, nontender, normal bowel sounds, no hepatosplenomegaly. Extremities: no edema. Neurologic: cranial nerves were intact. The patient had marked weakness with strength 2/5 in the hip flexors, 3/5 distal lower extremities, dorsiflexion, and plantar flexion. Strength was 4/5 in bilateral triceps and wrist flexion and extension. Sensation was intact. Deep tendon reflexes (DTRs) were normal, without evidence of hyperreflexia in both upper and lower extremities. No clonus or increased tone. Babinski were down going bilaterally.

Laboratory Studies

White blood cells 7.5, hemoglobin 15.8, hematocrit 46, and platelets 196. Na^+ 141, K^+ 2.8, Cl^- 109, Co_2 25, blood urea nitrogen 11, Cr 0.6, Ca 9.0, Mg 1.7, P 4.7. Thyroid-stimulating hormone (TSH) < 0.01, free T_4 1.8 ng/dL (normal 0.58–1.64 ng/dL), T_3 6.4 pg/mL (normal 2.3–4.2 pg/mL). Electrocardiogram (ECG) is shown in Fig. 60-1. Magnetic resonance imaging (MRI) of the brain and cervical, thoracic and lumbar spine were normal.

Case Resolution

The patient received 40 mEq of intravenous potassium chloride (KCl) with an increase in his serum K^+ from 2.8 to 3.7 and improvement in his symptoms. He was

Comment: Referred by: Unconfirmed

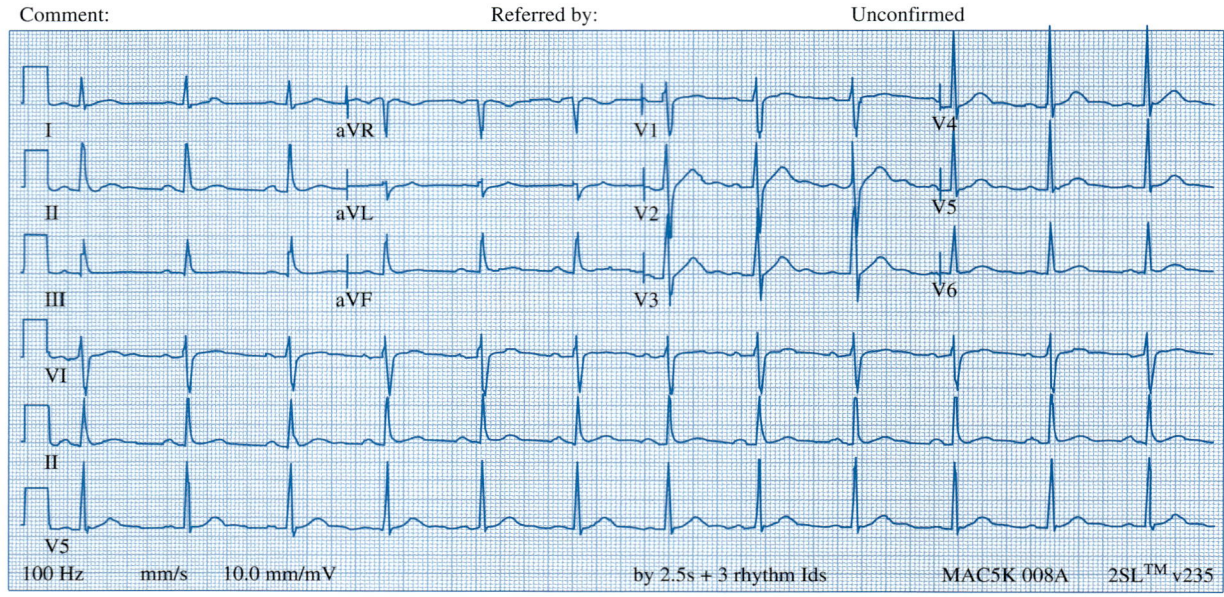

Figure 60-1 ECG with U waves.

observed overnight and then discharged home on oral propranolol with instructions for follow-up for a thyroid uptake scan the following week. Nuclear thyroid scan and uptake revealed a 24-hour iodine uptake calculated at 38% (normal range 10%–30%) with uniform uptake of radiotracer. No dominant nodules were seen. These findings were consistent with Graves disease. Endocrine follow-up was arranged.

Question

What is the most likely explanation of the patient's acute weakness?

Answer

Although the differential diagnosis of acute weakness is broad, the laboratory findings of a low serum potassium together with a low TSH are consistent with a diagnosis of thyrotoxic periodic paralysis (TPP).

Discussion

Despite subtle signs and symptoms of hyperthyroidism, TPP is a disorder characterized by thyrotoxicosis, hypokalemia, and predominantly lower limb paralysis.

TPP occurs most frequently in Asian males, including patients of Japanese, Chinese, and Korean ancestry. However it has been reported increasingly in other ethnic groups, particularly in American Indians and Hispanics. A disease once uncommon in the United States, physicians are becoming more familiar with this disorder as the population changes. Yet, it still is often overlooked on presentation and misdiagnosed as one of the other causes of paralysis, including Guillain-Barre syndrome.

TPP usually occurs in persons aged 20 to 40 years of age. This is in contrast to familial periodic paralysis (FPP) where the initial episode usually occurs at a much younger age. Many patients describe a prodrome consisting of muscle aches, cramps, or stiffness. Weakness usually begins symmetrically in the proximal muscles of the lower extremities and progresses to the upper torso. Bulbar, respiratory, and ocular muscles are rarely affected. The majority of episodes occur in the early morning or late evening. Precipitating factors include high-carbohydrate meals, alcohol, strenuous exercise, cold exposure, and even emotional stress. Attacks can be brief and recurrent, though between attacks, patients will be symptom free.

TPP is characterized by hypokalemia. Usually associated with a serum potassium of less than 3.0 mmol/lL, the hypokalemia is because of a massive intracellular shift rather than net loss from the body via urine or stool. Blood acid-base balance is maintained. The degree of hypokalemia is not indicative of the severity of the thyroid disease. Other electrolyte abnormalities seen include hypophosphatemia and hypomagnesemia. These abnormalities are also likely secondary to intracellular shifts that accompany the shift of potassium. Electrocardiographic findings associated with hypokalemia such as T-wave flattening and U waves are common.

The exact pathophysiology of TPP remains unclear, however, research points to several mechanisms. All etiologies of hyperthyroidism have been implicated in TPP, making it appear that the pathogenesis is related to the thyrotoxicosis per se. It appears that the thyroid hormone has a direct effect on both the number and activity of the Na-K-ATPase pump. The catecholamine surge seen with hyperthyroidism has also been found to increase the Na-K-ATPase pump activity, leading to increased potassium uptake. This may be why nonselective β-blockers are useful in the management of TPP. In addition, the adrenergic response may attribute to the hyperinsulinemia often observed in TPP patients, which can also indirectly stimulate Na-K-ATPase activity. This may explain the association between TPP and high-carbohydrate meals. Overall, it is the stimulation of the Na-K-ATPase pump either directly or indirectly leading to cellular potassium uptake. Whether there is a genetic predisposition to this increased activity remains unknown at this time.

The presentation of symptoms and overall picture of TPP is almost indistinguishable from other causes of hypokalemia and paralysis. The differential diagnosis of TPP includes other disorders leading to a transcellular shift of potassium or potassium wasting from either the kidneys or gastrointestinal tract (see Table 60-1). TPP can be distinguished from the other causes by a careful history, including family history of paralysis, physical examination, and assessment of serum and urine electrolytes and acid–base status.

The primary treatment of TPP is supplementation with either intravenous or oral KCl to hasten recovery and prevent cardiac and respiratory complications. Rebound hyperkalemia is a risk as potassium is shifted back in the intravascular component during recovery, as the overall body potassium stores are normal in patients with TPP. Therefore, potassium supplementation should be given at a slow rate with frequent potassium measurements unless there are severe complications that require more rapid correction. Potassium supplements are not useful in between attacks or for prophylaxis.

Besides potassium supplementation, nonspecific β-blockers have been proposed as an alternative therapy, based on the theory that hyperadrenergic activity is involved in the pathogenesis of TPP. More controlled studies are needed, however.

TABLE 60-1

Differential Diagnosis of Hypokalemia and Paralysis

Increased transcellular shift of potassium
  Familial periodic paralysis
  Thyrotoxic periodic paralysis
  Barium intoxication
  Theophylline toxicity
  β-Adrenergic agonist overdose
Renal potassium loss
  Renal tubular acidosis (distal or proximal)
  Primary hyperaldosteronism
  Licorice ingestion (secondary hyperaldosteronism)
  Diuretic use
Gastrointestinal potassium loss
  Celiac disease
  Profound diarrhea
  Short-bowel syndrome
  Ureteral diversion

Definitive therapy for TPP is identifying the cause of the hyperthyroidism and treating accordingly. The use of nonselective β-blockers is important during early treatment, when a euthyroid state is not yet achieved. Patients should also avoid precipitating factors including heavy carbohydrate loads, excessive exertion, and alcohol use until the thyrotoxicosis is controlled.

TPP is becoming more common in clinical settings across the country. As physicians, we must be familiar with the presentation to ensure early recognition and treatment to prevent more serious complications. Once TPP is diagnosed, slow repletion with KCl is the initial treatment of choice. Definitive therapy is aimed at controlling the hyperthyroidism.

Selected References

1. Barnabe C. Acute generalized weakness due to thyrotoxic periodic paralysis. *CMAJ*. 2005;172:471–472.
2. Kung A. Clinical review: thyrotoxic periodic paralysis: a diagnostic challenge. *J Clin Endocrinol Metab*. 2006;91:2490–2495.
3. Lin SH, Chiu JS, Hsu CW, et al. A simple and rapid approach to hypokalemic paralysis. *Am J Emerg Med*. 2003;21:487–491.
4. Lin S. Thyrotoxic periodic paralysis. *Mayo Clin Proc*. 2005;80(1):99–105.
5. Manoukian M, MA, Foote JA, Crapo LM. Clinical and metabolic features of thyrotoxic periodic paralysis in 24 episodes. *Arch Intern Med*. 1999;159:601–606.

2-Year-Old Female with Fever

CASE PRESENTATION

A 2-year-old girl was transferred to our hospital because of clinical deterioration during a febrile illness. She developed abdominal pain, fever, and vomiting 5 days prior to transfer. She was evaluated in a local emergency department (ED) on the third day of illness when she had developed an erythematous, maculopapular, blanching rash of the trunk, extremities, palms, and soles. Cultures of blood, urine, and throat were obtained at that time, and she was treated with Ceftriaxone. She was sent home on Augmentin. Over the following 2 days she developed diarrhea and worsening activity level, and the fever, abdominal pain, vomiting, and rash persisted. She presented to the ED again and was transferred to tertiary care for further evaluation.

Her past medical history was unremarkable. She lived with her family and was in a daycare with no specific sick contacts. Family denied known tick bite. Immunizations are up-to-date.

Physical Examination

Patient is alert but irritable, ill-appearing girl whose temperature is 38.8°C, heart rate 140 beats/min, respiratory rate 40 breaths/min, and blood pressure 62/32 mm Hg. Her skin is warm with an erythematous maculopapular blanching rash on the distal extremities as well as petechiae in the antecubital fossae. Her mouth is dry and without lesion. Her neck is supple. A cardiac gallop rhythm is present with capillary refill delayed to 4 seconds. Her lungs are clear with tachypnea but no increased work of breathing. Her abdomen is distended, diffusely tender, and devoid of bowel sounds. Her tone is markedly decreased.

Laboratory Studies

Her hemoglobin is 9.9 g/dL with hemarocrit 28.4%. Her platelets are very low at 20,000 per mcL, and white blood count is 3900 per mcL, with 82% neutrophils, 15% lymphocytes, and 3% monocytes. Serum sodium level is 123 mmol/L, HCO_3 is 18 mEq/L, and glucose is 242 mg/dL. Stool is positive for occult blood. Urinalysis is normal.

Abdominal radiograph does not show obstruction, and chest x-ray shows increased perihilar markings. Abdominal ultrasound shows hepatomegaly. A head CT shows diffuse cortical edema, with attenuation of the gray-white differentiation. Echocardiogram shows mildly dilated left ventricle with preserved systolic ventricular function.

Case Resolution

The patient was started on antimicrobials including vancomycin, ceftriaxone, doxycycline, and acyclovir. She was initially given intravenous fluids and required vaso-pressor support as well. She developed respiratory failure, which required mechanical ventilation and also disseminated intravascular coagulation, which was supported with blood products. Her rash developed into diffuse petechiae and purpura. She also developed seizures. The cerebrospinal fluid (CSF) contained 17 nucleated cells/mm[3] with a lymphocytic predominance, 2 erythrocytes/mm[3], a protein level of 597 mg/dL, and a glucose level of 122 mg/dL. Multiple cultures from various sites grew no organisms.

Despite appropriate antibiotics and supportive care, the child developed diffuse encephalopathy. Six weeks after her presentation, she was transferred to a rehabilitation center unable to speak, with contractures, and poor suck-swallow coordination that necessitated gastrostomy feedings.

Question

What infection explains this child's fever, rash, abdominal pain, and subsequent disseminated intravascular coagulation, myocardial dysfunction, and brain injury?

Answer

Rocky Mountain spotted fever (RMSF). Acute-phase Rocky Mountain spotted fever antibody titers were negative, but convalescent titers drawn after 2 weeks of hospitalization were 1:10,240, which is highly positive.

Discussion

Rocky Mountain Spotted Fever

RMSF is the most lethal tick-born illness in the United States. It most commonly presents in the summer in the southeastern United States, but can occur in any season and anywhere in the United States, Canada, Mexico, and Central and South America. The causative organism of RMSF, *Rickettsia rickettsii*, is transmitted through a tick bite from an *Ixodes* species tick, although up to half of patients with the illness will deny a known tick bite. Children less than 15 are most commonly affected. The illness usually occurs 2 to 12 days after the tick bite, and there is no evidence to support the use of prophylactic antibiotic treatment after tick bite to prevent the disease.

R. rickettsii infect the vascular endothelial cells and cause a small vessel vasculitis which can involve any organ. The skin, with petechial rash, is most often noted, but involvement of the heart, abdominal organs, brain, kidneys, liver, and lungs can also occur. Poorly perfused distal extremities may necrose. Other significant sources of morbidity from the disease include pulmonary hemorrhage, acute respiratory distress syndrome, myocarditis, and meningoencephalitis. Disseminated intravascular coagulation and shock develop in the worst cases and can lead to death.

Patients sick with RMSF always have history of fever. Rash is present during the course of illness in up to 80% of patients, but it is important to note that the absence of rash does not exclude the diagnosis. The classic RMSF rash begins on the ankles and wrists, and develops typically 2 to 6 days after the onset of fever. It may then move to the trunk, face, and extremities. Often, the rash starts as a maculopapular blanching exanthem that later becomes petechial. Involvement of the palms and soles is common. Delayed or absent rash can lead to delayed recognition and treatment of the disease and worsened outcomes.

Severe headache and myalgias are common in the clinical presentation. Nausea and vomiting occur in more than 50% of patients, and abdominal pain and diarrhea can also be prominent. Conjunctivitis and edema can occur.

The differential diagnosis includes many other infections such another tick-borne illness, ehrlichiosis, enteroviral and other viral infections, meningococcal disease, toxin-mediated illness from *Staphylococcus* or *Streptococcus*, leptospirosis, and measles. Kawasaki disease may also be considered.

Hyponatremia and thrombocytopenia are the classic laboratory findings in RMSF. These are caused by the vasculitis and emerge as the clinical disease progresses. The platelet count gradually falls during the course of worsening RMSF, but the initial platelet count measured may not fall outside the normal range. The white blood cell count usually is normal to slightly low, and mild anemia can occur. Other laboratory studies such as cardiac enzymes, transaminases, and creatinine may be abnormal, depending on organ involvement with the vasculitis.

The mortality rate in untreated cases is up to 25%, with death occurring most often 1 to 2 weeks after the onset of symptoms. The overall mortality rate is 1% to 4%, with the rate rising significantly if therapy is initiated after day 5 of illness. Delayed diagnosis and treatment is more common when the illness falls outside of the typical April-September time period and when patients lack rash.

Serologic testing demonstrating a fourfold or greater change between acute and convalescent titers is diagnostic of the illness. Indirect fluorescent antibody (IFA) testing, with a sensitivity of 90% is the most widely used test to confirm suspected RMSF. With IFA, antibodies to *R. rickettsii* usually are detected 7 to 10 days after the initial symptoms. Negative antibody results obtained during acute illness are expected and should not deter treatment.

PCR can be done on tissue samples (typically skin lesions) and is currently available as a referral test at the Centers for Disease Control and Prevention. Antibody testing of skin biopsy is also possible, but not available in every center.

First-line treatment of RMSF is with doxycycline, and outcomes are better the sooner that treatment is delivered, particularly by the fifth day of illness. Staining of teeth from doxycycline is dose related, and does not occur until after several courses of treatment in children. Therapy with doxycycline should be continued until the patient is afebrile for at least 3 days. The total duration of therapy is usually 7 to 10 days. Oral tetracycline is an alternative therapy but there is greater risk of teeth staining with this drug. Fluoroquinolones are also possible alternatives. Chloramphenicol is indicated in pregnant patients and those who have a tetracycline allergy, although it has been shown to be associated with a higher mortality rate than doxycycline in treating RMSF. It is also not effective against Ehrlichia, which is frequently difficult to differentiate from RMSF. Clinicians should note that cephalosporins, typically used to "rule out sepsis" in pediatric patients, are ineffective against RMSF.

In summary, RMSF is an infection that can have severe consequences. Clinicians should have a high suspicion for RMSF in the patient with persistent fever. Remember that a large fraction of these patients may not have rash, will deny history of tick exposure, and can present outside of the typical seasonal and geographic predictions. Promptly recognized RMSF can be effectively treated with doxycycline.

Selected References

1. Masters EJ, Olson GS, Weiner SH, et al. Rocky Mountain spotted fever: a clinician's dilemma. *Arch Intern Med*. 2003;163(7):769–774.
2. Abrahamian FM. Consequences of delayed diagnosis of Rocky Mountain spotted fever in children—West Virginia, Michigan, Tennessee, and Oklahoma, May–July 2000. *MMWR Morb Mortal Wkly Rep*. 2000;49(39):885–888.
3. Abramson JS, Givner LB. Rocky Mountain spotted fever. *Pediat Infect Dis J*. 1999;18(6):539–540.

1-Day-Old Infant with Bilious Emesis

CASE PRESENTATION

A term male infant was transferred from the newborn nursery to the neonatal intensive care unit when he had an episode of bilious emesis after breastfeeding. The patient was born at 38 weeks after a scheduled cesarean section for breech presentation. The mother is a primigravida, has no medical problems, and the pregnancy was uncomplicated. The baby appeared appropriate for gestational age at birth and was vigorous. The Apgar scores were 8 at 1 minute and 9 at 5 minutes. He was initially transferred from the delivery room to the newborn nursery for routine newborn care. The patient's mother attempted breastfeeding several times on the first day of life and the patient was noted to have a small volume emesis after each feeding attempt. The emesis was initially clear and whitish, but at 14 hours of life the patient had a larger volume emesis that was bilious. The neonatal intensive care unit was then called to transfer the patient for further evaluation and treatment. At the time of transfer the patient had not yet passed a stool, but had voided twice.

Physical Examination

The baby was resting comfortably in no acute distress. Vital signs: temperature 37.2°C, heart rate 144 beats/min, respiratory rate 32 breaths/min, blood pressure 86/50 mm Hg. Room air oxygen saturation was 100%. Head, eyes, ears, nose, and throat: anterior fontanelle was open, soft, and flat; ears: normally set and rotated; eyes: positive red reflex bilaterally; mouth: intact palate, vigorous suck, moist mucous membranes. Cardiovascular: regular rate and rhythm without murmur, femoral pulses 2+ bilaterally; lungs: clear bilaterally; abdomen: soft, mild distension, no apparent tenderness, and bowel sounds were present. Genitourinary: Tanner I male, uncircumcised left testicle palpable in the scrotum, right testicle was undescended but palpable in high in the inguinal canal. No inguinal hernias. Rectal: tight anal sphincter with expulsion of meconium following the examination. Musculoskeletal: negative Ortolani and Barlow maneuvers bilaterally.

Laboratory Studies

Initially no laboratory studies were performed, but the patient was taken emergently to radiology for an upper gastrointestinal (GI) series to rule out malrotation. The study did not reveal malrotation, but was notable for a markedly distended colon. A contrast enema was then performed and can be seen in Fig. 62-1. Subsequently, chemistries and complete blood count were performed and were within normal limits for age.

Case Resolution

The patient returned to the neonatal intensive care unit with a rectal tube in place for decompression. He was not permitted to eat and intravenous nutrition was initiated. A rectal biopsy was performed on day 4 of life and a definitive surgical procedure was performed on day 6.

Question

What is the cause of this patient's bilious emesis and colonic distension?

Answer

In this child the contrast enema was diagnostic for Hirschsprung disease (HD), given the small caliber rectum

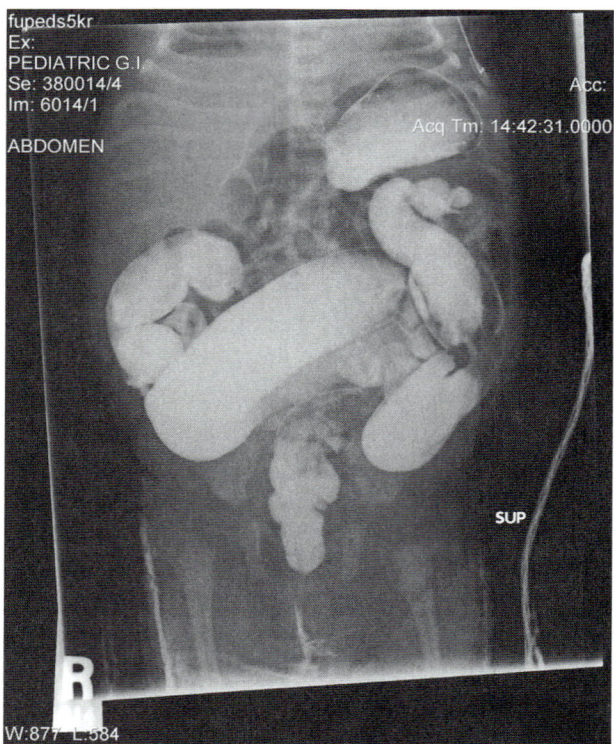

Figure 62-1 Contrast enema reveals a small caliber rectal segment and markedly dilated colon with a transition zone in the sigmoid colon.

TABLE 62-1

Differential Diagnosis of Intestinal Obstruction in the Neonate

Malrotation

Small bowel or colonic atresia

Hirschsprung disease

Meconium ileus

Meconium plug syndrome

Congenital band

Anorectal malformation

Intestinal motility disorder/pseudo-obstruction

Medical causes including sepsis, hypothyroidism, or electrolyte abnormalities

and transition zone visualized in the sigmoid colon. The diagnosis was confirmed prior to surgery by rectal suction biopsy, which demonstrated aganglionosis. Biopsies performed during surgery identified the transition zone 12 cm proximal to the dentate line.

Discussion

Bilious emesis in the neonate is an emergency and represents intestinal obstruction. A differential diagnosis of bowel obstruction in the neonate is listed in Table 62-1. In a neonate presenting with bilious emesis, malrotation with volvulus must be ruled out prior to pursuing other etiologies as it can result in total bowel necrosis if not identified and treated promptly. Other causes of bilious emesis, including intestinal atresias and HD, require surgical intervention in the postnatal period but do not carry the same grim prognosis as malrotation with volvulus without immediate surgical correction. Health care providers caring for newborns must recognize the clinical

importance of bilious emesis and promptly begin evaluation and surgical referral.

HD results from the absence of ganglion cells in the myenteric and submucosal plexuses of the distal intestine. Lack of innervation results in uncoordinated or absent peristalsis in the affected portion of bowel and commonly causes functional intestinal obstruction. HD was named after a Danish pathologist, who in 1887 described the condition among two children. However, a seventeenth century report of a young child who died of intestinal obstruction is regarded as the first description of the disease. Most affected children generally become symptomatic in the neonatal period and present with abdominal distension, feeding intolerance, and bilious emesis. Rarely, infants may present with colonic perforation. Even without symptoms of obstruction, suspicion for HD is raised when a term infant does not pass meconium in the first 24 hours of life. Few term infants with HD pass meconium in the first 24 hours of life, while nearly all normal term infants do. Children who present outside of the neonatal period can present with chronic constipation. Constipation from HD can be difficult to distinguish from functional constipation of childhood. Additionally HD can present with enterocolitis, which can be life threatening because of concomitant sepsis and dehydration. Bacterial overgrowth in the aganglionic bowel is thought to contribute to the enterocolitis, but the pathogenesis remains unclear.

The incidence of HD is approximately 1 in 5000 live born infants and is more common among African Americans and Asian infants. Additionally, HD has a male predominance of nearly 4:1. There is thought to be a genetic basis for the development of HD as there is an increased risk among siblings of affected children and around 10% children with HD have a positive family history. Research investigating the molecular pathology of HD has focused on the process of neural crest cell migration, which is thought to be arrested or delayed in affected patients. Other research has focused on identifying abnormalities in glycoproteins necessary for survival, proliferation, and differentiation of neural crest cells after they arrive at their destination. Genetic mutations associated with HD include the ret proto-oncogene, endothelin, and SOX-10, a gene known to be necessary in the development of neural crest lineages. The pattern of inheritance for HD and the contribution of known mutations to the clinical disorder are not well defined.

The presence of one congenital anomaly in a newborn is always a cause for concern, as birth defects often present in association with other anomalies and can represent named syndromes. HD presents as an isolated congenital anomaly in around 70% of cases. A list of syndromes and anomalies associated with HD can be found in Table 62-2. Of note, around 10% of children with Trisomy 21 have HD. Thus evaluation or at least careful consideration for HD is warranted in a child with Trisomy 21 presenting with constipation or intestinal obstruction. Additionally, there is an association between HD and multiple endocrine neoplasia type 2A (*MEN2A*). MEN2A is also associated with mutations in RET proto-oncogene located on chromosome 10. Approximately 1% of people with HD also have MEN2A. Mortality from MEN2A caused by medullary thyroid carcinoma is high, but can be reduced through prophylactic thyroidectomy if genetic testing in asymptomatic patients identifies the causative mutation. HD is more likely to be diagnosed prior to the onset of any manifestations of MEN2A. However, no clear recommendations for genetic screening for MEN2A among patients with HD exist.

The gold-standard for diagnosis of HD is a full-thickness rectal biopsy to evaluate for the presence of ganglion cells. Because this test requires general anesthesia, other modalities are generally used during diagnostic evaluation. A contrast enema is often the first test performed as it allows for evaluation of other possible causes of constipation or bowel obstruction. However, in preterm infants the change in colonic caliber from the aganglionic segment to the normally innervated segment can be difficult to demonstrate. Also, in children with total aganglionosis of the colon there can be no caliber change.

TABLE 62-2
Syndromes and Congenital Anomalies Associated with Hirschsprung Disease
Syndrome
Trisomy 21
Multiple endocrine neoplasia Type 2A (*medullary thyroid carcinoma, pheochromocytomas, parathyroid hyperplasia*)
Haddad syndrome (*congenital central hypoventilation, neuroblastoma*)
Waardenburg-Shah syndrome (*deafness, piebaldism, other neurologic deficits*)
Smith-Lemli-Opitz (*growth retardation, pedal syndactyly, mental retardation, hypospadias, dysmorphic facies*)
Mowat-Wilson (*abnormal facies, cardiac malformations, mental retardation, genitourinary anomalies*)
Bardet-Biedl (*obesity, retinal degeneration, polydactyly, gonadal and renal malformation*)
Nonsyndromic Congenital Anomalies
Hydrocephalus
Ventricular septal defect
Cystic deformities and renal agenesis
Imperforate anus
Meckel diverticulum
Polyposis of the colon
Cryptorchidism

Rectal suction biopsy is often used as a follow-up test after contrast enema because it provides a histologic diagnosis and does not require general anesthesia. False-negative tests can occur if the biopsy is too superficial, resulting in absence of the muscularis mucosa, where ganglion cells are located. Suction biopsy can be contraindicated in preterm infants, depending on weight and gestational age. Finally, anorectal manometry can be performed to evaluate for the rectoanal inhibitory reflex, which is absent in HD. This test is very difficult to interpret in children less than 1 year of age. A recent study evaluating diagnostic tests for HD found that the best predictor of HD on full-thickness biopsy was abnormal test results from at least two of the other diagnostic modalities.

The goal of surgical correction of HD is to allow for spontaneous and regular passage of stool while maintaining fecal continence. Several procedures have been developed, but the Soave procedure, or endorectal pull-through, is the performed most commonly. In this procedure, which does not require an abdominal incision, the aganglionic segment is removed and the normally innervated colon is anastomosed just above the dentate line. One-half to two-thirds of children with HD achieve the desired functional outcomes after surgical correction, but many children may have persistent obstructive symptoms or fecal incontinence after surgery. In addition, the risk of enterocolitis in children with repaired HD remains elevated. However, incontinence and obstructive symptoms appear to improve with time and the risk of enterocolitis decreases after 5 years of age in the absence of continued obstructive symptoms. Children with associated syndromes such as Trisomy 21, or those with a longer affected segment experience more complications and are less likely to have a good functional outcome.

In summary, HD commonly presents as a bowel obstruction during the neonatal period, but can present later in life as constipation or enterocolitis. The genetic basis of HD is intriguing, given its male predominance and association with other known syndromes. Study of the molecular

basis of HD is ongoing and will inform counseling of families regarding risk in subsequent children and the need for further genetic testing in children with HD. Surgical correction of HD continues to evolve, and functional outcomes are improving. However, achieving the desired functional outcome and limiting complications for all patients remains a challenge.

Selected References

1. Dasgupta R, Langer JC. Hirschsprung disease. *Curr Probl Surg.* 2004;41(120):942–988.
2. De Lorijn F, Reitsma JB, Voskuijl WP, et al. Diagnosis of Hirschsprung's disease: a prospective, comparative accuracy study of common tests. *J Pediatr.* 2005 Jun;146(6):787–792.
3. Feldman T, Wershil BK. In brief: Hirschsprung disease. *Pediatr Rev.* 2006;27(8):e56–e57.
4. Kapur RP. Multiple endocrine neoplasia type 2B and Hirschsprung's disease. *Clin Gastroenterol Hepatol.* 2005;3(5): 423–431.
5. Kessman J. Hirschsprung's disease: diagnosis and management. *Am Fam Physician.* 2006;74(8):1319–13122.

23-Year-Old with Easy Bruising

CASE PRESENTATION

A 23-year-old male presented to our emergency department complaining of easy bruising and gingival bleeding. The patient felt well until 2 days prior, when he developed a frontal headache that worsened with movement. He also began to experience profound weakness with presyncopal symptoms. One day prior to presentation, he awoke with spontaneous gingival bleeding. In addition, he began to have fevers as high as 38.6°C. On the day of admission, he went to the dentist for routine cleaning and has since had worsening of his gingival bleeding. His review of symptoms reveals a new rash. He did not travel outside of his home state. He denies any sick contacts, tick bites, unprotected sexual contacts, IV drug use, or transfusions. He does report being told he had hepatitis of unknown etiology 2 months prior. He currently takes no medication or uses any over-the-counter medications.

Past medical history includes the following:

- Jaundice 2 months ago, admitted for evaluation and no etiology identified, improved
- Nephrolithiasis 4 years ago, treated with lithotripsy
- Lone atrial fibrillation
- Enlarged right submandibular lymph node present for years, unchanged with antibiotics

Family history included mother with multiple sclerosis, and father who died of metastatic kidney cancer. He had a sister who was healthy.

Social history: He worked as a grade school physical education teacher and lived with his girlfriend. He had no children. He did have a sexual partner years ago who had some type of liver disease. Besides, he has a 7-pack/year history of smoking but quit 1 year ago. He quit drinking alcohol when diagnosed with liver disease 2 months ago, but prior to that he drank 10 beers every weekend and a binge twice a month. He denies any illicit drug use or herbal medications. He has several tattoos and one piercing done professionally.

C

63

Physical Examination

Vital signs: temperature 38.4°C, heart rate 100 beats/min, respiratory rate (RR) 16 breaths/min, and blood pressure 118/73 mm Hg. Oxygen saturation was 98% on room air. General: fatigued with blood oozing from gums; head, eyes, ears, nose, and throat: sclerae are anicteric; neck: right submandibular lymph node approximately 2 cm × 2 cm, mobile, and mildly tender; heart: regular rate and rhythm, normal S_1, S_2, no murmurs; lungs: clear to auscultation bilaterally, no wheezes. Skin: petechial rash throughout the extremities and in the trunk; large ecchymosis on left shoulder. Abdomen: soft, nontender, normoactive bowel sounds, no rebound or guarding, no hepatosplenomegaly. Neurologic: alert and oriented × 3, cranial nerves II through XII grossly intact. Strength is 5/5 in all extremities and axial groups, normal sensation throughout. Cerebellar function normal.

Laboratory Studies

White blood cells (WBC) 1.2, absolute neutrophil count (ANC) 0.2, absolute lymphocyte count (ALC) 0.9, absolute monocyte count (AMC) 0.0, absolute eosinophil count (AEC) 0.1, hemoglobin (Hgb)/hematocrit (Hct) 11.5/29.9, platelets less than 5. Total iron (Fe) 253, ferritin 709, reticulocyte percent 0.5; absolute retic count 16.6 (25.5–75), Na 138, K 3.6, Cl 102, HCO_3 27, blood urea nitrogen 21, Cr 1.1, glucose 110, Ca 8.5, Mg 1.8, and P 1.8. Albumin 3.7, total protein 6.6, total bilirubin 1.8, aspartate aminotransferase 22, alanine aminotransferase 86, alkaline phosphate 98, gamma-glutamyltransferase 37, lactate dehydrogenase LD 318, haptoglobin 185.

Complete blood count (CBC) 2 months prior: WBC 4.8 (ANC 2.3, ALC 1.6, AMC 0.5, AEC 0.2, ABC 0.0). Hgb/Hct 17.7/51.4, mean corpuscular volume 91, platelets 212, head CT showed no acute intracranial abnormality.

Question

What may be causing pancytopenia in this young patient?

Answer

Bone marrow aspiration and biopsy was performed and revealed a hypocellular bone marrow with 10% cellularity (normal cellularity is approximately 100-patient's age, approximately 75% for this patient) (see Fig. 63-1). It had normal cytogenetic studies and was consistent with aplastic anemia. This patient's aplastic anemia was found to be hepatitis-associated aplastic anemia. Hepatitis-associated aplastic anemia, a variant of aplastic anemia, occurs after an episode of acute hepatitis and often affects boys and young men. It is often fatal if untreated.

Discussion

Aplastic anemia is a rare process affecting two to four people per million per year with a bimodal age distribution affecting people in their twenties and then in their forties.

It is a specific entity describing a primary deficiency of stem cells. Aplastic anemia is defined by: pancytopenia (anemia, neutropenia, thrombocytopenia) with an inappropriately low reticulocyte count and aplastic bone marrow (hypocellular marrow with normal residual hematopoietic cells and no signs of malignancy, fibrosis, or megaloblastic hematopoiesis). It is important to define the severity of the aplastic anemia as outlined in Table 63-1 when addressing therapeutic and prognostic decisions, as severe aplastic anemia has a very low rate of spontaneous remission and a 70% mortality rate.

Patients often present, as this patient did, with fatigue and shortness of breath, thrombocytopenic bleeding including gingival bleeding, petechiae, oral blood blisters, hematuria, and heavy menses. They often have recurrent

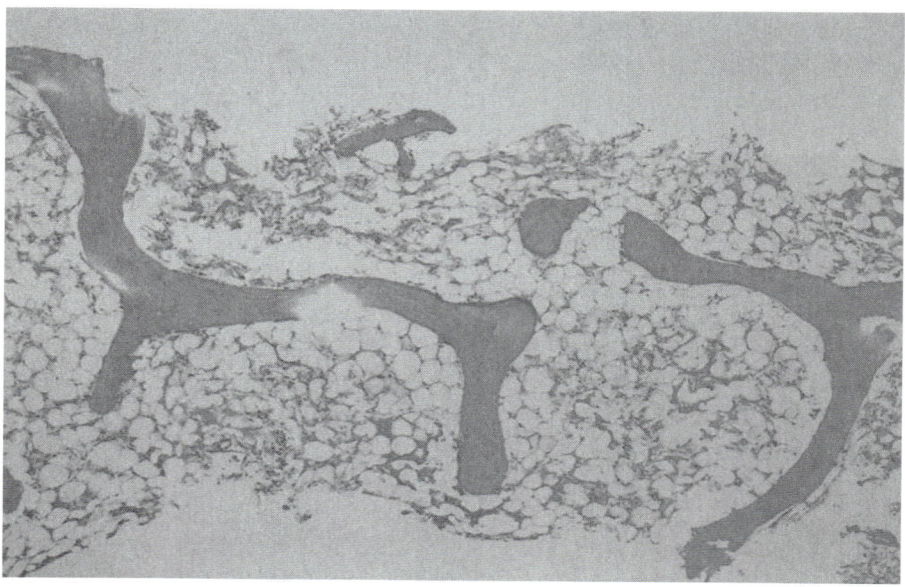

Figure 63-1 Hypocellular bone marrow.

TABLE 63-1

Definitions of Severity of the Aplastic Anemia

Severe aplastic anemia (SAA)

1. Marrow characteristics (one of the following):
   a. Less than 25% normal cellularity *or*
   b. Less than 50% normal cellularity with fewer than 30% of the cells being hematopoietic
2. Two of the following abnormal peripheral blood values:
   a. Absolute reticulocyte count < 40,000
   b. ANC < 500
   c. Platelets < 20,000

Very severe aplastic anemia (VSAA)

All of the above except ANC < 200

TABLE 63-2

Differential Diagnosis of Aplastic Anemia According to Presence or Absence of an Enlarged Spleen

Pancytopenia with splenomegaly: hypersplenism due to liver disease, CHF, etc

Pancytopenia without splenomegaly
– Aplastic anemia
  • Congenital: Fanconi anemia; dyskeratosis congenita; Shwachman-Diamond syndrome; Amegakaryocytic thrombocytopenia
  • Acquired: see Table 63-3
– Acute leukemia
– Large granular lymphocyte leukemia
– MDS
– Marrow replacement with tumor or fibrosis
– Severe megaloblastic anemia (folate or vitamin B_{12} deficiency)
– PNH
– Overwhelming infection HIV or viral hemophagocytic syndrome of EBV

bacterial infections or invasive fungal infectious caused by neutropenia. Examination typically demonstrates petechiae, ecchymosis, and pallor and no hepatosplenomegaly.

When faced with pancytopenia, it is important to evaluate the patient closely for hepatosplenomegaly. With hepatosplenomegaly, hypersplenism because of congestive heart failure, liver disease, and others may be to blame. And without hepatosplenomegaly one must consider malignancy, myelodysplastic syndromes, overwhelming infection, and severe megaloblastic anemia as listed in Table 63-2.

The cause of aplastic anemia is most often not identified, however it is important to consider all possible etiologies including both acquired and inherited causes (see Table 63-3). Irradiation, chemotherapeutics, certain drugs, and solvents may be responsible for bone marrow failure and should be discontinued. Aplasia may also occur during the prodrome of hairy cell leukemia, acute lymphoblastic leukemia (ALL), or rarely acute myelogenous leukemia (AML); or during the course of a myelodysplastic syndrome (MDS). In 2% to 5% of patients with aplastic anemia in the West, there will be history of hepatitis 2 to 3 months prior hepatitis-associated aplastic anemia. In the far East, hepatitis-associated aplastic anemia is accountable for 4% to 10% of all aplastic anemia cases. Hepatitis-associated aplastic anemia often affects boys and young men and often no identifiable etiology of the hepatitis is identified. The bone marrow failure is precipitous and often fatal if untreated. Knowing that patients with graft versus host disease (GVHD) have marrow aplasia; that immunosuppressive therapy improves success rates of bone

marrow transplant in patients with aplastic anemia; and that immunosuppressive therapy has been successfully used to treat aplastic anemia, one may argue that autoimmune processes may cause aplastic anemia. The blood of patients with aplastic anemia has an inhibitory hematopoietic response that may possibly be mediated by interferon-gamma or by its cytokine cascade. Interferon-gamma may lead to increased expression of the Fas receptor and antigen, which is involved in induction of apoptosis and T-cell-mediated killing, and is found in increased concentration in CD34+ bone marrow cells in patients with aplastic anemia. After immunosuppressive treatment, interferon-gamma levels have been shown to decrease. Additionally, there are fewer natural killer cells in patients with aplastic anemia and many autoimmune conditions are associated with lower NKT cell counts.

The key to diagnosis includes bone marrow aspirate and biopsy to confirm the diagnosis and then evaluation of possible etiologies as outlined above. A thorough history of exposures and testing for HIV, hepatitis, Epstein-Barr virus (EBV), and parvovirus should be obtained. If the history is suggestive, red cell CD55/59 may be performed to evaluate for paroxysmal nocturnal hematuria (PNH).

TABLE 63-3

Etiologies of Aplastic Anemia

Acquired

Radiation

Drugs and toxins

    Anticipated myelosuppression: cytotoxic chemotherapy,
    benzene

    Occasional myelosuppression: chloramphenicol, gold,
    NSAID, antiepileptics

Viruses: Hepatitis (non-A, non-B, non-C), EBV, parvovirus, HIV

Malignancy: Hairy-cell; ALL, AML (rarely); myelodysplastic
syndromes

Clonal disorders: paroxysmal nocturnal hemoglobinuria

Immune-mediated aplasia: eosinophilic fasciitis, SLE, GVHD

Pregnancy

Inherited

Fanconi anemia

Familial aplastic anemias

Dyskeratosis congenital

Reticular dysgenesis

ALL, acute lymphoblastic leukemia; AML, acute myelogenous
leukemia; EBV, Epstein-Barr virus; GVHD, graft versus host
disease; NSAID, nonsteroidal anti-inflammatory drug; SLE,
systemic lupus erythematosus.

TABLE 63-4

Therapies for Aplastic Anemia

Therapy	Response rate (%)	Relapse rate (%)
Antithymocyte globulin (ATG)	20–85	35
Cyclosporine A (CsA)	16–57	40–63
ATG/CsA	65–80	3–36
Cyclophosphamide	70	40
Bone marrow transplantation	66–90	10–36

Both the severity of the disease and the patient's age and health must be taken into consideration regarding treatment options for aplastic anemia. Treatment includes a combination of supportive care, immunosuppression, and, for some patients, curative therapy with bone marrow transplantation. Supportive care includes antibiotics, and platelet and red cell transfusions. Cytokine therapy, including G-CSF and GM-CSF, may be helpful in treating infection by improving neutrophil counts; however, they are most often successful when used in combination with immunosuppressive therapy. Immunosuppressive therapy is not curative. The goal is a sustained remission (see Table 63-4). About 20% to 36% of patients treated with immunosuppression have recurrent aplastic anemia, and up to 15% may develop a clonal disorder, PNH, MDS, or acute leukemia. Combination therapy appears to

work best with antithymocyte globulin (ATG), cyclosporine, and high-dose corticosteroids. Allogeneic bone marrow transplantation with a fully HLA-matched sibling has a 50% to 80% cure rate and a low incidence of clonal disorders. Outcomes are improved if patients are conditioned pre-transplant with ATG and cyclophosphamide. An unrelated donor may be considered, but survival is only half the rate of a matched sibling.

This patient had hepatitis-associated aplastic anemia. Supportive therapy with packed red blood cell (PRBC) and platelet transfusion, as well as antibiotics for neutropenic fever was initiated. Medication, leukemia, clonal disorders, and inherited disorders were ruled out as the etiology of aplastic anemia. He had a short course of immunosuppression with cyclosporine and ATG, but failed to improve. He subsequently underwent an allogeneic bone marrow transplant.

Selected References

Baggstrom MQ, TC Shea. Bone marrow failure states. In: Runge MS, Greganti MA, eds. *Netter's Internal Medicine*. Teterboro, NJ: Icon Learning Systems; 2003:393–396.

Brown KE, Tisdale J, Dunbar CE, et al. Hepatitis-associated aplastic anemia. *New Engl J Med*. 1997;336:1059–1064.

Schrier S. Anemia: production defects. In: David C. Dale and Daniel D. Federman, eds. *American college of Physicians (ACP) Medicine*. New York: Jun 2004:505–525.

Young NS, Maciejewski J. The pathophysiology of acquired aplastic anemia. *New Engl J Med*. 1997;336:1365–1372.

7-Year-Old with Left Eye Swelling

CASE PRESENTATION

A 7-year-old female presented with a 1-day history of left eye swelling, proptosis, and erythema preceded by 6 days of malaise, fatigue, and sore throat. The patient had been evaluated by her pediatrician 3 weeks prior to presentation and was diagnosed with *Streptococcal* pharyngitis by a rapid *Streptococcal* test. She had been treated with a 10-day course of amoxicillin. The patient developed a subjective low-grade fever 4 days after completion of her amoxicillin course, with increasing fatigue and malaise. In addition, she began to have mild swelling in the left eye 2 days later. She returned to her pediatrician and was placed on cefdinir. However, after 24 hours on therapy, the patient developed proptosis. She had no changes in vision. Because of treatment failure, she was admitted to the pediatric ward for further evaluation and IV antibiotics. Of note, the patient was up-to-date on her immunizations.

Physical Examination

Patient was a generally well appearing, pleasant, smiling, and conversant female in no acute distress. Vital signs: temperature 39.1°C, pulse 130 beats/min, blood pressure 114/69 mm Hg, and respiratory rate of 18 breaths/min. Ocular examination revealed mild proptosis OS (left eye), with swelling of the upper eyelid and partial eye closure. The patient could fully open OS 45% on command. Pupils were equal, round, and reactive to light and accommodation. Consensual papillary constriction was also intact. Significant left periorbital erythema and edema were also present. Extraocular movements were intact other than partially limited abduction OS. Visual fields were full to confrontation. OS-dilated funduscopic examination revealed cup to disk ratio of 0.2, pink optic nerve, sharp disk margin, flat macula, and normal retinal vessels. Ocular pressures were OD 19 mm Hg, OS 34 mm Hg, pharyngeal examination was unremarkable. Lung fields were clear to auscultation bilaterally. Heart was regular in rate and rhythm, with normal S_1, S_2, grade 2/6 systolic ejection murmur, musical in quality, heard best at the lower left sternal border (patient with verified previous diagnosis of benign murmur). Abdomen was soft, nondistended, and nontender, with normoactive bowel sounds

and no organomegaly. The remainder of the patient's examination was unremarkable.

Laboratory Studies

A complete blood count revealed white blood cells 10.4, absolute neutrophil count 9.4, hemoglobin 11.8, hematocrit 32.9, platelets 201, C-reactive protein 3.8 (normal range 0–1), Gram stain of left sinus drainage +1 polymorphonuclear neutrophils, no organisms, aerobic and anaerobic culture of left sinus drainage had no growth, blood culture has no growth at 5 days. CT of the orbit and sellae with contrast demonstrated presence of preseptal soft tissue thickening with inflammatory stranding of left orbit and proptotic left globe, thickened medial rectus, and surrounding inflammatory stranding. Sphenoid, ethmoid, and maxillary mucosal thickening were also present (Fig. 64-1).

Case Resolution

The patient was started immediately on IV ampicillin/sublactam. She was also placed on oxymetazoline nasal spray to decrease sinus inflammation. After 36 hours of IV

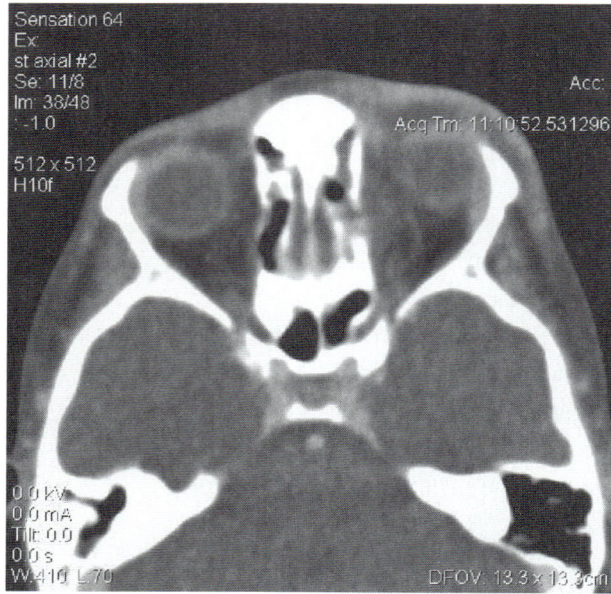 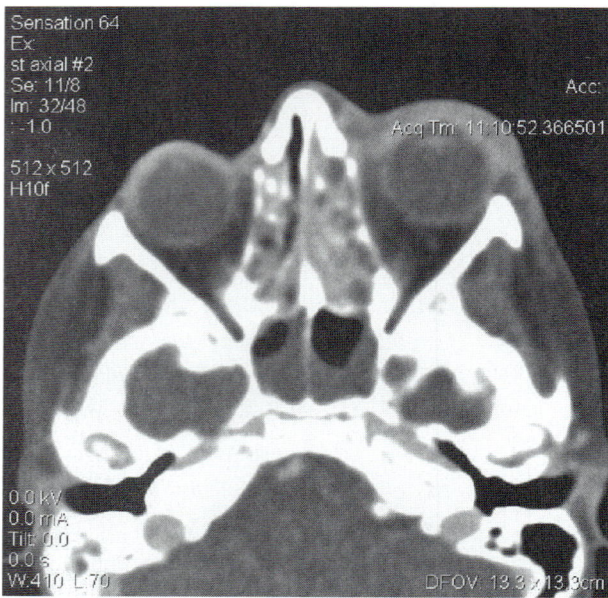

Figure 64-1 CT images obtained from patient described above show presptal soft tissue thickening with inflammatory stranding of left orbit with proptotic left globe, thickened medial rectus, and surrounding inflammatory stranding. Sphenoid, ethmoid, and maxillary mucosal thickening were also present.

antibiotic therapy, the patient had no clinical response of erythema and proptosis, even though her left ocular pressures normalized. At this point IV antibiotics were changed to clindamycin and ceftriaxone to cover community-acquired methicillin-resistant *Staphylococcus aureus* (CA MRSA). After this change, the patient's examination improved rapidly. Her proptosis and erythema resolved completely after 24 hours of therapy. Absence of culture growth prevented verification of the offending organism. The patient was discharged on oral clindamycin and oral cefdinir, for empiric coverage of CA MRSA, gram-negative organisms such as *Haemophilus influenza*, and anaerobes. She was treated with oral antibiotics for a total of 2-week course. It was felt that the patient had some MRSA involvement in her periorbital/orbital cellulitis evidenced by her marked clinical response to clindamycin.

Question

Which organisms are most prevalent offenders in periorbital cellulitis?

Answer

Gram-positive, gram-negative, anaerobic, or fungal organisms, or all of them can cause periorbital cellulitis.

Of positive culture isolates (ocular, sinus, and blood), approximately 40% of species are staphylococcal, 30% are streptococcal, 5% are *H. influenza* (Hib), 15% are related to other gram-negative organisms, and the remainder are anaerobic. Poly-microbial infections are quite common, validating the need for broad-spectrum antibiotics, as in the case of the aforementioned patient. Initial coverage with ampicillin/sublactam provided streptococcal, staphylococcal (non-MRSA), gram-negative and anaerobic coverage. Transition to ceftriaxone and clindamycin provided similar coverage and added effectiveness for some strains of CA MRSA. As sensitivity profiles of CA MRSA vary from region to region, with some strains demonstrating inducible clindamycin resistance for example, familiarity with local CA MRSA proves essential in choosing appropriate empiric coverage. The patient's home regimen oral cefdinir and clindamycin provided similar coverage and was instituted only after significant response was obtained from IV antibiotic therapy.

Prior to 1989, *H. influenzae* was the most common isolated organism. Now, gram-positive organisms are the most prevalent. Some studies have demonstrated higher rates of staphylococcal isolation; others have higher rates of streptococcal isolation. In light of this epidemiologic shift, general lack of positive blood and sinus cultures to guide therapy, and prevalence of MRSA, close attention must be given to initiation of appropriate MRSA antibiotic coverage with vancomycin, clindamycin, or TMP/SMX.

Discussion

Periorbital cellulitis (preseptal cellulitis) refers to infection of tissues outside the bony orbit, or anterior to the orbital septum. The diagnosis of periorbital cellulitis is limited palpebral infection only. Orbital cellulitis involves inflammation of tissues within the bony orbit (septal or postseptal cellulitis). Orbital cellulitis is much more serious than periorbital cellulitis because it can compromise the optic nerve and cause subsequent vision loss or impairment. Orbital cellulitis may often require surgical intervention. Orbital cellulitis is categorized using Chandler classification, which stratifies orbital cellulitis into categories I to V (Table 64-1). Although group II is subcategorized as orbital cellulitis, group I does not technically fall within the realm of periorbital cellulitis. Group I orbital cellulitis is differentiated from periorbital cellulitis by presence of mild proptosis of the globe and possible inflammation of the orbit, in addition to palpebral infection seen in periorbital cellulitis. Group V indicates extension of "phlebitis into the cavernous sinus." Intracranial abscess has also been described as a complication of orbital cellulitis. The patient above would be categorized as group II as

she had proptosis, intraorbital edema, and limitation of extraocular movements, but no abscess formation.

The overall incidence of orbital and periorbital cellulitis has dropped significantly in the last decade since the advent of *H. influenzae b* vaccination (Hib vaccine). As per retrospective analysis of databases at Massachusetts General Hospital, prior to 1990, approximately 12% of all cases of periorbital and orbital cellulitis were related to *H. influenzae b* infection. However, after the advent of Hib vaccination, only 3.5% of cases were related to Hib infection. Additionally, the total number of orbital and periorbital cellulitis cases has declined out of proportion to the reduction expected with prevention of Hib-related infections.

The routes of infection spread include bacteremia, sinusitis, and trauma. After the advent of Hib vaccination, there has been a sharp decline in bacteremic transmission of orbital and periorbital cellulitis. Currently, transmission of orbital and periorbital cellulitis is related most closely with presence of sinusitis.

The most common organisms currently implicated in orbital and periorbital cellulitis are *Staphylococcus* and *Streptococcus* species. Polymicrobial infections are common. In cases refractory to broad-spectrum antibiotic therapy, fungal infections must be considered. In cases of recurrent orbital cellulitis, malignancy (such as retinoblastoma and rhabdomyosarcoma) and chronic foreign body must be considered.

Periorbital and orbital cellulitis is twice more common among males than females. Evaluation of periorbital and orbital cellulitis requires close ocular examination to assess for proptosis, ptosis, decreased direct and consensual papillary reactivity, and restricted extraocular movements. If any of the above abnormalities are found, evaluation with noncontrast CT scan should be obtained for further evaluation and grading. Additionally, periorbital cellulitis not responsive to therapy after 24 hours should also be evaluated with CT scan. Use of CT scan in evaluation also proves helpful in assessing for underlying sinusitis. Additionally, in orbital cellulitis infections, formal ophthalmologic consultation should be considered to evaluate ocular pressures. These pressures should be monitored until normalization.

As stated above, therapy should be directed toward polymicrobial infection involving gram-positive, gram-negative, and anaerobic organisms. MRSA coverage should also be considered, perhaps initially, but certainly after 24 hours if no clinical improvement is seen on standard therapy. Initial IV antibiotic approaches could include ampicillin/sublactam or ceftazidime with clindamycin.

TABLE 64-1

Chandler Classification of Orbital Cellulitis

Chandler group		Criteria
I	Inflammatory edema	Affecting the eyelid with or without partial edema of the orbital contents; no limitation of extraocular movements. Presence of slight proptosis of the globe
II	Orbital cellulitis	Diffuse edema of orbital contents; no abscess formation
III	Subperiosteal abscess	Presence of a collection of pus between the periorbita and the bony wall of the orbit
IV	Orbital abscess	Presence of a discrete collection of pus within the orbital tissues
V	Cavernous sinus thrombosis	Extension of phlebitis posteriorly into the cavernous sinus

Adapted from Pereira F, Cruz A, Anselmo L, et al. Computed tomographic patterns of orbital cellulitis because of sinusitis. Arq Bras Oftalmol. 2006;69:513–518.

Oral antibiotics for outpatient therapy treating periorbital cellulitis or resolving orbital cellulitis include amoxicillin-clavulanate, or cefdinir with clindamycin. Trimethoprim-sulfamethoxazole may also be used for treatment of MRSA, but does not have the anaerobic coverage of clindamycin. Outpatient management with oral antibiotic therapy requires close (12–24 hours) follow up.

The average duration of therapy in orbital cellulitis is 21 days and periorbital cellulitis is 10 days. Orbital cellulitis generally requires longer IV antibiotic therapy (about 7 days compared to 3).

In cases of orbital cellulitis, surgical drainage is often required for full resolution/treatment in about 66% to 75%; especially in cases such as abscess drainage. Roughly 25% to 33% of infections fully resolve with antibiotics alone. Surgical drainage is imperative in cases of progressively worsening visual acuity and persistent ptosis. Vision loss from orbital cellulitis is a serious and relatively common complication, affecting about 5% of patients with infection. About 80% of patients with orbital cellulitis have full resolution of disease without complication. About 20% do experience residual complications such as vision loss, intracranial abscess extension, repeat infection, strabismus, or persistent ptosis.

Selected References

1. Ambati BK, Ambati J, Azar N, et al. Periorbital and orbital cellulitis before and after the advent of haemophilus influenzae type B vaccination. *Ophthalmology.* 2000;107:1450–1453.
2. American Academy of Pediatrics. Clinical practice guideline: management of sinusitis. *Pediatrics.* 2001;108:798–808.
3. Chaudhry CA, Shamsi FA, Elzaridi, E.et al. Outcome of treated orbital cellulitis in a tertiary eye care center in the Middle East. *Ophthalmology.* 2007;283:345–354.
4. K K Z Aabideen, Munshi V, Balasubramanian V, et al. Orbital cellulitis in children: a review of 17 cases in the UK. *Eur J Pediatrics.* 2006 Dec 22;165:189–197.
5. Nageswaran S, Woods CR, Benjamin DK, et al. Orbital cellulitis in children. *Pediatr Infect Dis J.* 2006;25:695–699.
6. Pereira F, Cruz A, Anselmo L, et al. Computed tomographic patterns of orbital cellulitis due to sinusitis. *Arq Bras Oftalmol.* 2006;69:513–518.
7. Starkey CR, Steele RW. Medical management of orbital cellulitis. *Pediatr Infect Dis J.* 2001;20:1002.
8. Uzcategui N, Warman R, Smith A, et al. Clinical practice guidelines for the management of orbital cellulitis. *J Pediatr Ophthalmol Strabismus.* 1998;35:73.
9. Vayalumkal JV, Jadavji T. Children hospitalized with skin and soft tissue infections: a guide to antibacterial selection and treatment. *Pediatr Drugs.* 2006;8:99–111.

76-Year-Old with Increasing Abdominal Girth

CASE PRESENTATION

A 76-year-old African American male presented to our emergency department with a chief complaint of vomiting and increasing abdominal girth. These symptoms were associated with progressive shortness of breath. Overall, his symptoms began approximately 3 weeks prior to presenting to the emergency department. On the day of presentation, he had three episodes of nonbloody, nonbilious emesis. He denied fevers, chills, and night sweats. He denied cough, hemoptysis, myalgias, and arthralgias at the time of presentation. He denied anorexia but did report weight loss, which he was unable to quantify.

His past medical history was significant for hypertension, gout, anemia, gastritis, gastric ulcer, diverticulosis, and chronic obstructive pulmonary disease. Current medications included clonidine, lisinopril, metoprolol, folic acid, esomeprazole, albuterol, tiotropium

His family medical history was significant for a mother who died at an unknown age of cancer (unknown what type of cancer). His father died of hypertension. His brother has hypertension and had several sisters who died of unknown causes. One of his sisters died of tuberculosis (TB) early in life. His social history is remarkable for a remote history of smoking cigars for approximately 2 to 3 years. He has a remote history of alcohol use, drinking 6-pack a day for about 2 years. He denied drug use. He reported two sexual partners and denied a history of sexually transmitted diseases. He reports being in prison for a year-and-a-half as a teenager. His review of systems was significant for a rash on his bilateral lower extremities, which is occasionally pruritic. He reported increased shortness of breath and abdominal swelling and emesis. Otherwise his review of systems was unremarkable.

C
65

Physical Examination

Vital signs: temperature 36.5°C, heart rate 79 to 86 beats/min, respiratory rate 18 breaths/min, blood pressure 141–154/74–82 mm Hg, room air oxygen saturation was 96% on room air.

General: He is a thin African American male, awake, alert, and in no apparent distress. His skin has nonblanching petechial rash on bilateral lower extremities. Head, eyes, ears, nose, and throat: sclerae clear and anicteric. Conjunctivae were without injection. Extraocular muscles are intact. Right eye is nonresponsive to light, secondary to trauma as a child. Oropharynx is without erythema or exudate. Poor dentition; nares without rhinorrhea.

Neck had small, soft mass in the left supraclavicular area with a pea-sized nodule in the left anterior chain. Chest: breath sounds were equal and symmetric; no wheezes or rhonchi. Rales at the bases bilaterally with right greater than left. Cardiac: regular rate and rhythm, no murmurs, gallops, or rubs. No carotid bruits. Abdomen: +distension, nonntender; + fluid wave; + tense abdominal wall; pea-sized inguinal lymph nodes bilaterally; right inguinal hernia.

Neurologic: the patient is alert and oriented × 3, mental status, mood and affect, and deep tendon reflexes were normal. Babinskis were absent bilaterally. Extremities: He has 1+ lower extremity edema bilaterally but no cyanosis or clubbing. Musculoskeletal: Dupuytren contracture of his left hand, gait normal.

Laboratory Data

White blood cell count 4.7, hemoglobin 10, hematocrit 30, platelet count 438 with 86% neutrophils, 9% lymphocytes, 5% monocytes, 0% eosinophils, and 0% basophils. Prothrombin time 10.1, international normalized ratio 1.01, partial thromboplastin time 35. Na 131, K 5.2, Cl 102, HCO_3 23, blood urea nitrogen 34, creatinine 1.4, glucose 126, Ca 8.5. Aspartate aminotransferase 28, alanine aminotransferase 14, alkaline phosphatase 54, total bilirubin 0.6, direct bilirubin 0.1, total protein 7.2, albumin 1.7. Urinalysis showed 1+ albumin, 10 red blood cells, 6 white blood cells, trace bacteria, moderate leukocyte esterase.

Case Resolution

Given the suspicion for ascites on clinical examination, the patient underwent abdominal ultrasonography. This revealed a large amount of free fluid within the abdominal cavity. A diagnostic paracentesis was then performed. The serum-ascites albumin gradient was below 1.1 g/dL. He was diagnosed after his peritoneal fluid grew *Mycobacterium tuberculosis*. He was subsequently treated with a four-drug regimen for TB, after which his ascites promptly resolved.

Question

How reliable is the physical examination for the presence or absence of ascites?

Answer

The physical examination is difficult for the detection and exclusion of ascites. Many different techniques are used, including shifting dullness to percussion, detection of a fluid wave, assessment for bulging flanks and peripheral edema. The interobserver reliability of these techniques is fair. The absence of peripheral edema and increased abdominal girth possess the lowest negative likelihood ratios in most reviews, 0.2 and 0.3 respectively. Detection of a fluid wave and shifting dullness to percussion are the best individual signs for confirming ascites. The reported positive likelihood ratios of these two signs range from 3 to 7.

Discussion

Ascites is defined as an abnormal (>25 mL) of fluid within the peritoneal cavity. It occurs as a consequence of portal hypertension, decreased plasma oncotic pressure, and avid sodium retention of the kidneys (1).

A detailed history regarding the onset of symptoms is helpful in distinguishing ascites from truncal obesity. Whereas a protuberant abdomen that has developed secondary to ascites typically occurs rather rapidly (ie, within a few weeks), patients often complain of early satiety and shortness of breath as compared to increasing abdominal girth from obesity, which often occurs gradually and patients are often tolerant of their progressive distension (2).

Physical examination findings that may be present in patients with chronic liver disease include signs of hyperbilirubinemia (icterus, jaundice, bilirubinuria), signs of increased systemic estrogen levels (gynecomastia, spider angiomata, testicular atrophy, palmar erythema), signs of hypoalbuminemia (lower extremity edema, ascites), signs of malnutrition (muscle wasting), leukonychia (white nails), and signs of portal hypertension (ascites, abdominal wall collaterals—Caput Medusae).

Physical examination findings that occur with ascites include abdominal distension, bulging flanks, presence of a fluid wave and/or shifting dullness, and the presence of inguinal or umbilical hernias. Of these, the most reliable technique for the detection of ascites is shifting dullness; a maneuver that relies on the premise that air-filled intestines will float on top of any fluid that is present.

Other physical examination findings in patients with ascites that may assist in determining the etiology include elevated JVP (suggesting heart failure or constrictive pericarditis), or palpation of an umbilical nodule (ie, Sister Mary Joseph nodule, suggesting cancer).

Pathophysiology

Ascites occurs most often as a complication of cirrhosis, particularly in the United States where it comprises approximately 85% of cases (13). A portal pressure greater than 12 mm Hg appears to be necessary for fluid retention (2, 16, 17), whereas it often will resolve if the portal pressure is reduced below 12 mm Hg (17). Portal hypertension is the most significant complication of cirrhosis as it is responsible for its most common sequelae, including variceal formation and hemorrhage, ascites, and hepatic encephalopathy. It occurs as the consequence of increased intrahepatic resistance and increased portal venous inflow. In addition, splanchnic and systemic vascular vasodilation and the hyperdynamic circulation that is characteristic of cirrhosis and portal hypertension play a pivotal role in the development of ascites (15).

Epidemiology

In the United States, cirrhosis is the most common cause of ascites and accounts for approximately 80% of cases (3). Causes of cirrhosis include the following:

- Viral hepatitis
- Alcoholic liver disease
- Autoimmune hepatitis
- Primary/secondary biliary cirrhosis
- Primary sclerosing cholangitis
- Hemochromatosis
- Wilson disease
- Alpha-1 antitrypsin deficiency
- Granulomatous disease (eg, sarcoidosis)
- Type IV glycogen storage disease
- Drug-induced liver disease (eg, methotrexate, alpha methyldopa, amiodarone)
- Venous outflow obstruction (eg, Budd-Chiari syndrome, veno-occlusive disease), chronic right-sided heart failure
- Tricuspid regurgitation (4)

Approach to Patient with Ascites

Patients with ascites should be extensively screened for risk factors associated with liver disease including the following:

- Alcohol consumption
- Hepatitis C infection (transfusions before 1990, needle sharing, substance use, cocaine snorting, tattoos, acupuncture, emigration from Japan or Southeast Asia)
- Hepatitis B infection (transfusion before 1971, persons in hyperendemic areas such as Africa, Southeast Asia including China, Korea, Indonesia, and the Philippines, the Middle East except Israel, southern and western Pacific Islands, the interior Amazon river basin, Haiti, and the Dominican Republic, men who have sex with men, injection drug users, individuals on dialysis, individuals with HIV infection, household and sexual contacts of HBV-infected persons)

- Nonalcoholic steatohepatitis (NASH) (obesity, diabetes, and hyperlipemia)
- Cancer
- Heart failure
- Tuberculosis,
- Hemodialysis
- Pancreatitis
- Nephrotic syndrome
- Systemic lupus erythematosus (SLE)
- Myxedema (2)

The International Ascites Club proposed a grading system for ascites as follows:

- Grade 1—mild ascites only detectable by ultrasound
- Grade 2—moderate ascites manifested by moderate symmetrical distension of abdomen
- Grade 3—large or gross ascites with marked abdominal distension (5)

An older system of characterizing ascites included the following:

- 1+ minimal and barely detectable
- 2+ moderate
- 3+ massive but not tense
- 4+ massive and tense

Imaging

Patients with ascites should undergo ultrasonography as it is cost-effective, does not involve radiation, does not require IV access, carries no risk of contrast allergy or nephropathy, is very sensitive as it can detect as little as 30 mL of fluid, and can help assess the patency of hepatic vessels.

Paracentesis

The most effective way to diagnose the cause of ascites and determine if the ascites fluid is infected is via fluid analysis after an abdominal paracentesis has been performed. Important components of ascitic fluid analysis include gross appearance, cell count with differential, serum-to-ascites albumin gradient, protein, glucose, lactate dehydrogenase, Gram stain, amylase, and culture.

Whereas uncomplicated ascites yields translucent yellow fluid, spontaneously infected fluid is often turbid or cloudy. Chylous ascites refers to milky white ascetic fluid that has elevated triglyceride content (ie, greater than serum and >200 mg/dL) and occurs in the setting of both cirrhosis and malignancy. Pink or frankly bloody samples occur most frequently in the setting of a traumatic tap with leakage of subcutaneous blood during the procedure. However, malignancy is another important cause of bloody ascites (ie, hepatocellular carcinoma and other malignancies). Brown-colored ascites can be secondary to increased bilirubin in deeply jaundiced patients but can also be seen in patients after a ruptured gallbladder, or a perforated duodenal ulcer. The cell count with differential is the most important test for the evaluation of peritonitis. Spontaneous bacterial peritonitis (SBP) is defined by the presence of greater than 250 polymorphonuclear cells in a specimen. However, if ascetic fluid has greater than 250 polymorphonuclear leukocytes (PMNs), but also has two of the three following criteria:

- Total protein greater than 1 g/dL
- Glucose less than 50 mg/dL
- LDH greater than the upper limit of normal,

then secondary peritonitis from gastrointestinal tract perforation into ascitic fluid has likely occurred (6, 7).

The serum-to-ascites gradient (SAAG) assists in the determining the etiology of the ascites, as it identifies the presence of portal hypertension. An SAAG greater than 1.1 g/dL indicates that the patient has portal hypertension with 97% accuracy and is superior to the concept of exudate (total protein of ascetic fluid ≥ 2.5 g/dL or 3 g/dL) versus transudate (8).

However, ascitic fluid total protein does have value in stratifying risk for SBP such that patients with a total protein less than 1 g/dL have a greater risk of SBP. Bacterial cultures of ascitic fluid should be obtained on all patients with new onset ascites, those with ascites and fever, abdominal pain, azotemia, acidosis, or confusion (9). The most sensitive technique for adequately identifying bacterial growth in ascitic fluid is to perform bedside inoculation of fluid in blood culture bottles. Ascitic fluid glucose should approximate the serum glucose concentration in most cases, but will be reduced in the presence of glucose consumers such as bacteria, white blood cells, or malignant cells in the peritoneal cavity (10). Furthermore, glucose concentrations can be minimal in the setting of gastrointestinal perforation (11, 12). Elevated levels of lactate dehydrogenase (ascitic fluid/serum ratio in uncomplicated cirrhosis ~0.4) in ascitic fluid occurs both in SBP (ascitic fluid/serum ratio ~1.0) and peritoneal carcinomatosis (ascitic fluid/serum ratio > 1.0). Elevated levels of amylase in ascitic fluid occur in the setting of pancreatitis and gut perforation into ascites.

When tuberculous peritonitis is suspected, the cell count can mimic SBP, but with a mononuclear predominance. In most patients with peritoneal TB, the ascitic fluid is proteinaceous with a protein content of the ascitic fluid greater than 3.0 mg/dL in more than 95% of patients (33). Adenosine deaminase is often used as a nonculture method for the detection of tuberculous peritonitis. However, patients with cirrhosis and tuberculous peritonitis usually have falsely low values. There is also literature to support the use of serum CA-125 levels for assistance with the diagnosis of tuberculous peritonitis, as it has been described as increased in patients with tuberculous peritonitis (30–33). The most useful method for diagnosing tuberculous peritonitis is laparoscopic exploration of the peritoneum with mycobacterial culture and histology of a biopsied tubercle. Biopsies of tubercle reveal caseating granulomas and may be positive for acid fast bacilli.

Peritoneal TB is a relatively uncommon manifestation of infection secondary to *M. tuberculosis* and occurs either after reactivation of latent TB in the peritoneum or from active pulmonary or miliary TB with hematogenous spread. Those at increased risk for the development of peritoneal TB include individuals with cirrhosis, diabetes mellitus, HIV infection, underlying malignancy, individuals who have received anti–tumor necrosis factor (TNF) agents or systemic corticosteroids, and in patients undergoing continuous ambulatory peritoneal dialysis (CAPD) (19–23). Tuberculous peritonitis usually develops in an insidious fashion and most patients present with ascites, abdominal pain, and fever (23–26). Physical examination findings often include abdominal distension with tenderness, ascites, and hepatomegaly (24–27). Laboratory analysis may reveal nonspecific findings such as leukocytosis and a normocytic, normochromic anemia (28, 29). Tuberculous peritonitis should be part of the differential diagnosis in patients presenting with insidious onset of abdominal pain with associated fever and weight loss. Furthermore, it should be considered in all patients presenting with unexplained lymphocytic ascites with a serum-ascites albumin gradient of less than 1.1 g/dL. Tuberculin testing with purified protein derivative (PPD) may be helpful as it may indicate previous exposure in nonanergic patients. Likewise, a chest x-ray may show evidence of old or active tuberculosis. Ultrasound characteristics include peritoneal thickening, omental caking, and the presence of ascites with fine mobile septations on ultrasound, whereas CT findings may include ascites, peritoneal lesions, and lymphadenopathy (34–36).

Selected References

1. Green G, Harris I, Lin G, Moylan K, eds. *The Washington Manual of Medical Therapeutics.* 31st ed. Philadelphia, PA: Lipincott Williams & Wilkins; 2004.

2. Gines P, Cardenas A, Arroyo V, Rodes J. Management of cirrhosis and ascites. N Engl J Med; 350:1646–1652.

3. Runyan BA. Care of patients with ascites. *New Engl J Med.* 1994;330:337.

4. Wolf DC, Cirrhosis. *eMed.* Available at: http://www.emedicine.com/med/topic3183.htm. Accessed Jan 16, 2006.

5. Moore KP, Wong F, Gines P, et al. The management of ascites in cirrhosis: report on the consensus conference of the International Ascites Club. *Hepatology.* 2003;38:258.

6. Runyon BA, Hoefs JC. Ascitic fluid analysis in the differentiation of spontaneous bacterial peritonitis from secondary bacterial peritonitis. *Gastroenterology.* 1990;98:127.

7. Akriviadis EA, Runyon BA. The value of an algorithm in differentiating spontaneous from secondary bacterial peritonitis. *Gastroenterology.* 1990;98:127.

8. Runyon BA, Montano AA, Akriviadis EA, et al. The serum-to-ascites gradient is superior to the exudate-transudate concept in the differential diagnosis of ascites. *Ann Intern Med.* 1992;117:215.

9. Runyon BA. Management of adult patients with ascites due to cirrhosis. *Hepatology.* 1998;27:264.

10. Runyon BA, Hoefs JC. Ascitic fluid analysis before, during and after spontaneous bacterial peritonitis. *Hepatology.* 1985;5:257.

11. Runyon BA, Hoefs JC. Ascitic fluid analysis in the differentiation of spontaneous bacterial peritonitis from secondary bacterial peritonitis. *Gastroenterology.* 1990;98:127.

12. Akriviadis EA, Runyon BA. The value of an algorithm in differentiating spontaneous from secondary bacterial peritonitis. *Gastroenterology.* 1990;98:127.

13. Runyon BA. Management of adult patients with ascites caused by cirrhosis. *Hepatology.* 2004;39:841.

14. Garcia-Tsao G. Portal hypertension. *Curr Opin Gastroenterol.* 2002 May;18(3):351–359.

15. Schrier RW, Arroyo V, Bernardi M, et al. Peripheral arterial vasodilation hypothesis: a proposal for the initiation of renal sodium and water retention in cirrhosis. *Hepatology.* 1988 Sep–Oct;8(5):1151–1157.

16. Gines P, Fernandez-Esparrach G, Arroyo V, et al. Pathogenesis of ascites in cirrhosis. *Semin Liver Dis.* 1997;17:175.

17. Morali GA, Sniderman KW, Deitel KM, et al. Is sinusoidal portal hypertension a necessary factor for the development of hepatic ascites? *J Hepatol.* 1992;16:249.

18. Reichle FA, Owen OE. Hemodynamic patterns in human hepatic cirrhosis: a prospective randomized study of the hemodynamic sequelae of distal splenorenal (Warren) and mesocaval shunts. *Ann Surg.* 1979;190:523.

19. Mehta JB, Dutt A, Harvill L, et al. Epidemiology of extrapulmonary tuberculosis. A comparative analysis with pre-AIDS era. *Chest.* 1991;99:1134.

20. Braun MM, Byers RH, Heyward WL, et al. Acquired immunodeficiency syndrome and extrapulmonary tuberculosis in the United States. *Arch Intern Med.* 1990;150:1913.

21. Rieder HL, Snider DE, Jr, Cauthen GM. Extrapulmonary tuberculosis in the United States. *Am Rev Respir Dis.* 1990;141:347.

22. Aguado JM, Pons F, Casafont F, et al. Tuberculous peritonitis: a study comparing cirrhotic and noncirrhotic patients. *J Clin Gastroenterol.* 1990;12:550.

23. Chow KM, Chow VC, Hung LC, et al. Tuberculous peritonitis-associated mortality is high among patients waiting for the results of mycobacterial cultures of ascitic fluid samples. *Clin Infect Dis.* 2002;35:409.

24. Jakubowski A, Elwood RK, Enarson DA. Clinical features of abdominal tuberculosis. *J Infect Dis.* 1988;158:687.

25. Demir K, Okten A, Kaymakoglu S, et al. Tuberculous peritonitis—reports of 26 cases, detailing diagnostic and therapeutic problems. *Eur J Gastroenterol Hepatol.* 2001;13:581.

26. Tanrikulu AC, Aldemir M, Gurkan F, et al. Clinical review of tuberculous peritonitis in 39 patients in Diyarbakir, Turkey. *J Gastro Hepatol.* 2005;20:906.

27. al-Quorain AA, Facharzt, Satti, MB, et al. Abdominal tuberculosis in Saudi Arabia: a clinicopathological study of 65 cases. *Am J Gastroenterol.* 1993;88:75.

28. Chow KM, Chow VC, Hung LC, et al. Tuberculous peritonitis-associated mortality is high among patients waiting for the results of mycobacterial cultures of ascitic fluid samples. *Clin Infect Dis.* 2002;35:409.

29. Marshall J. Tuberculosis of the gastrointestinal tract and peritoneum. *Am J Gastroenterol.* 1993;88:989.

30. Candocia SA, Locker GY. Elevated serum CA 125 secondary to tuberculous peritonitis. *Cancer.* 1993;72:2016.

31. Mas MR, Comert B, Saglamkaya U, et al. CA-125: a new marker for diagnosis and follow-up of patients with tuberculous peritonitis. *Dig Liver Dis.* 2000;32:595.

32. Younossian AB, Rochat T, Favre L, et al. Ascites and highly elevated CA-125 levels in a case of peritoneal tuberculosis. *Scand J Infect Dis.* 2006;38:216.

33. Manohar A, Simjee AE, Haffejee AA, et al. Symptoms and investigative findings in 145 patients with tuberculous peritonitis diagnosed by peritoneoscopy and biopsy over a five year period. *Gut.* 1990;31:1130.

34. Demirkazik FB, Akhan O, Ozmen MN, et al. US and CT findings in the diagnosis of tuberculous peritonitis. *Acta Radiol.* 1996;37:517.

35. Akhan O, Pringot J. Imaging of abdominal tuberculosis. *Eur Radiol.* 2002;12:312.

36. Vazquez Munoz E, Gomez-Cerezo J, Atienza Saura M, NET al. Computed tomography findings of peritoneal tuberculosis: systematic review of seven patients diagnosed in 6 years (1996–2001). *Clin Imaging.* 2004;28:340.

20-Year-Old with Shortness of Breath

CASE PRESENTATION

A 20-year-old Hispanic man presented to the emergency department with palpitations and nausea. The patient reported that for the past 2 years he had intermittent episodes of rapid heart rate and palpitations, which seemed to occur with exertion. Initially the episodes occurred every few weeks and only lasted a few minutes, but were now occurring more frequently and were lasting longer. They were associated with nausea and occasionally with vomiting. The patient had no other past medical history and denied taking any medications. He had not had consistent primary care for many years and reported only occasional ethanol use. He was a nonsmoker and did not use illicit drugs. Born in Mexico, he had illegally immigrated to the United States 5 years prior to this presentation. His family history was noncontributory.

Physical Examination

Vital signs: temperature 37°C, pulse 98 beats/min, blood pressure 120/76 mm Hg, respiratory rate 20 breaths/min, and oxygen saturation of 99% on room air. Physical examination revealed bibasilar crackles, grade 2/6 systolic ejection murmur, no clicks, normal S_1, S_2, no S_3 or S_4. No lower extremity edema. He had absent posterior tibial and dorsal pedis pulses bilaterally.

Laboratory Studies

His initial electrocardiogram showed sinus tachycardia and right atrial enlargement. On the telemetry monitor, however, he had long episodes of narrow complex tachycardia, not responsive to adenosine. He required digoxin, metoprolol and, eventually, amiodarone for rate control. His chest x-ray revealed cardiomegaly and pulmonary edema. Reevaluation later revealed rib notching, (Figs. 66-1 and 66-2). A bedside echocardiogram revealed severely decreased left ventricular systolic function, with an ejection fraction of 25%, moderate left ventricular hypertrophy, and a restrictive diastolic filling pattern. He had severe mitral regurgitation and a severely dilated left atrium. The aortic arch was not visualized. He was treated with furosemide and showed good initial improvement.

Case Resolution

Although initially normotensive, when his heart rate was controlled he had significant hypertension. Four extremity blood pressures revealed higher blood pressures in the upper extremities compared to the lower extremities. Given the differences in upper and lower extremity blood pressures, absence of lower extremity pulses and poor visualization of the aortic arch, a cardiac magnetic resonance imaging (MRI) was performed, (Fig. 66-3). The magnetic resonance angiogram showed a high-grade aortic coarctation 2 cm beyond the left subclavian origin. He also had an electrophysiology study done, which showed a slow atrial flutter conducting at a 1:1 rate. There were no retrograde pathways. He was transferred to a tertiary care center for surgical management. He eventually underwent balloon angioplasty with stent placement at the coarctated segment.

Question

When should secondary hypertension be suspected in patients?

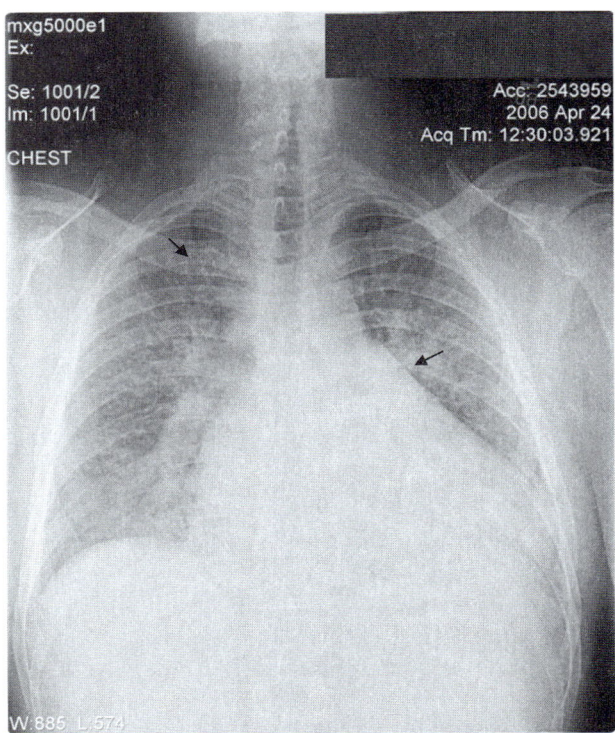

Figure 66-1 Chest radiography demonstrates cardiomegaly, cephalization of pulmonary vasculature, interstitial edema, and rib notching (arrows).

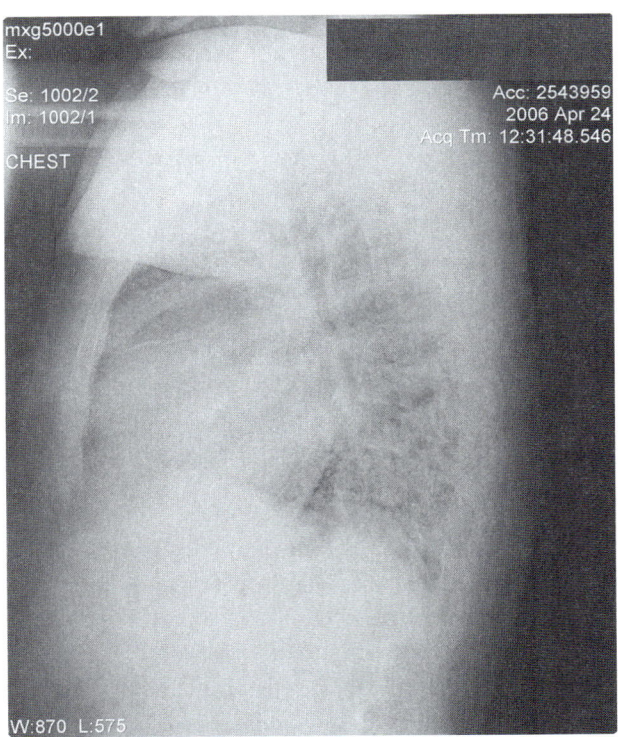

Figure 66-2 Lateral chest radiography reveals cardiomegaly, fluid filling the major fissure, and increased pulmonary vascular markings.

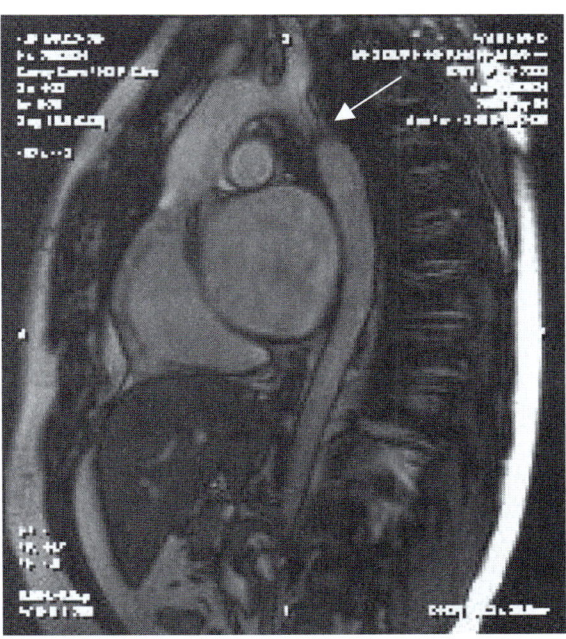

Figure 66-3 Magnetic resonance angiogram reveals coarctation of the aorta (arrow).

Answer

Several clinical scenarios warrant close evaluation for a secondary cause of hypertension. There are four major categories; severe or refractory hypertension; an acute rise in a previously stable blood pressure; age of onset before puberty or after age 50; and onset before age 30 in nonobese, nonblack patient with a negative family history. Our patient was young and had no family history of hypertension.

Discussion

Secondary hypertension is when elevated blood pressure is because of an underlying disorder. Children are more likely than adults to have secondary hypertension. Younger patients, patients with severe hypertension, patients without family history of hypertension, or without obesity are all at increased risk of secondary hypertension. The recommended work up for all patients with hypertension is shown in Table 66-1. The purpose of the workup is threefold: reveal identifiable causes of hypertension, identify comorbidities which may affect treatment, and evaluate for end-organ damage. Alcohol abuse and obesity are the most common causes of secondary

TABLE 66-1

Evaluation for a New Diagnosis of Hypertension§

Test	Target pediatric population	Target adult populations
BUN, creatinine	Children with BP > 95th percentile	All adults
Electrolytes	Children with BP > 95th percentile	All adults (potassium and calcium only)
Urinalysis, urine culture	Children with BP > 95th percentile	All adults (urinalysis only)
Urinary albumin/creatinine ratio	Children with BP > 95th percentile	Optional in adults
CBC	Children with BP > 95th percentile	All adults (hematocrit only)
Renal U/S	Children with BP > 95th percentile	
Fasting lipid panel, fasting glucose	Children with BP > 95th percentile, overweight children with BP 90th–94th percentile, family history of hypertension or cardiovascular disease. Children with chronic renal disease	All adults
Echocardiogram	Children with BP > 95th percentile, children with comorbid risk factors,* and BP 90th–94th percentile	
ECG		All adults
Retinal examination	Children with BP > 95th percentile, children with comorbid risk factors,* and BP 90th–94th percentile	
Plasma renin determination	Young children with Stage 1† hypertension and any child with Stage 2 hypertension.‡ Positive family history of severe hypertension	
Renovascular imaging	Young children with Stage 1† hypertension and any child with Stage 2 hypertension	
Plasma and urine steroid levels	Young children with Stage 1† hypertension and any child with Stage 2 hypertension	
Plasma and urine catecholamines	Young children with Stage 1† hypertension and any child with Stage 2 hypertension	

*Comorbid risk factors include diabetes mellitus and kidney disease.

†Stage 1 hypertension in children is systolic, or diastolic blood pressure 95th percentile to the 99th percentile plus 5 mm Hg.

‡Stage 2 hypertension in children is systolic, or diastolic blood pressure > 99th percentile plus 5 mm Hg.

§More extensive testing in adults for identifiable causes is not generally indicated unless BP control is not achieved or the clinical and routine laboratory evaluation strongly suggests an identifiable secondary cause.

hypertension. A more complete list of causes of secondary hypertension is in Table 66-2.

Coarctation of the aorta is an uncommon cause of hypertension, but should still be "ruled-out" in patients with a possibility of secondary hypertension. By definition, coarctation of the aorta is a congenital narrowing of the aorta between the distal aortic arch and the abdominal aortic bifurcation. In the past, lesions have been described as pre- or postductal; however, now 98% of lesions are classified as juxtaductal. The area that is narrowed may be discrete, with a shelf like structure, or it may be a long segment of the aorta that is affected. Typically, the segment of the aorta distal to the coarctation is dilated. Collateral vessels, connecting arteries from the upper part of the body to the lower part of the body are frequently seen. Hypertrophy of the intercostal arteries creates the pathognomonic rib notching seen on chest radiography. Other concomitant cardiac lesions are common, with bicuspid aortic valve

TABLE 66-2

Causes of Secondary Hypertension

Sleep apnea
Pheochromocytoma
Ethanol — excessive consumption
Cushing syndrome
Renovascular disease
Obesity
Coarctation of the aorta
Thyroid disease
Renal disease
Primary aldosteronism
Hyperparathyroidism
Drugs (NSAIDs, cocaine, amphetamines, decongestants, anorectics, steroids, cyclosporine, tacrolimus, erythropoietin, licorice/chewing tobacco)

waves in leads V5 and V6. An echocardiogram can confirm the diagnosis of aortic coarctation, but requires the sonographer to obtain a suprasternal notch view, which can be difficult in adults. Doppler flow velocities show an increase in the velocity at the coarctated segment. An MRI/MR angiogram can be considered if the diagnosis is in doubt, or if more information is needed to plan treatment. Cardiac catheterization with aortic angiography has traditionally been the diagnostic test of choice. It not only provides anatomic and pressure measurements but also allows for possible angioplasty and treatment.

Significant coarctation should be treated, particularly if the patient has hypertension or any evidence of heart failure. Optimal choice of treatment is still controversial. Surgical correction was first done in the mid-1940s. Surgical options include end to end anastomosis, subclavian flap angioplasty, prosthetic patch aortoplasty, and tubular bypass grafts. Surgical repair is preferred in patients with a long segment of aorta involved, complete or almost complete occlusion of the segment, or associated congenital defects which also need surgical treatment, such as ventricular septal defect or patent ductus arteriosus. Balloon angioplasty has proven to be safe and effective. A relatively frequent complication is restenosis of the previously stenosed segment, which is more common in younger patients. Less common complications include aortic perforation, dissection, and aneurism formation. Placement of a stent at the time of angiography is another treatment option. Indications include a long segment of coarctation, tortuous coarctation with misalignment of the proximal and distal segments, or recoarctation following previous surgical or balloon therapy.

being the most frequently observed lesion. Aortic coarctation makes up approximately 5% to 8% of all congenital heart defects. It is the most common lesion seen in Turner syndrome. A small male predominance has been observed, more often in adult studies than infant studies.

In adults, coarctation is most often discovered by an evaluation of secondary hypertension. Patients are typically asymptomatic when diagnosed, but may have lower extremity claudication. Infants with severe lesions can present with heart failure when the ductus arteriosus closes. These infants must be maintained on prostaglandin until a definitive procedure can be done. On examination, a radial-femoral delay may be noted. A systolic ejection click may indicate a bicuspid aortic valve. A blood pressure that is 20 mm Hg higher in the arm than in the leg supports the diagnosis of aortic coarctation. Case series of patients prior to the advent of surgical interventions documented the natural history of coarctation of children and adults. The median age of death was 31 years. Cardiac failure accounted for 26% of the deaths. Aortic rupture (21%), bacterial endarteritis (18%), and intracranial hemorrhage (12%) all significantly contributed to mortality. Only 24% of the patients' deaths were not attributable to the aortic coarctation. Initial evaluation typically involves a chest radiograph, which may be normal or show cardiomegaly. Significant collateral circulation may be evident by rib notching. An electrocardiogram may also be normal or show left ventricular hypertrophy, particularly with large S

Selected References

Jenkins NP, Ward C. Coarctation of the aorta: natural history and outcome after surgical treatment. *Q J Med.* 1999;92:365–371.
Rao PS. Coarctation of the aorta. *Curr Cardiol Rep.* 2005;7:425–434.
Burnstein D. Coarctation of the aorta. In: Behrmen RE, Kliegman R, Jenson HB, eds. *Nelson Textbook of Pediatrics.* 17th ed. St Louis, MO: Saunders; 2004: Section 420.6.
Chobanian AV, Bakris GL, Black HR, et al., National High Blood Pressure Education Program Coordinating Committee. The seventh report of the Joint National Committee on Prevention, Detection, Evaluation, and Treatment of High Blood Pressure: the JNC 7 report. *Hypertension.* 2003;42:1206–1252.
National High Blood Pressure Education Program Working Group on High Blood Pressure in Children and Adolescents. The fourth report on the diagnosis, evaluation, and treatment of high blood pressure in children and adolescents. *Pediatrics.* 2004;114:555–576.

75-Year-Old with Shortness of Breath

CASE PRESENTATION

A 75-year-old Caucasian female with a history of diabetes mellitus, hypertension, gout, and breast cancer, presents with $1^1/_2$ months of progressive shortness of breath. She complains of dyspnea on exertion and cough productive of yellow-orange sputum. She denies fevers, chest pain, hemoptysis, nausea, emesis, decreased urine output, or hematuria. About 4 to 5 weeks prior to admission, she was diagnosed clinically with pneumonia and treated for 10 days with a properly dosed oral fluoroquinolone. After these 10 days, she returned to her primary care provider with persistent symptoms and malaise. At that time, her chest radiograph revealed an infiltrate in the left lower lobe. She was again started on a fluoroquinolone, but at a higher dose, and completed a 14-day course. When she finished this course and followed up with her primary physician, she was found to be hypoxic and without improvement. She was then admitted for further workup. Her home medications include hydrochlorothiazide, glipizide, aspirin, ezetimibe, escitalopram, and gabapentin. She currently lives in a retirement community and previously worked as a homemaker. She has a 10-pack/years smoking history, but quit many years ago. She occasionally drinks alcohol. Her family history is significant for coronary artery disease in her father.

Physical Examination

Vital signs: temperature: 36.7°C, pulse: 72 beats/min, blood pressure: 162/64 mm Hg, respiratory rate: 20 breaths/min, Oxygen saturation was 90% on 4 L via nasal canula. She appears comfortable and in no apparent distress. head, Eyes, ears, nose, and throat: normocephalic, atraumatic, pupils equal, round, reactive to light, extraocular movement intact, sclera clear, oropharynx moist, no erythema or exudates, no oral lesion. Neck: supple, no lymphadenopathy no jugular venous distention. Cardiovascular: regular rate and rhythm with a 2/6 systolic murmur heard best at the left upper sternal border, no radiation, no rub or gallop, 2+ radial and dorsalis pedis pulses bilaterally. Lungs: bilateral rales left greater than right, no wheeze, and fair air movement. Abdomen: obese, soft, nontender, nondistended, normoactive bowel sounds, no hepatosplenomegaly. Extremities: no bilateral lower extremity edema. Neurologic: alert and oriented × 3, nonfocal.

Laboratory Studies

White blood cells 17.1, hemoglobin/hematocrit 10.1/30.7, platelets 647, absolute neutrophil count 15.0, absolute lymphocyte count 0.8, absolute eosinophil count 0.4, Na 136, K 4.4, Cl 100, CO_2 23, blood urea nitrogen 22, Cr 1.2, glucose 159, Ca 8.8, Mg 1.7, P 4.1. Arterial blood gas on 4 L NC: pH 7.41, P_{CO_2} 40, P_{O_2} 58, O_2 saturation 88.7%. Chest radiograph (CXR) is shown in Fig. 67-1 and demonstrated near complete opacification of the left lung fields with some right-sided alveolar airspace disease as well.

Case Resolution

The patient was started on broad spectrum antibiotics and initially admitted to a floor bed. Her chest CT (Fig. 67-2) showed consolidation involving the entire left lung and the right lower lobe, cardiomegaly, and extensive lymphadenopathy. Her sputum cultures remained negative

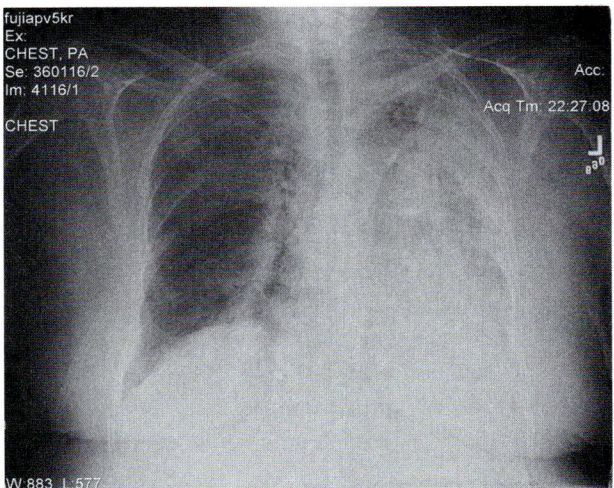

Figure 67-1 CXR demonstrated near complete opacification of the left lung fields with some right-sided alveolar airspace disease as well.

and she was gram-stain negative for any organisms. She went on to develop progressive hypoxia and worsening infiltrates on chest radiography. She required transfer to the medicine intensive care unit. Bronchoalveolar lavage of the right lower lobe revealed no organisms, no polymorphonuclear leukocytes (PMNs), and all subsequent viral, bacterial, fungal, and AFB cultures were negative.

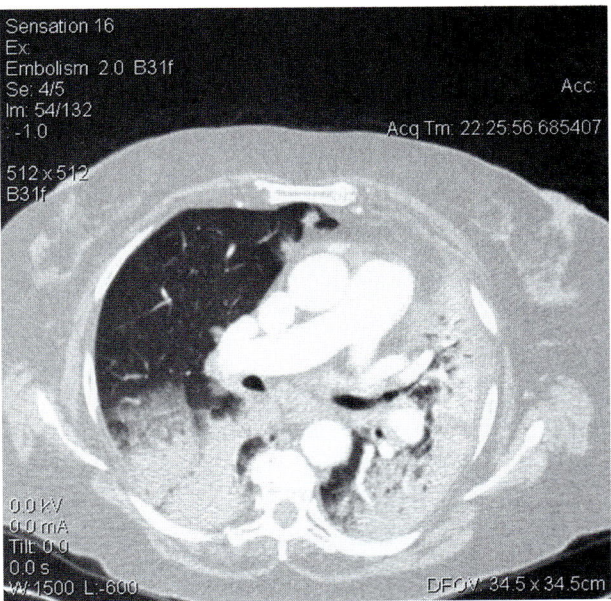

Figure 67-2 CT chest consolidation involving the entire left lung and the right lower lobe, cardiomegaly, and extensive lymphadenopathy.

Question

What is the cause of this patient's progressive pulmonary infiltrates and hypoxia?

Answer

She underwent video-assisted thoracoscopic surgery (VATS) to obtain a lung biopsy, which revealed bronchiolitis obliterans organizing pneumonia (BOOP)/cryptogenic organizing pneumonia (COP).

Discussion

Hypoxemia and pulmonary infiltrates on chest radiography are not uncommon features in patients obtaining admission to the hospital. This is a common scenario faced by clinicians. The differential diagnosis broadens, however, in patients who do not respond to typical therapies, especially broad spectrum antibiotics. A diagnosis of BOOP or COP should always be considered in these patients with progressive symptoms such as hypoxia, migratory pulmonary infiltrates, and worsening respiratory status.

BOOP is an inflammatory disorder of the lung that involves both the terminal bronchioles and the alveoli. It is defined by its histologic and pathologic features, which were first described in 1985, although the concept of an organizing pneumonia as a separate clinical entity was recognized on autopsy specimens at the beginning of the twentieth century. At that time the specimens studied were from patients who died from bacterial, usually pneumococcal pneumonia, and the end result of BOOP was thought to be a failure of that pneumonia to resolve. It is now known that BOOP can be caused not only by infection but many other etiologies as well (Table 67-1), although for the majority of cases the cause is unknown; hence the name cryptogenic organizing pneumonia (COP). Also, BOOP develops not as a result of a failure of infection to resolve, but rather from inflammation that organizes for unknown reasons. The process likely starts with injury to the alveoli and capillary endothelium that activates growth factors, coagulation factors, and soluble factors that promote angiogenesis. Inflammatory cells and fibroblasts deposit fibrin and connective tissue within the alveoli (organizing pneumonia) and bronchiolar lumen (bronchiolitis obliterans).

TABLE 67-1

Causes of Bronchiolitis Obliterans Organizing Pneumonia

Cryptogenic/Idiopathic

Infection

Bacterial: *Chlamydia, Legionella, Mycoplasma, Pseudomonas, Serratia, Staphylococcus, Streptococcus*
Viral: Adenovirus, cytomegalovirus, influenza, HIV, Herpes
Other: malaria, *Pneumocystis, Crypotococcus*

Drugs/Toxins

Amiodarone
Amphotericin
Bleomycin
Carbamazepine
Cephalosporins
Cocaine

Gold

Methotrexate
Minocycline
Nitrofurantoin
Phenytoin
Sulfasalazine
Ticlopid

Rheumatologic/Connective tissue disorders

Rheumatoid arthritis
Systemic lupus erythematosus
Sjogren syndrome
Dermatomyositis and Polymyositis
Behçet syndrome
Ankylosing spondylitis

Miscellaneous

Organ transplantation (lung, kidney, or bone marrow)
Radiation therapy
Inflammatory bowel disease
Myeloproliferative disorders

BOOP/COP typically affects patients aged 50 to 60 years, yet has been documented in patients ranging 29 to 80 years. Men and women are affected equally. No identifiable risk factors are known. Most patients will present with a flu-like illness. They will have some or all of the following symptoms: fever, malaise, cough, fatigue, dyspnea on exertion, and weight loss; symptoms not uncommon to other more common respiratory/cardiopulmonary conditions. Inspiratory rales will be present in more than half of patients, and more than 80% of patients will have hypoxemia.

No specific laboratory tests exist for diagnosing BOOP, which is actually a diagnosis of exclusion. Many nonspecific laboratory abnormalities have been identified, including leukocytosis, in about 50% of all patients, and elevated erythrocyte sedimentation rate or C-reactive protein, in up to 60% to 80% of patients. Pulmonary function testing in patients with COP reveals a mild to moderate restrictive pattern and a reduced diffusing capacity of carbon monoxide (DLCO), which are also nonspecific findings. Chest radiography usually reveals diffuse, bilateral alveolar opacities usually distributed peripherally. CT of the chest typically has patchy nodular opacities, ground glass opacities, and/or bronchial wall thickening, again, usually distributed in the lung periphery. These radiographic findings can help narrow the differential, but are not diagnostic of BOOP. Bronchoalveolar lavage can be helpful to rule out infection and other etiologies, but will not yield the diagnosis. The current gold standard for diagnosing BOOP/COP is obtaining a tissue sample by VATS. VATS is preferred over transbronchial biopsy because a sufficient amount of tissue is needed to exclude other entities.

Microscopic examination of lung tissue will yield the hallmarks of BOOP, which include granulation tissue and chronic inflammation within small airways and alveoli with the preservation of lung architecture (Fig. 67-3). With sufficient tissue samples, other pathologic processes can be excluded, such as granulomas, necrosis, vasculitis, interstitial fibrosis, or eosinophilic infiltration. Ruling out these entities is necessary to make the final diagnosis of BOOP or COP.

The mainstay of treatment for BOOP/COP is the administration of systemic steroids. Patients should receive 1 to 1.5 mg/kilogram/day, with a maximum dose of 100 mg, for 2 to 3 months. If patients are improved after this time period, the dose can be slowly tapered to 0.5 to 1 mg/kg/day for 1 to 2 more months. For patients with rapidly progressive disease, they can initially receive intravenous methylprednisolone dosed at 125 to 250 mg every 6 hours for the first 3 to 5 days of therapy. Almost all patients will respond quickly to steroid therapy with improvement in symptoms. Two-thirds of patients will

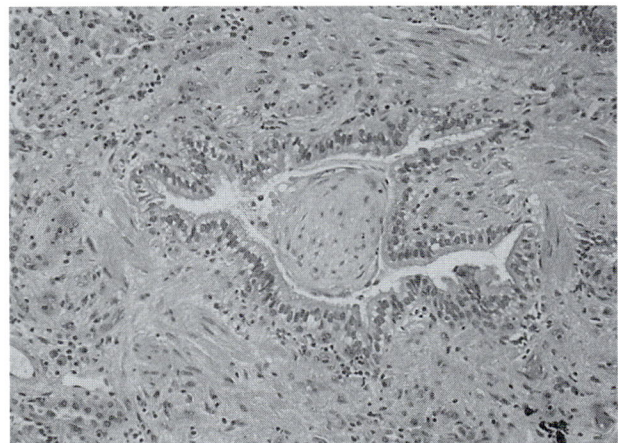

Figure 67-3 Lung architecture in bronchiolitis obliterans organizing pneumonia from the patient described in the vingette.

completely resolve. One-third of patient will have relapsing or persistent disease and may need long-term or even life-long steroids.

The diagnosis of bronchiolitis obliterans organizing pneumonia, or COP, can be difficult to make. It should always be included in the differential of patients with any of the symptoms described above and pulmonary infiltrates, as the case vignette included. As demonstrated in this case, patients can worsen clinically while receiving therapy for the most common diagnoses, such as lobar pneumonia, but can quickly improve on steroids once BOOP is recognized and diagnosed.

Selected References

Cordier JF. Organising pneumonia. *Thorax.* 2000;55:318–328.

Epler GR. Bronchiolitis obliterans organizing pneumonia. *Arch Intern Med.* 2001;161:158–164.

Krishna G, Berry G, Faul J, Kuschner W. A 24-year-old woman with bilateral pulmonary infiltrates, pericardial effusion, and bilateral pleural effusions. *Chest.* 2005;128:4013–4017.

14-Day-Old with Lethargy

CASE PRESENTATION

You are covering the intermediate nursery at night when you are called to see a 14-day-old ex-29-week premature infant. He was born at $29^1/_7$ weeks because of preterm labor of unknown etiology. The infant's mother had appropriate prenatal care, an otherwise normal pregnancy, and no concerning prenatal laboratory tests. She did admit to occasional cocaine use during pregnancy. At birth, the infant was briefly intubated because of respiratory distress, given one dose of surfactant, then quickly extubated, and weaned to a small amount of oxygen by nasal cannula. Because of low initial Apgar score of 1 at 1 minute (heart rate only) and 5 at 5 minutes, he was not fed enterally for the first 5 days of life, but was then slowly advanced to full feeds over the next 7 days. He has now been tolerating full enteral orogastric (OG) feeds well for 2 days without difficulty. You are now called to his bedside because his nurse reports that during this shift, he has not been as active as he was the previous night. She is also concerned about the appearance of his abdomen, and has gotten a large green residual from his OG tube.

Physical Examination

The patient is a toxic appearing African American male infant. He has poor tone and has a somewhat grayish tint to his skin. Vital signs: temperature 35.9°C, heart rate 160 beats/min, blood pressure 60/40 mm Hg, respiratory rate, heart, and lung examination is normal except for prolonged capillary refill (~5 seconds). The abdomen is tight and distended, and also grayish in appearance. On palpation, the infant makes a weak cry, and firm bowel loops can be felt directly under the skin. No other organomegaly is noted, and the rest of the examination, including genitals and extremities, is normal.

Laboratory Studies

Bedside arterial blood gas shows pH of 7.02, P_{CO_2} of 48, P_{AO_2} of 52. Complete blood count shows white blood cells count of 4.1, hematocrit of 28.1, and platelets of 53. Electrolytes are essentially normal with Na^+ 139, K^+ 4.5, Cl^- 104, HCO_3^- 11, blood urea nitrogen 20, Cr 0.3, and glucose 100. Blood and urine cultures were obtained. Abdominal left lateral decubitus radiograph shows free air in the abdomen and pneumatosis of the bowel (Fig. 68-1).

Case Resolution

The patient was diagnosed with necrotizing enterocolitis (NEC), started on ampicillin, gentamicin, and clindamycin, and taken immediately to the operating room owing to the intestinal perforation. During open laparotomy, a 30-cm section of dead bowel was removed, and a large portion of the remainder of the bowel looked marginal. The infant initially showed some improvement postoperatively, but platelet counts continued to fall, acidosis returned, and the infant became hypotensive. The pediatric surgeons felt that the infant would likely not tolerate further bowel resection, and the infant did not respond to pressors or volume resuscitation, and passed away.

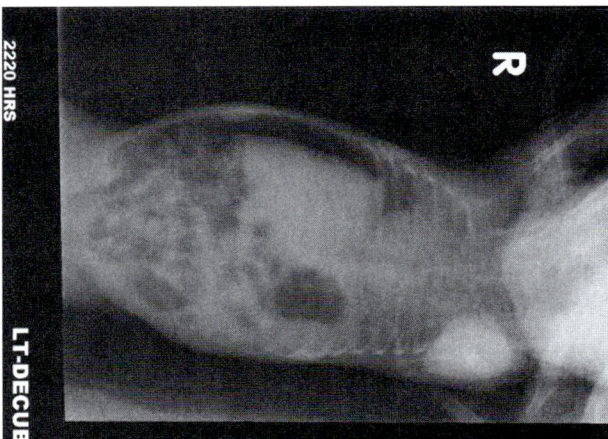

Figure 68-1 Left lateral decubitus abdominal radiograph. Note the large amount of free air between the liver and the abdominal wall, and the bubbly appearance of the small bowel inferior to the liver, consistent with pneumatosis cystoides intestinalis. There is also diffuse bowel wall edema.

Question

What is the pathogenesis of NEC, and what were this infant's risk factors?

Answer

The pathogenesis of NEC is still not completely understood, but it is likely that decreased bowel perfusion leads to ischemia and bacterial overgrowth. Known risk factors include prematurity, enteral feeds, and in utero cocaine exposure.

Discussion

NEC is a common source of morbidity and mortality in the neonatal ICU, and is one of the most common surgical emergencies in neonates. Overall mortality has been reported between 9% and 28%, but is significantly higher for very low birth weight (VLBW) infants (BW < 1500 gm), greater than 45%. There is also significant short- and long-term morbidity.

Known risk factors for NEC include prematurity (only 10% of infants with NEC are term), cocaine exposure in utero (2.5 times increased risk), enteral feeds (90% of infants with NEC have been fed enterally), and indomethacin use for closure of patent ductus arteriosus. Surprisingly, many suspected risk factors, such as maternal complications at birth, infant's postnatal course, and infant's postnatal management have not been consistently shown to be linked to NEC. Furthermore, risk of NEC is also independent of gender, race, and geography. Breast feeding provides some (but not complete) protection against NEC, presumably because of presence of antibodies in the milk.

The pathogenesis of NEC is not completely understood, but it is fairly clear that it is mediated by a complicated interaction between infectious, vascular, immunologic, and mucosal factors. Pathologic analysis often shows damage similar to adults with ischemic bowel, and this gives rise to the most popular theory regarding development of NEC. It is believed the a period of bowel ischemia is coupled with small mucosal tears and an immature immune system, allowing bacterial infection and inflammation, leading to further necrosis. Histopathology of NEC supports this process, but there is not always evidence for an instigating ischemic event. There is also increasing evidence that presence of platelet-aggregating factor (PAF) plays a significant role in the disease, supporting the idea of ischemia in part owing to local thrombosis and inflammation. A large number of infectious agents have been noted in NEC epidemics, but none has been proven causative. Terminal ileum and ascending colon is most commonly affected.

Presenting symptoms of NEC can be nonspecific, therefore a high index of suspicion must be present in cases of high-risk infants. While abdominal distension, tenderness, bilious gastric aspirates, and grossly bloody stools are the hallmark of the disease, it may begin with a sepsis-like picture of temperature instability, lethargy, or apnea with or without bradycardia. Initial signs may be as simple as irritability or poor feeding. Radiographic signs include bowel distension (including fixed, dilated loops on serial x-rays), bowel wall edema, and pneumatosis cystoides intestinalis, or air bubbles within the lumen of the bowel wall or portal venous air from fermentation by invasive bacteria (Fig. 68-1). Bowel wall perforation and free air may also be noted, and is an indication for emergent laparotomy. Laboratory findings may include significant and prolonged metabolic acidosis, thrombocytopenia, and hyponatremia, with or without a positive blood culture. Because of the difficulty of diagnosing NEC, a staging criterion was developed to help provide consistency in diagnosis and treatment. The Bell staging criteria is summarized in Table 68-1.

Much of the immediate treatment for NEC is supportive care and centers on what is known of the pathogenesis. Feeds should be held and nutrition should be given

TABLE 68-1

Bell Staging Criteria

Stage I: (suspected) clinical signs and symptoms, nondiagnostic radiographs	
Stage II: (definite) clinical signs and symptoms, pneumatosis on radiographs	a. Mildly ill b. Moderately ill, systemic symptoms
Stage II: (advanced) clinical signs and symptoms, pneumatosis on radiographs, critically ill	a. Impending intestinal perforation b. Proven intestinal perforation

parentally. Broad spectrum antibiotics should be started to cover gram-positives, gram-negatives, and anaerobes. Metabolic acidosis will often correct with volume resuscitation, but may occasionally require treatment with sodium bicarbonate in a critically ill neonate. Hypotension is a common complication and should be treated with volume resuscitation and if needed, pressors. Fresh frozen plasma is a good choice for volumes resuscitation, as coagulation factors are often low. Other hematologic abnormalities may require platelet or blood transfusions. Other immediate complications can include renal failure from hypoperfusion and neurologic sequelae from ischemia or meningitis.

Surgery consultation should be made at the suspicion of NEC. While intestinal perforation is an absolute indication for exploratory laparotomy, surgery may also be considered in a patient who is not responding to medical management. Perforation occurs in approximately 20% to 30% of cases, usually 12 to 48 hours after onset of NEC. The goal of surgery would be to remove any necrotic bowel, while maintaining as much live bowel as possible. An ostomy is made at the time of surgery, with reanastomosis occurring after the infant has recovered, and often, after significant weight gain.

Long-term morbidity from NEC includes feeding difficulties, failure to thrive, malabsorption, strictures, fistulas, hepatic dysfunction secondary to long-term parental nutrition, and long-term sequelae from neurologic or renal damage. Infants who have had bowel resection are also at risk for short gut syndrome, nutritional deficiencies (depending on which section of the bowel was resected), obstruction caused by adhesions, and long-term morbidity with ostomies.

Selected References

1. McAlmon KR. Necrotizing enterocolitis. In: Cloherty JP, Eichenwald EC, Stark AR, eds. *Manual of Neonatal Care.* 5th ed. Philadelphia, PA: Lippincott-Williams & Wilkins; 2004: chap 32.
2. Behrman RE. *Nelson's Textbook of Pediatrics.* 17th ed. Philadelphia, PA; Saunders: 2004.

22-Year-Old with Leg Pain

CASE PRESENTATION

A 22-year-old African American female with a 10-year history of poorly controlled insulin-dependent diabetes and multiple previous admissions for diabetic ketoacidosis (DKA) was admitted for left thigh pain. Her past medical history was significant for diabetic retinopathy, nephropathy, and gastroparesis, as well as depression.

Physical Examination

Vital signs: at presentation, she was febrile to 38.3°C with a pulse of 135 beats/min, blood pressure of 125/99 mm Hg, and an oxygen saturation of 99% on room air. Her physical examination at that time was only remarkable for the medial aspect of her left thigh being indurated, swollen, and extremely tender to touch and movement. She had marked limitation in her range of motion at the left knee only because of pain of the left medial thigh. In general, she appeared very anxious and uncomfortable.

Laboratory Studies

Laboratory studies on admission revealed an elevated white blood cell (WBC) count of 27.3×10^9/L, uncontrolled glucose at 267 mg/dL, and a hemoglobin A1C of 9.8%, a low albumin at 2.1 g/dL, thrombocytosis with a platelet count of 455×10^9/L, and an elevated erythrocyte sedimentation rate (ESR) at 113 mm/hr.

Question

What are the urgent conditions to consider as part of the differential diagnosis?

Answer

Due to the high morbidity and mortality the possibility of necrotizing fasciitis should be considered. Early operative intervention may be crucial to survival. Although unusual in the thigh, rhabdomyolysis with compartment syndrome must be considered. Fasciotomy may be required urgently. Lastly, pyomyositis should be considered early as incision and drainage of purulence may aid resolution.

Case Resolution

She was begun empirically on broad spectrum antibiotics with no improvement in her fever curve, symptoms, or ESR. An aggressive workup for other sources of fever was unrevealing and included a chest radiograph, pelvic MRI, transesophageal echocardiogram, upper and lower extremity venous Dopplers to assess for deep venous thrombosis (DVT), and multiple blood and urine cultures.

The pain and swelling progressed with surrounding warmth of the entire left thigh. There was no rash or knee effusion. She could no longer bear weight on the left leg secondary to pain and required escalating doses of narcotic pain control. This progressed over the next several days, and repeat MRI of the left leg showed significant inflammation of the adductor compartment musculature. Serial blood cultures remained negative, but she continued on intravenous antibiotics.

Approximately 1 week after the development of left thigh swelling, the medial aspect of her right thigh began the same process. Beginning with the medial aspect of the right thigh, there was swelling, induration, warmth, and exquisite pain. Again, there was limited range of motion at the hip and knee joints because of discomfort. Laboratory evaluation was unrevealing as blood and right thigh muscle aspirate cultures were negative, as were Epstein-Barr virus, cytomegalovirus, toxoplasma, and human immunodeficiency virus serologies.

MRI of bilateral lower extremities first suggested the diagnosis. It showed extensive abnormal signal intensity throughout the musculature bilaterally. The T2-weighted images demonstrate a gross degree of abnormal signal intensity throughout multiple muscle bellies, suggesting ischemia and necrosis. The muscles involved included the bilateral gluteus, quadriceps, and hamstring compartments, but it particularly affected the adductors (Fig. 69-1).

She was then taken to the operating room for an open muscle biopsy of the right thigh adductors. No fluid or pus collection was detected, but the muscle was found to be grossly necrotic and very light brown in appearance. Swabs for aerobic, anaerobic, acid fast bacilli, and fungi cultures were all sent and showed no growth. A biopsy was taken from one of the adductor compartment muscles and sent for histologic review.

Examination of the histologic specimen revealed large focal areas of muscle necrosis. Infarcted myocytes and ghost myotubes with absent cross striations are seen, surrounded by nonnecrotic muscle fibers of varying caliber. Regenerating muscle cells with prominent nucleoli are also identified (Figs. 69-2 and 69-3). The microvasculature appeared normal.

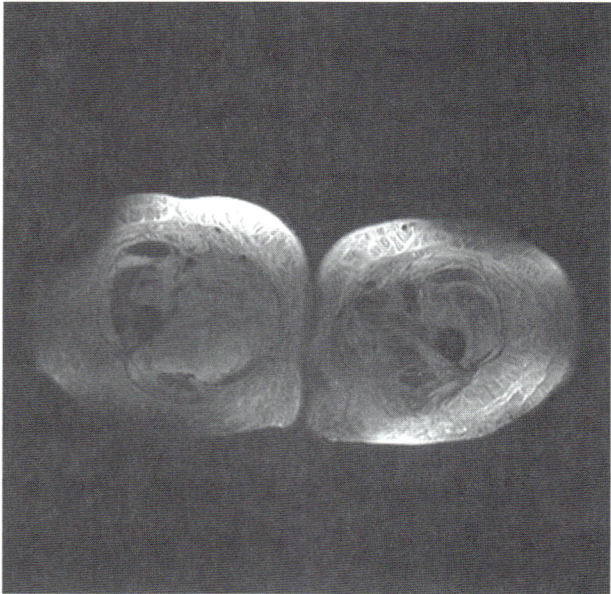

Figure 69-1 T2-weighted MRI image of the bilateral lower extremities showing necrosis of muscle bellies in the medial thigh compartments.

Discussion

Introduction

Diabetic muscle infarction (DMI) is a rare and incompletely understood complication of poorly controlled diabetes. It is characterized by the abrupt onset of exquisite pain, swelling, and inflammation in the absence of trauma or systemic signs of infection, most commonly in the thigh muscles. There is infarction and necrosis of muscle as a result of diabetic microvascular disease. First described by Angervall and Stener in 1965 as "tumoriform focal muscular degeneration," it is now thought to be a harbinger of severe underlying vascular disease in poorly controlled diabetic patients and is associated with a 5-year mortality rate above 50% from complications related to diabetes. DMI is likely under-reported because of lack of recognition and misdiagnosis as it is not yet described in most standard medical textbooks

Younger diabetic patients are more commonly affected with a mean age of approximately 40 years and a slight female predominance. More than 70% are type I diabetics with the majority of type II patients requiring insulin for control. The average duration of diabetes at the time of diagnosis is around 15 years with a high associated prevalence of end-organ microvascular complication such as nephropathy in about 70% of patients, and up to 50% having retinopathy or neuropathy. Recurrence of muscle infarction is seen within weeks to months in the same or contralateral muscle groups in up to 50% of cases.

Multiple etiologies for DMI have been proposed, as the exact mechanism is not known. Often, there are large confluent areas of muscle infarction and necrosis with more than 80% of cases involving the thigh muscles and up to 40% having bilateral lower extremity involvement. Only one previous case involving an upper extremity has been reported in the literature.

Etiology

The exact mechanism of action underlying DMI is still unknown. Ischemic infarction of the peripheral nerves, retina, and kidneys is well-described in diabetic patients, but rarely does muscle tissue undergo this type of infarction because of its rich collateral blood supply. Multiple etiologies have been proposed by numerous authors, but there are five pathways that have garnered the most attention in the literature: (1) arteriosclerosis obliterans, (2) atheroembolism,

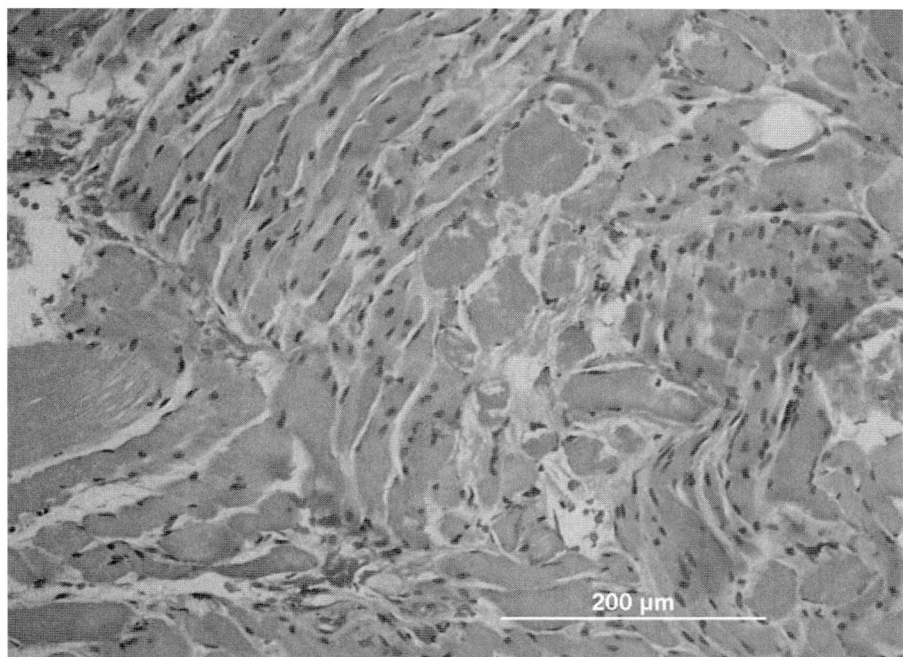

Figure 69-2 H&E stain of open muscle biopsy of adductor compartment of right thigh at 20× power. A focal area of necrotic myocytes is identified in the center of the image. These ghost myotubes are surrounded by non-necrotic muscle fibers of varying caliber and regenerating muscle cells with prominent nucleoli.

(Courtesy of Dr Funkhouser, MD PhD, UNC Hospitals Department of Pathology.)

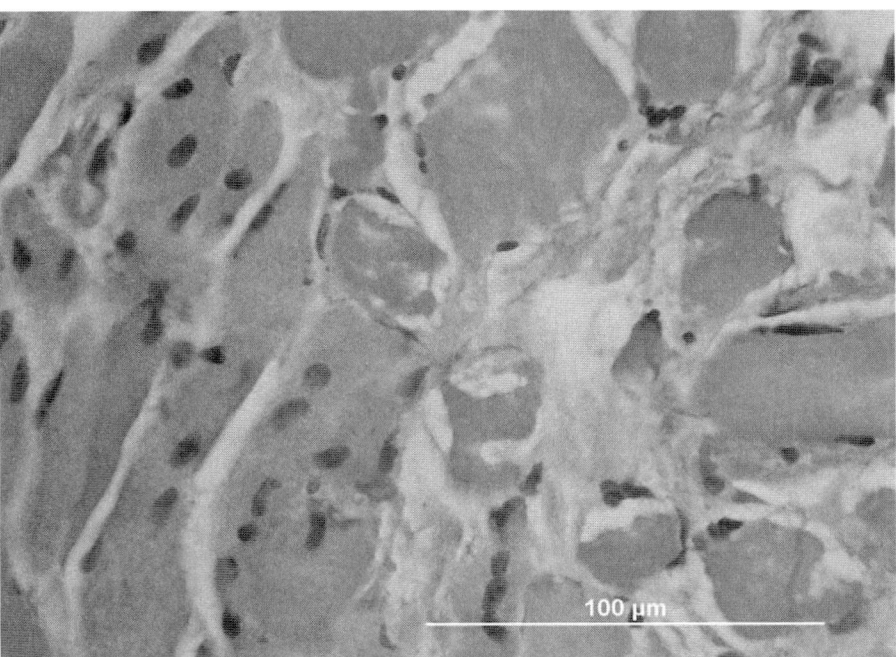

Figure 69-3 High-power (60×) view of Figure 69-2. On the right are necrotic muscle cells with loss of skeletal muscle striations and cellular architecture. The adjacent myotubes show normal nuclei with retained cytoplasmic skeletal striations. Again seen is the extensive variation in muscle fiber size.

(Courtesy of Dr Funkhouser, MD PhD, UNC Hospitals Department of Pathology.)

(3) compartment syndrome, (4) acquired hypercoagulability, and (5) hypoxia-reperfusion injury

Arteriosclerosis obliterans. Accelerated arthrosclerosis is a known complication of diabetes, and histologic examination of the vasculature within the infracted muscle of DMI supports diabetic microangiopathy as the causative mechanism. Multiple studies have demonstrated small-vessel walls that are thickened and hyalinized with luminal narrowing. They are often thrombosed by calcium, fibrin, and fat. Medium-sized arteries have been found to be occluded by loose connective tissue and often are recanalized. Similarly, microvascular abnormalities have been described with thickened capillary basement membranes, swelling of endothelial cells, and luminal narrowing.

Atheroembolism. In patients in whom there is advanced small-vessel disease, the muscle compartment which normally has a rich collateral blood supply changes to an end-vessel circulatory pattern. An embolic occlusive insult to a medium-sized vessel could result in large areas of infarction as the small vessels distal to that embolus, which are already damaged by thickened walls, receive insufficient blood supply. An early report supported this with the finding of aortic ulcers as the source of emboli; however this has since been inconsistently found. The frequency with which this occurs in a bilateral manner would also support an embolic cause; however, postmortem studies rarely identify a source, nor can they demonstrate emboli within the vasculature on histologic examination

Compartment syndrome. An initial ischemic event can cause enough tissue swelling, cell breakdown, and edema within a fascial compartment to produce a compartment syndrome. These high pressures in an area with already compromised blood supply lead to significant muscle infarction within that compartment. There is one case report, where the pressure within the affected fascial compartment was measured using a needle unit and found to be more than four times that of the surrounding compartments and was successfully treated with simple fasciotomy.

Acquired hypercoagulability. It has been suggested that in diabetes mellitus there is an acquired hypercoagulability state and impaired fibrinolytic process that may contribute to DMI. Carmassi et al compared coagulation and fibrinolytic parameters in insulin-dependent diabetic persons and nondiabetics and found that those with diabetes had elevated levels of factor VII, fibrinogen, plasminogen activator inhibitor–1 (PAI-1), along with diminished tissue plasminogen activator (tPA). Others have found an association between DMI and antiphospholipid antibody

syndrome. Whether anticoagulation would help prevent or treat DMI has not been studied, as few patients in this age demography have been tried on anticoagulation such as coumadin or aspirin.

Hypoxia-reperfusion injury. In this proposed mechanism, an initial ischemic insult causes inflammation and swelling with diminished blood supply. During reperfusion, oxygen-free radicals are generated that may cause direct myotoxicity and indirect injury via vascular leak that could worsen edema.

There may be other factors involved that precipitated this event. There have been reports that have correlated the development of DMI temporally with surgery, immobilization, and the use of compression wraps. It is felt that stasis of blood flow in an area, immobilization, and compression, in combination with the factors listed above, leads to the formation of micro-thromboemboli.

Clinical Presentation

DMI begins with the abrupt onset of pain, tenderness, and swelling in the affected muscle groups as a result of spontaneous muscular infarction. There is usually no antecedent history to suggest trauma or systemic signs such as fever or elevated WBC to indicate infection. Surrounding erythema and warmth are usually absent, but they can be present. Over the course of days, it typically progresses to a firm, palpable, fusiform mass that was initially described as "tumoriform focal muscular degeneration" by Angervall and Stener in 1965. The mass eventually changes to diffuse swelling with induration and exquisite pain that is present at rest and exacerbated by the slightest movement. Range of motion at the proximal and distal joints is limited by pain, and patients such as ours typically are unable to bear weight on that extremity.

It most commonly presents with abrupt swelling and pain in the medial aspect of the anterior thigh, with the most common muscles being the thigh adductors, biceps femoris, and vastus muscle group. All other cases, except for two reports including ours, involve the calf muscle groups, as there has only been one prior case involving the upper extremity reported until now. The symptoms of DMI slowly resolve spontaneously, usually taking several weeks to months for complete resolution. As in our report, approximately 50% of patients have a recurrence of DMI within the same or contralateral limb within weeks of the initial event. The etiology of the recurrent event, or how muscle infarction can be migratory, is unknown.

Laboratory studies are often unhelpful in the initial evaluation of these patients. Elevation in creatinine phosphokinase (CPK), ESR, and WBC count have been inconsistently found in the cases reported. In patients where an elevated WBC was found, fevers were also typically present, but there was usually no response to antibiotics. The fevers persisted intermittently for weeks until the muscle swelling and inflammation resolved, but the elevation in WBC and subsequent decline was independent of the resolution of muscle infarction. CPK levels are often checked in these patients and have been found to be both normal and very high. This disparity is felt to be because of the time in the clinical course when the CPK is checked, as muscle infarction is often not considered until late, after the acute infarction has occurred and the elevated CPK levels have resolved.

Differential Diagnosis

DMI is likely under-recognized and often misdiagnosed because of the many other conditions it mimics, which contributes to its relative rarity. The differential diagnosis one should consider in evaluating a patient with DMI can be grouped under the categories of infectious, neoplastic, vascular, and neurologic. Table 69-1 contains a detailed list of conditions that may present like DMI. The most common infectious etiologies that should not be missed include pyomyositis, cellulitis, and fasciitis. Benign and malignant tumors such as lipomas, fibromas, and sarcomas can have a similar clinical appearance to DMI, but often do not develop as acutely. Thrombophlebitis and DVT are two vascular conditions that may present as acute thigh swelling with pain and induration very similar to that seen with DMI and should always be considered. Diabetic amyotrophy is a severe neurologic deficit that is also a complication of diabetes and can present with acute thigh pain. It differs from DMI in that it more likely is associated with diffuse back, hip, and buttock pain with significant sensory impairment, weakness, and atrophy of the proximal muscles without swelling or induration. Acute hemorrhage and lymphedema also mimic the presentation of DMI but are usually easily distinguished from DMI. Lastly, there are a number of other conditions such as muscle rupture, acute compartment syndrome, and myositis ossificans that should be considered in the differential diagnosis.

Histology

Histologic findings within muscle biopsies of the affected areas have been generally consistent among the cases

TABLE 69-1

Differential Diagnosis Painful Extremity Swelling

Infectious

Pyomyositis, abscess, cellulitis, osteomyelitis, septic arthritis, tuberculosis, cat-scratch disease, fasciitis, parasitic myositis

Neoplastic

Metastatic tumors, lipoma, chondroma, fibroma, leiomyoma, sarcoma

Vascular

Thrombophlebitis, DVT, vasculitis, arterial occlusion, hemangioma, hemorrhage, lymphedema

Neurologic

Diabetic amyotrophy, diabetic neuropathy

Other

Trauma, muscle strain/rupture, proliferative or focal nodular myositis, pseudothrombophlebitis, calcific myonecrosis, myositis ossificans, bursitis, sarcoidosis, amyloidosis, granulomatous disease, acute compartment syndrome

reported. Large areas of focal muscle necrosis with loss of muscle fibers are the most striking feature (Fig. 69-2). Infarcted myocytes and ghost myotubes with absent cross striations are found, usually surrounded by atrophy of the adjacent muscle fibers (Fig. 69-3). Within the area of infarction, various stages of degeneration are seen. Acutely infarcted muscle contains hemorrhagic changes and polymorphonuclear infiltrate, while older infarcts have been found to contain mononuclear infiltrates and increased fibrous connective tissue with collagen-replacing muscle. Regenerating myocytes of different stages with prominent nucleoli were almost universally found along the periphery of the infarcted area or intermixed among the ghost tubules. Edema, inflammatory infiltrates, and microvasculopathy with arteriolar and capillary occlusions containing fibrin and calcium have been observed. Many of the small blood vessels are often thickened with hyalin and have narrowed lumens. However, in some biopsy samples, the vessels have appeared normal. In a review of 52 patients it was found that while 100% of the biopsy specimens showed muscle fiber necrosis, only 70% demonstrated inflammatory cell infiltrate, and just more than 50% had microvascular abnormalities.

Radiographic Findings

Magnetic resonance imaging (MRI) is simply the most accurate and useful radiographic tool in establishing the diagnosis of DMI, as it is 100% sensitive in detecting the muscular changes. Standard T2-weighted imaging shows increased signal intensity (increased brightness) in the intramuscular compartments and surrounding areas, secondary to increased water content from edema accompanying the infarction, and is the modality of choice. Diffuse swelling of the affected muscle groups is detected without a focal fluid collection. Gadolinium is not necessary to identify DMI, but should be used if pyomyositis or abscess is thought to be likely. On the other hand, T1-weighted images show low signal intensity changes and are less sensitive. T2-weighted MRI has been suggested to be the first and only imaging performed when DMI is suspected, but caution must be taken as the findings are not very specific for this process as infectious, inflammatory, and autoimmune myopathies can mimic its appearance. MRI can be used to limit the differential diagnosis, determine muscle groups involved, and establish the extent of disease. It has been reported that MRI findings may precede symptoms by several weeks, and in two patients reimaged after the resolution of symptoms, the hyper-intense signals disappeared and only atrophic muscle was found.

Other imaging modalities have been tried with limited usefulness. CT scans will show increased muscle size owing to swelling and lower attenuation secondary to edema. Ultrasonography shows loss of ultrasonic myofascial landmarks and mass-like changes of the swollen muscle that may be hypo or hyperechoic. Bone scans typically show increased blood flow to the involved muscle groups but is very nonspecific. Plain films are of limited value except to rule out bony abnormalities or soft-tissue calcification.

Treatment

Supportive, conservative care with pain management, activity restriction, and aggressive glucose control is the treatment method of choice. Initiation of physical therapy must be slow, as overzealous resumption of activity and ambulation will exacerbate the pain and has led to repeated hemorrhagic transformation with delayed muscle regeneration. There is much controversy as to the role of muscle biopsy in the management of patients with DMI. In those with typical features of DMI, such as long-standing insulin-dependent diabetes mellitus, other diabetic microvascular disease, and consistent MRI findings, a diagnosis should be made without the use of biopsy, as

the risks of biopsy are too great in an area of poor healing potential. For patients in whom there is a suspicion of infectious etiology, or in those with atypical presentations or inconclusive MRI findings, a biopsy is recommended. Needle biopsy is sufficient for histologic diagnosis and is associated with fewer complications such as hemorrhage, infection, delayed healing, or fewer injuries as compared to open surgical biopsy. For those who do not respond to conservative measures, surgical decompression of involved muscle compartments has been shown to be effective in at least one case, who was able to return to complete physical therapy in 3 weeks. The issue of the role of anticoagulation has been raised by several authors, but there is insufficient evidence at this time to asses its effectiveness or recommend its routine use.

Selected References

1. Banker BQ, Chester CS. Infarction of thigh muscle in the diabetic patient. *Neurology.* 1973;23(7):667–677.
2. Lentine KL, Guest SS. Diabetic muscle infarction in end-stage renal disease. *Nephrol Dial Transplant.* 2004;19:664–669.
3. Angervall L, Stener B. Tumoriform focal muscular degeneration in two diabetic patients. *Diabetologia.* 1965;1:39.
4. Wintz RL, Pimestone KR, Nelson SD. Detection of diabetic myonecrosis. *Postgrad Med Online.* January 2002;111. www.postgradmed.com. Accessed Sept 5, 2004.
5. Rocca PV, Alloway JA, Nashel DJ. Diabetic muscular infarction. *Semin Arthritis Rheum.* 1993;22(4): 280–287.
6. Grigoriadis E, Fam AG, Starok M, et al. Skeletal muscle infarction in diabetes mellitus. *J Rheumatol.* 2000;27:1063–1068.
7. Trujillo-Santos AJ. Diabetic muscle infarction: an underdiagnosed complication of long-standing diabetes. *Diabetes Care.* 2003;26:211–215.
8. Khoury NJ, El-Khoury GY, Kathol MH. MRI diagnosis of diabetic muscle infarction: report of two cases. *Skeletal Radiol.* 1997;26(2):122–127.
9. Gee R, Munk PL, O'Connell JX, et al. Diabetic muscle infarction: case report. *Can Assoc Radiol J.* 2003;54(5):296–298.
10. Bjornskov EK, Carry MR, Katz FH, et al. Diabetic muscle infarction: a new perspective on pathogenesis and management. *Neuromusc Disord.* 1995;5(1):39–45.
11. Umpierrez G, Stiles RG, Kleinbart J. Diabetic muscle infarction. *Am J Med.* 1996;101(3):245–250.
12. Eady JL, Cobbs KF. Diabetic muscle infarction. *J South Orthop Assoc.* 1997;6:250–255.
13. Chason DP, Fleckenstein JL, Burns DK, et al. Diabetic muscle infarction: radiologic evaluation. *Skeletal Radiol.* 1996;25(2): 127–132.
14. Chester CS, Banker BQ. Focal infarction of muscle in diabetes. *Diabetes Care.* 1986;9:623–630.
15. Pamoukian VN, Rubino F, Iraci JC. Review and case report of idiopathic lower extremity compartment syndrome and its treatment in diabetic patients. *Diabetes Metab.* 2000;26(6):489–492.

16. Carmassi F, Morale M, Puccetti R, et al. Coagulation and fibrinolytic system impairment in insulin dependent diabetes mellitus. *Thromb Res.* 1992;67(6):643–654.

17. Silberstein L, Britton KE, Marsh FP, et al. An unexpected cause of muscle pain in diabetes. *Ann Rheum Dis.* 2001;60:310–312.

18. Scully RE, Mark EJ, McNeely WF, et al. Case records of the Massachusetts General Hospital. Case 29-1997. *N Engl J Med.* 1997;337(12):839–845.

19. Barohn RJ, Kissel JT. Case-of-the-month: painful thigh mass in a young woman: diabetic muscle infarction. *Muscle Nerve.* 1992;15(7):850–855.

20. Lafforgue P, Janand-Delenne B, Lassman-Vague V, et al. Painful swelling of the thigh in a diabetic patient: diabetic muscle infarction. *Diabetes Metab.* 1999;25(3):255–260.

21. Hinton A, Heinrich SD, Craver R. Idiopathic diabetic muscular infarction: the role of ultrasound, CT, MRI, and biopsy. *Orthopedics.* 1993;16(5):623–625.

22. Sagar M, Bowerfind WM, Wigley FM. A man with diabetes and a swollen leg. Lancet 1999;353(9147):116.

23. Kiers L. Diabetic muscle infarction: magnetic resonance imaging (MRI) avoids the need for biopsy. *Muscle Nerve.* 1995;18(1):129–130.

24. Boulman N, Schapira D, Militianu D, et al. Diabetic muscle infarction. *Isr Med Assoc J.* 2003;5(9):669–670.

25. Bodner RA, Younger DS, Rosoklija G. Diabetic muscle infarction. *Muscle Nerve.* 1994;17(8):949–950.

26. Barohn RJ, Bazan C, III, Timmons JH, et al. Bilateral diabetic thigh muscle infarction. *J Neuroimaging.* 1994;4(1):43–44.

27. Van Slyke MA, Ostrov BE. MRI evaluation of diabetic muscle infarction. *Magn Reson Imaging.* 1995;13(2):325–329.

28. Chason DP, Fleckenstein JL, Burns DK, et al. Diabetic muscle infarction: radiologic evaluation. *Skeletal Radiol.* 1996;25:127–132.

29. Keller DR, Erpelding M, Grist T. Diabetic muscular infarction: preventing morbidity by avoiding excisional biopsy. *Arch Intern Med.* 1997;157(14):1611–1612.

8-Year-Old with Diarrhea

CASE PRESENTATION

An 8-year-old male presented with 5 days of nausea, 4 days of nonbloody/nonbilious emesis, and 3 days of nonbloody diarrhea. He had experienced fevers of 38.8°C to 40°C, chills, sore throat, epigastric pain, and decreased oral intake as well as decreased urine output. The patient's medical history is significant for pressure-equalizing (PE) tubes and asthma. He is up-to-date on immunizations. He lives in "the country" where the family has a pony and two outside dogs. The primary care pediatrician felt the patient was dehydrated and warranted admission for IV fluids and a direct admission to the pediatrics floor was arranged. At the time of admission, the patient was febrile and tachycardic. He was noted to have pharyngeal erythema and a sparse maculopapular rash over the anterior chest and upper extremities, with central clearing and questionable vesicles present on several of the lesions. His abdominal examination was benign. Laboratories were consistent with dehydration and notable for serum sodium of 129. A complete blood count was unremarkable and stool sample was negative for fecal leukocytes. The patient was discharged home following less than 24 hours of IV hydration and the ability to tolerate clears.

Within 24 hours of discharge, the patient experienced vomiting, diarrhea, and recurrence of fever to 40°C. He continued to have sore throat, malaise, headache, and developed symptoms of orthostasis. At the time of second presentation, he now had 7 days of fever, nausea, vomiting, and diarrhea which was loose but not watery. He tolerated only sips of clears. His parents had noted rash on his trunk/back/thighs, which was nonpruritic and nonprogressive. He was evaluated in the pediatric emergency department (ED) and admitted because of length of illness, persistence of symptoms, and hypotension in the ED.

Physical Examination

Patient was ill-appearing, pale young male with low energy. Vital signs: temperature: 39.4°C, heart rate: 130 beats/min, blood pressure: 90/47 mm Hg, respiratory rate: 26 breaths/min with 97% oxygen saturations on room air. Bilateral PE tubes were noted. Tonsillar erythema with white exudate was noted bilaterally. The abdomen was diffusely tender to palpation in the right upper quadrant, right lower quadrant, and epigastric regions. There was no rebounding or guarding and no hepatosplenomegaly. Skin examination was remarkable for a maculopapular rash with 5 to 7 lesions on the abdomen, 2 to 3 on the anterior thighs, and several on the posterior right shoulder. All were noted to have a 0.5 to 1 cm macular base with a papule present on some lesions. There was no cervical, axillary, or inguinal adenopathy appreciated. The remainder of the examination was unremarkable.

Laboratory Studies

For comparison purposes, laboratory studies from first admission: white blood cells (WBC) 5.4, hemoglobin (Hgb) 12.8, platelets 213, Na 129, K 3.4, Cl 99, CO_2 17, blood urea nitrogen (BUN) 14, Cr 0.7, no fecal leukocytes, rapid strep test was negative. From second admission: WBC 7.3 (61% segs), Hgb 11.7, platelets 171, Na

128, Cl 95, CO_2 19, BUN 7, Cr 0.5, Albumin 2.6, C-reactive protein 14.6, negative urinalysis, rapid strep and strep screen negative, monospot negative. Blood, urine, and stool cultures were sent. Rocky Mountain spotted fever titers, Epstein-Barr virus titers, rotavirus Ag were also sent.

Case Resolution

On hospital day 2, patient remained febrile and had two loose, nonwatery, nonbloody stools. On hospital day 3, there was concern for conjunctivitis, markedly erythematous tongue, and continued rash. Patient remained febrile and continued to have abdominal pain and loose stools. Clinical concerns included RMSF infection, Kawasaki or other vasculitis, and enteric pathogens. Eventually stool culture revealed heavy *Salmonella* species. All other cultures and abdominal screens were negative. On further discussion with the patient and his family, it was discovered that there were several "pet" chickens present on the family's land. The patient and his brothers had a game of crushing the chicken eggs in the dirt and then throwing this mixture at one another, despite frequent instruction to stay away from the eggs. The patient continued to receive supportive care until he defervesced and could tolerate consistent PO intake.

Question

What are the indications to use antimicrobial agents to treat salmonella-type infections?

Answer

Antibiotic treatment for acute gastroenteritis is a controversial area. The empiric use of antibiotics for a clinical syndrome of emesis and diarrhea is usually unwarranted. The vast majority of these syndromes is caused by a viral agent and is self-limited (Table 70-1). Stool cultures from patients with an acute diarrheal illness yield a specific bacterial pathogen in 2% to 10% of cases. Gastroenteritis caused by bacterial agents can either be worsened, improved, or have prolonged shedding by the use of an antibiotic depending on the causative agent. Gastroenteritis caused by *Shigella* is usually self-limited and lasts 7 days.

TABLE 70-1

Common Causative Agents of Acute Infectious Diarrhea

Bacteria

Salmonella
Campylobacter
Shigella
Escherichia coli
Clostridium difficile

Viruses

Calciviruses (Norovirus and related)
Rotavirus
Adenovirus
Astrovirus

Protozoa

Cryptosporidium
Giardia
Cyclospora
Entamoeba histolytica

However, antibiotic therapy is recommended to shorten the clinical syndrome and reduce fecal shedding. Antibiotic therapy for enterohemorrhagic *Escherichia coli* has been associated with an increased incidence of the hemolytic uremic syndrome. As will be discussed below, antibiotic therapy for *Salmonella* gastroenteritis varies depending on the clinical scenario and species type.

Discussion

Acute gastroenteritis is a common childhood affliction with significant associated time and financial burdens. In the United States alone, gastroenteritis accounts for at least 1.5 million outpatient visits annually as well as 200,000 hospitalizations. Worldwide, the statistics are staggering, with 123 million outpatient visits, 9 million hospitalizations, and 1.8 millions deaths. It remains to be seen what impact vaccination against Rotavirus may have on these numbers. An overwhelming proportion of these infections are caused by viral pathogens.

The mainstay of therapy for acute gastroenteritis is supportive care. Assessment of dehydration and therapy to ensure adequate hydration is critical. Oral rehydration therapy with commercially available or home-made oral rehydration solutions has become the treatment of choice for mild and moderate illness. Oral rehydration solutions take advantage of the physiology of intestinal water absorption. Water is passively absorbed. This absorption is dictated by the osmotic gradient created by sodium transport out of the intestinal lumen. Sodium is transported via three mechanisms: First, sodium-hydrogen exchanger actively moves sodium out of the intestinal lumen. Second, sodium also follows an electrochemical gradient. Third, sodium is transported by coupled movement with organic solutes (glucose). This sodium-coupled transport with organic solutes remains intact even with epithelial damage observed in various types of gastroenteritis. The preservation of this transport method is the basis of oral rehydration therapy. Beginning in the 1960s, solutions containing equimolar concentrations of glucose and sodium were used as supportive therapy for cholera patients. Solutions with too high a concentration of either glucose or sodium will exacerbate diarrhea by increasing the osmotic load within the intestines. Many studies have demonstrated reduced costs and similar outcomes (hospitalization, length of stay,

complications of therapy, and mortality) for oral rehydration therapy and intravenous therapy.

Salmonella organisms are flagellated gram-negative bacilli, belonging to the Enterobacteriaceae family. More than 2000 serovars have been identified; however 99% of disease-causing strains in humans come from S. *enterica* subspecies I. These are responsible for the culture-confirmed 50,000 nontyphoid infections in the United States annually. *Salmonella typhi* and *S. paratyphi* account for enteric or typhoid fever, with only 400 cases in the United States per year; however this is endemic to many other areas of the world. Please see Table 70-2 to compare/contrast features of typhoid versus nontyphoidal infection. Attack rates are highest in those less than 5 and greater than 70 years old, with invasive disease and mortality highest in infants, elderly, and immunosuppressed individuals.

This case raised a question regarding antibiotic treatment for *Salmonella* infection. The 2006 Red Book guidelines were used to answer this question, see Table 70-3 for summary. For nontyphoidal gastroenteritis no therapy is indicated for healthy, uncomplicated infection as antibiotics have not been shown to shorten duration of disease, and in some cases have prolonged shedding of *Salmonella*

TABLE 70-2

Characteristics of Typhoid and Nontyphoidal Salmonella Infections

Characteristics	Nontyphoidal salmonella	Typhoid salmonella
Clinical	Diarrhea, abdominal cramps, fever Focal infections: osteomyelitis, meningitis Sustained *or* intermittent bacteremia Focal infections in up to 10% of patients with bacteremia	Gradual onset of fever, malaise, anorexia, lethargy, possible abdominal pain, HSM, rose spots, mental status changes in severe form May have early constipation Diarrhea very common in children May have few GI symptoms even though infection starts in small intestine
Pathogenesis	Invasion of small gut epithelium with adjacent mesenteric lymph node involvement	Spreads from epithelium to Peyer patches to liver/gallbladder/spleen to bloodstream (bacteremia) Survives within phagocytic cells and the gallbladder which can lead to carrier state
Epidemiology	Incubation period of 12–36 hours (6–72 range reported) 50,000 confirmed infections in United States annually	Incubation period of 7–14 days (3–60 range reported) 400 cases annually in United States, endemic worldwide
Mode of infection	Reservoirs: poultry, livestock, reptiles, pets Infection via contact with contaminated food, water, infected animals, or animal products	*Humans* are the only carriers

TABLE 70-3

Treatment Guidelines

Patient population	Treatment	Agents
Nontyphoidal gastroenteritis in healthy, uncomplicated individuals	No. Antibiotics have not been shown to limit disease process and in some cases have prolonged shedding in stool	None
Nontyphoidal gastroenteritis in < 3 months of age, chronic GI disease, hemoglobinopathy, malignancy, or immunosuppressive illness	Unproven, but recommended	Ampicillin, amoxicillin, or TMP-SMX usually; may require ceftriaxone, cefotaxime, or fluoroquinolones (if > 18 years) in areas with frequent resistance
Localized invasive disease such as osteomyelitis, abscess, meningitis	Yes	Empiric treatment with cefotaxime or ceftriaxone while awaiting susceptibilities. Treat for at least 4 weeks (6 weeks in meningitis)
Bacteremia with nontyphoidal strain	Yes	10–14 days of therapy based on susceptibility
Enteric fever with *S. typhi*	Yes	10–14 days of therapy based on susceptibility

Adapted from Committee on Infectious Diseases. The Red Book, *27th ed. Elk Grove Village, IL: American Academy of Pediatrics; 2006:579–584.*

in the stool. Although unproven, antibiotic therapy is empirically recommended for infants less than 3 months of age, individuals with chronic gastrointestinal disease, and the immune compromised.

Although infrequent in the pediatric population, chronic carriage (>1 year) is possible with *S. typhi*. Eradication may require high-dose ampicillin or amoxicillin or ciprofloxacin in adult patients. Additionally, chronic carriage can be related to gallstones, leading to cholecystectomy to eliminate carrier state. For those patients with severe forms of enteric fever with delirium or shock, corticosteroids may be beneficial. Dexamethasone is recommended with a 3 mg/kg loading dose, followed by 1 mg/kg every 6 hours for 48 hours.

Selected References

1. Amieva M. Important bacterial gastrointestinal pathogens in children: a pathogenesis perspective. *Pediatr Clin North Am.* 2005;52:749–777.
2. Farmer, CN. Typhoid Fever. CDC/Armed Forces Institute of Pathology. 2007. Available at: http://www.wrongdiagnosis.com/phil/html/typhoid-fever/2215.html. Accessed Mar 27, 2008.
3. Levinson W, Jawetz E. *Medical Microbiology & Immunology,* 7th ed. New York: Lange; 2002:115–118, 121–124.
4. Sirinavin S, Garner P. Antibiotics for treating salmonella gut infections. *Coch Database Syst Rev.* 1999;1:art no:CD001167. DOI: 10.1002/14651858.CD001167.
5. Committee on Infectious Diseases. *The Red Book,* 27th ed. Elk Grove Village, IL: American Academy of Pediatrics; 2006:579–584.

28-Year-Old with Hemoptysis

CASE PRESENTATION

A 28-year-old white male, whose past medical history was significant for bilateral slipped capital femoral epiphysis and depression, presented to our emergency department (ED) with a 1-year history of intermittent hemoptysis occurring approximately once a month and most often associated with coughing spells. He also endorsed intermittent fevers, chills, and myalgias. He also noted intermittent episodes of diarrhea and had been hospitalized 4 months prior with a pneumonia for which he received IV levofloxacin and azithromycin. One week prior to his current presentation, he developed cough productive of clear, yellow sputum and mild shortness of breath and began feeling a "rattling" in his chest every 3–4 hours. On the day of his presentation, he had an episode of "large" hemoptysis during which he coughed up several tablespoons of thick bloody secretions and thus presented to the ED. On presentation, his vital signs were stable and the medicine team was called for further evaluation and management. Upon further questioning, he denied any history of tobacco, alcohol, or illicit drug use. He was employed by a company that stocked vending machines. His assigned route included machines located in doctor's offices, homeless shelters, and nursing homes.

Physical Examination

Patient was an alert, nontoxic-appearing adult male in no acute distress, with weight of 114 kg. Vital signs: temperature 38.5C°, pulse 94 beats/min, respirations 18 breaths/min, blood pressure 144/80 mm Hg, and oxygen saturation of 95% on room air. Head, eyes, ears, nose, and throat examination only revealed 3-dime size dark spots on his tongue, and his neck was supple without lymphadenopathy. His right upper lung field revealed decreased breath sounds, positive egophony, and few crackles. His lungs were otherwise clear. His heart had regular rate and rhythm without murmurs, rubs, or gallops. His abdomen was obese, soft, nontender, nondistended, and had normoactive bowel sounds. He had no hepatosplenomegaly or other palpable masses. His extremities had no clubbing, cyanosis, or edema. His neurologic examination was within normal limits with grossly normal sensation and strength, intact cranial nerves, and symmetric 2+ deep tendon reflexes bilaterally.

Laboratory Studies

White bood count count was 11, hemoglobin 13.5, hematocrit 38.3, and platelet count was 322,000. Na$^+$ 140, K$^+$ 3.6, Cl 102, HCO$_3$ 27, blood urea nitrogen 8, Cr 1.0, glucose 104, and calcium 9.3. D-dimer was 3.42. Prothrombin time was 11.0, international normalized ratio was 1.0, and partial thromboplastin time was 32.3. Chest radiograph (Fig. 71-1) showed a large right upper lobe opacity. Chest CT with contrast showed right upper lobe opacity versus a mass in the bronchus and a small right pleural effusion.

Case Resolution

After consultation with a pulmonary specialist, the decision was made to pursue a flexible bronchoscopy, which revealed a smooth nonulcerated mass almost completely obstructing the right upper lobe bronchus. Tissue biopsy

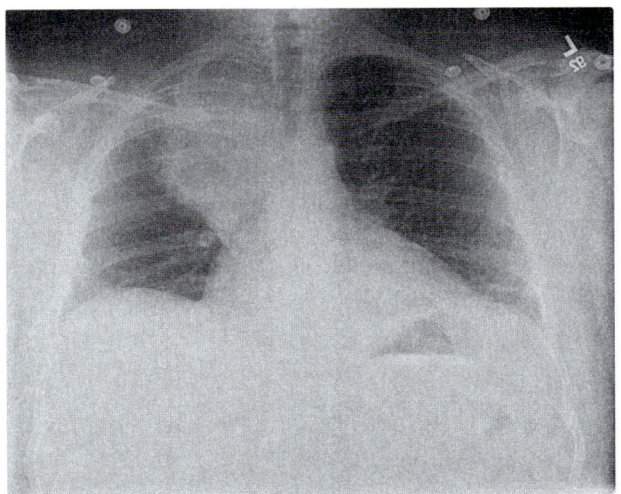

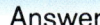

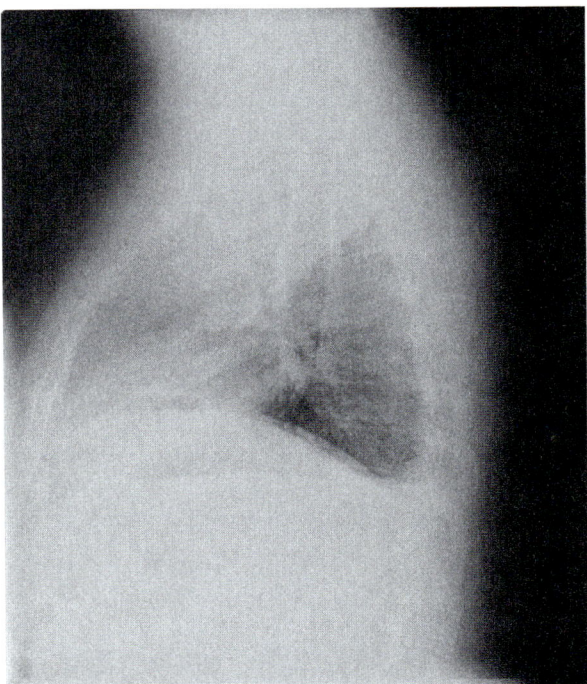

Figure 71-1 Chest radiograph at presentation reveals a large right upper lobe opacity.

and immunohistochemical staining were obtained. No bacteria were grown from the bronchial alveolar lavage (BAL); however, the patient's fever and cough were attributed to postobstructive pneumonia secondary to this mass. Sputum acid-fast bacillus smears were negative ×3, and the patient's purified protein derivative was also negative.

Question

What is the most likely diagnosis of a bronchial mass in an otherwise healthy 28-year-old male?

Answer

Although the differential diagnosis is quite broad, the pathology is the key. Pathology revealed organized clusters of cells with moderate amounts of cytoplasm and minimal cytologic atypia. The cells stained positively for chromogranin and synaptophysin. These are all characteristics diagnostic of typical bronchial carcinoid.

Discussion

A 28-year-old otherwise healthy male with hemoptysis is a diagnostic dilemma as the differential diagnosis is broad. There are several categories to be considered including anatomic, infectious, neoplastic, autoimmune, and iatrogenic (Table 71-1). The most likely diagnoses were tuberculosis, community-acquired pneumonia with or without pulmonary abscess, bronchogenic carcinoma, and autoimmune disease. In the end, the bronchoscopy and biopsy was the key to the diagnosis of bronchial carcinoid.

Carcinoid tumors in any location occur in 1–2 of every 100,000 people. The clinical features most often reflect the tumor's location, such as bowel obstruction in the intestines and hemoptysis and pneumonia in the lungs. These tumors occur in the GI tract 55% of the time and in the lungs 30% of the time. Other possible locations include ovary, testicle, and GU tract. All carcinoid tumors have the potential to cause the carcinoid syndrome which is caused by the release of numerous bioactive substances, most often including serotonin, kallikrein, histamine, and prostaglandins. The symptoms include flushing, secretory diarrhea, wheezing, venous telangiectasias, palpitations, and cardiac valvular lesions.

Diagnosis of carcinoid tumors involves detection of biochemical markers and tumor localization. Analysis of a 24-hour urine collection for 5-HIAA is the most common initial test. The carcinoid cells metabolize tryptophan to 5-HIAA, which is excreted in the urine. In the presence of carcinoid cells, urinary excretion is often at least tenfold normal. Serum serotonin level is often used if the 5-HIAA

TABLE 71-1

Differential Diagnosis

Anatomic/structural	Infectious	Neoplastic	Inflammatory/autoimmune	Iatrogenic
Aortopulmonary fistula	Tuberculosis	Bronchogenic carcinoma	Bronchiectasis/bronchitis	S/p lung biopsy
	Aspergillus		Goodpasture syndrome	
Airway foreign body				Pulmonary
	Pneumonia		Wegener granulomatosis	artery
				perforation via
Trauma				Swan-Ganz
Pulmonary AVM	Pulmonary abscess	Lupus pneumonitis		catheter
			Idiopathic pulmonary	
			hemosiderosis	

test is equivocal. Epinephrine and pentagastrin provocation testing is also used to diagnose carcinoid. Scans used to localize tumors include indium-111 octreotide imaging, CT scan, positron-emission tomography (PET) scan, and metaiodobenzylguanidine (MIBG) scintigraphy. Though the above tests are helpful, diagnosis can only be definitively made by biopsy and biochemical staining. On pathology, the tumors are made of neuroendocrine cells containing numerous membrane-bound secretory granules, which can contain numerous substances including serotonin, histamine, dopamine, and prostaglandins. The cells stain positively for neuron-specific enolase, synaptophysin, and chromogranin.

Pulmonary carcinoid represents 2% of primary lung tumors and is most often endobronchial, but can be parenchymal. The tumor cells arise from Kulchitsky cells in the bronchial mucosa. It can present with cough, hemoptysis, wheeze, chest pain, and recurrent pneumonia; however, it is usually asymptomatic and only detected on routine chest radiography. Pulmonary carcinoid is not related to cigarette smoking or other environmental exposures. It is more common in women and Caucasians. The mean size of tumors is between 2 and 5 cm.

Tissue diagnosis of pulmonary carcinoid is most often performed via bronchoscopic biopsy for central tumors and CT-guided needle aspiration for peripheral tumors. Biopsy is not without its own risks as it can lead to carcinoid crisis secondary to release of bioactive substances causing hypotension, bronchoconstriction, acidosis, myocardial infarction, and even death. The treatment for this condition is IV octreotide.

There are several paraneoplastic syndromes associated with bronchial carcinoid. There is a bronchial variant of

carcinoid syndrome, which occurs in less than 5% of patients. It can occur without liver metastases because pulmonary tumors have direct access to the systemic circulation, whereas substances released from gastrointestinal tumors are filtered through the liver and may never reach the systemic circulation. The symptoms of bronchial carcinoid syndrome include severe and prolonged flushing, disorientation, tremor, tachycardia, oliguria, asthma, and hypotension. Carcinoid tumors can also secrete adrenocorticotropic hormone (ACTH), causing Cushing syndrome, and growth hormone releasing hormone leading to acromegaly.

There are two categories of bronchial carcinoid tumors, typical and atypical (Table 71-2). The classification is based on histologic appearance. Typical carcinoids

TABLE 71-2

Typical versus Atypical Carcinoid

	Typical	Atypical
Pathology	Small cells containing regular, well-rounded nuclei; minimal atypia and rare mitotic figures	Poorly differentiated, nuclear atypia, increased mitotic activity, some necrosis
Clinical course	Indolent	Aggressive
Location	Perihilar	Peripheral
Metastasis	< 15%	30%–50%
Average age	45 year	55 year
5-year survival	> 90%	30%–70%

are well-differentiated, most often perihilar, and usually have a good prognosis. Atypical carcinoids, on the other hand, are more poorly differentiated, more often peripherally located, and have an aggressive clinical course.

The primary treatment for bronchial carcinoid is resection, either surgical or bronchoscopic. Surgical resection is preferred as it allows for the ability to obtain clear margins. The specifics of the resection depend on the tumor histology. Patients with typical carcinoid most often undergo bronchial sleeve resection with mediastinal lymph node dissection, sparing all normal lung parenchyma. Patients with atypical carcinoid often have more extensive surgeries because this type of tumor more often has satellite lesions undetectable during surgery. Thus, these patients often undergo complete lobectomy with complete mediastinal lymph node dissection or pneumonectomy if necessary. Bronchoscopic resection is only performed in poor surgical candidates or emergently in the case of complete airway obstruction. The carcinoid syndrome can be treated with somatostatin analogues including octreotide or lantreotide. Adjuvant chemotherapy can also be used in advanced disease most often occurring with atypical carcinoid.

In the above case, the patient was referred to a cardiothoracic surgeon once the diagnosis was confirmed. He underwent a right upper lobe sleeve resection with mediastinal lymph node dissection without complication. Surgical pathology revealed mature carcinoid tumor (2.1 cm × 1.3 cm × 1.0 cm) with slight invasion into the bronchial wall. All surgical margins and lymph nodes were negative. He returned to see the surgeons approximately 1 month later with recurrent complaints of myalgias, fatigue, and diarrhea. An octreotide scan was performed with concern for recurrent carcinoid. The scan revealed no areas of focal uptake and thus no metastases. He has since done well.

In summary, this case illustrates the importance of formulating a broad differential diagnosis in order to ensure appropriate diagnostic testing. In this case, timely diagnosis and resection allowed the patient to quickly return to his previous life.

Selected References

1. Kulke MH, Mayer RJ. Carcinoid tumors. *N Engl J Med.* 1999;340: 858–868.
2. Chughtai TS, Morin JE, Sheiner NM, et al. Bronchial carcinoid—twenty years' experience defines a selective surgical approach. *Surgery.* 1997;122:801–808.
3. Marty-Ane CH, Costes V, Pujol JL, et al. Carcinoid tumors of the lung: do atypical features require aggressive management? *Ann Thorac Surg.* 1995;59:78–83.
4. Rea F, Rizzardi G, Zuin A, et al. Outcome and surgical strategy in bronchial carcinoid tumors: single institutional experience with 252 patients. *Eur J Cardiothorac Surg.* 2007 Feb;31(2):186–191.
5. Thomas CF, Jett JR. Bronchial carcinoid tumors. *Up to Date.* 2006.
6. Sitaraman SV, Goldfinger SE. The carcinoid syndrome. *Up to Date.* 2006.

80-Year-Old Man with the Worst Headache of His Life

CASE PRESENTATION

An 80-year-old man with a history of prostate cancer and hypertension presents to the local university urgent care clinic with complaints of weakness and headache. He was feeling in his usual state of fairly good health until 3 days prior to presentation, when he had a fever of 39.4°C. That night, he got up from bed and slowly collapsed to the floor. He was not able to get up; his muscles felt "weak, like they were paralyzed." After about an hour, he was able to use his arms to raise himself back to his feet, using furniture as support. Since then, he says that it has been difficult to "swing his legs out of bed" and get up in the morning; he also says that he is unsteady when he walks. He feels that the major area of weakness is in his hips, with some decrease in strength in his upper legs. On further questioning, the patient says that his shoulders and upper arms have been sore for 5 or 6 weeks, and his hips have been stiff for the same amount of time, especially in the morning. He denies weakness or numbness in any other muscle group. The patient has also been experiencing headaches in the past few days. The pain is located bilaterally at the temples; he rates the pain as 7 to 8 out of 10. He says that he does not recall ever having headaches like this before. He reports no changes in his vision and denies jaw pain during chewing food. He had gone to another urgent care center the day prior to presentation, where urinalysis revealed a UTI, which is currently being treated with ciprofloxacin. The patient's hypertension is well controlled on hydrochlorothiazide/triamterene and atenolol. He does not smoke, and he drinks alcohol socially. He is a retired newspaper publisher and lives alone in a retirement community. He has no known tick exposures.

Physical Examination

Patient is a well-nourished male lying in bed comfortably. Vital signs: temperature 36.4°C, blood pressure 132/67 mm Hg, respiratory rate 20 breaths/min, pulse 78 beats/min, SPO_2 96% on room air. Head, eyes, ears, nose, and throat are normocephalic, atraumatic, extraocular muscle intact, pupils equal, round, reactive to light, no scleral icterus, no nasal discharge, mucous membranes moist, no scalp tenderness, although there is mild/moderate tenderness to palpation in temporal areas. Neck is supple with no carotid bruits. Cardiovascular examination reveals distant heart sounds, with regular rate and rhythm, normal S_1/S_2, no murmurs, gallops, or rubs, radial pulses 2+ bilaterally. Lungs are clear to auscultation bilaterally. Skin has no rash. Abdomen is soft, nontender, and without distension; bowel sounds are active and no organomegaly is identified. Extremities show no edema. Musculoskeletal examination reveals no joint effusions, range of motion intact in elbows, wrists, knees, and ankles; flexion and abduction of the shoulders are mildly limited by stiffness. No muscle or joint tenderness. Neurologically alert and oriented to person, place, and time, CN II to XII intact grossly, strength is 5 or 5/5 in all muscle groups, sensation is normal throughout. The patient weighs 77.5 kg.

Laboratory Studies

Serum chemistries show Na 130, K 3.8, Cl 91, HCO_3 27, blood urea nitrogen 36, creatinine 1.3, glucose 143.

A complete blood count shows white blood cells (WBC) 11.4, hemoglobin 15.8, hematocrit 43.3, platelets 182, creatine kinase 1969, CK-MB 8.9, troponin T less than 0.029, thyroid-stimulating hormone level is 1.14. Urinalysis shows specific gravity 1.010, pH 5.0, leukocyte esterase negative, nitrite negative, trace protein, no glucose , ketones +2, blood +1, urobilinogen normal, bilirubin negative , WBC 2, red blood cells 2, occasional bacteria. Erythrocyte sedimentation rate is 55 mm/hr. CT scan of the head was normal. Gross visual acuity was normal.

Case Resolution

The patient was admitted to the hospital for further workup of his weakness. He was given 1 mg/kg of prednisone per day, and his headaches and weakness resolved over the ensuing 48 to 72 hours. The remainder of his workup including cardiac and neurologic, was negative, and he was discharged home in good condition on an extended steroid taper.

Question

What is the best treatment for this patient's underlying illness?

Answer

The patient's symptoms, physical examination, and laboratory studies are consistent with a diagnosis of polymyalgia rheumatica (PMR) and possible giant cell arteritis (GCA). The mainstay of treatment of these related conditions is corticosteroids.

Discussion

PMR and GCA are two interrelated inflammatory conditions that in general affect persons over the age of 50. Although they are clinically distinct, the two entities may represent divergent manifestations of a single disease process. The clinical features of each condition required for diagnosis are listed below in Table 72-1. While GCA is a vasculitis that affects medium and large-sized vessels,

TABLE 72-1

Diagnostic Criteria for GCA and PMR

Giant cell (temporal) arteritis (must have 3 of 5)*	Polymyalgia rheumatica (must have all 4)
Age > 50	Age > 50
New headache	Bilateral aching/stiffness for at least a month in two of the following: neck/torso, shoulders/upper arms, hips/upper thighs
Erythrocyte sedimentation rate > 50	Erythrocyte sedimentation rate > 40
Temporal artery tenderness or decreased pulsation	Exclusion of all alternative diagnoses except giant cell arteritis
Abnormal artery biopsy†	

*The presence of any 3 or more criteria yields a sensitivity of 93.5% and a specificity of 91.2%.

†Predominance of mononuclear cell infiltration or granulomatous inflammation, usually with multinucleated giant cells.

Adapted from Hunder GG, Bloch DA, Michel BA, et al. The American College of Rheumatology 1990 criteria for the classification of giant cell arteritis. Arthritis Rheum. 1990;33:1122–1128; Chuang TY, Hunder GG, Ilstrup DM, et al. Polymyalgia rheumatica: a 10-year epidemiologic and clinical study. Ann Intern Med. 1982 Nov;97(5):672–680.

PMR is a systemic inflammatory syndrome that is often associated with GCA. The most commonly affected arteries in GCA are those in the vascular beds of the cranial nerves and the aorta and its primary and secondary branches. Typically this includes branches of the internal and external carotid arteries. Involvement of these large vessels oftentimes leads to the symptomatology seen in the disease—headache, scalp tenderness, blindness, and so on. Histologically, GCA is characterized by granulomatous inflammation of the arterial wall; the involved cells are typically activated macrophages and CD4+ T cells. The inciting event leading to this inflammation is not known.

The prevalence of GCA and PMR is increased in people of Scandinavian descent, women, and those over the age of 50. In those over 50, the incidence of either condition is approximately 15 to 25 per 100,000. Of patients meeting criteria for GCA, approximately 50% also have

PMR; of those meeting criteria for PMR, 10% also have GCA. The outcomes for patients with either condition are generally very good, especially if steroids are administered promptly. However it is vital that practitioners be able to recognize GCA and distinguish between the two entities since GCA can lead to permanent visual loss. When properly treated, most patients will have relief from symptoms within 24 to 48 hours of starting steroids. Of those who require extended therapy, most require treatment for no longer than 3 to 4 years. Life expectancy is not shortened by either disease.

The diagnosis of both conditions is largely clinical. There are no specific laboratory tests for either disorder except for an arterial biopsy in the case of GCA. A high index of suspicion for either disease in the absence of other conditions should warrant treatment. One laboratory test that may be helpful in ruling out GCA is a normal ESR. It should be noted that in general, ESR is elevated in both disorders as well as C-reactive protein levels.

In the case of PMR, treatment consists largely of oral prednisone in doses from 10 to 20 mg/day. Treatment responses vary but usually patients respond within 1 to 2 weeks. Because of this, if persons do not respond to steroid treatment, it may lead to a reassessment of the diagnosis. Tapering of the dose over time occurs slowly as symptoms resolve. A PMR disease activity scale may be useful in determining length of treatment, response to treatment such as induction of remission, or treatment dose adjustments (Table 72-2).

In the case of GCA, also referred to as temporal arteritis, steroids should be administered as soon as possible after the diagnosis is suspected. Treatment should not be delayed in order to make a definitive diagnosis via biopsy, as blindness may result if the condition is left untreated. Biopsy of the temporal artery should be done however to confirm the diagnosis. Because arteries other than the temporal artery can be involved, a negative biopsy does not rule out the disease. It may however lead to a reassessment of the differential diagnosis.

For treatment of GCA, initial doses of 40 to 60 mg of prednisone per day are typically used (some suggest 1 mg/kg/day), with a taper extending over at least several weeks. Recurrence of symptoms after steroid withdrawal is common; the disease activity is usually monitored using clinical symptoms and inflammatory markers (C-reactive protein, erythrocyte sedimentation rate) during the taper. In refractory cases, the steroid taper must be continued for several months to years.

TABLE 72-2

PMR Disease Activity Score with Newly Proposed State of Remission*

Disease activity category	Total score
Newly proposed remission	0–1.5
Low disease activity	1.5–7
Medium disease activity	7–17
High disease activity	> 17

*Calculate disease activity score for patient suffering from PMR (PMR-AS) by adding serum C-reactive protein level in mg/dL + patients visual analogue pain scale (1–10) + physician-assessed visual analogue pain scale (1–10) + morning stiffness time in minutes × 0.1 + ability to elevate upper limbs (0 points = above shoulder girdle, 1 point = up to shoulder girdle, 2 points = below shoulder girdle, 3 points = unable to elevate upper limbs) Adapted from Figure 1 in Leeb BF, Rintelen B, Sautner J, et al. The polymyalgia rheumatica activity score in daily use: proposal for a definition of remission. Arthritis Rheum. 2007 May 25;57(5):810–815.

Long-term steroid use frequently leads to serious side effects, most notably osteoporotic fractures and diabetes mellitus. Patients should be monitored for complications of long-term steroid therapy. For this reason, alternative treatments have been investigated, but none of these have been conclusively shown to be better than conventional therapy. Multiple studies have been conducted comparing concurrent methotrexate (MTX) and prednisone therapy versus the conventional prednisone doses alone. The outcomes measured in these studies included disease relapse rates and cumulative steroid doses needed for treatment. One recent study concluded that adding MTX decreased both outcomes; two other studies found no difference between the interventions. Cyclosporine A has been shown to be ineffective in sparing steroid use in GCA, due to its many side effects. Other drugs under investigation but without definitive evidence for or against them include the tumor necrosis factor alpha inhibitors infliximab, etanercept, and adalimumab.

In summary, PMR and GCA are inflammatory disorders primarily of older persons over the age of 50. Although ESR and other laboratory tests are useful adjuncts to diagnosis, the diagnosis of either is largely based on clinical grounds including history and physical examination combined with a high index of suspicion. In GCA, temporal artery biopsy should be pursued in patient suspected of having the disease but treatment should not be delayed due to the potential sequelae of visual loss. Treatment for both consists mainly of oral or systemic corticosteroids with higher doses and longer courses being given for those with GCA.

Selected References

1. Weyand CM, Goronzy JJ. Giant-cell arteritis and polymyalgia rheumatica. *Ann Intern Med*. 2003 Sep 16;139(6):505–515.
2. Salvarani C, Cantini F, Boiardi L, et al. Polymyalgia rheumatica and giant-cell arteritis. *N Engl J Med*. 2002;347(4):261–271.
3. Jover J, Hernandez-Garcia C, Morado I, et al. Combined treatment of giant cell arteritis with methotrexate and prednisone. A randomized, double-blind, placebo-controlled trial. *Ann Intern Med*. 2001;134:106–114.
4. Hoffman GS, Cid MC, Hellman DB, et al. A multicenter, randomized, double-blind, placebo-controlled trial of adjuvant methotrexate treatment for giant cell arteritis. *Arthritis Rheum*. 2002;46:1309–1318.
5. Spiera RF, Mitnick HJ, Kupersmith M, et al. A prospective, double-blind, randomized, placebo-controlled trial of methotrexate in the treatment of giant cell arteritis. *Clin Exp Rheumatol*. 2001;19:495–501.
6. Schaufelberger C, Mollby H, Uddhammar A, et al. No additional steroid-sparing effect of cyclosporine A in giant cell arteritis. *Scand J Rheumatol*. 2006 Jul–Aug;35(4):327–329.
7. Hunder GG, Bloch DA, Michel BA, et al. The American College of Rheumatology 1990 criteria for the classification of giant cell arteritis. *Arthritis Rheum*. 1990;33:1122–1128.
8. Chuang TY, Hunder GG, Ilstrup DM, et al. Polymyalgia rheumatica: a 10-year epidemiologic and clinical study. *Ann Intern Med*. 1982 Nov;97(5):672–680.
9. Leeb BF, Rintelen B, Sautner J, et al. The polymyalgia rheumatica activity score in daily use: proposal for a definition of remission. *Arthritis Rheum*. 2007 May 25;57(5):810–815.
10. Unwin B, Williams CM, Gilliland W. Polymyalgia rheumatica and giant cell arteritis. *Am Fam Physician*. 2006 Nov 1;74(9):1547–1554.
11. Smetana GW, Shmerling RH. Does this patient have temporal arteritis? *JAMA*. 2002 Jan 2;287(1):92–101.

43-Year-Old with Syncope

CASE PRESENTATION

A 43-year-old female with no significant past medical history presents to the emergency department (ED) with syncope. She was in her usual state of health until the day of admission when she felt palpitations while running. She describes this sensation as "feeling her heart racing" without any accompanying symptoms of chest pain or shortness of breath. Within approximately a minute after the start of her palpitations she felt lightheaded and subsequently fainted. She suffered loss of consciousness lasting about 2 minutes that was witnessed by her running partner. According to witnessed reports, there was no bowel or bladder incontinence, generalized motor activity, or head trauma. At the time of assessment, the patient was without any complaints and resting comfortably in the ED bed. She reports experiencing three similar episodes of syncope over the past 2 years, all involving exertional activities. This is the first time the patient has sought medical attention. She denies alcohol or illicit drug use. She does not take any medicine.

Physical Examination

Patient is a healthy appearing female in no acute distress and is answering questions appropriately. Vital signs: temperature 36.4°C, pulse 72 beats/min and regular, respiratory rate 16 breaths/min, blood pressure 120/70 mm Hg, oxygen saturation is 100% on room air. Cardiovascular examination revealed regular rate and rhythm without any murmurs, gallops, or rubs. No carotid or abdominal bruit was detected. Jugular venous distention was measured at 8 cm. She was not orthostatic by blood pressure or heart rate criteria between supine and standing. Remainder of the examination was unremarkable.

Laboratory Studies

Serum chemistry studies were essentially normal with Na 139, K 4.6, Cl 102, HCO_3 26, blood urea nitrogen 18, creatinine 0.9, glucose: 86, Ca 9.1, Mg 2.0, P 4.6. Creatine kinase: 52, creatine kinase MB: 2.9, troponin T less than 0.029. A complete blood count showed a white blood cell count of 9.5, hemoglobin 13.0, hematocrit 37.7, platelets 289. A chest x-ray and head CT were normal. A urine drug screen was normal. Electrocardiogram is shown below in Fig. 73-1.

Case Resolution

Delta waves seen on the ECG along with her history of syncope and palpitations is concerning for rapid atrioventricular (AV) conduction via an accessory pathway. This can potentially result in fatal ventricular tachycardias. Once the possibility of vasovagal and orthostatic syncope was quickly ruled out by history and physical examination, the patient was taken for an electrophysiological (EP) study because of a diagnosis of Wolff-Parkinson-White (WPW) syndrome. Atrial fibrillation was induced during her EP study. The AV conduction was 1:1 over the accessory pathway. During the procedure, the accessory pathway was ablated. Her overnight observation following the procedure was uneventful, and she remains symptom-free at her 1-year follow-up.

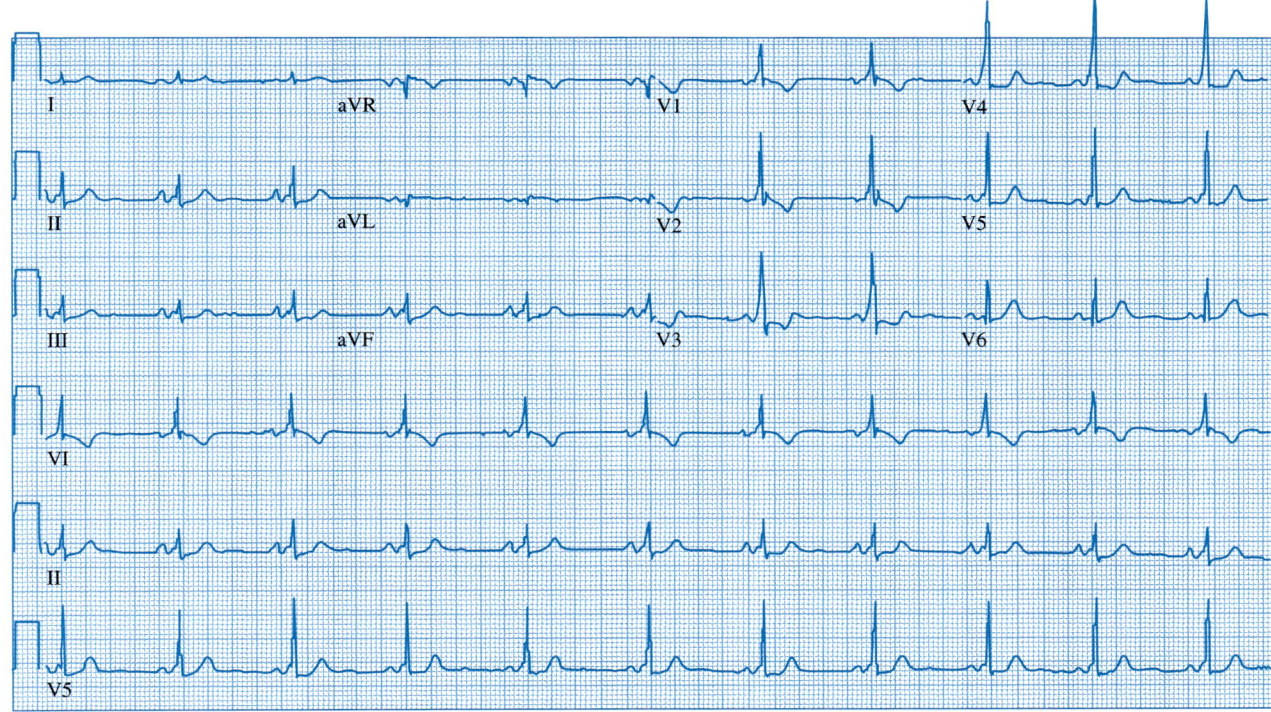

Figure 73-1 ECG tracing from patient described in vignette above. Notice marked delta waves and shortened PR interval prominent in lead II.

Question

Which medications are considered contraindicated in patients with WPW and atrial fibrillation?

Answer

Any medication that blocks AV node can precipitate AV condition via the accessory tract. These medications include β-blockers, calcium channel blockers (especially verapamil), and adenosine. Unlike the AV node, which has an inherent ability to slow conduction from atria to the ventricles, the accessory tract lacks this insurance mechanism. Therefore, rapid atrial impulses can be transmitted to the ventricles via the accessory tract if the AV node is medically blocked.

Discussion

Syncope, defined as transient loss of consciousness, is a frequent chief complaint in patients presenting to physicians offices and up to 1.5% of all ED visits and 6% of hospital admissions. Although the differential diagnosis of syncope includes multiple etiologies that can lead to sudden death, it is thought that history, physical examination, and an ECG alone in majority of cases are enough to elucidate the diagnosis (when one can be made) and determine whether a patient need be admitted. Fortunately, vasovagal—also called neurocardiogenic syncope—is the most commonly made diagnosis and is a relatively benign condition. An overview of frequent causes of syncope is summarized in Table 73-1.

It is important to recognize red flags during the initial evaluation of syncope and palpitations in order to distinguish high-risk patients from those whose workup can be continued as an outpatient basis (Fig. 73-2). A hospital admission should be considered in a patient present with syncope with any of the following:

A wide QRS complex on an ECG with a history of structural or ischemic heart disease

Symptoms of previously undiagnosed convulsive disorder

Elderly patient with signs of injury as a result of falling secondary to syncope

TABLE 73-1

Common Causes of Syncope with Typical Presentation, Pathophysiology, and Treatment

Type	Presentation	Pathophysiology	Diagnosis and treatment
Vasovagal (neurocardiogenic) syncope	Patients presents with syncope following micturition, defecation, or coughing. Feeling of lightheadedness, diaphoresis, nausea, warmth, pallor, or vision changes may precede syncope. Patient spontaneously recovers within minutes	Syncope results from increased parasympathetic tone. Hyperactive baroreceptors in carotid sinus activate vagal efferent fibers to sinus and AV node, leading to bradycardia. Similar physiology occurs with Bezoid-Jarish reflex: mechanoreceptors in atria and left ventricle respond to stretch resulting in activation of vagal efferents	Diagnosis is made by history that may also identify the trigger of syncope such as micturition, defecation, pain, and fever. Physician must exclude arrhythmia, seizures, intracranial injury, and hypoglycemia. Chemistry and CBC are generally normal. ECG may show AV node block, bradycardia. Tilt table test, done to induce neurocardiogenic reflex, is specific. Nitroglycerin and isoproterenol prior to tilt table test increases its sensitivity Treatment: Although not intuitive, β-blockers are effective in decreasing the frequency of vasovagal syncope in patients with recurrent episodes. The use of pacemakers can be considered
Orthostatic hypotension	Patients present with hypotension, tachycardia, and lightheadedness	Diabetics: Patients have autonomic dysfunction and are not able to increase systemic vascular resistance (SVR) to compensate for drop in BP	Look for signs of dehydration on physical examination: poor skin turgor, dry mucus membranes, flat JVD, poor capillary flush. Check for orthostasis. Orthostatic hypotension is defined as drop in systolic BP > 20 mm Hg or drop in diastolic BP > 10 mm Hg from supine to standing
		Intravascular depletion: Patient who are dehydrated either because of decreased PO intake of fluids or are on diuretics or have active hemorrhage do not have adequate volume to maintain mean arterial pressure (MAP)	In a patient with dehydration, blood work is reflective of hemo-concentrated CBC and chemistries suggestive of BUN to creatinine ratio > 20:1. Hyponatremia accompanied with hyperkalemia and metabolic acidosis in setting of orthostatic hypotension should raise suspicion for adrenal insufficiency. The next step will be to check renin:aldosterone ratio
		Adrenal insufficiency: Because of dysfunctional renin-angiotensin-aldosterone, patients are unable to increase renal reabsorption of Na and water	Treatment: centered on the underlying cause of orthostatic hypotension. For example, IV fluids for volume repletion, glycemic control for autonomic dysfunction caused by diabetes, mineralocorticoids and glucocorticoids for adrenal insufficiency
Stokes-Adams attack	Syncope occurs without warning. Flushed face may occur in recovery	Transient ventricular fibrillation or transient asystole in setting of AV block	Sudden, transient loss of consciousness in a patient with AV block, sinoatrial block, paroxysmal tachycardia, or fibrillation should raise suspicion of Stokes-Adams. Between attacks patients usually have sinus rhythm with wide QRS complex. Thus, diagnosis is made based on Holter monitor recording during recordings or EP study. Pacemaker or defibrillator implantation is treatment of choice

(continued)

TABLE 73-1

Common Causes of Syncope with Typical Presentation, Pathophysiology, and Treatment (*continued*)

Type	Presentation	Pathophysiology	Diagnosis and treatment
Seizure disorder	Convulsive movements, urinary incontinence, postictal confusion, prodromal aura. (Persons with cardiogenic syncope can have seizures further complicating the diagnosis)	Seizures occur as a result of abnormal neuronal activity. By definition, seizures in which consciousness is impaired are classified as complex partial seizure. (In contrast, consciousness is preserved in simple partial seizures.)	Diagnosis is made by history and EEG. Approximately one out of three patients with complex partial seizures will not have any EEG changes. A classing EEG for complex seizure will reveal a rhythmic sinusoidal activity or repetitive spike discharges Treatment: the type of antiseizure medication will depend on the type of seizure
Vascular/valvular disease	Syncope is often precipitated by exertion. Patients may also have a history of generalized fatigue	Decrease cardiac output caused by outflow obstruction results in cerebral hypoperfusion leading to syncope. Examples include aortic stenosis (AS), hypertrophic obstructive cardiomyopathy (HOCM), subclavian steal, atrial myxoma, pulmonary embolism	Diagnosis is made by physical examination (ie, specific murmur of HOCM). Further testing includes ECG, echocardiogram, and exercise testing. Treatment is directed toward the etiology
Arrhythmia	Patients may present with palpitations, as shown in this case, chest pains, and dyspnea. Alternatively, they may also be asymptomatic	Arrhythmia leads to decreased cardiac output, which in turn causes cerebral hypoperfusion. Examples include ventricular tachycardia (VT), high-grade AV block, prolonged QT syndrome, WPW, sick sinus syndrome, atrial fibrillation with rapid ventricular response	As with valvular disease, diagnosis is made by examination and ECG findings. Sometimes a holter or loop monitor may be required if arrhythmia is not captured on 12-lead ECG. Treatment options range from antiarrhythmic drugs to EP procedures and pacemaker placements

As illustrated by this case, a patient's history is often more helpful in excluding the major causes of syncope, rather than identifying specific etiologies. The patient's history of syncope with exertion and complaint of palpitations accompanied with preceding lightheadedness points to a cardiac etiology. A widened QRS complex on the ECG confirms this suspicion. The differential diagnosis of wide QRS narrows the diagnoses to the following:

(1) Ectopic ventricular beat

(2) Bundle branch block (either right or left)

(3) WPW or

(4) Metabolic or medications such as hyperkalemia, flecainide, propafenone, phenothiazine, tricyclic antidepressants, and quinidine

The presence of (1) wide QRS, (2) delta wave, and (3) short PR interval confirms the diagnosis of WPW. It is important to understand that this patient with history WPW and atrial fibrillation is at risk of sudden cardiac death. This is because the ventricles are depolarized by a combination of two distinctive pathways from the atrium to the ventricle. Simultaneous conduction from the normal AV node and the bypass tract, also called accessory tract,

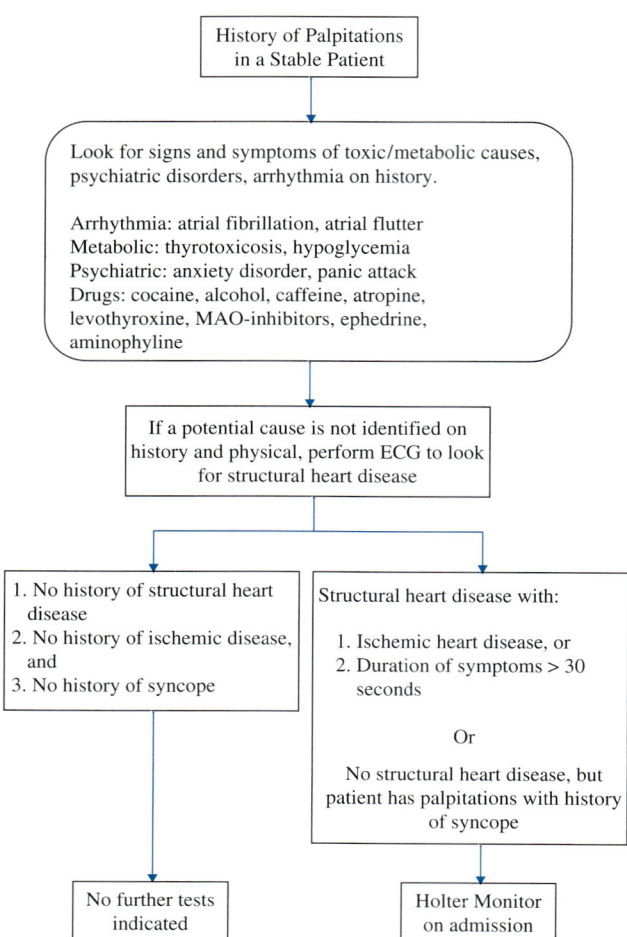

Figure 73-2 Approach to the patient with a history of palpitations.

contributes to the ventricular depolarization. Thus, the QRS complex with its delta wave is a composite of two conduction pathways, resulting in a fusion beat.

The clinical signification of the bypass tract is its propensity to lead to paroxysmal supraventricular tachycardia (PSVT). Rapid atrial impulses that occur in atrial flutter and atrial fibrillation are conducted to the ventricles without being blocked by the accessory pathway. This extremely fast ventricular rate can result in ventricular fibrillation and sudden cardiac arrest.

The management of WPW depends on the patients' symptoms and whether there is a history of atrial fibrillation or flutter. Asymptomatic patients without underlying arrhythmia should be referred for exercise testing. Resolution of WPW during exercise in these patients indicates that the accessory pathway cannot conduct fast impulses. No further testing or interventions are needed. By contrast, WPW in a symptomatic patient with a history of atrial arrhythmia is cured by radiofrequency ablation of the accessory pathway.

In summary, although this case was atypical in that the syncope experienced by this otherwise healthy individual was not because of neurocardiogenic causes, it illustrates the centrality of why a good history and physical is combined with laboratory and diagnostic data such as an ECG in making the appropriate diagnosis.

Selected References

1. McCorry D, McCorry A. Collapse with loss of awareness. *BMJ.* 2007 Jan 20;334(7585):153.
2. Huff JS, Decker WW, Quinn JV, et al.; American College of Emergency Physicians. Clinical policy: critical issues in the evaluation and management of adult patients presenting to the emergency department with syncope. *Ann Emerg Med.* 2007 Apr;49(4):431–444.
3. Fuster V, Ryden LE, Cannom DS, et al. ACC/AHA/ESC guidelines for the management of patients with atrial fibrillation. A report of the American College of Cardiology/American Heart Association Task Force on Practice Guidelines and the European Society of Cardiology Committee for Practice Guidelines (Writing committee to revise the 2001 guidelines for the management of patients with atrial fibrillation). *J Am Coll Cardiol.* 2006 Aug 15;48(4):854–906.

23-Year-Old Female with Abdominal Pain

CASE PRESENTATION

A 23-year-old Hispanic female presented to the emergency department with a 48-hour history of worsening lower abdominal pain, nausea, vomiting, and diarrhea. The diarrhea had accelerated to 10 bowel movements in 24 hours with the appearance of blood. Five days prior to this presentation, the patient had been admitted to the same facility after being diagnosed with intrauterine fetal demise following the stillbirth of a 20- to 24-week fetus. The woman had received no prenatal care and had no reported medical conditions other than the fetal demise. She was discharged home after overnight observation. The abdominal pain started soon after discharge and was followed by fever, chills, rigors, and the aforementioned vomiting and diarrhea. The patient also noted darkening of her urine, a decrease in urine output, lightheadedness with standing, and feeling short of breath. She specifically denied dysuria, flank pain, or pleuritic chest pain. She had noted foul discharge from her vagina in the last 48 hours and the appearance of a rash on her chest and inflammation of her conjunctiva.

Physical Examination

The patient is an anxious but well-developed female in moderate distress. Vital signs: temperature on presentation was 39.05°C, respiratory rate 40 breaths/min, pulse 140 beats/min, blood pressure (supine) 65/35 mm Hg, and oxygen saturation 99% on 5 L of O_2 via nasal cannula. Patient was alert and oriented × 3. Mucous membranes are tacky and sclera is injected bilaterally without limbic sparing. Neck is supple without lymphadenopathy or JVD. Heart is regular but tachycardic with a hyperdynamic precordium, S_1/S_2 clearly audible without murmur/gallop/rub. Patient is tachypneic but clear bilaterally with faint crackles at bases. Skin examination reveals a diffuse erythematous rash about the neck and face. Abdominal examination reveals nearly absent bowel sounds with a firm lower abdomen with guarding and rebound. Right upper quadrant (RUQ) and epigastrium are also tender with guarding and rebound. Rectal examination recreates abdominal tenderness and reveals heme-positive stool. Pelvic examination revealed purulent drainage from cervix with diffuse tenderness to palpation. The rest of the examination, including musculoskeletal and neurologic examinations, is unremarkable.

Laboratory Studies

Initial laboratory results included a white blood cell count of 9.4; hemoglobin 9.7 g/dL, hematocrit 28, and platelets 158. Chemistries were notable for Na 137, K 2.6, Cl 106, HCO_3 12, blood urea nitrogen 29, creatinine 2.6, glucose 94. Lipase was normal at 21. Total bilirubin was 3.3 with normal transaminases. Arterial blood gas showed a pH of 7.18, PCO_2 of 19, PaO_2 of 89, and saturation of 94% on 5 L of O_2 per minute. Lactate was 4.7. Gram stain of vaginal and cervical discharge revealed gram-positive cocci in chains and pairs. Erythrocyte sedimentation rate was 66. Urinalysis was notable for pH of 6 with specific gravity of 1.030, 118 WBC/hpf, large leukocyte esterase, and 2+ protein without sediment. Three views of the abdomen revealed no free air, but a nonspecific pattern suggestive of ileus. Chest x-ray demonstrated developing bilateral diffuse opacities.

Case Resolution

The patient was admitted to the medical intensive care unit (ICU) following administration of 4 L of IV normal saline in the emergency department. Urine output was established, but the patient's low blood pressure remained unresponsive to IV fluids. A lower extremity central line was inserted and vasopressin and neosynephrine were started. Within 2 hours, respiratory failure ensued and the patient was intubated. Broad spectrum antibiotics were administered including vancomycin, clindamycin, levaquin, and piperacillin/tazobactam. An arterial line as well as a right internal jugular triple lumen catheter was inserted for hemodynamic monitoring. Mean arterial pressures (MAP), central venous pressure (CVP), and mixed venous oxygen saturations were checked periodically in the initial 6 to 8 hours. In the following 12 hours, the patient received activated protein C. Intravenous immunoglobulin (IVIG) was also administered for suspected severe toxic shock syndrome. Blood cultures grew group A *Streptococcus* within 12 hours. Culture of vaginal discharge demonstrated identical culture results. Despite aggressive fluid resuscitation, the patient remained hypotensive and developed the acute respiratory distress syndrome. On day 5 of hospitalization, the patient's necrotic uterus was removed. With renal replacement therapy and careful monitoring for secondary and nosocomial infection, the patient made a full recovery from her postpartum sepsis and was discharged to acute rehabilitation.

Question

On the spectrum of disease severity, how could this patient's sepsis be classified and what is the best initial treatment of patients that have similar presentation?

Answer

The patient is suffering from severe sepsis and later septic shock, probably from gram-positive organisms infecting her uterus. The surviving sepsis campaign published guidelines in 2004 that made evidence-based recommendations for the treatment of severe sepsis.[1] These recommendations were implemented in the form of treatment bundles. One prominent component of this bundle includes the use of aggressive fluid resuscitation as an initial measure using specific hemodynamic parameters or goals. The use of early goal-directed therapy, when possible, has been shown to reduce mortality in severe sepsis.[2]

Discussion

Sepsis is a significant cause of morbidity and mortality in the United States. Over the last 5 years of available data, septicemia has been the tenth leading cause of death.[3-7] Incidence of sepsis increases with increasing age. As the average age of the population in the United States increases, the incidence of sepsis is expected to increase as well. Martin et al found that between 1979 and 2000, incidence of sepsis increased from 82.7 to 240.4 cases per 100,000 population.[8] Angus et al analyzed discharge data from seven states in 1995.[9] Overall mortality during a hospitalization where severe sepsis was coded on the discharge summary was 28.6%. Mortality in all pediatric age groups was close to 10%. After the age of 19, mortality rose steadily with age to a maximum of 38.4% in those patients greater than 85 years of age. While some strides have been made in decreasing mortality from sepsis, it remains unacceptably high. Martin et al analyzed hospital discharge data for adult patients with diagnostic codes suggestive of sepsis from approximately 500 hospitals between 1979 and 2000.[8] Overall mortality rates decreased from 27.8% in the years from 1979 to 1984 to 17.9% in the years from 1995 to 2000. Differences in mortality rates were further analyzed by severity of illness. They found that patients with sepsis and no organ failure had a 15% mortality compared to 70% in patients with failure of three or more organ systems. Both of these studies were limited by the fact that data was collected from hospital discharge records. The results depended on accurate coding and it was not possible to determine if mortality could be directly attributed to sepsis.

In 1992, the American College of Chest Physicians and the Society of Critical Care Medicine published a consensus statement defining sepsis.[10] The previously broad term of "sepsis" was divided into four more specific diagnoses: (1) systemic inflammatory response syndrome (SIRS), (2) sepsis, (3) severe sepsis, and (4) septic shock (Table 74-1).

SIRS is defined as two or more of the following: (1) temperature greater than 38°C or less than 36°C; (2) heart rate greater than 90 beats/min; (3) respiratory rate greater than 20 breaths/min or $PaCO_2$ less than 32 mm Hg; or (4)

TABLE 74-1

Diagnostic Entities Related to Sepsis

Term	Definition
Systemic inflammatory response syndrome (SIRS)	Two or more of the following: Temperature > 38°C or < 36°C Heart rate > 90 beats/min Respiratory rate > 20 breaths/min or P_{CO_2} < 32 mm Hg WBC > 12,000 cells/μL or < 4,000 cells/μL
Sepsis	SIRS with a source of infection
Severe sepsis	Sepsis with organ dysfunction
Septic shock	Severe sepsis in which the patient remains hypotensive in spite of adequate fluid resuscitation

Adapted from Levy MM, Fink MP, Marshall JC, et al. 2001 SCCM/ESICM/ACCP/ATS/SIS International Sepsis Definitions Conference. Crit Care Med. 2003;31(4):1250–1255.

a white blood cell count greater than 12,000 cells/μL or less than 4000 cells/μL. As the name implies, SIRS represents the body's inflammatory response to an insult. Common causes of SIRS include trauma, infection, burns, and other inflammatory causes, such as pancreatitis. Sepsis is defined as SIRS plus infection, either documented or suspected. Therefore if SIRS is caused by infection, the patient is then categorized as sepsis rather than SIRS. Severe sepsis is sepsis with organ dysfunction. Organ dysfunction may include cardiovascular (hypotension), renal (low urine output or elevated creatinine), hematologic (decrease in platelets, disseminated intravascular coagulation), hepatic (elevated bilirubin or transaminases), respiratory (PaO_2/FIO_2 < 300), metabolic (increased plasma lactate or decreased pH), or neurologic (altered mental status) failure. Septic shock is defined as severe sepsis with persistent hypotension once adequate volume status has been attained.

Current treatment of sepsis consists of goal-directed therapy based on objective measures. In 2004, the Surviving Sepsis guidelines were published by the Society of Critical Care Medicine.[5] These guidelines emphasize that therapy needs to be initiated as soon as sepsis is recognized.

Initial resuscitation should begin immediately using the following goals:

CVP of 8 to 12 mm Hg

MAP of greater than or equal to 65 mm Hg

Urine output of greater than or equal to 0.5 mL/kg/hr

Central venous or mixed venous oxygen saturation greater than or equal to 70%

In a partially blinded, randomly controlled study of 263 patients with severe sepsis or septic shock, Rivers et al showed that if these goals were used to guide therapy during the initial 6 hours after presentation, in-hospital mortality was reduced from 46.5% to 30.5% and 60-day mortality from 56.7% to 44.3%.[2] Early studies of goal-directed therapy for sepsis enrolled patients up to 72 hours after admission to the ICU. These studies did not report a decrease in morbidity or mortality with goal-directed therapy. The decrease in mortality found by Rivers et al is thought to be because of early implementation and has resulted in the current standard of care of early goal-directed therapy for patients with severe sepsis or septic shock.

The initial step in treatment of severe sepsis or septic shock is placement of central venous access, monitoring of CVP, and aggressive IV hydration. If the CVP is below 8 mm Hg, fluid boluses should be initiated until the CVP is within the target range. No difference has been found between the efficacies of crystalloid or colloid solutions. If the patient also has a mixed venous oxygen saturation less than 70% or is profoundly anemic, red blood cell transfusion should be considered to increase oxygen-carrying capacity in addition to volume resuscitation.

If the MAP target range cannot be attained using fluid and/or blood therapy alone, vasopressor therapy should be initiated. First-line vasopressors are dopamine and norepinephrine. Either may be selected, however mechanism of action should be considered. Dopamine primarily acts by increasing heart rate and stroke volume, while norepinephrine acts by vasoconstriction. If hypotension persists, more than one vasopressor may be required. Vasopressor selection should be based on the specific indications of the patient. In patients with low cardiac output and adequate volume resuscitation, dobutamine may be added as an inotrope. In patients with low blood pressure, dobutamine should be combined with a vasopressor.

In addition to hemodynamic support, appropriate cultures should be obtained. All patients should have blood and urine samples collected. In patients with central venous lines in place for longer than 48 hours, blood cultures should be obtained from each port in addition to a peripheral blood sample. Samples of sputum, cerebrospinal fluid, wound, and/or other body fluids should be collected as indicated by the clinical presentation. All cultures should be collected prior to antibiotic administration. Once cultures have been obtained, broad-spectrum antibiotics should be started immediately. Ideally, IV antibiotics should be started within 1 hour of identification of sepsis. Antibiotic coverage can be narrowed once culture and sensitivity data is available. If a focus of infection is identified, such as an infected central line or abscess, action should be taken to remove the focus.

Additional recommendations in the Surviving Sepsis guidelines include hydrocortisone therapy in patients who are suffering from relative adrenal insufficient and activated protein C therapy for patients who are critically ill. Hydrocortisone treatment should be considered in patients who are vasopressor dependent in spite of adequate hydration. An ACTH stimulation test is recommended prior to initiation of hydrocortisone, although treatment should not be delayed for results. If a stimulation test is unable to be performed, dexamethasone can be used without interfering with stimulation test results. Hydrocortisone treatment should be discontinued in patients who respond appropriately to the stimulation test. However, more recent studies have concluded that hydrocortisone may not improve survival or reversal of shock in patients with septic shock, both overall or in patients who did not have a response to the ACTH stimulation test. However hydrocortisone hastened reversal of shock in patients in whom shock was reversed by steroid administration. Caution should be used in this setting until more definitive conclusions can be made.[11] Some severely ill patients may be candidates for activated protein C therapy, which has been shown to reduce mortality in severe sepsis patients that are at high risk of death (APACHE score ≥25, ARDS, multiple-organ failure). There are numerous contraindications to activated protein C, primarily related to an increased risk of bleeding. Once a patient is identified as a candidate for activated protein C, therapy should be initiated as soon as possible.

While tight glucose control (blood glucose level ≤ 150 mg/dL) has been shown to improve outcome in critically ill surgical patients, studies in ICU patients with sepsis receiving tight glycemic control would suggest that there is tendency towards significant hypoglycemia with no clear benefit in morbidity and mortality. Additional interventions, which may be necessary to support patients with severe sepsis, include dialysis for those patients with sepsis-induced acute renal failure and mechanical ventilation in patient with respiratory failure.

In order for the treatment of sepsis to be effective, aggressive therapy must be started as soon as the diagnosis is established to prevent further end-organ damage. This means that initial therapy will often take place on the hospital ward or in the emergency room, prior to transfer to the ICU.

Selected References

1. Dellinger RP, Carlet JM, Masur H, et al. Surviving Sepsis Campaign guidelines for management of severe sepsis and septic shock. *Crit Care Med.* 2004;32(3):858–873.
2. Rivers E, Nguyen B, Havstad S, et al. Early goal-directed therapy in the treatment of severe sepsis and septic shock. *New Eng J Med.* 2001;345(19):1368–1377.
3. Heron MP, Smith BL. Deaths: leading causes for 2003. *Natl Vital Stat Rep.* 2007;55(10):1–92.
4. Anderson RN. Deaths: leading causes for 1999. *Natl Vital Stat Rep.* 2001;49(11):1–87.
5. Anderson RN. Deaths: leading causes for 2000. *Natl Vital Stat Rep.* 2002;50(16):1–85.
6. Anderson RN, Smith BL. Deaths: leading causes for 2001. *Natl Vital Stat Rep.* 2003;52(9):1–85.
7. Anderson RN, Smith BL. Deaths: leading causes for 2002. *Natl Vital Stat Rep.* 2005;53(17):1–89.
8. Martin GS, Mannino DM, Eaton S, et al. The epidemiology of sepsis in the United States from 1979 through 2000. *New Engl J Med.* 2003;348:1546–1554.
9. Angus DC, Linde-Zwirble WT, Lidicker J, et al. Epidemiology of severe sepsis in the United States: analysis of incidence, outcome and associated costs of care. *Crit Care Med.* 2001;29 (7): 1303–1310.
10. Levy MM, Fink MP, Marshall JC, et al. 2001 SCCM/ESICM/ ACCP/ATS/SIS International Sepsis Definitions Conference. *Crit Care Med.* 2003;31(4):1250–1255.
11. Sprung CL, Annane D, Keh D, et al. Hydrocortisone therapy for patients with septic shock. *N Engl J Med.* 2008 Jan 10;358(2):111–24.
12. van den Berghe G, Wouters P, Weekers F, et al. Intensive insulin therapy in the critically ill patients. *New Engl J Med.* 2001;345:1359–1367.
13. Brunkhorst FM, Engel C, Bloos F, et al. Intensive Insulin Therapy and Pentastarch Resuscitation in Severe Sepsis. *N Engl J Med.* 2008; 358:125–39.

Page numbers followed by *f* indicate figure; those followed by *t* indicate table.

Cellulitis (*Cont.*):
    infecting organisms, 284–285
    treatment, 285–286
Central nervous system tuberculosis, 47
CHADS2 scoring system, for stroke, 212, 212*t*
Chandler classification, of orbital cellulitis, 285, 285*t*
Chemotherapy, neutropenia due to, 243–245
Chest pain
    symptom in cardiomyopathy, 168
    symptom in endocarditis, 6
    symptom in variant angina, 17
Chromobacterium violaceum, sepsis due to, 12–13, 13*f*
Chronic cough. *See* Cough, chronic
Chronic granulomatous disease (CGD), 12–16
    diagnosis of, 15
    presentation of, 14–15
    treatment, 15–16
Churg-Strauss syndrome, 27*t*
Cirrhosis
    in ascite development, 288–289
    etiology, 289
Clopidogrel
    actions of, 225
    aspirin combined with
        for stroke, 197, 198*t*
        for unstable angina, 225–226, 226*t*
    bleeding related to, 226–227, 226*t*
    percutaneous coronary intervention and,
        226, 226*t*
    for stroke, 197
Clotting factors, disease state patterns, 79, 79*t*
Coarctation of the aorta
    in adults, 295
    diagnosis of, 295
    heart murmur in, 122*t*
    in infants, 295
    pathogenesis of, 294–295
    secondary hypertension due to, 294–295
Compartment syndrome, in diabetic muscle infarction, 306
Complement system, in immune system, 14
Congenital heart disease. *See also* Cyanotic
        congenital heart disease
    diagnosis of, 121, 123–124
    heart murmur in, 120–124, 121*t*, 122*t*–123*t*
    incidence, 121
Congestive heart failure (CHF)
    cardiomyopathy in, 169–170
    etiology, 84, 84*t*, 169
Conjunctivitis, symptom in Kawasaki disease, 133
Coombs test
    direct, 186, 186*t*
    indirect, 186, 186*t*

Corticosteroids, in PCP treatment, 218, 218*t*
Cough
    chronic, 253–256
        defined, 254
        diagnostic examination, 255–256, 256*f*
        etiology, 255, 255*t*
    symptom in Goodpasture syndrome, 25
Cryptogenic organizing pneumonia (COP). *See* BOOP/COP
CT scan, angiogram, in thoracic aortic aneurysms,
        71, 71*f*, 73
Cyanosis
    symptom in methemoglobinemia, 30
    symptom in tetralogy of Fallot, 49–50
Cyanotic congenital heart disease
    common, 51*t*, 106*t*
    differential diagnosis, 105
    tetralogy of Fallot, 49–54, 51*t*, 106*t*
    truncus arterious, 104–107, 106*t*
Cystic fibrosis, 257–259
    management, 259
    newborn screening, 258
    presentation in infant, 257–258, 258*t*

D
Dactylitis, defined, 93
Deep venous thrombosis (DVT), 87–90
    diagnosis of, 88–89
    pediatric, 149–150
    presentation of, 88
    treatment, 89–90
    Wells criteria for, 89, 89*t*
Dementia, HIV-related, 206–210
    presentation of, 209
    screening tool for, 210, 210*t*
Diabetes mellitus, stroke risk and, 199
Diabetic muscle infarction, 303–308
    differential diagnosis, 307, 307*t*
    etiology, 304, 306
    histology, 305*f*, 307
    overview, 304
    presentation of, 306–307
    radiographic findings, 308
    treatment, 308
Diarrhea
    acute infectious, causative agents in, 311, 311*t*
    in neuroblastoma, 65–66
    rehydration therapy for, 312
    in *Salmonella* infections, 310
Dipyridamole, aspirin combined with, for
        stroke, 197
Disc herniation, treatment, 5
Diskitis, lumbar, 2, 2*f*

Rickettsia, 38*t,* 40, 40*t*
Rickettsia africae, 40
Rickettsia rickettsi, 273
Rocky Mountain spotted fever, 22, 272–274
    diagnosis of, 273–274
    presentation of, 273–274, 273*f*
    treatment, 274
Ross procedure, 7

S
S. aureus bacteremia, 2
Salmonella infections, 312–313
    nontyphoidal, 312*t*
    treatment, 313, 313*t*
    typhoid, 312*t*
Sarcoidosis, in pleural effusion, 180–181
Schistocytes, etiology, 22
Sciatica, pain due to, 3
Secondary hypertension
    diagnosis of, 292, 294*t*
    etiology, 293–294, 295*t*
    pediatric, 292–295
        coarctation of the aorta, 294–295
        diagnosis of, 292–293
Seizure disorder, syncope in, 325*t*
Sepsis
    Chromobacterium violaceum, 12–13, 13*f*
    defined, 329
    incidence, 328
    septic shock
        defined, 329
        treatment, 329–330
    severe, 327–330
        defined, 329
        treatment, 328, 329–330
    Surviving Sepsis guidelines, 328, 330
    systemic inflammatory response syndrome (SIRS), defined, 328–329
    treatment, 329–330
Sequestration, acute splenic, 93–94
Serum-to-ascites gradient (SAAG), 290
Shortness of breath
    symptom in BOOP/COP, 296
    symptom in myxedema coma, 233
    symptom in pleural effusion, 179
    symptom in secondary hypertension, 292
Sickle cell disease, 91–94, 265, 267*t*
    acute chest syndrome in, 91, 92*f,* 93
    acute splenic sequestration, 93–94
    pain episodes, 92–93
    pathogenesis of, 92
    screening for, 92, 93*t*

Skin reactions. *See also* Rash
    drug-induced, 247, 248*t*
Sore throat, symptom in pericarditis, 260–262
Splenic sequestration, acute, in sickle cell disease, 93–94
Splenomegaly, in aplastic anemia, 281, 281*t*
Spontaneous bacterial peritonitis, 290
Staphylococcus aureus
    in lymphadenitis, 96, 97*t*
    methicillin-resistant (MRSA), in periorbital cellulitis, 284
Staphylococcus pyogenes, in lymphadenitis, 96, 97*t*
Statins, for stroke, 197–198
Stenosis
    aortic valve, 122*t*
    critical pulmonic, 107*t*
    peripheral pulmonic, 122*t*
    pulmonary valve, 122*t*
Stevens-Johnson syndrome, 248*t,* 249
Stokes-Adams attack, syncope due to, 324*t*
Streptococcus pneumoniae, hemolytic uremic syndrome, 125–127
Streptococcus viridans, in endocarditis, 7
Stroke, 192–199
    acute treatment, 194
    antiplatelet drugs for prevention, 196–197
    atrial fibrillation and, 212
    CHADS2 scoring system for, 212, 212*t*
    defined, 194
    diabetes mellitus and, 199
    dyslipidemia in, 197–198
    Framington stroke prediction tool, 194
    hemorrhagic, defined, 194
    hypertension in, 198–199
    incidence, 194
    ischemic
        defined, 194
        prevention of, 193–194
    risk factors for, 194–195, 195*f,* 212
    in sickle cell disease, 94
    statins for, 197–198
    transient ischemic attack, 194
Surviving Sepsis guidelines, 328, 330
Swelling
    abdominal, symptom in Burkitt lymphoma, 164
    eye, symptom in periorbital cellulitis, 283
    hand, symptom in polyarthritis, 108
Syncope, 322–326
    defined, 323
    diagnostic approach for, 323, 325, 326*f*
    etiology, 323, 324*t*–325*t*
    red flags with, 323
    symptom in hypoglycemia, 151
    vasovagal, 324*t*
    due to Wolff-Parkinson-White syndrome, 325–326